EXERCISE TESTING and EXERCISE PRESCRIPTION
for SPECIAL CASES
Theoretical Basis and Clinical Application

Third Edition

EXERCISE TESTING and EXERCISE PRESCRIPTION for SPECIAL CASES

Theoretical Basis and Clinical Application

Third Edition

EDITOR

James S. Skinner, PhD

Professor, Department of Kinesiology
Indiana University
Bloomington, Indiana

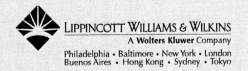

LIPPINCOTT WILLIAMS & WILKINS
A **Wolters Kluwer** Company

Philadelphia • Baltimore • New York • London
Buenos Aires • Hong Kong • Sydney • Tokyo

Acquisitions Editor: Peter J. Darcy
Managing Editor: Linda S. Napora
Marketing Manager: Christen D. Murphy
Production Editor: Jennifer D. Glazer
Designer: Risa Clow
Illustrator: Kimberly Battista
Compositor: TechBooks
Printer: R.R. Donnelley—Willard

351 West Camden Street
Baltimore, MD 21201

530 Walnut Street
Philadelphia, PA 19106

Printed in the United States of America

First Edition, 1985
Second Edition, 1993

Library of Congress Cataloging-in-Publication Data

Exercise testing and exercise prescription for special cases: theoretical basis and clinical application/editor, James S. Skinner.—3rd ed.
     p. ; cm.
   Includes bibliographical references and index.
   ISBN 978-0-7817-4113-2 ISBN 0-7817-4113-0
    1. Exercise therapy.   2. Exercise tests.
   [DNLM: 1. Exercise Therapy.   2. Exercise Test.   WB 541 E955 2005]
   I. Skinner, James S., 1936-
RM725.E94 2005
615.8′2—dc22

2004027772

To purchase additional copies of this book, call our customer service department at **(800) 638-3030** or fax orders to **(301) 824-7390**. International customers should call **(301) 714-2324**.

Visit Lippincott Williams & Wilkins on the Internet: http://www.LWW.com.
Lippincott Williams & Wilkins customer service representatives are available from 8:30 am to 6:00 pm, EST.

Preface

The sedentary lifestyle so prevalent today in most developed countries is associated directly or indirectly with a number of health problems (e.g., obesity and coronary heart disease). There is a need for a reference source book that discusses the theoretical and applied aspects of exercise testing and prescription for many of these special problems. One must search for and read numerous articles to: (1) understand why certain exercise tests were used, (2) understand why certain types of exercise were used, and (3) determine the efficacy of exercise programs relative to the special health state. Scientists and clinicians in the rapidly growing fields of exercise science and sports medicine have provided the research and experience needed for such a compendium. The authors of the chapters within this book were selected because they have been responsible for much of this information.

First presented (Section I) are the general principles of exercise testing and exercise prescription for muscle strength and general conditioning. This is followed by a discussion of general factors such as age, gender, and environment, as well as adherence to and effectiveness of exercise programs. Finally, there are chapters on the specific health states within sections on neuromuscular and skeletal, metabolic, respiratory, cardiovascular, and other conditions (Sections II to VI, respectively). Where applicable, authors were asked to discuss the health state and its general treatment, risk factors and associated health states, how the health state may affect and be affected by exercise, how to modify exercise testing procedures, how to prescribe exercise (especially the types of exercise that should be emphasized or avoided and why), and the effects to be expected from exercise programs.

Most physicians have studied various diseases and health states but are not as well versed in exercise testing and exercise prescription. Conversely, most physical educators and exercise specialists learn about exercise but know far less about medical problems and their signs and symptoms. Because many people seek the advice of physicians and exercise specialists as to what to do and what to avoid, both groups need information on what role exercise testing and exercise programs might play in modifying a person's health status. The goal of this book is to provide information for all professional groups interested in the interaction between exercise and health.

Two important findings from research in exercise science are: (1) optimal exercise tests and exercise programs are those that are individualized and personalized and (2) the effects of training are specific to the systems that are stimulated to adapt. Thus, even though the basic principles of exercise testing and exercise prescription are the same for everyone, these principles can be and may have to be modified because of the restrictions or limitations imposed by the particular health state involved. The understanding of these restrictions and the modifications that should be made form the basis for adequate functional evaluations and exercise programs that are safe and effective. It should be mentioned that although exercise testing and exercise prescriptions are based on scientific facts, the leading of *enjoyable* exercise programs is still an art.

The proper selection of activities requires communication and cooperation among the physician, the exercise specialist, and the patient. The physician should have basic information concerning exercise and should recommend exercise programs led by competent and qualified professionals. Exercise specialists should have basic information about the medical aspects of various health states so that they can receive and understand results from the medical screening (e.g., special problems and medications) and the exercise test. It is hoped that this book will help to bridge the gap, assisting professionals to understand their roles better, as well as the place that exercise testing and exercise prescription have in preventive and rehabilitative exercise programs.

This third edition reflects the continued growth of exercise science and sports medicine and their application to special populations. Although the basic principles and programs have changed little over the years, new developments and refinements have been reported and incorporated in the revised chapters. Also, reflecting this growth is the fact that the third edition has 26 chapters, whereas the first edition had 18 and the second edition had 21 chapters. These revisions and additions should give the reader an even broader and deeper understanding of how exercise testing and exercise prescription can be applied to the general population and to special cases.

James S. Skinner
Bloomington, Indiana

Contributors

Kirsten Ambrose, MS (Chapter 12)
Research Associate in Clinical Trials
Chronic Pain and Fatigue Research Program
University of Michigan
Ann Arbor, Michigan

Oded Bar-Or, MD (Chapter 5)
Professor Emeritus
Department of Pediatrics
McMaster University
Director, Children's Exercise and
  Nutrition Centre
Hamilton Health Sciences
Chedoke Hospital
Hamilton, Ontario, Canada

Frank J. Cerny, PhD (Chapter 17)
Professor Emeritus
Department of Exercise and Nutrition
  Science, Pediatrics
State University of New York at Buffalo
Buffalo, New York

**Samuel N. Cheuvront, PhD, RD
  (Chapter 7)**
Principal Investigator
Thermal and Mountain Medicine Division
U.S. Army Research Institute of
  Environmental Medicine
Natick, Massachusetts

Daniel J. Clauw, MD (Chapter 12)
Assistant Dean, Clinical & Translational
  Research
Director, Chronic Pain and Fatigue Research
  Program
Professor of Medicine, Division of
  Rheumatology
Center for the Advancement of Clinical
  Research
University of Michigan
Ann Arbor, Michigan

J. Larry Durstine, PhD (Chapter 18)
Associate Professor
Department of Exercise Science
University of South Carolina
Columbia, South Carolina

Bo Fernhall, PhD (Chapter 26)
Associate Dean for Research and
  Academic Affairs
College of Applied Life Sciences
University of Illinois
Champaign-Urbana, Illinois

Kenneth D. Fitch, MD (Chapter 16)
Adjunct Professor
Department of Human Movement
  and Exercise Science
University of Western Australia
Nedlands, Western Australia

Steven J. Fleck, PhD (Chapter 3)
Professor and Chair
Sports Science Department
Colorado College
Colorado Springs, Colorado

Victor F. Froelicher, MD (Chapter 1)
Professor of Medicine
Stanford University School of Medicine
Cardiology Division
Palo Alto VA Medical Center
Palo Alto, California

Andrew W. Gardner, PhD (Chapter 20)
Professor
Department of Health and Sport Sciences
The University of Oklahoma
Norman, Oklahoma

William L. Haskell, PhD (Chapter 18)
Professor of Medicine
Stanford Prevention Research Center
Division of Cardiovascular Medicine
Stanford University School of Medicine
Palo Alto, California

Helge U. Hebestreit, MD (Chapter 5)
Priv.-Doz., Director
Pediatric Pulmonology and Sports Medicine
University of Wuerzburg
Wuerzburg, Germany

Maria T.E. Hopman, PhD (Chapter 13)
Department of Physiology
University Medical Center
University of Nijmegen
Institute for Fundamental and Clinical
    Human Movement Sciences
Nijmegen, The Netherlands

Thomas W.J. Janssen (Chapter 13)
Assistant Professor
Vrije Universiteit
Research Coordinator, Rehabilitation Center
Institute for Fundamental and Clinical
    Human Movement Sciences
Amsterdam, The Netherlands

William J. Kraemer, PhD (Chapter 3)
Professor of Kinesiology, Physiology,
    and Neurobiology
Professor of Medicine
The Human Performance Laboratory
Department of Kinesiology
The University of Connecticut
Storrs, Connecticut

Kirstin Lane, MS (Chapter 24)
School of Human Kinetics and
    Division of Sports Medicine
The University of British Columbia
Vancouver, British Columbia, Canada

Arthur S. Leon, MD (Chapter 14)
H. L. Taylor Professor of Exercise
    and Health Enhancement
Department of Kinesiology
University of Minnesota
Minneapolis, Minnesota

Angela K. Lyden, MS (Chapter 12)
Research Associate in Clinical Trials
Chronic Pain and Fatigue Research Program
University of Michigan
Ann Arbor, Michigan

Robert S. McKelvie, MD, PhD (Chapter 21)
Professor of Medicine
Division of Cardiology
McMaster University
Staff Cardiologist
Hamilton Health Sciences
Hamilton, Ontario, Canada

**Donald C. McKenzie, MD, PhD
    (Chapter 24)**
Professor
School of Human Kinetics
Division of Sports Medicine
The University of British Columbia
Vancouver, British Columbia, Canada

Alan R. Morton, EdD (Chapter 16)
Emeritus Professor
Department of Human Movement
    and Exercise Science
The University of Western Australia
Nedlands, Western Australia

Neil B. Oldridge, PhD (Chapter 9)
Visiting Professor and Interim Director
Indiana Center for Rehabilitation Sciences
    and Engineering Research
School of Health and Rehabilitation Sciences
Indiana University—Purdue
University at Indianapolis
Indianapolis, Indiana
Senior Scientist
College of Health Sciences
University of Wisconsin—Milwaukee
Milwaukee, Wisconsin

David M. Orenstein, MD (Chapter 17)
Associate Professor of Pediatrics
Director, Pediatric Pulmonary/Cystic Fibrosis
Children's Hospital of Pittsburgh
Pittsburgh, Pennsylvania

Scott G. Owens, PhD (Chapter 15)
Assistant Professor of Exercise Science
Department of Health, Exercise Science,
   and Recreation Management
Western Carolina University
Cullowhee, North Carolina

Patricia L. Painter, PhD (Chapter 23)
Associate Adjunct Professor
Department of Physiological Nursing
Transplant Rehabilitation Director
University of California at San Francisco
San Francisco, California

Kent B. Pandolf, PhD, MPH (Chapter 7)
Senior Scientist
Office of the Commander
U.S. Army Research Institute of
   Environmental Medicine
Natick, Massachusetts

**Kenneth H. Pitetti, PhD, FACSM
   (Chapter 26)**
Professor
Department of Physical Therapy
College of Health Professions
Wichita State University
Wichita, Kansas

John S. Raglin, PhD (Chapter 8)
Department of Kinesiology
Indiana University
Bloomington, Indiana

Nicholas A. Ratamess, Jr, PhD (Chapter 3)
Health and Physical Education Department
The College of New Jersey
Ewing, New Jersey

Otto A. Sánchez, MD, PhD (Chapter 14)
Research Fellow
Radiology Department
Vanderbilt University
Nashville, Tennessee

Michael N. Sawka, PhD (Chapter 7)
U.S. Army Research Institute of
   Environmental Medicine
Natick, Massachusetts

**James S. Skinner, PhD (Chapters 2, 6,
   19, 20)**
Professor
Department of Kinesiology
Indiana University
Bloomington, Indiana

Christine M. Snow, PhD (Chapter 11)
Professor
Exercise and Sports Science
Oregon State University
Corvallis, Oregon

Stephen G. Stahr (Chapter 1)
Student, Department of Biophysical
   Chemistry
Dartmouth College
Hanover, New Hampshire

Ilkka M. Vuori, MD, PhD (Chapter 10)
Professor Emeritus and Former Director
UKK-instituutti Centre for Health Promotion
   Research
University of Tampere
Tampere, Finland

Reginald L. Washington, MD (Chapter 22)
Associate Clinical Professor
Department of Pediatrics
University of Colorado
Denver, Colorado

Jack H. Wilmore, PhD (Chapter 4)
Professor Emeritus
Department of Health and Kinesiology
Texas A&M University
College Station, Texas

Gregory S. Wilson, PED (Chapter 8)
Professor and Director of Exercise Science
Department of Human Kinetics and
   Sport Studies
University of Evansville
Evansville, Indiana

Kerri M. Winters-Stone, PhD (Chapter 11)
Assistant Professor and Scientist
School of Nursing SN-ORD
Oregon Health and Science University
Portland, Oregon

Larry A. Wolfe, PhD, FACSM (Chapter 25)
Professor
School of Physical and Health Education
Queen's University
Kingston, Ontario, Canada

Contents

General Considerations

General Principles of Exercise Testing

Victor F. Froelicher and Stephen G. Stahr

Exercise can be considered one of the true tests of a person's health because it is the most common everyday stress that we undertake. The exercise test can be one of the most practical and useful procedures in the clinical evaluation of a wide variety of medical conditions, as discussed in other sections of this book.

Despite the many recent advances in technology, the exercise test remains an important diagnostic modality. Its many applications, widespread availability, and high yield of clinically useful information continue to make it an important gatekeeper for more expensive and invasive procedures. Excellent guidelines have been updated by organizations on the basis of a multitude of research studies over the last 30 years and have led to greater uniformity in methods. Before moving on to a discussion of exercise tests themselves, however, one must have a basic understanding of the physiologic basis of exercise.

Physiologic Principles of Testing the Oxygen Transport Systems

OXYGEN TRANSPORT AND MUSCULAR EFFORT

The transport of oxygen from the external environment to the mitochondria of the contracting muscle cell requires the coupling of blood flow and ventilation to cellular metabolism (1). This transport chain is normally capable of supporting a level of metabolism 10- to 12-fold greater than that at rest. Because this coupling is not tight enough to support rapid increases in muscular activity, however, anaerobic metabolism temporarily compensates for these transitions in energy demands. Similarly, anaerobic processes make an increasing contribution to metabolism as the limit of oxygen transport is approached and is briefly exceeded at maximal exercise.

Respiratory contributions to oxygen transport involve an increased minute ventilation ($\dot{V}_E$) resulting from increases in both rate (f) and tidal volume (TV). Diffusion and the ratio of alveolar ventilation ($\dot{V}_A$) to lung perfusion ($\dot{Q}_L$) also determine gas exchange. Cardiovascular adjustments include an increase in cardiac output ($\dot{Q}$), which is a function of heart rate (HR) times stroke volume (SV). $\dot{V}O_2$ depends on $\dot{Q}$ and the extraction of oxygen from the blood, the arteriovenous oxygen difference (AVD-O_2). With exercise, blood flow is directed away from inactive organs to the active skeletal muscle. The $\dot{V}O_2$ of muscle then depends upon vascularity, diffusion, muscle fiber distribution, and the total oxidative potential of these muscle fibers. In normal individuals, the limitation in oxygen transport probably lies in the delivery of oxygen to active muscle by the circulation (2,3).

When cardiovascular adjustments to dynamic exercise for a hypothetical 25-year-old, nonathletic man are depicted (Fig. 1-1) (4), there is a linear rise in $\dot{Q}$ versus $\dot{V}O_2$, with HR contributing most to this rise because SV increases minimally above 40 to 50% $\dot{V}O_{2max}$. Systolic blood pressure (SBP) increases with $\dot{V}O_2$, but diastolic pressure (DBP) changes are small and Korotkoff sounds can be heard all the way down to zero, particularly in normals. The mean arterial pressure (MAP) increases modestly. Predicting or directly measuring $\dot{V}O_{2max}$ during graded exercise testing provides a noninva-sive method of estimating $\dot{Q}_{max}$ because AVD-O_2 has a physiologic limit.

In contrast to dynamic exercise, static or isometric exercise results in disproportionate increases in ventilatory and cardiovascular variables relative to the external work performed. The proportional increases in $\dot{Q}$, SV, and HR and minimal change in MAP for dynamic exercise indicate a volume load for the heart. Static exercise produces a marked elevation in MAP, with relatively small increases in HR and $\dot{Q}$. This pressure load on the heart occurs in proportion to the relative muscle tension and the muscle mass involved (5,6).

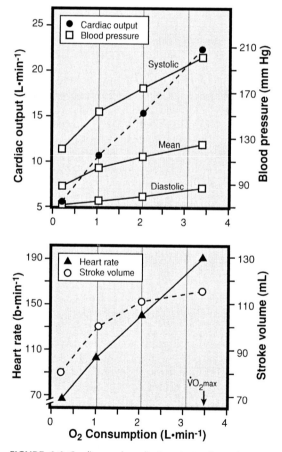

FIGURE 1-1 Cardiovascular adjustments to dynamic exercise for a 25-year-old man. (Modified from Bar-Or O, Buskirk ER. The cardiovascular system and exercise. In: Johnson WR, Buskirk ER, eds. Science and Medicine of Exercise and Sport. 2nd ed. New York: Harper & Row, 1974.)

GENERAL PRINCIPLES OF CHALLENGING THE OXYGEN TRANSPORT SYSTEMS

All exercise tests designed to measure functional capacity, $\dot{V}O_2$, or both should meet the following general requirements suggested by Åstrand and Rodahl (7).

1. Work must involve large muscle groups.
2. Work must be measurable and reproducible.
3. Test conditions must be such that the results are comparable and repeatable.
4. Testing must be tolerated by the individuals being evaluated.
5. Mechanical efficiency (skill) required to perform the task should be as uniform as possible in the population to be tested.

Considerations for Testing the Oxygen Transport System

INDICATIONS

The most common clinical applications of exercise testing are diagnosis and prognosis. Both of these are discussed in good detail in later sections. An exercise test can be used to determine the appropriateness or effects of rehabilitation programs, medications, and coronary artery bypass surgery. It can be used to evaluate patients with arrhythmias or to induce such arrhythmias as premature ventricular contractions, sick sinus syndrome, paroxysmal tachycardia, and heart block (8). The exercise test can be used to evaluate the safety of participation in an exercise program or the performance of other activities; it can be used to formulate an individualized exercise prescription based on a person's actual maximal HR rather than on an estimated value. In addition, the successful performance of a test after an acute myocardial infarction can be reassuring and is the first step in rehabilitation (9). In all exercise test applications, the ACC/AHA Guidelines should be followed (10).

CONTRAINDICATIONS

Just as there are times when an exercise test should be administered, there are times when a test should be avoided. Table 1-1 lists the absolute and relative contraindications to performing an exercise test as well as the factors to consider in assessing the degree of exercise. Good clinical judgment should be foremost in deciding the indications and contraindications for exercise testing. In selected cases with relative contraindications, testing can provide valuable information even if performed submaximally.

TABLE 1-1 CONTRAINDICATIONS TO EXERCISE TESTING

Absolute
- Acute myocardial infarction (within 2 days)
- Unstable angina not stabilized by medical therapy
- Uncontrolled cardiac arrhythmias causing symptoms or hemodynamic compromise
- Symptomatic severe aortic stenosis
- Uncontrolled symptomatic heart failure
- Acute pulmonary embolus or pulmonary infarction
- Acute myocarditis or pericarditis

Relative[a]
- Left main coronary stenosis or its equivalent
- Moderate stenotic valvular heart disease
- Electrolyte abnormalities
- Severe arterial hypertension[a]
- Tachyarrhythmias or bradyarrhythmias
- Hypertrophic cardiomyopathy and other forms of outflow tract obstruction
- Mental or physical impairment leading to inability to exercise adequately
- High-degree atrioventricular block

[a] Relative contraindications can be superseded if benefits outweigh risks of exercise

TYPE OF EXERCISE

An exercise test can involve any of a wide range of different types of exercise. Following is a look at some of the different types and comments about the uses of each.

Isometric versus Isotonic Exercise

Evaluating the cardiovascular responses to the pressure load of isometric exercise as well as to the volume load of isotonic exercise may be warranted in some clinical and occupational exercise testing. Results of several investigations reveal that isometric exercise alone fails to elicit the myocardial ischemia produced by dynamic exercise (11–13). When isometric was added to dynamic exercise, the threshold for ischemia occurred at a higher $M\dot{V}O_2$ (11,13). This result was attributed to a higher coronary perfusion pressure produced by the isometric elevation of DBP.

Although induction of arrhythmias by isometric and dynamic exercise was not different in some coronary artery disease (CAD) patients, a significantly greater incidence has been reported during isometric effort (11,14,15). In normal men, isometric exercise was effective in inducing ventricular premature beats, while their induction by treadmill exercise was highly variable (16).

Arms versus Legs

Dynamic exercise responses of individuals with lower-extremity impairments or who normally engage in arm work may be evaluated by arm ergometry (17–19). Arm ergometry effectively elicits myocardial ischemia (17,20,21). In one group of patients, electrocardiographic (ECG) ischemic responses occurred more frequently for leg than arm ergometry, but ventricular premature beats occurred more frequently with arm exercise (15). Both arm and wheelchair ergometry have effective applications in testing and rehabilitating the disabled person (22).

Treadmill versus Cycle Ergometry

In clinical testing, the type of exercise can influence the diagnostic value of the exercise test. For example, in exercise-induced bronchospasm, treadmill running has proven to be more asthmogenic than treadmill walking or cycle ergometry (23).

Physiologic monitoring, however, is easier to perform during cycling.

For coronary patients, Niederberger and colleagues found that bicycle exercise constituted a greater stress on the cardiovascular system at any given $\dot{V}O_2$ than did treadmill exercise; HR, rate pressure product or RPP (HR × SBP), MAP, and peripheral vascular resistance values were higher (24). Forty post-myocardial infarction (MI) patients achieved a 17% higher $\dot{V}O_{2max}$ on the treadmill than on a cycle ergometer, but the RPP was similar (HR was higher and SBP was lower) (25). ECG changes consistent with myocardial ischemia were similar. Leg ergometry was somewhat more effective in eliciting ischemia but was less arrhythmogenic than arm ergometry (15). Posture can also influence the diagnostic value of an exercise test because body position alters central hemodynamics and the ventilatory and metabolic responses to dynamic exercise (26–28).

Maximal Oxygen Intake ($\dot{V}O_{2max}$)

During a progressive exercise test, $\dot{V}O_{2max}$ is defined as the greatest $\dot{V}O_2$, in spite of an increase in the external power output (PO). This value represents an objectively defined limit of aerobic performance but requires additional equipment and technical support. Reasonable estimates of $\dot{V}O_{2max}$ can be obtained from the external PO, provided that standard testing methods are used. The highest values for $\dot{V}O_{2max}$ have been obtained during grade walking and running. Lower values were recorded for stepping (–3%), bicycling upright (–4 to –7%), bicycling supine (–15 to –18%), and arm cranking (–30 to –35%) (29,30). $\dot{V}O_2$ is commonly expressed in METS, which represent multiples of the metabolic requirements at rest (31,32).

Methods

PATIENT PREPARATION

Preparations for exercise testing include the following:

1. The patient should be instructed not to eat or smoke at least 2 to 3 hours prior to the test and to come dressed for exercise.

2. A history and physical examination (particularly for systolic murmurs) should be accomplished to rule out any contraindications to testing.

3. Specific questioning should determine which drugs are being taken, and potential electrolyte abnormalities should be considered. Labeled medication bottles should be brought along so that they can be identified and recorded. Because of the life-threatening rebound phenomena associated with β-blockers, they should not be completely stopped prior to testing. However, if testing is performed for diagnostic purposes, they can be stopped gradually if a physician or nurse supervises the tapering process carefully.

4. If the reason for the exercise test is not apparent, the referring physician should be contacted.

5. A 12-lead ECG should be obtained in both the supine and standing positions. The latter is important, particularly in patients with known heart disease, since an abnormality may prohibit testing.

6. There should be careful explanations of (*a*) why the test is being performed, (*b*) the testing procedure including its risks and possible complications, and (*c*) how to perform the test. If the treadmill will be used, this should include a demonstration of getting on and off as well as walking on the treadmill. The patient should be told that he or she can hold onto the rails initially, but later on should use the rails only for balance.

SAFETY PRECAUTIONS AND RISKS

Exercise testing should be an extension of the history and physical examination. A physical examination should always be performed to rule out significant obstructive aortic valvular disease. In some instances, such as when asymptomatic, apparently healthy subjects are being screened or a repeat treadmill test is being done on a patient whose condition is stable, a physician need not be present but should be in close proximity and prepared to respond promptly. The reaction to signs or symptoms should be moderated by the information the patient gives regarding his or her usual activity. If abnormal findings occur at levels of exercise that the patient usually performs, then it may not be necessary to stop the test. Also, the patient's activity history should help determine appropriate work rates and work levels for testing.

The safety precautions outlined by the American Heart Association are very explicit in regard to the requirements for exercise testing. Everything necessary for cardiopulmonary resuscitation must be available, and regular drills should be performed to ascertain that both personnel and equipment are ready for a cardiac emergency. The classic survey of clinical exercise facilities by Rochmis and Blackburn (33) showed exercise testing to be a safe procedure, with approximately one death and five nonfatal complications per 10,000 tests. Perhaps because of an expanded knowledge concerning indications, contraindications, and endpoints, maximal exercise testing appears safer today than 20 years ago. Gibbons et al. (34) reported the safety of exercise testing in 71,914 tests conducted over a 16-year period. The complication rate was 0.8 per 10,000 tests. Even with this excellent safety record, the risk of exercise testing in CAD patients cannot be disregarded.

Most problems can be avoided by having an experienced physician, nurse, or exercise physiologist standing next to the patient, measuring blood pressure, and assessing patient appearance during the test. The exercise technician should operate the recorder and treadmill or ergometer, take the appropriate tracings, record data, and alert the physician to any abnormalities that may appear on the monitor scope. If the patient's appearance is worrisome, if SBP drops or plateaus, if there are alarming ECG abnormalities, if chest pain occurs and becomes worse than the patient's usual pain, or if a patient wants to stop the test for any reason, the test should be stopped, even at a submaximal level. In most instances, a symptom-limited maximal test is preferred, but it is usually advisable to stop if 0.2 mV of additional ST-segment elevation occurs or if 0.2 mV of flat or down-sloping ST depression occurs. For some patients estimated to be at high risk because of their clinical history, it may be appropriate to stop at a submaximal level since it is not unusual for severe ST-segment depression, dysrhythmias, or both to occur only in recovery. If the measurement of maximal exercise capacity or other information is needed, it is better to repeat the test later, once the patient has demonstrated a safe performance of a submaximal PO.

SELECTION OF EXERCISE TESTING DEVICES

The most commonly used devices for testing are the bicycle ergometer, treadmill, step, and arm ergometer (35). Bicycle ergometry is favored in Europe and Scandinavia, whereas the treadmill is most often used in North America (36,37). Arm ergometry offers a suitable means for testing individuals with lower-extremity impairment (19,21).

PROTOCOLS

A number of testing protocols have been used to evaluate functional capacity. Protocol considerations should be consistent with testing objectives and should consider maximal versus submaximal testing, single versus multiple-stage testing, continuous versus intermittent effort, and stage duration.

Protocols suitable for clinical testing should include a low-intensity warm-up phase, 8 to 10 min of continuous progressive exercise during which the myocardial oxygen demand is elevated to the patient's maximal level, and a suitable recovery or cool-down period. The most widely used treadmill test used in clinical settings has been the Bruce protocol. Its significant disadvantages for functional testing, especially among patients with low exercise capacities or orthopedic problems, have led to other protocols. The MET increments in the Bruce protocol are large and uneven, and it limits the number of submaximal responses that may be observed in relation to exercise states. The Balke-Ware protocol is a particularly attractive alternative because of its constant treadmill speed of either 2.0 or 3.3 mph and grade increments of 5% applied every 2 to 3 min. A constant treadmill speed requires only an initial adaptation in stride and produces less ECG and blood pressure artifacts than do protocols involving increasing speeds (38).

A relatively new and very useful protocol, the ramp protocol, in which work increases constantly and continuously, is being used more and more. The advisability of "optimizing" exercise testing appears to be facilitated by the ramp approach, since work increments are small, and since it allows for individualized increases in work, a given test duration can be targeted. To investigate this, our laboratory compared ramp treadmill and bicycle tests with protocols more commonly used clinically. Ten patients with chronic heart failure, 10 with CAD who were limited by angina during exercise, 10 with CAD who were asymptomatic during exercise, and 10 age-matched normal subjects performed three bicycle tests (25 W/2-min stage, 50 W/2-min stage, and ramp) and three treadmill tests (Bruce, Balke, and ramp) in randomized order on different days. For the ramp tests, ramp rates on the bicycle and treadmill were individualized to yield a test duration of approximately 10 minutes for each subject. $\dot{V}O_{2max}$ was significantly higher (18%) on the treadmill protocols than on the bicycle protocols collectively, confirming previous observations. However, only minor differences in $\dot{V}O_{2max}$ were observed between the treadmill protocols themselves or between the cycle ergometer protocols themselves. We presently perform all our clinical and research testing using a ramp protocol.

Deciding on an exercise protocol that will optimize test duration for each patient is important, whether the approach used involves ramping or staging. Errors in this step can advance the patient toward maximal exertion too rapidly or too slowly. The consequence of early test termination is an inadequate opportunity to observe clinically important responses, whereas the consequence of a prolonged procedure is muscular fatigue, which may limit performance before a myocardial challenge adequate for diagnosis can be obtained. Thus, the protocol should be individualized to accommodate the patient's limitations. Performance should be estimated on the basis of $\dot{V}O_2$ ($mL \cdot kg^{-1} \cdot min^{-1}$) or METs associated with the maximal PO achieved, rather than on total treadmill time (39,40). Estimates of $\dot{V}O_2$ should be based on values derived for the patient population tested.

Finally, as mentioned in the section on patient preparation, in all cases in which an exercise test involves the use of a treadmill, patients should be discouraged from grasping the rails of the treadmill. This is because doing so causes the work to decrease, the exercise time to increase, and muscle artifacts to result (41). It is helpful to have patients close their fists and extend one finger, which

by touching the rail can help to maintain balance while walking.

Data Analysis

HEMODYNAMIC RESPONSES TO EXERCISE TESTING

When deciding on a suitable protocol, it is not advisable to use age-predicted maximal HR targets. Population studies have documented a relatively poor relationship of maximal HR to age, with correlation coefficients of −0.4 and a standard error of the estimate of 10–25 beats·min^{-1}.

Exertional hypotension, best defined as a drop in SBP below standing rest or a drop of 20 mm Hg after a rise, is very predictive of severe angiographic CAD and a poor prognosis. Until automated devices are adequately validated, we strongly recommend that blood pressure be taken manually with a cuff and stethoscope.

ST ANALYSIS

The analysis of an exercise test's results requires careful study and interpretation of the ECG. While the interpreter must have a good knowledge of the multitude of possible ECG characteristics, ST analysis is one that is of paramount importance.

ST-segment depression represents global subendocardial ischemia, with a direction determined largely by the placement of the heart in the chest. ST depression does not localize coronary artery lesions. V5 is the lead predominating in significant ST depression. Depression isolated to other leads is usually due to Q-wave distortion of the resting ECG. ST depression in the inferior leads (II, AVF) is most often due to the atrial repolarization wave, which begins in the PR segment and can extend to the beginning of the ST segment. When ST depression is isolated to these leads and there are no diagnostic Q waves, it is usually a false positive. ST-segment depression limited to the recovery period does not generally represent a "false-positive" response. Inclusion of analysis during this time period improves the diagnostic yield of the exercise test.

When the resting ECG shows Q waves of an old MI, ST elevation is due to wall motion abnormalities. When the resting ECG is normal, ST elevation is due to severe ischemia (spasm or a critical lesion). Such ST elevation is uncommon and very arrhythmogenic and localizes the involved coronary artery. Exercise-induced ST elevation (not over diagnostic Q waves) and ST depression both represent ischemia, but they are quite distinctive: *elevation* is due to transmural ischemia, is arrhythmogenic, has a 0.1% prevalence, and localizes the artery in which there is spasm or a tight lesion, while *depression* is due to subendocardial ischemia, is not arrhythmogenic, has a 5 to 50% prevalence, is rarely due to spasm, and does not localize. Figure 1-2 illustrates the various patterns. The standard criterion for abnormal is 1 mm of horizontal or down-sloping ST depression below the PR isoelectric line or 1 mm further depression if there is baseline depression. Ninety-five percent of the information is available in lead V5, with maximal exercise and 3 min into recovery being the most important times to look for ST depression (42). ECG recordings should continue for 5 min in recovery or until any new changes from baseline stabilize.

Nonsustained ventricular tachycardia is uncommon during routine clinical exercise testing (prevalence less than 2%), is well tolerated, and its prognosis is determined by the accompanying ischemia and left ventricular damage (43).

Diagnostic Use of the Exercise Test

ACC/AHA GUIDELINES FOR DIAGNOSTIC USE OF THE STANDARD EXERCISE TEST

The task force to establish guidelines for the use of exercise testing met and produced guidelines in 1986, 1997, and 2002 (44). Over the years, some dramatic changes have occurred, including the recommendation that the standard exercise test be the first diagnostic procedure in women and in most patients with resting ECG abnormalities rather than imaging studies. The following is a synopsis of these evidence-based guidelines.

Class I (Definitely appropriate). Conditions for which there is evidence and/or general agreement that the standard exercise test is useful and helpful to diagnose CAD. This class includes:

Adult male or female patients (including those with complete right bundle-branch block or with <1 mm of resting ST depression) with an *intermediate pretest probability* of CAD based on gender, age, and symptoms (specific exceptions are noted under class II and III below). *Note:* Pretest probability was determined from the Diamond-Forrester estimates tabulated in the guidelines as in Table 1-2.

Class IIa (Probably appropriate). Conditions for which there is conflicting evidence and/or a divergence of opinion that the standard exercise test is useful and helpful for diagnosis, but the weight of evidence for usefulness or efficacy is in favor of the exercise test. Patients with vasospastic angina often fall into this class.

Class IIb (May be appropriate). Conditions for which there is conflicting evidence and/or a divergence of opinion that the standard exercise test is useful and helpful for the diagnosis of CAD, but the usefulness/efficacy is less well established. This class includes:

1. Patients taking digoxin with <1 mm of baseline ST depression
2. Patients with ECG criteria for left ventricular hypertrophy with <1 mm of baseline ST depression
3. Patients with a high pretest probability of CAD by age, symptoms, and gender
4. Patients with a low pretest probability of CAD by age, symptoms, and gender

Class III (Not appropriate) — Conditions for which there is evidence and/or general agreement that the standard exercise test is not useful and helpful for the diagnosis of CAD and in some cases may be harmful.

1. To use the ST-segment response in the diagnosis of CAD in patients who demonstrate the following baseline ECG abnormalities:
   • Preexcitation (Wolff-Parkinson-White) syndrome
   • Electronically paced ventricular rhythm
   • >1 mm of resting ST depression
   • Complete left bundle-branch block
2. To use the ST-segment response in the diagnosis of CAD in patients who have had a well-documented MI. Although the diagnosis of CAD is established by the MI, ischemia and risk can be determined by testing.

TEST PERFORMANCE DEFINITIONS

Sensitivity and *specificity* are the terms used to define how reliably a test distinguishes diseased from nondiseased individuals. They are parameters of the accuracy of a diagnostic test. Sensitivity is the percentage of times that a test gives an abnormal ("positive") result when those with the disease are tested. Specificity is the percentage of times that a test gives a normal ("negative") result when those without the disease are tested. This is quite different from the colloquial use of the word *specific*. The method of calculating these terms is shown in Table 1-3, and the effects of prevalence change on the test performance values is shown in Table 1-4.

When the ST level begins at or above the isoelectric line (A & B):

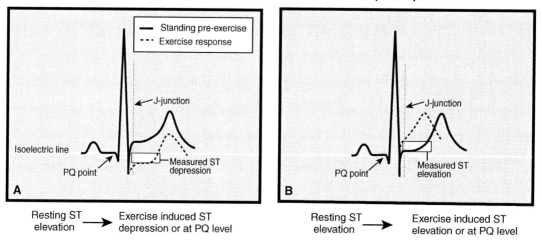

When the ST level begins below the isoelectric line (C & D):

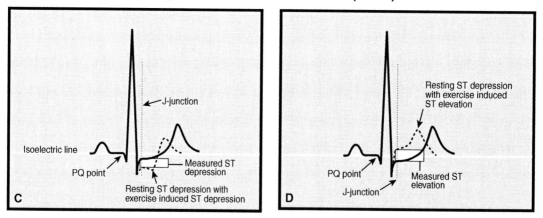

FIGURE 1-2 Various patterns of exercise-induced ST elevation and depression. ST level begins at or above the isoelectric line (**A and B**) and below the isoelectric line (**C and D**). ST deviation assessment *(continued)*

ST deviation assessment (E):

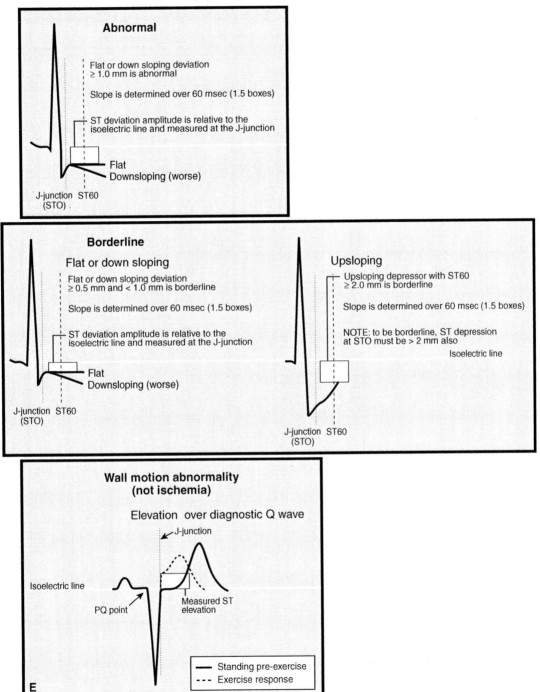

FIGURE 1-2 (*Continued*) (E) includes abnormal, borderline, and wall motion abnormality.

TABLE 1-2   PRETEST PROBABILITY OF CORONARY DISEASE BY SYMPTOMS, GENDER, AND AGE

Age	Gender	Typical/Definite Angina Pectoris	Atypical/Probable Angina Pectoris	Nonanginal Chest Pain	Asymptomatic
30–39	Males	Intermediate	Intermediate	Low (<10%)	Very low (<5%)
	Females	Intermediate	Very low (<5%)	Very low	Very low
40–49	Males	High	Intermediate	Intermediate	Low
	Females	Intermediate	Low	Very low	Very low
50–59	Males	High (>90%)	Intermediate	Intermediate	Low
	Females	Intermediate	Intermediate	Low	Very low
60–69	Males	High	Intermediate	Intermediate	Low
	Females	High	Intermediate	Intermediate	Low

There are no data for patients <30 years or >69 years, but it can be assumed that CAD prevalence increases with age.
  High, >90%; intermediate, 10–90%, low, <10%; very low, <5%.

FEINSTEIN'S METHODOLOGICAL STANDARDS FOR STUDIES OF DIAGNOSTIC TEST PERFORMANCE

Feinstein proposed seven methodological standards for research design when conducting exercise testing. However, only the requirement for an adequate variety of anatomic lesions received general

TABLE 1-3   DEFINITIONS AND CALCULATION OF THE TERMS USED TO QUANTIFY TEST DIAGNOSTIC ACCURACY

Sensitivity = (TP/TP + FN) × 100
Specificity = (TN/FP + TN) × 100
- TP = those with abnormal test result and disease (true positives)
- TN = those with a normal test result and no disease (true negatives)
- FP = those with an abnormal test result but no disease (false positives)
- FN = those with a normal test result but disease (false negatives)
- TP + TN + FP + FN = total population
- PV+ = percentage of those with an abnormal (positive) test result who have disease
- PV– = percentage of those with a negative test result that do not have disease
- Predictive accuracy = percentage of correct classifications, both + and –
- ROC = range of characteristics curve; plot of sensitivity vs. specificity for the range of measurement cut-points

compliance. Only one study met as many as five of the seven standards. Reid, Feinstein, and colleagues updated these criteria for "methodologic standards" for diagnostic tests in 1995 (45).

Most of the standards for evaluating diagnostic tests (e.g., blinding to test interpretation, exclusion of patients with prior MIs, and chest pain classification) are very logical and easy to appreciate. The two subtle standards that are least understood but affect test performance drastically and are most commonly not fulfilled are *limited challenge and work-up bias*. Limited challenge actually could be justified as the first step of looking at a new measurement or test. An investigator may choose healthy persons and sick persons, test them using the new measurement, and see if they are different. If no differences are noted, then further investigation is not indicated. Such a subject choice favors the measurement, but its true test is when consecutive patients present for evaluation. A measurement or test may function well to separate the extremes but fail in a clinical situation. Workup bias means that the decision of who goes to catheterization is based on the clinical acumen of the physician using the test. The patients in the study differ from patients presenting for evaluation before this selection process occurs. This can be avoided only in studies describing test characteristics by having patients agree to both procedures before any testing is performed.

Populations chosen for test evaluation that fail to avoid limited challenge will result in predictive

TABLE 1-4 EXAMPLE OF CALCULATING TEST PERFORMANCE AND EFFECT OF DIFFERENCES IN POPULATION TESTED

CAD Prevalence	Subjects	Test Characteristics	Number with Abnormal Test Result	Number with Normal Test Result	Predictive Value of a Positive Result
5%	500 with CAD	50% sensitive	250 (TP)	250 (FN)	250/250 + 950 = 21%
	9500 w/o CAD	90% specific	950 (FP)	8550 (TN)	
50%	5000 with CAD	50% sensitive	2500 (TP)	2500 (FN)	2500/3000 = 83%
	5000 w/o CAD	90% specific	500 (FP)	4500 (TN)	

	Predictive Value of an Abnormal Test Result		Risk	Ratio
Disease Prevalence	5%	50%	5%	50%
Sensitivity/specificity				
70/90%	27%	88%	27×	3×
90/70%	14%	75%	14×	5×
90/90%	32%	90%	64×	9×
66/84%	18%	80%	9×	3×

Note: Calculation of the predictive value of an abnormal test result (positive predictive value) using a test with a sensitivity of 50% and a specificity of 90% in two populations of 10,000 patients: one with a CAD prevalence of 5% and the other with 50% prevalence. This demonstrates the important influence that prevalence has on the positive predictive value.

accuracies and ROC curves greater than those truly associated with the test measurement. The two studies that have removed workup bias by protocol have included 2000 patients and have considerably different test characteristics (46).

CLINICAL META-ANALYSIS OF EXERCISE TESTING STUDIES

Following Feinstein's approach but considering more of the clinical and test methodologic issues, Gianrossi et al. investigated the variability of the reported diagnostic accuracy of the exercise ECG by applying a meta-analysis (47). One hundred forty-seven consecutively published reports, involving 24,074 patients who underwent both coronary angiography and exercise testing were summarized and the results entered into a computer spreadsheet. Details regarding population characteristics and methods were entered, including publication year, number of ECG leads, exercise protocol, preexercise hyperventilation, definition of an abnormal ST response, exclusion of certain subgroups, and

blinding of test interpretation. Wide variability in sensitivity and specificity was found (the mean sensitivity was 68%, with a range of 23–100% and a standard deviation of 16%; the mean specificity was 77%, with a range of 17–100% and a standard deviation 17%). The median predictive accuracy (percentage of total true calls) was approximately 73%.

To more accurately portray the performance of the exercise test, only the results in 41 studies of the original 147 were considered. These 41 studies removed patients with a prior MI from this meta-analysis, fulfilling one of the criteria for evaluating a diagnostic test, and provided all of the numbers for calculating test performance. These 41 studies, including nearly 10,000 patients, demonstrated a lower mean sensitivity of 68% and a lower mean specificity of 74%; this means that there also is a lower predictive accuracy of 71%. In several studies in which workup bias was lessened (which fulfills the other major criterion), the sensitivity is approximately 50% and the specificity 90%, and the predictive accuracy stays at 70% (48). This demonstrates that the key feature of the standard exercise test for clinical use is its high specificity and that its low sensitivity is a problem.

EFFECTS OF DIGOXIN, LEFT VENTRICULAR HYPERTROPHY (LVH), AND RESTING ST DEPRESSION

To resolve the issues of LVH, resting ST depression, and digoxin, the results from the meta-analysis were considered. Of the appropriate studies, only those that provided sensitivity, specificity, and total patient numbers and included more than 100 patients were considered. The conclusion from this analysis was that only digoxin had a major effect on test performance.

GENDER

There has been controversy regarding the use of the standard exercise ECG test in women. In fact, some experts have recommended that only imaging techniques be used for testing women because of the impression that the standard exercise ECG did not perform as well in them as it did in men. The recent ACC/AHA guidelines reviewed this subject in detail and came to another conclusion. This position was based on evidence and used information from meta-analyses as well as 15 studies that considered only women. The recent guidelines have definitely stated that exercise testing for diagnosing significant obstruction CAD in adult patients including women, with symptoms or other clinical findings suggesting CAD is a class I indication

(i.e., definitely indicated). Women in the intermediate classification are those from 30 to 59 years with typical or definite angina pectoris, those from 30 to 69 years with atypical or probable pectoris, and those 60 to 68 years with nonanginal chest pain.

COMPARISON WITH OTHER DIAGNOSTIC TESTS

Investigators from the University of California at San Francisco reviewed the contemporary literature to compare the diagnostic performance of exercise echocardiography (ECHO) and exercise nuclear perfusion scanning (NUC) in CAD diagnosis (49). Studies published between January 1990 and October 1997 identified from a MEDLINE search included bibliographies of reviews, original articles, and suggestions from experts in each area. Articles were included if they discussed exercise ECHO and/or exercise NUC imaging with thallium or sestamibi to detect and/or evaluate CAD, if data on coronary angiography were presented as the reference test, and if the absolute numbers of true-positive, false-negative, true-negative, and false-positive observations were available or derivable from the data presented. Studies performed exclusively in patients after an MI, after percutaneous transluminal coronary angioplasty, after coronary artery bypass grafting, or with recent unstable coronary syndromes were excluded. The results are presented in Table 1-5. In models comparing the discriminatory abilities of exercise ECHO and

---

TABLE 1-5   COMPARISON OF EXERCISE TESTING SUBGROUPS AND DIFFERENT TEST MODALITIES.

Grouping	No. of Studies	Total No. of Patients	Sensitivity	Specificity	Predictive Accuracy
Meta-analysis of standard ET	147	24,047	68%	77%	73%
Meta-analysis without MI	58	11,691	67%	72%	69%
Meta-analysis of treadmill scores	24	11,788			80%
Electron beam computed tomography	4	1,631	90%	45%	68%
Thallium scintigraphy	59	6,038	85%	85%	85%
SPECT without MI	27	2,136	86%	62%	74%
Persantine thallium	11		85%	91%	87%
Exercise ECHO	58	5,000	84%	75%	80%
Exercise ECHO without MI	24	2,109	87%	84%	85%
Dobutamine ECHO	5	869	88%	4%	86%

exercise NUC to exercise testing without imaging, both ECHO and NUC performed significantly better than the exercise ECG. While the nonexercise stress tests are very useful, the results shown in Table 1-5 are probably better than their actual performance because of patient selection.

EXERCISE TEST SCORES

The exercise testing studies that have considered information in addition to the ST response have been reviewed and demonstrate the improved test characteristics obtained using this approach (50). The DUKE prognostic score has been extended to diagnosis (51).

"SIMPLIFIED" SCORE DERIVATION

Simplified scores derived from multivariable equations have been developed to determine the probability of disease and prognosis. All variables were coded with the same number of intervals so that the coefficients would be proportional. For instance, if 5 is the chosen interval, dichotomous variables are 0 if not present and 5 if present. Such continuous variables as age and maximal HR were coded in five groups associated with increasing prevalence of disease. The relative importance of the selected variables is obvious, and the health care provider merely compiles the variables in the score, multiples by the appropriate number, and then adds up the products. Calculation of the "simple" exercise test score can be done using Figure 1-3 (52) for men and Figure 1-4 (53) for women.

PREDICTIVE ACCURACY

Some test results are dichotomous (normal vs. abnormal, positive vs. negative) rather than continuous like a score. Predictive accuracy (true positives plus true negatives divided by the total population studied) can be used to compare dichotomous test results. Any score can also be dealt with as a dichotomous variable by choosing a cut-point. An advantage of predictive accuracy is that it provides an estimate of the number of patients correctly classified by the test out of 100 tested. However, when predictive accuracy is used to compare tests, populations with roughly the same prevalence of disease

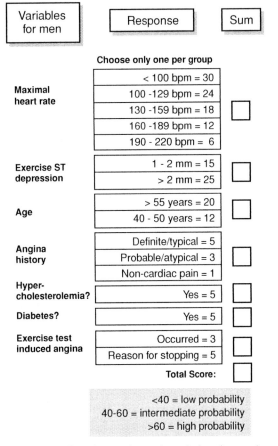

FIGURE 1-3 Chart that can be used to calculate the exercise score for men. (From Raxwal V, Shetler K, Do D, Froelicher V. A simple treadmill score. Chest 2000;113:1933–1940.)

should be considered. Table 1-5 is based on published meta-analyses and summarizes the predictive accuracy of the major diagnostic tests for CAD currently available (54).

SUMMARY OF THE DIAGNOSTIC USE OF EXERCISE TESTING

With patients subgrouped according to β-blocker administration that was initiated by their referring physician, no differences in test performance were found in a consecutive group of males being evaluated for possible CAD. Though perhaps optimal, it appears unnecessary with routine exercise

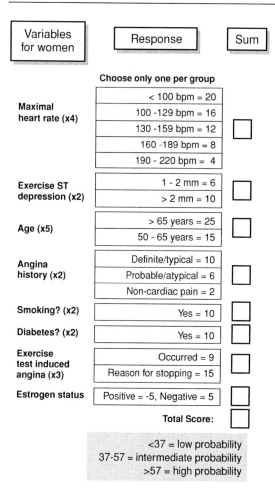

Variables for women	Response	Sum

Choose only one per group

Maximal heart rate (x4)	< 100 bpm = 20
	100 -129 bpm = 16
	130 -159 bpm = 12
	160 -189 bpm = 8
	190 - 220 bpm = 4
Exercise ST depression (x2)	1 - 2 mm = 6
	> 2 mm = 10
Age (x5)	> 65 years = 25
	50 - 65 years = 15
Angina history (x2)	Definite/typical = 10
	Probable/atypical = 6
	Non-cardiac pain = 2
Smoking? (x2)	Yes = 10
Diabetes? (x2)	Yes = 10
Exercise test induced angina (x3)	Occurred = 9
	Reason for stopping = 15
Estrogen status	Positive = -5, Negative = 5

Total Score:

<37 = low probability
37-57 = intermediate probability
>57 = high probability

FIGURE 1-4 Chart that can be used to calculate the exercise score for women. (From Morise AP, Lauer MS, Froelicher VF. Development and validation of a simple exercise test score for use in women with symptoms of suspected coronary artery disease. Am Heart J 2002;144:818–825.)

testing for physicians to accept the risk of stopping β-blockers before testing when patients exhibit possible symptoms of ischemia or when they are used to treat hypertension.

To obtain the best diagnostic characteristics with the exercise test, clinical and non-ECG test responses should be considered. Computerized ECG measurements and ECG scores are not superior to visual analysis but can duplicate the results of expert readers. Multivariate scores using computers to make the calculations from logistic regression equations appear to significantly improve on test characteristics.

The summary from the guidelines are well stated regarding testing women: concern about false-positive ST responses may be addressed by careful assessment of posttest probability and selective use of a stress imaging test before proceeding to angiography.

Prognostic Use of the Exercise Test

ACC/AHA GUIDELINES FOR THE PROGNOSTIC USE OF THE STANDARD TEST

Indications for exercise testing to assess risk and prognosis in patients with symptoms or a prior history of CAD:

Class I (Definitely appropriate). Conditions for which there is evidence and/or general agreement that the standard exercise test is useful and helpful to assess risk and prognosis in patients with symptoms or a prior history of CAD.
1. Patients undergoing initial evaluation with suspected or known CAD. Specific exceptions are noted below in class IIb.
2. Patients with suspected or known CAD previously evaluated, with significant change in clinical status

Class IIb (May be appropriate). Conditions for which there is conflicting evidence and/or a divergence of opinion that the standard exercise test is useful and helpful to assess risk and prognosis in patients with symptoms or a prior history of CAD but the usefulness/efficacy is less well established.
1. Patients who demonstrate the following ECG abnormalities:
   • Preexcitation (Wolff-Parkinson White) syndrome
   • Electronically paced ventricular rhythm
   • >1 mm of resting ST depression
   • Complete left bundle-branch block
2. Patients with a stable clinical course who undergo periodic monitoring to guide management

Class III (Not appropriate). Conditions for which there is evidence and/or general agreement that the standard exercise test is not useful and helpful to assess risk and prognosis in patients with symptoms or a prior history of CAD and in some cases may be harmful.

Patients with severe comorbidity likely to limit life expectancy and/or candidacy for revascularization

DUKE TREADMILL SCORE AND NOMOGRAM

Mark et al. studied 2842 consecutive patients who underwent cardiac catheterization and exercise testing and whose data were entered into the Duke computerized medical information system (55).

The median follow-up for the study population was 5 years and 98% complete. All patients underwent a Bruce protocol exercise test and had standard ECG measurements recorded. A treadmill angina index was assigned a value of 0 if angina was absent, 1 if typical angina occurred during exercise, and 2 if angina was the reason the patient stopped exercising. Before the test, 54% of the patients had taken propranolol and 11% had taken digoxin. ST measurements considered were the sum of the largest net ST depression and elevation, sum of the ST displacements in all 12 ECG leads, the number of leads showing ST displacement of 0.1 mV or more, and the product of the number of leads showing ST displacement and the largest single ST displacement in any lead. This nomogram and an example are shown in Figure 1-5.

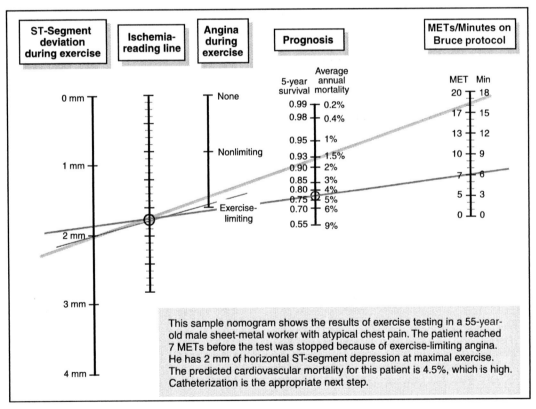

FIGURE 1-5 Duke treadmill score nomogram with an example. The *grey line* shows how prognosis would be improved by a higher exercise capacity with the same other responses. One printing of this for the ACC/AHA guidelines evened the vertical lines, ruining the prognostic estimates.

On the basis of clinical and exercise test data, patients with signs and symptoms of CAD can be classified into low- and high-risk categories. The latter clearly should be considered for cardiac catheterization, while the former should not, unless their symptoms dictate otherwise. The problem lies in justifying intervention to improve survival for patients whose symptoms are satisfactorily managed medically. Our study demonstrates that simple clinical indicators can stratify these patients with stable CAD into high- or low-risk groups. Cardiac catheterization is not needed to do so for most such patients. In our VA population, we consider a history of congestive heart failure or digoxin administration and responses to three exercise tests as the most important predictors of cardiovascular death (56). Clinical judgment must be applied to decide whether intervention is likely to improve survival in our high-risk patients. The DUKE and VA predictive equations appear to be the best and represent the "state of the art" in prognostication.

RECOVERY HEART RATE

HR usually falls rapidly at the end of a bout of progressive exercise. While the rate of the drop in HR is related to fitness, more recently it has been shown to be inversely related to survival (57). In general, a decline in HR of less than 20 beats·min^{-1} by the first or second minute of recovery is associated with an increased risk of death (58).

Legal Implications of Exercise Testing

The legal aspects of exercise testing include several considerations. Establishing good communication between tester and patient before and after the exercise test should be the first consideration. A test should not be performed without first obtaining the patient's informed consent, preferably in writing. The patient should be made aware of the potential risks and benefits of any procedure. Even if the test is carefully performed, a tester may be held responsible for a major untoward effect if consent was not first obtained. The position can be taken that a patient would not have undergone the procedure had he or she been aware of the associated

risks. After the test is completed, the physician is responsible for prompt interpretation and considering the implications of the test. Communication of these results to the patient is essential and advice concerning adjustments in lifestyle should be made without delay. It would be of major concern if an untoward event occurred during such a delay.

The second consideration should be adherence to proper standards of care during the test. Every test should be preceded by a physical examination and an ECG performed by the supervising or referring physician. Testing should be carried out only by persons thoroughly trained in the administration of exercise tests, in recognizing signs and symptoms that may arise, and in cardiopulmonary resuscitation. The patient must be instructed to report symptoms (e.g., angina or lightheadedness) that may require test termination. A physician trained in exercise testing and resuscitation should be immediately accessible during the test to make the judgment to stop. Resuscitative equipment and medications should always be available.

The purpose of this chapter is to provide an overview of many factors of exercise testing. The reader is referred to several other references for a more extensive review (10,59,60).

Summary

- The results of standard exercise tests are greatly influenced by the condition of a person's oxygen transport system. This system is governed by factors including heart rate, stroke volume, ventilation, tidal volume, and the ratio of alveolar to lung perfusion.
- The clinical applications of the exercise test are many and varied. Two common uses include prognostic and diagnostic applications. Each of these is governed by specific guidelines established by the ACC, AHA, and ACSM.
- A number of contraindications exist of which a test administrator must be aware. Failure to observe a critical contraindication could result in complications.
- There are a number of different types of exercises that an exercise test could involve. The condition and special needs of the individual being testing

should be taken into consideration when determining which type is used.

- There are specific guidelines that should be followed when preparing a patient for an exercise test and a number of safety precautions that must be taken. As with the type of exercise used, the type of protocol used should consider the condition and special needs of the individual being tested.
- Accurate analysis of the ST segment is of crucial importance to the interpretation of the results. There are specific guidelines one must follow in the analysis.
- A set of specific standards for the diagnostic studies of test performance has been developed, and they should be followed.
- As for the prognostic value of the exercise test, on the basis of clinical and exercise test data, patients with signs and symptoms of CAD can be classified into low- and high-risk categories. Also, the recovery heart rate has been shown to be related to mortality.

REFERENCES

1. Wasserman K, Whipp BJ. Exercise physiology in health and disease. Am Rev Respir Dis 1975;112:219–227.
2. Saltin B, Rowell LB. Functional adaptations to physical activity and inactivity. Fed Proc 1980;39:1506–1513.
3. Gonzalez-Alonso J, Calbet J. Reductions in systemic muscle blood flow and oxygen delivery limit maximal aerobic capacity in humans. Circulation 2003;107:824–830.
4. Bar-Or O, Buskirk ER. The cardiovascular system and exercise. In: Johnson WR, Buskirk ER, eds. Science and Medicine of Exercise and Sport. 2nd ed. New York: Harper & Row, 1974.
5. Michell JH, Wildenthal K. Static (isometric) exercise and the heart: physiological and clinical considerations. Annu Rev Med 1974;25:369–376.
6. Mitchell JH, Payne FC, Saltin B, et al. The role of muscle mass in the cardiovascular response to static contractions. J Physiol (Lond) 1980;309:45–54.
7. Åstrand PO, Ekblom B, Saltin B, et al. Intra-arterial blood pressure during exercise with different muscle groups. J Appl Physiol 1965;20:253–260.
8. Goldschlager N, Cohn K, Goldschlager A. Exercise-related ventricular arrhythmias. Mod Concepts Cardiovasc Dis 1979;48:67–72.
9. Sivarajan ES, Lerman J, Mansfield LW, et al. Progressive ambulation and treadmill testing of patients with acute myocardial infarction during hospitalization: a feasibility study. Arch Phys Med Rehabil 1977;58:241–252.
10. Froelicher VF, Myers J. Exercise and the Heart. 4th ed. Philadelphia: Saunders/Mosby Year Book Medical Publishers, 1999.
11. DeBusk R, Pitts W, Haskell WL, et al. Comparison of cardiovascular responses to static-dynamic effort and dynamic effort alone in patients with chronic ischemic heart disease. Circulation 1979;59:977–984.
12. Haissly J, Messin R, Degre S, et al. Comparative response to isometric (static) and dynamic exercise tests in coronary disease. Am J Cardiol 1974;33:791–796.
13. Kerber RE, Miller RA, Najjar SM, et al. Myocardial ischemic effects of isometric, dynamic and combined exercise in coronary artery disease. Chest 1975;67:388–394.
14. Atkins JM, Mathew OA, Blomqvist CG, et al. Incidence of arrhythmias induced by isometric and dynamic exercise. Br Heart J 1976;38:465–471.
15. DeBusk R., Valdez R, Houston N, et al. Cardiovascular responses to dynamic and static effort soon after myocardial infarction. Circulation 1978;58:368–377.
16. DeBacker G, Jacobs DR Jr, Prineas RJ, et al. Ventricular premature beats: screening and induction tests in normal men. Cardiology 1980;65:23–30.
17. Balady GJ, Weiner DA, Rothendler JA, et al. Arm exercise-thallium imaging testing for the detection of coronary artery disease. J Am Coll Cardiol 1987;9:84–93.
18. Fletcher GF, Lloyd A, Waling JF, et al. Exercise testing in patients with musculoskeletal handicaps. Arch Phys Med Rehabil 1988;69:123–129.
19. Glaser RM., Sawka MN, Brune MF, et al. Physiological responses to maximal effort wheelchair and arm crank ergometry. J Appl Physiol 1980;48:1060–1064.
20. Lazarus B, Cullinane E, Thompson PD. Comparison of the results and reproducibility of arm and leg exercise tests in men with angina pectoris. Am J Cardiol 1981;47:1075–1079.
21. Schwade J, Blomqvist CG, Shapiro W. A comparison of the response to arm and leg work in patients with ischemic heart disease. Am Heart J 1977;94:203–210.
22. Sawka MN. Upper body exercise: physiology and practical considerations. Med Sci Sports Exerc 1989;21:S119–125.
23. Cropp GJ. The exercise bronchoprovocation test: standardization of procedures and evaluation of response. J Allergy Clin Immunol 1979;64:627–635.

24. Niederberger M, Bruce RA, Kusumi F, et al. Disparities in ventilatory and circulatory responses to bicycle and treadmill exercise. Br Heart J 1974;36:377–382.

25. Wicks JR, Sutton JR, Oldridge NB, et al. Comparison of the electrocardiographic changes induced by maximum exercise testing with treadmill and cycle ergometer. Circulation 1978;57:1066–1070.

26. Bevegård S, Holmgren A, Jonsson B, et al. The effect of body position on the circulation at rest and during exercise, with special reference to the influence on the stroke volume. Acta Physiol Scand 1960;49:279–286.

27. Lear JL. Effect of exercise position during stress testing on cardiac and pulmonary thallium kinetics and accuracy in evaluation of coronary artery disease. J Nucl Med 1986;27:788–795.

28. Wetherbee JN, Bamrah VS, Ptacin MJ, et al. Comparison of ST segment depression in upright treadmill and supine bicycle exercise testing. J Am Coll Cardiol 1988;11:330–337.

29. Åstrand PO. Quantification of exercise capability and evaluation of physical capacity in man. Prog Cardiovasc Dis 1976;19:51–60.

30. Shephard RJ, Allen C, Benade AJ, et al. The maximum oxygen intake. Bull WHO 1968;38:757–764.

31. American College of Sports Medicine. Guidelines for Graded Exercise Testing and Exercise Prescription. 6th ed. Philadelphia: Lippincott Williams & Wilkins, 2000.

32. Subcommittee on Exercise Testing. Guidelines for exercise testing: a report of the American College of Cardiology/American Heart Association Task Force on Assessment of Cardiovascular Procedures. J Am Coll Cardiol 1986;8:725–730.

33. Rochmis P, Blackburn H. Exercise tests: a survey of procedures, safety, and litigation experience in approximately 170,000 tests. JAMA 1971;217:1061–1066.

34. Gibbons L, Blair SN, Kohl HW, et al. The safety of maximal exercise testing. Circulation 1989;80:846–852.

35. Andersen KL, Shephard RJ, Denolin H, et al. Fundamentals of Exercise Testing. Geneva: World Health Organization, 1971.

36. Atterhog J, Jonsson B, Samuelsson R. Exercise testing in Sweden: a survey of procedures. Scand J Clin Invest 1979;39:87–93.

37. Stuart RJ, Ellestad MH. National survey of exercise stress testing facilities. Chest 1980;77:94–101.

38. Callaham PR, Froelicher VF, Klein J, et al. Exercise-induced silent ischemia: age, diabetes mellitus, previous myocardial infarction and prognosis. J Am Coll Cardiol 1989;14:1175–1182.

39. Froelicher VF, Brammell H, Davis G, et al. A comparison of three maximal treadmill exercise protocols. J Appl Physiol 1974;36:725–734.

40. Tonino RP, Driscoll PA. Reliability of maximal and submaximal parameters of treadmill testing for the measurement of physical training in older persons. J Gerontol 1988;43:M101–104.

41. Pina IL, Karalis DG. Comparison of four exercise protocols using anaerobic threshold measurement of functional capacity in congestive heart failure. Am J Cardiol 1990;65:1269–1271.

42. Lachterman B, Lehmann KG, Abrahamson D, Froelicher VF. "Recovery only" ST-segment depression and the predictive accuracy of the exercise test. Ann Intern Med 1990;112:11–16.

43. Yang JC, Wesley RC, Froelicher VF. Ventricular tachycardia during routine treadmill testing: risk and prognosis. Arch Intern Med 1991;151:349–353.

44. Gibbons RJ, Balady GJ, Bricker JT, et al. ACC/AHA 2002 guideline update for exercise testing: a report of the American College of Cardiology/American Heart Association Task Force on Practice Guidelines (Committee on Exercise Testing). Circulation 2002;106:1883–1892.

45. Reid M, Lachs M, Feinstein A. Use of methodological standards in diagnostic test research. JAMA 1995;274:645–651.

46. Froelicher VF, Lehmann KG, Thomas R, et al. The electrocardiographic exercise test in a population with reduced workup bias: diagnostic performance, computerized interpretation, and multivariable prediction. Veterans Affairs Cooperative Study in Health Services #016 (QUEXTA) Study Group. Quantitative exercise testing and angiography. Ann Intern Med 1998;128(12 Pt 1):965–974.

47. Gianrossi R, Detrano R, Froelicher VF, et al. Exercise-induced ST depression in the diagnosis of coronary artery disease: a meta-analysis. Circulation 1989;80:87–98.

48. Morise A, Diamond GA. Comparisons of the sensitivity and specificity of exercise electrocardiography in biased and unbiased populations of men and women. Am Heart J 1995;130:741–747.

49. Fleischmann KE, Hunink MG, Kuntz KM, et al. Exercise echocardiography or exercise spect imaging: a meta-analysis of diagnostic test performance. JAMA 1998;280:913–920.

50. Yamada H, Do D, Froelicher VF, et al. Review of studies utilizing multi-variable analysis of clinical and exercise test data to predict angiographic coronary artery disease. 1997;39:457–481.

51. Shaw LJ, Peterson ED, Shaw LK, et al. Use of a prognostic treadmill score in identifying diagnostic coronary disease subgroups. Circulation 1998;98:1622–1630.

52. Raxwal V, Shetler K, Do D, Froelicher VF. A simple treadmill score. Chest 2000;113:1933–1940.

53. Morise AP, Lauer MS, Froelicher VF. Development and validation of a simple exercise test score for use in women with symptoms of suspected coronary artery disease. Am Heart J 2002;144:818–825.

54. O'Rourke RA, Brundage BH, Froelicher VF, et al. American College of Cardiology/American Heart Association expert consensus document on electron-beam computed tomography for the diagnosis and prognosis of coronary artery disease. J Am Coll Cardiol 2000;36:326–340.

55. Mark DB, Hlatky MA, Harrell FE, et al. Exercise treadmill score for predicting prognosis in coronary artery disease. Ann Intern Med 1987;106:793–800.

56. Morrow K, Morris CK, Froelicher VF, et al. Prediction of cardiovascular death in men undergoing noninvasive evaluation for CAD. Ann Intern Med 1993;118: 689–695.

57. Cole CR, Blackstone EH, Pashkow FJ, et al. Heart-rate recovery immediately after exercise as a predictor of mortality. N Engl J Med 1999;341:1351–1357.

58. Shetler K, Marcus R, Froelicher VF, et al. Heart rate recovery: validation and methodologic issues. J Am Coll Cardiol 2001;38:1980–1987.

59. Atwood JE, et al. Exercise testing in patients with aortic stenosis. Chest 1988;93:1083–1089.

60. Fletcher GF, Froelicher VF, Hartley LH, et al. Exercise standards. A statement for health professionals from the American Heart Association. Circulation 1990;82:2286–2293.

RELATED WEB SITES

Cardiology division at the VA Palo Alto Health Care System
www.cardiology.org

American Heart Association
www.americanheart.org

American College of Cardiology
www.acc.org

American College of Sports Medicine
www.acsm.org

2

General Principles of Exercise Prescription

James S. Skinner

According to the American College of Sports Medicine (ACSM), an exercise prescription is "the process whereby a person's recommended regimen of physical activity is designed in a systematic and individualized manner"(1). This chapter outlines some of the knowledge required and the basic components of good programs, as well as general principles and factors to consider when prescribing exercise in a "systematic and individualized manner."

General Knowledge

Physicians and exercise leaders find variations in motivation, attitude, and responses to exercise in any group of persons they encounter and advise. These variations may be due to such factors as age, health status, race, social class, genetic background, personal goals, and previous experience. Therefore, physicians and allied health professionals need to be knowledgeable about many factors and the potential of each for modifying an exercise prescription.

EXERCISE PHYSIOLOGY

A good understanding of exercise physiology is necessary to prescribe individualized exercise programs. This knowledge includes such factors as steady-state exercise, efficiency, sources of energy, and mechanisms of energy production; differences and similarities between kilocalories and metabolic equivalents (METs); and the relationship between work performed and oxygen intake ($\dot{V}O_2$) or heart rate (HR). The person prescribing exercise should also know how prescriptions can be affected by specific characteristics of an activity, i.e., whether it is static or dynamic, brief or prolonged, intermittent or continuous, and whether it is done with the arms or legs or while supine, sitting, or standing. It is assumed that the reader has this knowledge, as it is the basis for an important aspect in exercise prescription—the measurement and quantification of exercise.

EFFECTS OF AGE, GENDER, AND ENVIRONMENT

Physiologic (functional) age is more important than chronologic age in the type of activity chosen, but age is a risk factor in itself and must be considered. Physiologically, there is little difference in the mechanisms used by men and women to respond to exercise or to adapt to training. Any differences are more likely to be quantitative (partly related to body size). There also may be differences in the types of exercise men and women select. Because environment (heat, cold, pollution, and altitude) can affect the capacity to perform exercise, it can also modify an exercise prescription. Each of these factors, discussed in more detail in subsequent chapters, can modify the selection and performance of activities.

KNOWLEDGE ABOUT HEALTH AND FITNESS

Health Status

Exercise may be contraindicated for some persons who have certain diseases or medical conditions. For more detailed information related to persons to be tested and the tests to be performed, the reader is referred to other chapters in this book and to publications by the ACSM, the American Association of Cardiovascular and Pulmonary Rehabilitation, and other organizations (2–5). If there is any doubt about a person's health status, a comprehensive medical examination should be performed, especially for individuals who plan to increase their activity level significantly. Musculoskeletal status is as important as cardiovascular–respiratory health because orthopedic problems are common in adults and are a major reason why participants drop out in the initial stages of an exercise program. A person's health status also influences the frequency, intensity, duration, type, and progression of exercise.

Fitness Profile

After a medical examination has been performed for those persons at possible risk, a comprehensive fitness profile can be given. This profile could include such variables as body composition, physical working capacity, responses to a series of submaximal power outputs (POs), flexibility, strength and muscle endurance, as well as information on each person's needs, interests, and objectives. As is detailed below, persons who are more active and fitter tend to be able to exercise more often, at higher intensities, and for longer durations (i.e., they do more total exercise) and will probably progress more rapidly.

Health and Fitness

Evaluating a person's health and fitness and subsequent consultations with them about their results can be a useful tool to teach about the benefits and risks of exercise and to motivate persons to begin or to continue exercising. Specific and reasonable goals can then be given to each individual. Information regarding a person's health status and re-

sponse to exercise forms the basis for prescribing an exercise program that will be safe and effective. Another important factor, enjoyment, can be promoted by understanding the needs, interests, and goals of the individual. Thus, a comprehensive approach is needed to promote regular and continued participation in safe, effective, and enjoyable programs.

Need for Exercise Prescription

Once a person's functional capacity, medical status, and interests are known, individualized exercise prescriptions can be given. The physician or exercise leader should define the major purposes of the exercise program and plan accordingly. Because the reasons for exercising can vary greatly, however, the need for precision in exercise testing and prescribing exercise will also vary.

As suggested by Balke (6), only two categories of persons need careful and precise prescriptions: athletes and those who have a disease or medical condition that adversely affects their ability to exercise (e.g., coronary heart disease, arthritis, or emphysema). Figure 2-1 is a schematic representation of the need for precision in prescribing exercise for different types of persons according to their reasons for exercising.

Although health, fun, and fitness may result from intense training, the primary goal of most athletes is to improve performance. The exercise leader is more involved than the physician with this type of person. The exercise leader should determine the specific characteristics of the activity in which the athlete competes, decide on the relative importance of pertinent physiologic factors, and design a detailed program geared specifically to develop those factors in particular, so that athletes can perform as closely as possible to their genetic potential.

At the other end of the fitness continuum, disease-limited persons or those with a medical condition that affects their ability to exercise are probably most interested in improving their health. Fun and fitness are generally secondary, and performance per se is less important. The physician is more involved with these persons because of the medical nature of their problems and because they need guidance on how to improve their functional reserves and possibly to counteract further

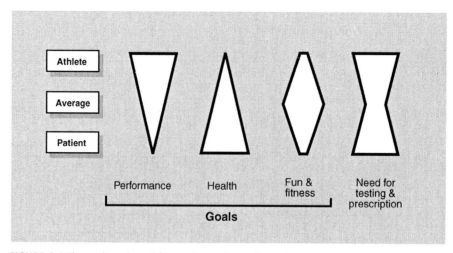

FIGURE 2-1 The goals and need for precise testing and exercise prescription in different types of persons.

degeneration. As well, medications can affect responses to exercise and training. Not only do patients need precise prescriptions to know the types of exercise to emphasize and avoid, they may have to exercise under varying degrees of supervision. It appears that persons of below-average health and fitness are often the ones who (*a*) need exercise most, (*b*) do less, (*c*) are less motivated to exercise, (*d*) have more problems and limitations when they do exercise, (*e*) need more guidance, and (*f*) have been studied less (7).

Between these two extremes are the "average" persons. Fun and fitness are generally the main reasons why they exercise, although performance, health, and appearance may be important considerations. Often, the health status of this group is not known, i.e., they may have no signs or symptoms and may not know or recognize any limitations. Only when average persons migrate to either end of the continuum do they need more assistance. In other words, the more risk factors these apparently healthy adults have, the longer they have been inactive, the more sedentary they have been, or the more they wish to compete, the more important is their need for exercise testing and precise prescriptions. If it is assumed that these individuals are healthy, however, precision is rarely needed, and general principles of exercise and training are adequate. Most such persons select activities that they enjoy or that allow them to have social, recreational, or competitive interactions.

The important point to remember is that the same principles of training apply to everyone. Modifications are usually associated with the absence or presence of medical restrictions or contraindications, types of activities to emphasize or avoid, the initial level of fitness, the intensity of participation, and the rate of improvement expected or desired.

Principles of Training

No one program or set of programs is best for everyone or even for the same person over time, as interests, needs, goals, and capabilities change. People also respond differently to exercise and adapt differently to training. Nevertheless, programs can be individualized if the prescriptions are modified using the general principles outlined in this chapter.

The body tries to adapt to the habitual demands placed on it. Training is a form of adaptation to the repeated stimulation of exercise. When one has no difficulty adjusting to these demands, adaptation is said to be complete. When the demands placed on the body are too great or are applied too rapidly, too often, or too long, the adaptation will then be incomplete; this partial adjustment usually manifests itself in the form of fatigue, soreness, pain, or injury.

The two major principles of training that apply to all individuals are overload and specificity. Related to overload are the principles of reversibility and maintenance (8).

OVERLOAD

If the body is not required to adapt, it will not. For adaptation to occur, the body and its various parts and systems must be stimulated at higher levels than they habitually encounter. A safe and effective training program is one that progressively overloads the body and allows adequate time for adaptation to each level of stimulation. There is a minimal amount (threshold) of activity that is effective. There is also an upper limit that may require more adaptation than is possible and may be unsafe. The key is to find the upper and lower limits for each individual. As persons adapt to a higher level of activity, these limits may also rise. The lower limit may increase because they have to do more to maintain their higher level of fitness or performance, while the upper limit may increase because they now can work at higher intensities, frequencies, or durations.

SPECIFICITY

The effects of training are specific to those parts and systems of the body that are overloaded. As an example, weight lifting produces muscle hypertrophy and strength, whereas distance running produces cardiorespiratory endurance but no hypertrophy. Adaptation is specific to the muscle groups that are stimulated (e.g., arms vs. legs). Adaptation is also specific to the energy-producing systems that are stimulated. For example, running sprints stimulates the anaerobic system, running middle distances uses a combination of aerobic and anaerobic energy, and running marathons principally involves the aerobic system. In other words, the effects of training depend greatly on the activities that are selected. The principle of specificity is probably most important for persons with specific goals (e.g., to lose weight or to run 10 km) and becomes less important for those who exercise for fun, health, and general fitness.

REVERSIBILITY

Because the body adapts to its habitual level of stimulation, the changes brought about by training reverse if the individual becomes more sedentary. In other words, the effects of training are transient and reversible. The opposite of overload, this principle states that the body can also adapt to inactivity.

MAINTENANCE

It generally takes less time and effort to maintain an improved level of fitness than it does to attain it. Once persons adapt to a level of stimulation and there is no overload, further adaptation is not required. If they are satisfied with their current level of fitness, they may be able to maintain it by continuing to do the same amount of training per week and even by slightly reducing their training for brief periods. The higher the level of fitness or performance, the higher the amount of exercise required to maintain it will be.

Basic Components of Exercise Programs

The five components of exercise programs are frequency, duration, intensity, type of exercise, and progression. Training is the product of frequency, duration, and intensity of exercise, i.e., the total amount of stimulation or overload. Type of activity is associated with the principle of specificity, as are duration and intensity, because high-intensity activities tend to be brief and anaerobic and low-intensity activities tend to be prolonged and aerobic.

With all the possible combinations of the first four components, training can be as general or as specific as is desired. The key to a good exercise program is to select activities that the individual enjoys and will do often enough, long enough, and at an intensity sufficient to produce a training effect. For the general population, cardiorespiratory endurance and control of body weight are important objectives of an exercise program, followed by strength, muscular endurance, and flexibility (9). With the proper selection of activities, all of these objectives can be attained.

FREQUENCY

The inactive person should exercise one to three times per week during the first few weeks to allow adequate time for adaptation. Exercise should not be done on consecutive days because the chances of soreness, fatigue, and possible injury are greatest during the first few weeks of overload. If there are no problems, frequency can be gradually increased to three to four times per week over the next few months. The eventual goal should be three to five times per week, as this frequency is associated with significant gains in fitness and loss of body fat (3).

Frequency may be reduced after reaching the desired fitness level. How much of a reduction depends primarily on the fitness level one wishes to maintain. An athlete who has been training daily may be able to maintain a very high level on four to six times per week, whereas a below-average level of fitness may be maintained by exercising one to two times per week. For the general population, it appears that three to four times per week is optimal. Twice per week is the minimum for maintaining a good level of fitness but only for brief periods (e.g., 2 to 4 weeks) or the fitness level may drop (2,3).

DURATION

Sedentary asymptomatic and symptomatic persons tolerate low-intensity exercise for a long duration better than they tolerate high-intensity exercise for brief periods. They are also less likely to have musculoskeletal problems. Therefore, exercise sessions should last 20 to 30 min, gradually increasing to 40 to 60 min. An optimal program has three phases: warm-up (5–10 min), overload (15–40 min), and cool-down (5–10 min), for a total of 25 to 60 min.

The warm-up phase includes walking, slow jogging, stretching exercises, and moderate exercises for muscular strength and endurance. This phase allows the body to increase its metabolism gradually and to prepare for the more strenuous exercise to follow. The older and less fit the individual, the more important is this phase, and the longer it should be (8).

Activities during the overload phase should be at intensities that are safe and effective, i.e., high enough to provide an overload but not so high that they are unsafe or cannot be done for 15 to 20 min. Once a person has worked up to it, the minimal duration of the overload phase should be 20 min; this amount is especially important in programs designed to increase maximal aerobic power ($\dot{V}O_{2max}$) and to control body weight. Although 20 min is considered by many to be a minimal duration, there is research demonstrating that multiple short bouts of moderate-intensity exercise training are also effective. DeBusk et al. (10) found that three 10-min sessions per day were as effective as one 30-min session for improving the $\dot{V}O_{2max}$ of middle-aged

men. For many individuals, short bouts of exercise training may fit better into a busy schedule than a single long bout, thus making it easier for exercise to become a part of one's lifestyle.

The cool-down phase should include slow movements, similar to those used in the warm-up. Less fit and older persons require more time to recover from exercise. The cool-down time will also be longer if the overload exercises were difficult, were done for a long time, or were done in a hot or humid environment.

INTENSITY

Exercise intensity is a critical factor in exercise prescriptions and is the most difficult to adjust. Duration and frequency are absolute values that can be the same for persons differing greatly in fitness, whereas exercise intensity may be absolute or relative. Exercise intensity can be expressed in absolute terms (e.g., PO in watts [W], speed and grade on the treadmill, or METs); this would be the same for everyone. Exercise intensity can also be a relative term, i.e., the energy required to do an activity relative to the maximal amount of energy that can be provided aerobically; this relative intensity is expressed as a percentage of $\dot{V}O_{2max}$). Even though two persons may run at the same absolute intensity (e.g., 7 mph), the same exercise will be relatively more stressful for the person who is less fit. While a general exercise prescription can be given using absolute intensities, a more precise prescription presumes a determination or estimation of a person's $\dot{V}O_{2max}$, i.e., that an exercise tolerance test has been given.

During the 5 to 15 min of the warm-up and cool-down phases, intensity should be 30 to 50% $\dot{V}O_{2max}$. For many, this will be walking at a slow to moderate pace. Because this level of exercise can be done for up to 8 hours daily, it can be easily done for these brief periods. To overload the cardiorespiratory systems, however, the minimal relative intensity should be higher.

For sedentary persons with low fitness levels, improvements have been obtained with intensities of 50 to 60% $\dot{V}O_{2max}$ (3). Although there is a suggestion that the threshold intensity is about 40% $\dot{V}O_{2max}$ in unfit subjects (3), 50% appears to be the threshold for most adults and is a good level of intensity during the first weeks of increased activity.

If there are no problems, the average intensity during the overload phase can be gradually increased to 60 to 70% and then to 70 to 85%. At intensities above 90%, the anaerobic system provides significant amounts of the required energy. The resulting fatigue and lactic acid accumulation reduce exercise duration to <15 to 20 min. For the general population, the optimal intensity is about 60 to 80% (3,8,9).

According to the ACSM, this relative intensity can be lower (~40% $\dot{V}O_{2max}$) in "quite unfit" persons (3). However, remember that walking requires 3 to 4 METs or a $\dot{V}O_2$ of 10.5 to 14 mL · kg^{-1} · min^{-1} and may already be ~50% $\dot{V}O_{2max}$ for those with below-average fitness levels whose $\dot{V}O_{2max}$ is 6 to 8 METs or 21 to 28 mL · kg^{-1} · min^{-1}. Therefore, unfit persons and patients should be encouraged to walk at moderate speeds on most days of the week. The lower intensity level suggested by ACSM also may not apply to patients in whom a given intensity is associated with signs and symptoms. Because their safety is more important than exercising at an arbitrary percentage of their $\dot{V}O_{2max}$, patients are often advised to exercise at intensities that are below their thresholds for symptoms.

Especially for those who are just beginning an exercise program, the intensity should be kept at a moderate level. High-intensity exercise has been associated with a higher risk for orthopedic injury, cardiac arrest, anaphylaxis, upper respiratory tract infection, and exercise-induced bronchospasm than either duration or frequency of exercise (11). One result of this is that high-intensity activities tend to be associated with a higher rate of dropout, especially during the first few months.

Results from large-scale epidemiologic studies suggest that regular participation in light or moderate exercise reduces the risk of developing coronary heart disease (12–15). Similarly, training programs requiring no more than 55% of initial functional capacity have produced significant increases in the $\dot{V}O_{2max}$ of men whose initial fitness levels were low (16). More research is needed to determine threshold levels for stimulating adaptations and for improving health.

TOTAL AMOUNT OF EXERCISE

Training is the product of frequency, duration, and intensity of exercise, i.e., the total amount of exercise done. Table 2-1 shows how these components might be increased to overload the aerobic system. By gradually increasing one or two components during each 2-week period, a sedentary person can adapt over 3 to 4 months. Depending on how each person reacts and feels, the rate at which the total is increased can be modified. Interestingly, once the frequency, duration, and intensity are above certain levels and the total amount of exercise done per week is similar, the effects of aerobic training are also similar (3,9). The importance of this fact is that training programs and sessions within these programs can vary widely and apparently still produce similar results. This is especially important for those who are active for fun, fitness, and/or health, because it means that they can vary

TABLE 2-1 EXAMPLE OF GRADUALLY INCREASING OVERLOAD WITH AEROBIC TRAINING

	Week Since Onset of Training							
	0	2	4	6	8	10	12	14
Frequency (sessions/week)	2	3	3	3	3	4	4	4
Duration (min)								
Warm-up	5	5	6	6	7	7	7	8
Overload	10	10	15	15	20	20	25	25
Cool-down	5	5	5	6	6	7	7	7
Total	20	20	26	27	33	34	39	40
Intensity (% $\dot{V}O_{2max}$)	50	55	60	60	65	65	70	70

their exercise sessions according to the season of the year, the availability of facilities or equipment, or their own personal interests. Knowing that one can vary the program and still attain one's goals should help them to maintain their interest in exercise and enhance their compliance to their program.

TYPE OF EXERCISE

Work is defined as force times distance. For example, if 132 lb (60 kg) are lifted 33 ft (10 m), then $132 \times 33 = 5082$ ft-lb, or $60 \times 10 = 600$ kg-m of work is done. Power is work done per unit time. As an example, 600 kg-m done in 30 sec or in 1 min is 1200 and 600 kgM $\cdot$ min^{-1}, respectively. Because there are ~ 6 kg-m $\cdot$ min^{-1} in 1 W, the corresponding POs are 200 and 100 W.

A given PO requires a given amount of energy, even though the source of that energy may differ. As an example, 100 W requires 40 to 50% $\dot{V}O_{2max}$ in an average young man and is primarily aerobic. On the other hand, 200 W requires 80 to 90% $\dot{V}O_{2max}$ in the same person, a part of which comes from anaerobic sources.

The same number of kilocalories are needed to run 10 miles, whether a person runs the 10 miles in 1 day or runs 1 mile per day for 10 days. Speed of running has little effect on total energy expenditure per mile, i.e., the same amount of energy is required to run each mile, even though the intensity or PO will vary with the speed. Thus, the total amount of work done (in this case, distance run) is more important for weight loss, whereas PO (in this case, running speed) is more important for training because it affects the intensity and duration of exercise and the relative stimulation of the aerobic and anaerobic systems.

To overload the aerobic system specifically, it is best to use prolonged, continuous, and moderate-intensity activities involving rhythmic contractions of large muscle groups. Strength and speed tend to be anaerobic and are best developed by brief, intermittent, and high-intensity activities.

EXERCISE PROGRESSION

The older participants are, the longer they have been sedentary, and the more limitations they have, the slower should be the rate of progression in the total amount of exercise done per week (frequency $\times$ duration $\times$ intensity). The main goals when beginning an exercise program are to avoid injuries, to allow the participants to tolerate and adapt to each increase in activity, and to make exercise part of their lifestyle. Once participants have adjusted to a regular program (e.g., week 8 in Table 2-1), a good rule of thumb is to increase the total amount of exercise done per week by no more than 10%. This can be done by keeping two factors constant and slightly increasing the third factor (e.g., maintaining frequency and intensity while increasing duration).

At the onset of an exercise program, it is important for each individual to set a number of small steps toward realistic goals that can be evaluated periodically. Participants should also be instructed to pay attention to how they are feeling so that they can look for signs and symptoms suggesting that they stop exercising or that another evaluation is needed before they continue.

Refinements and Individualization of Exercise Programs

LEVEL OF FITNESS

Persons who are older, less fit, less healthy, and less active generally have more problems when beginning an exercise program. As noted above, relative exercise intensity is usually expressed as a percentage of each person's functional capacity (e.g., %$\dot{V}O_{2max}$). However, the percentage of $\dot{V}O_{2max}$ that a given person can sustain for a given duration is quite variable and is associated with the level of fitness and genetic background (17). For example, well-trained endurance athletes can often exercise at 80 to 90% $\dot{V}O_{2max}$ for 2 hours, whereas less fit, inactive persons may become fatigued after only 5 to 15 min at these same relative intensities (18). For this reason, Balke suggested a sliding scale for prescribing average training intensities: Average intensity (%$\dot{V}O_{2max}$) = $(60 + \dot{V}O_{2max}$ in METs$)/100$ (6). According to this scale, sedentary persons with a maximum of 10 METs should exercise at $(60 + 10)/100 = 70$% of their capacity, or 7 METs, while endurance athletes with a maximum of 20 METs should work at $(60 + 20)/100 = 80$%, or 16 METs.

Another method for estimating exercise intensity and for possibly equating the exercise stimulus among people with different levels of fitness is available. This method uses the concept of the lactate threshold (LT), which is identified by the PO at which blood lactate levels rise markedly. Because ventilation also increases at or about this same PO, the ventilatory threshold also can be used. These thresholds generally occur from 50 to 90% $\dot{V}O_{2max}$, with the higher percentages being more prevalent in well-trained endurance athletes. If one assumes that the PO associated with this threshold represents a similar stimulus for change in cellular homeostasis, then exercise requiring the same $\dot{V}O_{2max}$ may produce a different stimulation in people with similar $\dot{V}O_{2max}$ values but different thresholds (18). As an example, Baldwin et al. (19) had trained and untrained men exercise at intensities relative to their $\dot{V}O_{2max}$ and to their LT. They found that the untrained men had significantly higher plasma lactate and HR at 70% $\dot{V}O_{2max}$ but similar values at 95% LT.

The ventilatory threshold can be used to monitor intensity using the so-called talk test. If exercise intensity is below the threshold, then one can talk while exercising. However, once the threshold is surpassed, then ventilation increases markedly and it is more difficult to talk. By adjusting the exercise intensity to stay at or slightly above the point where ventilation rises, one can generally exercise for 20 to 30 min.

Although well-trained athletes can and should train regularly at higher percentages of their maximum, sedentary and less-fit individuals are better off working at low-to-moderate intensities for longer durations, especially during the initial part of their program.

CONTROLLING INTENSITY

The intensity of an exercise program should be above the threshold for effectiveness but below some upper value to ensure safety and adequate duration.

Energy Cost Estimates

One way to control intensity is to prescribe exercise on the basis of energy required for an activity. Reasonable estimates of energy cost are available for a whole range of such standardized activities as walking, running, rowing, and cycling, at which the exercise can be done for a long enough period and at a constant speed to reach a metabolic steady state (2,8). When there are changes in wind or water resistance, in the slope or firmness of the terrain, or in mechanical efficiency, these estimates are less accurate. Similarly, accurate estimates are not available for activities that are anaerobic, intermittent, done at variable speeds, or have wide variations in skill and efficiency (e.g., games). In these cases, averages and ranges are usually presented (2,8,9).

Relationship between HR and $\dot{V}O_2$

Intensity can also be controlled by the linear relationship between HR and $\dot{V}O_2$ for each individual (20). If HR and $\dot{V}O_2$ have been measured during a progressively increasing exercise test, participants can estimate their $\dot{V}O_2$ by measuring their steady-state HR. With this method, they can stay within the prescribed range of intensity (e.g., 60–80% $\dot{V}O_{2max}$) by knowing the HRs associated with this range. When HR and $\dot{V}O_2$ have not been measured, participants can measure their HR after 4 to 5 min of walking or running at constant speeds or doing any standardized activity in which $\dot{V}O_2$ can be estimated with reasonable accuracy.

Once the HR/$\dot{V}O_2$ relationship has been established for each person, it does not change over time. Skinner et al. (21) analyzed data from 653 subjects in the HERITAGE Family Study who had been classified by age, sex, race, initial $\dot{V}O_{2max}$, and $\dot{V}O_{2max}$ response after 20 weeks of a standardized training program. These analyses showed that there was a significant decrease in HR at the same absolute intensity (PO in W) but no difference in HR at the same relative intensity (%$\dot{V}O_{2max}$) after training. This was true for all subjects, for both sexes (men and women), for both races (black and white), for three age groups (17–29, 30–49, and 50–65 years), for four levels of initial $\dot{V}O_{2max}$ (14–57 mL · kg^{-1} · min^{-1}), and for four groups classified by their increase in $\dot{V}O_{2max}$ with training (0–50%). Figure 2-2 shows the results from two of the groups classified by sex and age. These results demonstrate that once $\dot{V}O_{2max}$ and the relationships among HR and $\dot{V}O_2$ are known for each individual, then HR is a good estimate of relative exercise intensity. In addition, HR can be used to estimate relative exercise intensity over the course of an exercise training program; this is important because it suggests that

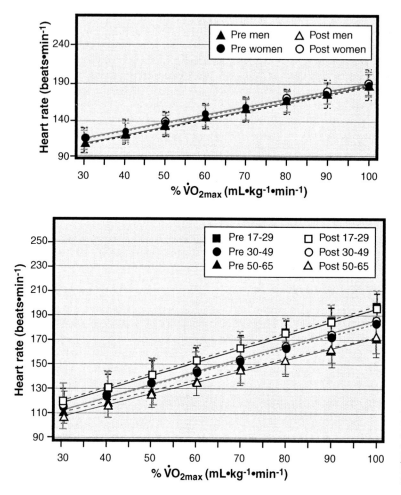

FIGURE 2-2 Heart rates at fixed relative intensities (%$\dot{V}O_{2max}$) for 293 men and 360 women *(top)* and for 295 young (17–29 years), 229 middle-aged (30–49 years),) and 129 older (50–65 years) subjects *(bottom)* pre- and posttraining in the HERITAGE Family Study (see ref 21).

frequent testing is not necessary to adjust the exercise prescription.

Even if exercise testing has not been performed, a fair estimate of intensity can be made by using a percentage of the maximal HR reserve or HRR (8, 22):

$$\text{Intensity}(\%\dot{V}O_{2max})=\frac{(\text{Exercise HR} - \text{resting HR})}{(\text{Maximal HR} - \text{resting HR})}$$

Using a person with a maximal HR of 200 beats · min^{-1} and a resting HR of 80 beats·min^{-1} as an example, an exercise requiring a HR of 164 beats·min^{-1} represents an intensity of (164 − 80)/(200 − 80) = 84/120 = 0.70, or 70%.

Whereas resting HR is easy to obtain, most persons have little idea of their maximal HR unless they have been tested to maximum or have pushed themselves to exhaustion and measured their HR. As a rule of thumb, maximal HR decreases 1 beat·min^{-1} each year after age 20 to 25 years and can be estimated by subtracting present age from 220. Thus, the average 40-year-old individual has a maximal HR of 220 − 40 = 180 beats·min^{-1}. This estimate may not be accurate, however, because maximal HR varies by about 10%, i.e., although the average for 40-year-old persons is 180 beats·min^{-1}, values may vary from 160 to 200 beats·min^{-1}. As with any estimate, one should obtain accurate measurements under standardized conditions and realize their limitations.

Another method to determine the training HR range is to take a fixed percentage of the estimated or determined maximal HR. For comparative purposes, it has been shown that 60 to 80% $\dot{V}O_{2max}$ corresponds to approximately 60 to 80% HRR and 70 to 85% of the maximal HR (2).

If a given HR is associated with a given intensity for each person (21), exercise HR is a useful and convenient way to control intensity. For example, HR at a given PO usually drops with aerobic conditioning. Because relatively minor changes occur in maximal and resting HRs with training, it appears that $\dot{V}O_{2max}$ has risen and that the PO represents a lower relative intensity. The PO should then be raised to reach the desired HR and intensity. With increasing altitude or temperature, HR will increase at a given level of exercise. Using the same training HR range as a guide, a person can do less exercise but will still be at the same relative stress. Similarly, persons who stop training because of such factors as lack of interest, injury, or job pressures can use a lower PO to exercise at the same HR and %$\dot{V}O_{2max}$ when they resume exercise.

Ratings of Perceived Exertion

Even though such objective physiologic indices as HR and $\dot{V}O_2$ change minimally from day to day during standard exercise, subjective feelings of psychologic strain may vary and should also be considered. Borg developed a scale for rating perceived exertion (RPE) associated with a given amount of exercise (23). This RPE scale can be helpful in exercise prescription when ratings are obtained with HR and $\dot{V}O_2$ during exercise testing or with HR during standardized exercise tasks for which the energy costs are known. Once persons perceive the effort associated with various exercise intensities, they may have a better understanding of how hard they should exercise. After training regularly at a prescribed intensity, the subjective feelings can then be transferred to other activities, e.g., used to estimate fatigue and the varying intensities associated with games or other non-steady-state activities (9,23,24).

Exercise intensity can be controlled reasonably well throughout an exercise session without having to stop, just on the basis of subjective RPEs (9,23). Using Borg's 15-point scale, RPEs of 12 to 13 (somewhat hard) and 16 (hard) correspond to 60 and 85% of the HR reserve, respectively (2). The

respective ratings on the Borg 10-point scale are 4 and 6.

Use of All Three Factors

As mentioned above in this chapter, the same principles apply to all but can be modified according to the needs, interests, status, etc. of the particular persons involved. A brief review of a recent study should give the reader a better idea of how these factors can be used to prescribe exercise for a specific population.

The author was asked to prescribe exercise in a large multicenter study of patients with Gulf War veterans' illnesses (GWVI), a multisymptom illness characterized by persistent pain, fatigue, and cognitive symptoms (25). The design of the exercise program for GWVI required careful planning to enhance tolerability and to ensure long-term compliance.

A submaximal cycle ergometer exercise test was used to determine physical fitness at baseline and to develop individualized prescriptions for a low-intensity aerobic exercise program. A submaximal exercise test was used because chronic fatigue and pain are common symptoms with GWVI, and it was unclear whether the veterans would be able to exercise to a high enough level to obtain a valid measure of $\dot{V}O_{2max}$.

Veterans exercised 1 hour per week in the presence of an exercise therapist for 12 weeks. During this time, therapists used the HR, PO, and RPE data from the exercise test to select an appropriate range of exercise intensities. The therapists then instructed veterans about exercise, how to use the HR monitor that was given to each, and how to select activities using RPE, HR, and a table of energy cost in METS that corresponded to the appropriate intensities. Participants were also asked to exercise independently two to three times per week during the 12-week treatment phase and three times a week for the remainder of the year. Veterans were encouraged to select activities from the METs table that they enjoyed or were able to do easily each day, as well as to use the HR monitor to stay within the target range of intensity. However, because of the fatigue and pain associated with GWVI, because of the variability in amount and occurrence of fatigue and pain from one day to another, and because the purpose of the program was to make exercise a part of their lifestyle, they were also encouraged to use the RPE scale when exercising. Thus, on the days that they did not feel like exercising and might have had difficulty doing the same amount of exercise or reaching their target HR, they were still encouraged to do some exercise at an RPE of 12–14 (somewhat hard).

Using all three factors made the exercise prescription easily modifiable and gave the participants a great deal of flexibility in choosing how to be active. It was felt that this flexibility would lead to better compliance and increase the chances that exercise would become a regular part of their lifestyle.

RESPONSE TO TRAINING

It is a commonly observed that some persons have less and some have more difficulty adapting to a training program and that some progress more slowly or more rapidly than others. As a result, there is considerable individual variation in the rate of adaptation to, and the physiologic responses of, participants to the same training program. A good example of this variability can be seen in Figure 2-3, which shows the change in $\dot{V}O_{2max}$ in response to a standardized 20-week endurance exercise training program (26). Of the 633 subjects, 64, or 10%, had little or no change (i.e., ± 2 mL·kg^{-1}·min^{-1}) and 63 or 10% had increases of 10 mL·kg^{-1}·min^{-1} or

more. Further data analyses revealed that age, sex, race and initial fitness level had little or no effect on the response of $\dot{V}O_{2max}$ in this large heterogeneous, biracial, sedentary population. Figure 2-4 combines the data from 633 subjects in the HERITAGE Family Study (26) with those from 110 subjects in a similar training study by Kohrt et al. (27) and shows the response to training of black and white subjects from the age of 17 to 71 years. There appear to be high, medium, and low responders to training at all ages in both races. Although not shown here, there also were high, medium, and low responders in both sexes and at all levels of initial fitness studied. In fact, there was a nonsignificant relationship ($r = 0.08$) between where the subjects began ($\dot{V}O_{2max}$ in mL·kg^{-1}·min^{-1}) and their absolute change in $\dot{V}O_{2max}$ (mL·kg^{-1}·min^{-1}) (26). Genetic factors may help to explain the large variation in training response.

PERIODIC EVALUATION

Periodic testing is useful to assess the effectiveness of an exercise program, to modify an exercise prescription, and to motivate persons to continue. A trained exercise leader may observe small signs and symptoms (changes in fatigue, gait, or comments) that suggest the need for reevaluation, resulting in

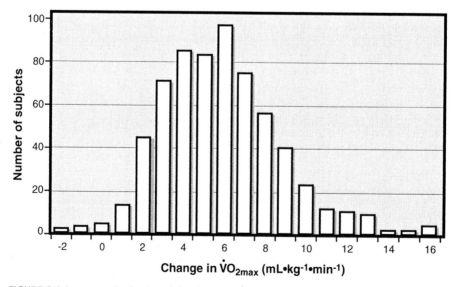

FIGURE 2-3 Frequency distribution of the change in $\dot{V}O_{2max}$ of 633 subjects in response to a standardized 20-week endurance exercise training program (see ref 26).

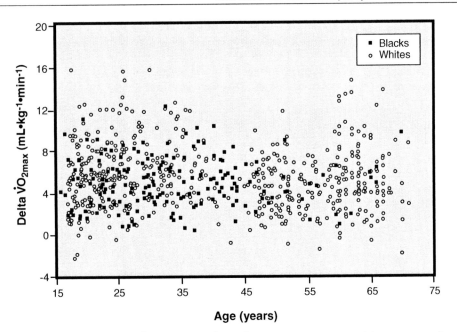

FIGURE 2-4 The response of $\dot{V}O_{2max}$ ($mL\cdot kg^{-1}\cdot min^{-1}$) to endurance exercise training programs of black and white subjects from the age of 17 to 71 years. The data include 633 subjects from the study by Skinner et al. (26) and 110 subjects from the study by Kohrt et al. (27).

a modified prescription and, in a few cases, termination of the exercise program. All exercise staff should be aware of the signs and symptoms suggesting that participants should modify their activities.

How often persons should be reevaluated depends on their need for a precise prescription. As shown in Figure 2-1, athletes and patients may need to be evaluated more often than the average person. As the needs, interests, and goals of these three groups change, however, so might the need for evaluation. For example, the average person who decides to run a marathon or who develops chest pain should be evaluated more than the average person who continues to exercise for fun, health, and general fitness. Likewise, patients who improve their health status or athletes who stop or reduce training may need less evaluation than was previously required.

Exercise for Health

It is well documented that regular physical activity makes positive contributions to health and well-being (12–15). In recent physical activity

guidelines, various health-related organizations recommend that people "obtain 30 minutes of moderate intensity physical activity, such as brisk walking, on most days of the week" (12–15). Epidemiologic and experimental studies indicate that regular physical activity is associated with lower morbidity and mortality rates from cardiovascular disease (CVD), lower levels of several major CVD risk factors, and lower rates of all-cause mortality. Greater health benefits appear to occur between low and moderate levels of activity or cardiorespiratory fitness (2,11,28) than between moderate and high levels of activity or fitness. In other words, the biggest drop in risk occurs when people go from doing little or nothing to being moderately active on a regular basis. Further increases in activity give more protection, but the person must do more for less gain. The promotional message in terms of public health is that one does not have to be an athlete or exercise at high levels to obtain a protective or beneficial effect.

From the standpoint of an exercise prescription, this suggests that general advice on being active on a regular basis is sufficient for many healthy, sedentary people. However, knowledge is not always followed by action and there is still a need for guidance so that participants will have a better chance of choosing a safe and enjoyable program. With proper guidance, there is also a better chance that the program will be more effective for increasing fitness.

One should remember, however, that activity and fitness are not synonymous. Two persons can have the same $\dot{V}O_{2max}$ but have quite different levels of activity. For example, the first person might be sedentary but has inherited a higher level of fitness, while the second person is genetically less fit but is regularly active.

As mentioned above, people can respond quite differently to the same amount of exercise. For those in a program who are low responders (or worse, nonresponders), this presents a special challenge to the physician and exercise leader. Evidence from the HERITAGE Family Study suggests that even though a person may not respond to training in terms of fitness, this does not mean that he or she will not respond in terms of particular risk factors for various diseases. In other words, exercise might help one person to reduce serum cholesterol and body weight but not blood pressure or serum triglycerides. This can be explained partly by the fact that different genes are involved and that the genetic background of each person is different.

Most health problems today are associated with lifestyle and not heredity. As Corbin suggests, "the process of being active is more important than the product of being fit." Many persons who become more active also stop smoking, improve their weight, and may reduce their high blood pressure. Thus, persons need to think less that training results in better fitness and should think more that a higher level of physical activity will improve their health.

Other Considerations

PROBLEMS ASSOCIATED WITH OVERUSE

Many problems associated with exercise programs arise from overuse, i.e., overstimulation from exercise that is more intense, more frequent, or longer than the demands to which the body has adapted. The signs and symptoms of this inadequate adaptation are fatigue, soreness, pain, and injury.

Fatigue

Fatigue is a general feeling of weariness that can produce performance decrements due to slower reaction and movement times and reduced levels of speed, agility, strength, and neuromuscular coordination. Thus, persons who are tired are more prone to injury. Because the amount of fatigue and its onset are related to the relative intensity of exercise, proper training can reduce the chance of injury by increasing a person's maximum. Some fatigue is normal after exercise, especially during the first few weeks of increased activity. If fatigue persists, the individual should stop exercising for several days or exercise at a lower intensity or duration until the body has recovered.

Soreness

Soreness is a dull ache that comes on gradually due to overuse. General soreness lasts 4 to 8 hours, followed by localized, specific soreness that may last for several days. The degree of overuse and the resulting soreness is associated with a person's present level of adaptation. Persons who are older, less fit, less healthy and who have been sedentary longer tend to have more soreness after exercise.

The type and amount of exercise is also a contributing factor, i.e., too much of the same or even a different type of exercise can cause overstrain and soreness. As a general rule, one should continue to exercise at a lower frequency, duration, and/or intensity. One can also change the type of exercise for a few days to reduce soreness. Remember, however, to start at a lower intensity and duration to avoid soreness in the new muscle groups.

Pain

Pain is a localized, sharp feeling of discomfort that usually comes on rapidly. If pain develops, one should stop immediately and attempt to determine whether it is due to muscle, joint, or cardiovascular problems. It is neither necessary nor advisable to continue with pain. Although "no pain, no gain" may be an acceptable motto for an elite athlete committed to excellence who is willing to put forth the time and effort needed to attain it, the same principle is not valid for the average person or patient.

Injury

The severity of an injury is associated with the past history of injury, the type and speed of the movement causing the injury, and the present level of fitness and habitual activity. The risk of injury is usually greatest during the first few months of exercise or whenever there are abrupt increases in the total amount of exercise done (2,3). First, beginning exercisers may be overweight and unfit, such that their low VO_{2max} and excess weight increase the relative intensity of exercise. Second, beginners often have inadequate strength, endurance, and flexibility, making them more prone to injury. Third, beginners may not know what exercises to do or how to do them; this fact emphasizes the need for and importance of individualized exercise prescriptions, as well as qualified people to lead exercise programs.

EXERCISING ALONE OR WITH OTHERS

Exercise is a social activity for many persons. Belonging to a group may fill a strong social need and is an excellent way to receive the positive reinforcement that is so critical in the initial stages of increased exercise. Qualified instructors can lead, educate, and motivate individuals to ensure that the appropriate exercises are done properly to avoid problems of overuse and to improve the chances of progress. Another advantage of group programs is that there is usually a fixed routine that may help some persons make exercise a regular part of their lifestyle.

There are, however, disadvantages to group exercise. Some persons prefer to exercise alone, may have difficulty with regular schedules, or may not know what to do when they are away from the group. If a group program attempts to have one program for persons with varying degrees of fitness and ability, the intensity is not optimal for all participants. As a result, the rate of progress also varies. Individualized exercise prescriptions, flexibility within the programs, and qualified leadership can minimize some of these problems.

One compromise that has been found useful, easier to schedule, and more individualized is to exercise with one or two other persons. This approach works best when the members of the group have similar interests and fitness levels.

DEGREE OF SUPERVISION

Whether supervision is required or suggested depends mainly on the degree of risk associated with exercise. The important thing is to provide effective and enjoyable programs that are also safe but not too restrictive in terms of the participants' work schedules or economic situations (2). Individuals who have a functional capacity of less than 8 METs, who are known to be at high risk for coronary heart disease, or who have CVD (regardless of their functional capacity) should exercise in a group under the supervision of a qualified leader (2).

Qualified and creative instructors can make the program more diversified, more individualized, more interesting, and safer by demonstrating appropriate exercises and their proper sequences. Instructors can provide a degree of health surveillance, can monitor changes in intensity and duration of exercise, and can educate the group so that its members know what to do, how to do it, and why. For example, the group can be taught how to measure HR and then can be informed that their highest training HR during nonsupervised exercise should not exceed the mean HR attained during supervised exercise (2). Another advantage of supervised exercise programs is that persons with similar medical problems or risks can help each other understand and cope with the restrictions imposed by their medical condition.

STARTING VERSUS CONTINUING AN EXERCISE PROGRAM

Research shows that among those who begin an exercise program, an average of 50% will fail to adhere (30). The highest dropout occurs in the first few months, which is before most participants see any changes in fitness or other desired outcomes (31). Although the highest incidence of injuries also occurs at this time, it is not the only or major factor. Factors that influence an individual to begin exercising are usually quite different from those associated with continuing an exercise plan (32). In oversimplified terms, many persons begin because others (physician, family, or friends) think it is the best thing to do, they want to improve their appearance, it is the "in" thing to do, or they want to improve their health. The same persons continue to exercise, however, because of themselves and how they perceive that the program helps them, e.g., the program has an effective leader who makes the activities enjoyable, they feel better, and they can see improvements.

There are so many reasons why persons decide to start or to continue to exercise that health professionals should not try to impose their own reasons. Instead, health professionals should give as many reasons as possible and let the participants decide which are important in their particular case. As well, participants should set short-term, realistic goals to increase the chances of having many small successes that will motivate them to continue. Periodic evaluations also can be used to monitor progress and to motivate continued participation.

At the onset of training, games and sports are not the ideal choice for those who are older and less fit because these activities tend to be more intermittent and less well controlled. Persons beginning an exercise program should train to play a sport and not use sports as the main way to train. Sports and games are better used during the maintenance phase when the fitness level is adequate and when enjoyment is more important for continued participation.

Summary

- Successful exercise programs are based on sound exercise prescription and qualified leadership. This statement implies that there is communication and cooperation among exercisers, physicians, and exercise leaders so that the exercisers are taught what to do and why and are then motivated to follow through on their own initiative.
- The best activities during any phase of a program are those that are safe, effective, and enjoyable.
- There are many ways that one can increase physical activity and obtain similar results for health. If the frequency, duration, and intensity of exercise are adequate to stimulate adaptation but are not high enough to cause incomplete adaptation or be unsafe, then it makes little difference which activities are selected.
- Programs can and should vary, because no one program is correct for all or even for the same person over time, as interests, needs, goals, health, or fitness change. A more important factor is whether the activity is fun so that it will be continued and become part of one's lifestyle.

REFERENCES

1. American College of Sports Medicine. Guidelines for Graded Exercise Testing and Exercise Prescription. 4th ed. Philadelphia: Lea & Febiger, 1991.

2. American College of Sports Medicine. ACSM's Guidelines for Exercise Testing and Prescription. 6th ed. Philadelphia: Lippincott Williams & Wilkins, 2000.

3. American College of Sports Medicine. ACSM's position stand. The recommended quantity and quality of exercise for developing and maintaining cardiorespiratory and muscular fitness, and flexibility in healthy adults. Med Sci Sports Exerc 1998;30:975–991.

4. American Association of Cardiovascular and Pulmonary Rehabilitation: Guidelines for Cardiac Rehabilitation and Secondary Prevention Programs. 3rd ed. Champaign, IL: Human Kinetics, 1999.

5. American College of Sports Medicine. Exercise Management for Persons with Chronic Diseases and Disabilities. 2nd ed. Champaign, IL: Human Kinetics, 2003.

6. Balke B. Prescribing physical activity. In: Ryan AJ, Allman F, eds. Sports Medicine. New York: Academic Press, 1974.

7. Skinner JS. Exercise research on persons of below-average health and fitness: a commentary. In: Skinner JS, Corbin C, Landers DM, et al., eds. Future Directions in Exercise and Sport Science Research. Champaign, IL: Human Kinetics, 1986.

8. Skinner JS. Physiology of exercise and training. In: Strauss RH, ed. Sports Medicine, 2nd ed. Philadelphia: WB Saunders, 1991:282–298.

9. Pollock ML, Wilmore JH, Fox SM. Exercise in Health and Disease. Philadelphia: WB Saunders, 1984.

10. DeBusk RF, Stenestrand U, Sheehan M, et al. Training effects of long versus short bouts of exercise in healthy subjects. Am J Cardiol 1990;65:1010–1013.

11. Haskell WL. Health consequences of physical activity: understanding and challenges regarding dose-response. Med Sci Sports Exerc 1994;26:649–660.

12. US Department of Health and Human Services. Physical activity and health: a report of the Surgeon General. Atlanta: US Department of Health and Human Services, Centers for Disease Control and Prevention, National Center for Chronic Disease Prevention and Health Promotion, 1996.

13. NIH Consensus Development Panel on Physical Activity and Cardiovascular Health. NIH consensus conference: physical activity and cardiovascular health. JAMA 1996;276:241–246.

14. Pate RR, Pratt M, Blair SN, et al. Physical activity and public health: a recommendation from the Centers for Disease Control and Prevention and the American College of Sports Medicine. JAMA 1995;273:402–407.

15. Fletcher GF, Balady G, Blair SN, et al. Statement on exercise: benefits and recommendations for physical activity programs for all Americans: a statement for

health professionals by the Committee on Exercise and Cardiac Rehabilitation of the Council on Clinical Cardiology, American Heart Association. Circulation 1996;94:857–862.

16. Gossard D, Haskell WL, Taylor C, et al. Effects of low- and high-intensity home-based exercise training on functional capacity in healthy middle-aged men. Am J Cardiol 1986;57:446–449.

17. Gaskill SE, Rice T, Bouchard C, et al. Familial resemblance in ventilatory threshold: the HERITAGE Family Study. Med Sci Sports Exerc 2001;33:1832–1840.

18. McLellan TM, Skinner JS. Submaximal endurance performance related to the ventilatory thresholds. Can J Appl Sport Sci 1985;10:81–87.

19. Baldwin J, Snow RJ, Febbraio MA. Effect of training status and relative exercise intensity on physiological responses in men. Med Sci Sports Exerc 2000;32:1648–1654.

20. Wilmore JH, Haskell WL. Use of the heart rate–energy expenditure relationship in the individual prescription of exercise. Am J Clin Nutr 1971;24:1186.

21. Skinner JS, Gaskill SE, Rankinen T, et al. Heart rate vs %VO$_2$ max: age, sex, race, initial fitness & training response—HERITAGE. Med Sci Sports Exerc 2003;35:1908–1913.

22. Karvonen MJ, Kentala K, Musta O. The effects of training on heart rate: a longitudinal study. Ann Med Exp Biol Fenn 1957;35:308–315.

23. Borg GA. Borg's Perceived Exertion and Pain Scales. Champaign, IL: Human Kinetics, 1998.

24. Noble BJ. Clinical applications of perceived exertion. Med Sci Sports Exerc 1982;14:406–411.

25. Donta ST, Clauw DJ, Engel CC, et al. Cognitive behavioral therapy and aerobic exercise for Gulf War veterans' illnesses: a randomized controlled trial. JAMA 2003;289:1396–1404.

26. Skinner JS, Krasnoff J, Jaskólski A, et al. Age, sex, race, initial fitness and response to training: the HERITAGE Family Study. J Appl Physiol 2001;90:1770–1776.

27. Kohrt WM, Malley MT, Coggan AR, et al. Effects of gender, age and fitness level on response of VO$_2$ max to training in 60–71 yr olds. J Appl Physiol 1991;2004–2011.

28. Blair SN, Kampert JB, Kohl III HW, et al. Influences of cardiorespiratory fitness and other precursors on cardiovascular disease and all-cause mortality in men and women. JAMA 1996;276:205–210.

29. Corbin CB. Physical activity for everyone: what every physical educator should know about promoting lifelong physical activity. J Teach Phys Educ 2002;21:128–144.

30. Morgan WP. Prescription of physical activity: a paradigm shift. Quest 2000;53:366–382.

31. Dishman RK. Advances in exercise adherence. Champaign, IL: Human Kinetics, 1994.

32. Heinzelmann F. Social and psychological factors that influence the effectiveness of exercise programs. In: Naughton J, Hellerstein H, eds. Exercise Testing and Exercise Training in Coronary Heart Disease. New York: Academic Press, 1973.

3

General Principles of Exercise Testing and Exercise Prescription for Muscle Strength and Endurance

William J. Kraemer, Steven J. Fleck, and Nicholas A. Ratamess, Jr.

It is well-known that resistance training (RT) is an effective exercise modality to increase muscle strength and local muscle endurance. Traditionally, RT was performed by athletes to improve muscle strength, hypertrophy, power, and sports-specific fitness. As well, RT has profound effects on general health and performance (Table 3-1) and is now recommended by national health organizations, e.g., the American College of Sports Medicine (ACSM), in conjunction with other exercise modalities (e.g., aerobic, flexibility) to maintain and improve health and performance for virtually everyone (1). The key qualities of RT programs are proper program design and evaluation. An RT program consists of variables (e.g., load, volume, rest intervals, exercise selection and order, lifting velocity, and frequency) that may be systematically varied according to goals. This systematic variation, along with specificity of training and progressive overload, is paramount to progression.

Individualized Resistance Training

Prior to initiating an RT program, it is important to obtain medical clearance to ensure that RT is bene-ficial rather than injurious to those individuals with predisposing injuries or illnesses. Once an individual is deemed healthy to participate, the next step in RT prescription is goal setting via a *needs analysis*. A needs analysis consists of answering questions on the basis of what is expected from RT. It also ensures that the program is individualized. Individualized RT programs are most effective because they ensure that all goal-oriented facets are included within the design. Some common questions that need to be addressed are (2)

- Are there health/injury concerns (e.g., arthritis, cardiovascular) that may limit the exercises performed or the exercise intensity?
- What type of RT equipment (e.g., free weights, machines, bands/tubing, medicine balls, functional, etc.) is available?
- What is the targeted training frequency and are there any time constraints that might affect workout duration?
- What muscle groups need to be trained? Generally, all major muscle groups are trained, but some may require prioritization based upon strengths/weaknesses or the demands of the sport or activity.
- What are the targeted energy systems (e.g., aerobic or anaerobic)?

TABLE 3-1 HEALTH- AND PERFORMANCE-RELATED IMPROVEMENTS DUE TO RESISTANCE TRAINING (106)	
Increases	**Decreases**
Muscle strength	Blood pressure
Muscle power	Cardiovascular demands to exercise
Local muscle endurance	LDL and total cholesterol
Muscle size	Sarcopenia
Motor performance (e.g., jumping ability, sprinting speed, sports performance)	Risk of osteoporosis and colon cancer
	Body fat
Flexibility	Low back pain
Balance and coordination	
Functional capacity (e.g., stair climbing, walking)	
Aerobic capacity (circuit training programs)	
Basal metabolic rate and energy expenditure	
HDL cholesterol	
Glucose tolerance and insulin sensitivity	
Left ventricular and septal wall thickness	
Bone mass and connective tissue strength	

- What types of muscle actions (e.g., concentric [CON], eccentric [ECC], isometric [ISOM]) are needed?
- If training for a sport or activity, what are the most common sites of injury?
- What are the goals of this RT program? Is it to increase muscle size, strength, power, speed, local muscular endurance, balance, coordination, and/or flexibility? Is it to reduce percentage body fat, or to improve general health (e.g., lower blood pressure, strengthen connective tissue, reduce stress), or is it a combination of these factors?

An individualized program may be designed once these questions have been addressed. An individual's strengths/weaknesses need to be identified. This is accomplished through proper testing and evaluation, which along with the needs analysis, form the basis of RT program design.

Resistance Exercise Prescription for Muscle Strength

ROLE OF MUSCLE ACTION

Most RT programs consist predominantly of dynamic muscle actions (e.g., a CON and ECC component). Greater force is produced during ECC actions (3), and ECC actions are more neuromuscularly efficient (3,4), less metabolically demanding (5), and more conducive to hypertrophy (6) and delayed-onset muscle soreness (7) than CON actions. Maximizing dynamic muscular strength is most effective when ECC actions are included (8). The ACSM recommends including CON and ECC actions during strength training for novice to advanced programs (1,9).

Isometric (ISOM) exercise increases muscular strength (10) and is a popular testing modality during RT (11). ISOM training is useful because it elicits range-of-motion (ROM)-specific strength increases and is inexpensive to perform. ISOM training increases strength most specifically at the joint angles trained (known as *angular specificity*) (10,12), with some strength carryover to nontrained angles within approximately ±30° of the trained angle. When ISOM training is performed, it is generally recommended that maximal or near-maximal contractions be performed for at least 3 to 5 sec, using at least 15 to 20 contractions daily at multiple joint angles (2).

LOAD AND REPETITION PRESCRIPTION

Load represents the amount of weight lifted per repetition or set and is highly dependent upon such variables as exercise order, volume, frequency, muscle action, repetition speed, and rest period length. Altering the training load can significantly affect the acute metabolic (13,14), hormonal (15,16), neural (17,18), and cardiovascular (19) responses to training. Training status is an important determinant of load prescription. Loads <45 to 50% of one-repetition maximum (1 RM) increase dynamic strength in untrained individuals (20) because of improved motor learning and coordination (21). However, greater loading (>80% of 1 RM) is needed to progress to intermediate and advanced levels of training (17). Neural adaptations are crucial to strength training as they precede hypertrophy during intense training periods. Fewer motor units are recruited for a given load following RT when hypertrophy occurs (22). Progressively heavier loads are needed to continually recruit these higher-threshold motor units. Proper loading during RT encompasses either (*a*) increasing load based on a load-repetition continuum (e.g., performing 8 repetitions with a heavier load as opposed to 12 repetitions with a lighter load) or (*b*) increasing loading within a prescribed zone, e.g., 8 to 12 RM.

There is an inverse relationship between the amount of weight lifted and the number of repetitions performed. Training with loads corresponding to 1 to 6 RM is most specific to increasing maximal dynamic strength (23,24). Although significant increases have been reported using loads corresponding to 7 to 12 RM (25–27), this load range appears to be less effective for increasing muscular strength in highly trained lifters. Loads lighter than this have only small effects on maximal strength in previously-untrained individuals (28). Although training with high loads and low repetitions is most specific to increasing maximal strength, optimal RT requires the systematic use of various loading strategies (29). The ACSM recommends that novice-to-intermediate individuals train with loads corresponding to 60 to 70% of 1 RM for 8–12 repetitions and that advanced individuals use 80 to 100% of 1 RM in a periodized fashion. For progression in those individuals training at a specific RM load (8–12 repetitions), it is recommended that a 2 to 10% increase be applied based on muscle group size and involvement when the individual can perform the current workload for 1 to 2 repetitions over the desired number in two consecutive training sessions (9).

RESISTANCE TRAINING VOLUME

Training volume is estimated by summing the total number of repetitions performed during a workout session. Volume depends upon such variables as loads used, number of exercises selected, frequency, and muscle actions used and is inversely related to training intensity. Volume affects the neural (30), hypertrophic (31), metabolic (13), and hormonal (15,16,32) responses and adaptations to RT.

Training volume can be varied by changing the number of exercises performed per session, changing the number of repetitions performed per set, or changing the number of sets per exercise. Studies using 2 (33), 3 (23,26,27), 4 to 5 (8), and 6 or more (34,35) sets per exercise have all produced significant increases in both trained and untrained individuals. In direct comparison, studies report similar strength increases between 2 and 3 sets (36), and 2 and 4 sets (37), whereas 3 sets were superior to 1 and 2 (38). There is little or no difference between variation in set number within multiple-set RT programs. Each set within a multiple-set paradigm will serve a specific purpose. Other variables (e.g., intensity, the number of exercises performed, rest periods, frequency, and training goals) are important to determine the number of sets per workout and/or per exercise.

Single- and multiple-set RT programs have been investigated, with studies comparing one set per exercise performed for 8 to 12 RM at a slow velocity to both periodized and nonperiodized multiple-set programs (i.e., several studies have examined general program comparisons as opposed to isolating the number of sets per exercise). In untrained individuals, several studies report similar increases between single- and multiple-set programs (39–41), whereas others report that multiple sets are superior (38,42–45). In resistance-trained individuals, multiple-set programs are superior to enhance strength (27,46,47) and high-intensity endurance (27,48). To date, no study has found single-set training superior to multiple-set training in either trained or untrained individuals. Both program types effectively increase strength in untrained individuals during short-term training (e.g.,

6–12 weeks). Long-term studies support the contention that a higher volume of training is needed for a greater rate of improvement (49). The ACSM (9) recommends that novice individuals use a general RT program (with either single or multiple sets) initially and that intermediate-to-advanced individuals use multiple-set programs with systematic variation of training volume and intensity over time for optimal progression. A dramatic increase in training volume is not recommended to reduce the risk of overtraining.

SELECTION OF EXERCISES

Exercises should be selected specific to training goals. It is generally recommended that exercises stress all major muscle groups to maintain muscular balance. Single-joint exercises target one general muscle group or joint action, whereas multiple-joint exercises target more than one muscle group or involve multiple joint actions and interactions. Multiple-joint exercises may be further classified as basic strength and Olympic lifts. Basic strength exercises involve mostly two to three joints (e.g., squat, bench press), whereas Olympic lifts are total body power exercises that involve most major muscle groups.

There has been little research concerning the efficacy of performing different exercises on various assessments. Both single- (50) and multiple-joint exercises (27,30,51–54) are effective for strengthening the targeted muscle groups. Multiple-joint exercises are generally regarded as most effective in increasing overall strength in trained individuals because more weight can be lifted (55). Performing multiple-joint exercises may have greater impact on multiple-joint activities involved in daily living (2). Thus, multiple-joint exercises should form the core of an RT program. Single-joint exercises are effective primarily when isolating specific muscle groups and are commonly used. Both types of exercises (with free weights and machines) should be included in an RT program targeting strength (9).

EXERCISE SEQUENCING

The sequence of exercises performed during an RT session significantly affects performance and subsequent adaptation. Sequencing is based upon training goals and is highly dependent upon energy metabolism and fatigue. Improper exercise sequences can compromise the lifter's ability to perform the desired number of repetitions with the desired load (56). For strength training, priority is given to multiple-joint and/or large-muscle-mass exercises. The ACSM (9) provides the following guidelines and suggestions in their most recent position stand:

> *When training all major muscle groups in a workout:* large muscle-group exercises before small muscle-group exercises, multiple-joint exercises before single-joint exercises, or alternation of upper- and lower-body exercises
>
> *When training upper-body muscles on one day and lower-body muscles on a separate day:* large muscle-group exercises before small muscle-group exercises, multiple-joint exercises before single-joint exercises, or alternation of opposing exercises (agonist-antagonist relationship)
>
> *When training individual muscle groups:* multiple-joint exercises before single-joint exercises, higher-intensity exercises before lower-intensity exercises

REST INTERVALS

The amount of rest between sets and exercises significantly affects performance and subsequent adaptation to RT. Rest period length depends on training intensity, goals, fitness level, and the targeted energy system. Few studies have compared RT performance with various rest intervals. The length of the rest period significantly affects the metabolic (57), hormonal (15,16), and cardiovascular (19) responses to an acute bout of resistance exercise, as well as performance of subsequent sets (27). Long-term adaptations may also be affected by rest interval length (58–59). Rest period length will vary based on the goals of that particular exercise, i.e., not every exercise will use the same rest interval. Muscle strength may be increased using short rest periods but at a slower rate. The ACSM (9) recommends rest intervals of at least 2 to 3 min for multiple-joint exercises using heavy loads that stress a relatively large muscle mass for novice, intermediate, and advanced training. For assistance exercises (e.g., leg extension, leg curl), a shorter rest period of 1 to 2 min may suffice.

LIFTING VELOCITY

Lifting velocity used to perform dynamic muscle actions affects adaptations to RT. Lifting velocity depends upon the loads used, fatigue, and goals of the exercise and affects the neural (17), hypertrophic (34,60), and metabolic (61) adaptations to RT. Force production and lifting velocity directly interact during exercise performance. Generally, CON force production is greatest at slower velocities and lowest during high-velocity isokinetic (ISOK) movements (2). Studies examining CON ISOK RT have shown strength increases specific to the training velocity, with some carryover above and below the training velocity (2). Several researchers have trained individuals from 30°/s (10) to 300°/s (60,62) and report significant increases. However, training at moderate velocity (180–240°/s) appears to produce the greatest strength increases across all testing velocities (62). Otherwise, training at fast, moderate, and slow velocities may produce the greatest strength increases across all testing velocities (2).

Dynamic constant external RT poses a different stress, as velocity is not controlled. The rate of lifting affects the magnitude of force production. Significant reductions in force production are observed when the intent is to perform the repetition slowly. Two types of slow-velocity contractions exist during dynamic constant external RT, *unintentional* and *intentional*. Unintentional slow velocities are used during high-resistance repetitions in which either the loading and/or fatigue are responsible for the velocity of movement. Thus, the lifter exerts maximal force, but a fast lifting velocity cannot be attained because of the magnitude of loading. Fatigue can also affect lifting velocity (63).

Intentional slow-velocity contractions are used with submaximal loads in which the individual has greater control of the velocity. CON force production and integrated electromyogram (IEMG) are significantly lower for an intentionally slow lifting velocity (5 sec CON: 5 sec ECC) than for a traditional (moderate) velocity (64). These data suggest that motor-unit activity is limited when intentionally lifting at a slow velocity. In addition, the lighter loads required for slow velocities of training may not provide an optimal stimulus for strength enhancement in resistance-trained individuals. When performing a set of 10 repetitions using a very slow velocity (10-sec CON: 5-sec ECC) compared with a slow velocity (2-sec CON: 4-sec ECC), required a 30% reduction in training load; this resulted in less strength gain in most of the exercises tested after 10 weeks of training (65). Compared with slow velocities, moderate (1-2 sec CON: 1-2 sec ECC) and fast (<1 sec CON: 1 sec ECC) velocities are more effective for enhanced muscular performance, e.g., number of repetitions performed, work and power output, volume (66), and for increasing the rate of strength gain (67). Recent studies examining training at fast velocities with moderately high loading have shown this to be more effective for advanced training than traditionally slower velocities (68–70).

Slow-to-fast lifting velocities appear to be important for maximizing strength. Training goals and the level of strength fitness will be key determinants for selecting velocities during program design. The ACSM (9) recommends that intentionally slow and moderate velocities be used primarily for individuals with limited RT experience. This allows individuals to learn proper exercise technique while establishing a lifting base for future modifications. For intermediate training, a moderate velocity should be used. For advanced training, a continuum of velocities from unintentionally slow to fast velocities is recommended to maximize strength (9). Proper technique should be used for any exercise velocity to reduce risk of injury.

FREQUENCY

The number of RT sessions performed during a specific period time may affect subsequent training adaptations and depends upon such factors as the volume and intensity of exercise, exercise selection, level of conditioning and/or training status, nutrition, and goals. Numerous RT studies used frequencies of 2 to 3 alternating days per week in untrained individuals (8,71). This is an effective initial frequency, whereas 1 to 2 days per week appears to be an effective maintenance frequency for those already engaged in an RT program (72). In a few studies (*a*) 3 days per week were superior to 1 (73) and 2 days per week (72); (*b*) 4 days per week were superior to 3 (74); (*c*) 2 days were superior to 1 (75); and (*d*) 3 to 5 days per week were superior to 1 and 2 days (76) for increasing maximal strength. The recommended training frequency for beginning lifters is 2 to 3 total body workouts per week (9).

The progression from novice to intermediate status does not necessitate a change in training frequency for each muscle group but may depend more on alterations in such variables as the selection of exercises, volume, and intensity. Increasing training frequency allows greater specialization. Performing upper-body exercises during one workout and lower-body exercises during a separate workout or training specific muscle groups during a workout, as well as total-body workouts, are common at this level of training (2). Considering that similar increases in strength have been observed between upper/lower- and total-body workouts (77), the ACSM (9) recommends a similar frequency of 2 to 3 days per week be used for total-body workouts for progression to intermediate training. For persons desiring a change in training structure, the ACSM recommends a frequency of 3 to 4 days per week, such that each muscle group is trained only 1 to 2 times per week. Frequency for advanced or elite athletes may vary considerably as higher frequencies are recommended (9,78–80).

Resistance Exercise Prescription for Muscle Endurance

Local muscular endurance is the ability of a muscle or group of muscles to perform repeated maximal or submaximal contractions for a certain period of time. It also entails the ability to resist fatigue and maintain a certain level of force or power for as long as possible. During RT, this entails the maximal number of repetitions performed with a specific load, the ability to maintain a specific number of repetitions per load when rest intervals are reduced, or the ability to generate a certain level of ISOM tension for an extended period of time.

Local muscular endurance improves during RT (28,48,49,81). There are two general types of local muscle endurance: *high-intensity* and *submaximal*. High-intensity (also called strength endurance) endurance refers to the ability to maintain maximal or near-maximal force production for a period of time, whereas submaximal endurance refers to the

ability to maintain low-to-moderate levels of force for a substantial period of time. Traditional RT increases absolute muscular endurance (assessed by the maximal number of repetitions performed with a specific pretraining load) (27,28,81), but limited effects are observed in relative local muscular endurance (endurance assessed at a specific relative intensity, or percentage of 1 RM pre- and posttesting) (82). Moderate-to-low RT with high repetitions is most effective for improving absolute and relative submaximal local muscular endurance (28,81). High-intensity local muscle endurance improves with moderate-to-heavy RT, especially with short rest intervals. A relationship exists between increases in strength and local muscle endurance, such that RT alone may improve local muscular endurance. However, because following the principle of training specificity produces the greatest improvements, the primary strategies for designing RT programs targeting local muscular endurance are to (*a*) perform high repetitions or long-duration sets (i.e., long-duration implies increasing the time muscles are stressed via a slow lifting velocity or extending the time during ISOM muscle actions) and (*2*) minimize recovery between sets.

EXERCISE SELECTION AND SEQUENCING

Exercises stressing multiple or large muscle groups elicit the greatest short-term metabolic responses during RT (61). Metabolic demand is an important stimulus concerning the adaptations within skeletal muscle necessary to improve local muscular endurance. The sequencing of exercises may not be as important as with strength training because fatigue is a necessary component of endurance training, i.e., performing an exercise in a semifatigued condition may improve local muscle endurance, and variation in exercise order may be beneficial. The ACSM (9) recommends that both multiple- and single-joint exercises be included in a program targeting improved local muscular endurance using various sequencing combinations for novice, intermediate, and advanced training. For progression, proper training records should be kept to examine short-term performance for each exercise when it is performed at different intervals throughout a series of workouts.

INTENSITY AND VOLUME

Light loads coupled with high repetitions (15–20 or more) are most effective (28,83). However, moderate-to-heavy loading (coupled with short rest periods) is also effective for increasing high-intensity and absolute local muscular endurance (28,48). Program goals will specify the loading. High-volume programs are superior for endurance enhancement (27,49,71), especially when multiple sets per exercise are performed (27,49). The ACSM (9) recommends using relatively light loads (10–15 repetitions) with moderate-to-high volume for novice and intermediate training. For advanced training, various loading strategies should be used for multiple sets per exercise (10–25 repetitions or more) in a periodized manner. The key quality for optimal progression in advanced training is to vary volume and intensity.

REST INTERVALS

The duration of rest intervals during RT affects muscular endurance. Body builders (who typically train with short rest periods) have a significantly lower fatigue rate than power lifters (who typically train with longer rest periods) (57). The lack of full recovery between sets, and subsequent training in a semifatigued state, appears to be a critical component of optimal local muscle endurance training. Various strategies may be used to vary rest interval length depending on the number of repetitions performed and loads use. For example, one may use a specified weight and repetition number. Each week, one may reduce rest interval length gradually while maintaining repetition number until a minimal rest interval is attained (i.e., 30 sec). At this point, the individual may increase the weight and maintain repetition number or decrease weight and increase repetition number. In either case, the rest interval will increase and a similar pattern will be used. The ASCM (9) recommends short rest periods, i.e., 1 to 2 min for high-repetition sets (15–20 repetitions or more) and <1 min for moderate (10–15 repetitions) sets.

FREQUENCY

Training frequency depends on the number of muscle groups trained per workout. While RT stud-

ies examining frequency have focused on strength and not local muscle endurance per se, it appears that similar recommendations may apply to local muscle endurance training. Training 2 to 3 days per week is effective in novice and intermediate men and women when training the total body per workout. Higher frequency of training (as well as overall training volume) is suggested for advanced local muscle endurance training. However, only certain muscle groups are trained per workout, not the whole body. The ACSM (9) recommends using frequencies similar to those with strength training during novice, intermediate, and advanced training.

LIFTING VELOCITY

Lifting velocity affects the amount of enhancement as it relates highly to the duration of the set. Because extending duration is paramount to local muscle endurance training, this may be accomplished by selecting a slow lifting velocity or by increasing repetition number within a certain time period. Studies examining ISOK exercise find that a fast training velocity ($180°/s^{-1}$) is more effective than a slow training velocity ($30°/s^{-1}$) (84,85). Thus, fast lifting velocities are recommended for ISOK training. However, it appears that both fast and slow velocities are effective during dynamic constant external RT. Intentionally slow velocity training with light to moderate loads (5-sec CON: 5-sec ECC and slower) places continued tension on the muscles for an extended period and is more metabolically demanding than moderate and fast velocities (61). However, it is difficult to perform a large number of repetitions using intentionally slow speeds. Thus, repetition number must be adjusted accordingly. The ACSM (9) recommends intentionally slow velocities when a moderate number of repetitions (10–15) are used. If performing a large number of repetitions (15–25 or more) is the goal, then moderate-to-faster velocities are recommended. In this manner, increasing the repetition number offsets the faster lifting velocity but contributes to extending set duration.

Methods of Progression

Once the RT program has been properly designed and initiated, progression becomes a primary consideration for those seeking to enhance performance. The three most important concepts in RT progression are progressive overload, specificity, and variation. *Progressive overload* refers to gradually increasing the stress placed on the body during training; this increased demand is paramount for progression. The following are some common overloading strategies:

1. Increase the load
2. Add repetitions to the current workload
3. Alter lifting velocity according to goals
4. Shorten rest periods for local muscle endurance improvements
5. Increase volume within reasonable limits (i.e., 2.5–5%) (2)

Specificity is an important concept, as all training adaptations are specific to the stimulus applied. The physiologic adaptations to RT are specific to the

1. Muscle actions involved
2. Velocity of movement
3. Range of motion
4. Muscle groups trained
5. Energy systems involved
6. Intensity and volume of training (2)

Although there is some carryover of training effects, the most effective RT programs are those designed to target specific goals. *Variation* is also an important concept (29), which becomes increasingly important over long-term training periods when progression is the ultimate goal. Variation implies that alterations in one or more of the short-term program variables are systematically included in the program design. Lastly, proper supervision during RT is important (82). The rate of progression is greater when each workout is supervised by a competent strength and conditioning professional (82).

Importance of Strength and Endurance Testing

The most important reason to assess muscle strength and local muscle endurance is to assist in the evaluation and progression of RT programs.

Presently, RT is performed by most segments of the population, from children to the elderly (including clinical populations), and is recommended by the ACSM for general health and fitness exercise programs in adults (1,9). The programs, as well as the goals for training, are quite diverse, i.e., no single program structure will benefit everyone to the same degree. Infinite variations in program design are available, and each program should be tailored to the individual's needs. The amount of strength and local muscle endurance development depends on the initial level of muscular fitness, exercise prescription, time availability, and objectives of the program (i.e., progression or maintenance). Regular assessment of muscular strength and endurance enables proper evaluation of the exercise prescription and modifications when appropriate.

Testing Modalities

Perhaps the most common tools for assessing muscle strength and endurance are free weights, machines, and body weight. Although free weights and machines are commonly used for testing, free weights present a number of different testing challenges. Free weights require greater motor coordination primarily because they must be controlled through all spatial dimensions, whereas machines generally involve control through only one plane of movement (86). This can be an advantage or a disadvantage, depending on the motor skill level of the individuals being tested. Those with poor balance and impaired motor function (e.g., frail elderly) may require machine-based testing. Machines offer another advantage in that some exercises may be used during evaluations that are difficult to perform using free weights. A practical reason for using free weights is their low cost and availability. Single-joint exercises may be performed with free weights or machines, although they may be performed in a more restricted manner by use of machines when isolated muscle function is of interest.

TEST SPECIFICITY

Muscular strength and endurance testing show the greatest improvement when the assessment modality is similar to the training modality. This concept of testing specificity is especially valid with ISOM tests that are not highly correlated with dynamic performance (87,88). The chance of underestimating the effects of the RT program is greater when inappropriate tests are used.

IMPORTANCE OF FAMILIARIZATION

Without proper familiarization, values for strength gains from RT can be inflated. Before testing begins, all individuals (especially those with limited experience) must be thoroughly instructed and indoctrinated in the proper lifting methods. Some free-weight exercises may require a longer familiarization period, whereas others may require only a short period to eliminate the effects of learning and improved motor coordination. Participants must learn how to produce maximal effort, which requires proper familiarization. Two weeks of RT, including four practice/training sessions for each exercise, will achieve appropriate familiarization and reliability for strength testing (89). Familiarization is crucial in such populations as children or the elderly, e.g., elderly women require more familiarization (nine sessions vs. four for younger women) (90). The test conditions are unique to the methods used and developed for the population being evaluated. Familiarization includes (*a*) practice of the exercises; (*b*) a "dry run" through the test protocol; and (*c*) repeated practice of the protocol under actual test conditions until a stable, reproducible baseline for strength performance is achieved.

IMPORTANCE OF AROUSAL AND ENCOURAGEMENT

Performance on strength and endurance tasks can be enhanced if individuals are optimally aroused (91). Verbal encouragement is suggested for all testing to ensure optimal results. It was recently shown that merely the presence of an audience can affect 1 RM performance (92). Care must be taken that the form of encouragement is consistent. A factor such as yelling during testing can affect arousal and the resulting strength scores (93). Such factors must be controlled.

SAFETY CONSIDERATIONS

Safety is an important consideration when performing strength evaluations, especially those with free weights. All testing equipment must be in proper working order, inspected prior to use to avoid accidental injury, and capable of withstanding heavy use. This includes properly rotating barbells, properly functioning collars, solidly secured weights, and calibration of all weights to be used. The presence of properly trained spotters is mandatory. Emergency procedures should be identified and posted before testing is performed. Prudent methods and procedures will help avoid litigation due to negligence and enhance the efficacy of testing. Maximal strength tests are safe if proper technique and instruction are used.

The safety of maximal strength testing in special populations (e.g., the elderly) has been questioned. Shaw et al. (4) examined the safety of machine 1 RM strength testing in 83 elderly men and women. Only two individuals were injured during testing, and they had no previous lifting experience. No one with lifting experience was injured. Similar results were obtained by Barnard et al. (95) who reported no injuries during 1 RM testing in 74 men and women enrolled in a cardiac rehabilitation program. These data demonstrate that 1 RM strength testing is safe in the clinical setting but also stress the importance of prior familiarization and proper instruction prior to testing. If it is decided to include 1 RM testing, then staff should be trained in safety and testing protocols. Other assessments such as a multiple RM, estimation of 1 RM via regression equations, or close examination of training logs may be useful alternatives for some populations.

PROPER POSITIONING WITH FREE WEIGHTS

Proper positioning is critical to testing. Factors such as grip style and position, foot stance, body position, and bar position can all affect the mechanics and results. The starting position of the limbs and exercise ROM are also very important. Often there is a natural tendency to reduce ROM when loading is maximal. Thus, exercise ROM and the actual positions used should be standardized and controlled over all testing situations. Consistency of test procedures is vital to establish good test reliability. The use of free weights can make reliability difficult to attain if confounding variables are not controlled.

RESISTANCE EXERCISE MACHINES

Strength testing with machines is most appropriate when RT is performed using machines. If training has been performed using a different modality, such a machine may not be appropriate for evaluation. Many machines operate in only one plane of motion, resulting in different requirements for motor coordination and lifting technique (19). By ruling out technique factors, strength testing with machines may more accurately assess pure strength changes; this is important when evaluating individuals with little RT experience. Also, machines are readily available at many facilities, even though their cost may be prohibitive. A popular aspect for many is greater safety. Generally, spotters are not necessary, although someone knowledgeable should be present. Equipment must be closely inspected for safety factors. Machines must operate smoothly because improper lubrication or a misalignment of the trainee with the device may add unknown resistance. Machine strength testing may provide certain advantages such as the ability to assess exercises difficult to perform with free weights and use of a testing modality for those with severely limited motor skills.

BODY POSITIONING IN MACHINES

Weight machines can isolate muscle groups/joints while minimizing extraneous body movements. Although most are adjustable, some individuals may have problems determining the proper fit. With properly adjusted equipment, the individual must be positioned each time according to a predetermined protocol to meet the needs of the test. Small position deviations on a machine can affect resultant force production (97). Quantifying and recording the starting positions of the machine is mandatory. The weight increments possible with some machines may be a limiting factor. When evaluating individuals with low levels of strength, an increase of 10 lb (as is commonly found with many weight stacks) may be too great. If a weight stack is used, it might be necessary to attach smaller weights. This

is true when exceptionally strong individuals are tested and there is not enough resistance on the machine. Plate-loaded machines offer a distinct advantage for these situations.

DYNAMIC STRENGTH TESTING PROTOCOLS

Strength assessments using free weights and machines are commonly cited. A 1 RM effort is the "gold standard" for evaluating strength, although RM testing can involve any number of repetitions. Some researchers have attempted to predict maximal strength from submaximal efforts, but this has resulted in mixed effectiveness, as higher RMs may better indicate local muscle endurance (98). Although several protocols for strength testing are effective, the following is one that has commonly been used in our laboratory (96):

1. A light warm-up of 5–10 repetitions at 40–60% of perceived maximum
2. After a 1-min rest with light stretching, 3–5 repetitions at 60–80% of perceived maximum
3. Step 2 will take the individual close to the perceived 1 RM. A conservative increase in the resistance is made, and a 1 RM lift is attempted. If the lift is successful, a rest period of 2–3 min is allowed. One of the most costly errors is not allowing enough rest before the next maximal attempt. A 1 RM should be obtained within 3–5 sets to avoid excessive fatigue. The process of selecting the weight can be enhanced by prior familiarization and by expertise of the investigator in evaluating performance. This process continues until a failed attempt occurs, after which the weight is adjusted accordingly.
4. The 1 RM value is reported as the weight of the last successfully completed lift

Communication between the individual and tester is paramount. Questioning the individual about readiness and the magnitude of load increase is vital to testing. The number of preliminary repetition attempts (warm-up) and rest intervals is important. To some extent, these factors need to be individualized, as individuals lifting very heavy weights will require more warm-up sets and longer rest intervals than someone lifting a lighter weight. Sufficient recovery needs to be given. Stress that each individual must rest 48 hours prior to testing and ensure proper nutrition (e.g., adequate caloric intake, proper hydration) (99). If more repetitions are attempted, fewer warm-up sets should be used. Higher RMs (e.g., 10 and 20) produce greater muscle disruption, thereby indicating that one trial may be necessary or that additional trials require a much longer recovery period (100). The following protocol is suggested for testing a 6 RM and could be modified to test other RM numbers (96).

1. Warm-up with 5–10 repetitions at 50% of the estimated 6 RM
2. After 1 min of rest and light stretching, 6 repetitions at 70% of the estimated 6 RM
3. Step 2 is repeated at 85–90% of the estimated 6 RM
4. After a 2-min rest, 6 repetitions with 100 to 105% of the estimated 6 RM
5. After a 2-to 3-min rest (if step 4 is successful), increase the resistance by 2.5–5% for another 6-RM attempt. If 6 repetitions were not completed, subtract 2.5–5% of the resistance used in step 4 and attempt another 6 RM.
6. If weight was removed for step 5 and 6 repetitions were performed, this is the 6 RM. If not successful, retest after at least 24 hours of rest.

There are estimations of 1 RM capabilities from a multiple-RM performance. Several prediction equations have been developed and, although attractive, their validity has been questioned, especially when higher RMs are used (101). For example, conversion factors have been developed that allow a 10 RM resistance to be equated with a 1 RM resistance (102), but these can lead to erroneous results (101). For field settings involving large numbers of untrained individuals, a case may be made to estimate 1 RM, but definitely not for research purposes. Nevertheless, such equations can help target the actual 1 RM.

Isometric Testing

Devices for ISOM strength assessment have been in existence for many years. Early work commonly used devices such as the hip and back dynamome-

ter. Strength of isolated joints can be tested using cable tensiometers. The handgrip dynamometer is used to evaluate grip strength. Modern testing has used force transducers (load cells), force plates, and strain gauges that allow interfacing with computerized data storage and analysis systems. ISOK devices can be used for ISOM testing by selecting zero velocity. In addition to peak force, the rate of force development may be obtained. When testing ISOM strength, at least a 5-sec maximal contraction should be used to ensure maximal force production.

Fatigue tests are commonly used with ISOM devices to assess local muscular endurance. These tests generally involve maintaining a certain level of force over a period of time. If a fatigue curve is to be developed, the individuals must exert maximal effort and not pace themselves. Evaluation of the mean force over a specific time period provides a measure of ISOM endurance and the total amount of fatigue. Other ISOM tests can be quantified in several ways, with fatigue defined as the time that the individual can maintain a certain percentage of maximum torque. The percentage decline (fatigue rate) can be determined over a set period.

ISOMETRIC TESTING CONSIDERATIONS

The ISOM testing device should be calibrated with known masses before testing and at periodic intervals. Calibration should be performed through the entire range of measurement of the device. Before testing, a general warm-up with activities using the musculature to be tested is performed. Caution is necessary to not "prefatigue" the individual. The actual test requires approximately three maximal voluntary efforts (or more if individuals continue to improve). Generally, the peak force of the best trial is recorded.

For every test protocol, one must properly isolate the joint and position the individual. To enhance reliability, positioning must be carefully quantified with regard to the specific joint angles used. Individuals must be comfortable. and all surfaces being pushed against must be comfortably padded. Individuals must be securely stabilized in the desired position, as this affects the magnitude of force production. The use of restraining straps is critical, although these may give way or shift, resulting in a change in body position.

Specificity of testing must be considered. Studies that use dynamic RT but assess strength changes only with static methods are not evaluating specific dynamic improvements (87). The testing tool must be identical to that used in RT to give a valid assessment of functional changes. Individuals performing an ISOM test should be provided concurrent feedback about their performance; this is especially important for unfamiliar tasks. Local muscular endurance may decrease in the absence of feedback (103). Visual feedback is critical, but verbal encouragement can also be given. These factors can contribute to optimal reproducibility.

Isokinetic Testing

ISOK testing is performed on specially constructed dynamometers that control the velocity of movement. The cost of an ISOK dynamometer can be prohibitive, but many laboratories, training rooms, and clinical facilities have them. There are a number of important considerations when assessing ISOK strength. Of primary importance is the specificity of angular limb velocities. The velocity used for CON testing should be carefully considered because the resulting forces can increase at slower velocities (104). Specificity of the joint being tested is important because different muscle groups exhibit different ISOK performance characteristics (105). The reliability of the testing device must be high for acceptable data to be collected. All ISOK dynamometers should be calibrated according to the manufacturer's guidelines on a regular basis and monitored for test–retest reliability.

Proper positioning of the individual is essential for accurate testing. As with other types of strength testing, various limb positions can result in altered torque production (97). Joints that have a large ROM in many directions must be carefully secured in the proper position. Because only one joint is tested at a time, it is necessary to stabilize all body parts that may affect the torque measurement. All securing straps must be snug but comfortable, without interfering with the exercise ROM and should be regularly inspected for safety.

Numerous protocols are used for ISOK testing. Once the test has been performed appropri-ately, measures that can be monitored include peak torque, angle-specific peak torque, mean torque, total work (area under the curve), time to peak torque, angle of peak torque, and torque at various time intervals (96). Fatigue tests can be performed, with a greater number of repetitions resulting in a fatigue index or percentage decline (96). The variables available will depend on the brand and model of dynamometer used, as well as the software package accompanying it. The actual test should be preceded by several submaximal warm-up efforts and individuals should be instructed to perform their repetitions as forcefully and quickly as possible. It is common to attain the greatest torques on the second or third repetition.

Assessing Local Muscle Endurance

Local muscle endurance tests are performed specifically to evaluate repetitive muscular capabilities. Although there is some relationship between 1 RM and muscle endurance, it is generally poor; this is the rationale against using multiple RM testing to estimate 1 RM. An important consideration is what resistance to use. For free-weight and machine testing, the maximal number of repetitions performed with a specific load is typically used. Relative loading is based on a percentage of an individual's RM (e.g., 60% 1 RM), whereas absolute loading entails performance of the test with the same load before, during, and after the training intervention. It is important to standardize lifting velocity, as a faster speed leads to greater performance (66). Local muscular endurance may be assessed during standard multiple-set protocols in which repetition number with a specific resistance and cadence is assessed using various rest intervals. Verbal feedback and encouragement should be provided during such tests.

Summary

- RT has many benefits for improving health and performance, and it is recommended by major health organizations for inclusion into an overall fitness program for most adults.

- Success in RT depends on the proper manipulation of program variables in accordance with the specific training needs and goals of the individual.
- The most important concepts for progression during RT are progressive overload, specificity, and variation. Their inclusion is important for improving health and performance.
- It is important to assess muscle strength and local muscle endurance to assist in the evaluation and progression of RT programs. Several protocols are used with equipment such as free weights, machines, ISOK dynamometers, and ISOM devices.
- Tests selected for evaluation should be specific to the training modality.

REFERENCES

1. American College of Sports Medicine. Position stand: The recommended quantity and quality of exercise for developing and maintaining cardiorespiratory and muscular fitness, and flexibility in healthy adults. Med Sci Sports Exerc 1998;30:975–991.
2. Fleck SJ, Kraemer WJ. Designing Resistance Training Programs. 2nd ed. Champaign, IL: Human Kinetics, 1997.
3. Komi PV, Kaneko M, Aura O. EMG activity of leg extensor muscles with special reference to mechanical efficiency in concentric and eccentric exercise. Int J Sports Med 1987;8(suppl):22–29.
4. Eloranta V, Komi PV. Function of the quadriceps femoris muscle under maximal concentric and eccentric contraction. Electromyogr Clin Neurophysiol 1980;20:159–174.
5. Bonde-Peterson F, Knuttgen HG, Henriksson J. Muscle metabolism during exercise with concentric and eccentric contractions. J Appl Physiol 1972;33:792–795.
6. Hather BM, Tesch PA, Buchanan P, Dudley GA. Influence of eccentric actions on skeletal muscle adaptations to resistance training. Acta Physiol Scand 1991;143:177–185.
7. Ebbeling CB, Clarkson PM. Exercise-induced muscle damage and adaptation. Sports Med 1989;7:207–234.
8. Dudley GA, Tesch PA, Miller BJ, Buchanan MD. Importance of eccentric actions in performance adaptations to resistance training. Aviat Space Environ Med 1991;62:543–550.
9. Kraemer WJ, Adams K, Cafarelli E, et al. American College of Sports Medicine. Position stand: pro-

gression models in resistance training for healthy adults. Med Sci Sports Exerc 2002;34:364–380.
10. Knapik JJ, Mawdsley RH, Ramos MU. Angular specificity and test mode specificity of isometric and isokinetic strength training. J Orthop Sports Phys Ther 1983;5:58–65.
11. McDonagh MJN, Davies CTM. Adaptive response of mammalian skeletal muscle to exercise with high loads. Eur J Appl Physiol 1984;52:139–155.
12. Bandy WD, Hanten WP. Changes in torque and electromyographic activity of the quadriceps femoris muscles following isometric training. Phys Ther 1993;73:455–467.
13. Collins MA, Cureton KJ, Hill DW, Ray CA. Relation of plasma volume change to intensity of weight lifting. Med Sci Sports Exerc 1989;21:178–185.
14. Willoughby DS, Chilek DR, Schiller DA, Coast JR. The metabolic effects of three different free weight parallel squatting intensities. J Hum Move Stud 1991;21:53–67.
15. Kraemer WJ, Marchitelli L, Gordon SE, et al. Hormonal and growth factor responses to heavy resistance exercise protocols. J Appl Physiol 1990;69:1442–1450.
16. Kraemer WJ, Gordon SE, Fleck SJ, et al. Endogenous anabolic hormonal and growth factor responses to heavy resistance exercise in males and females. Int J Sports Med 1991;12:228–235.
17. Häkkinen K, Alen M, Komi PV. Changes in isometric force- and relaxation-time, electromyographic and muscle fibre characteristics of human skeletal muscle during strength training and detraining. Acta Physiol Scand 1985;125:573–585.
18. Sale DG. Neural adaptations to strength training. In: Komi PV, ed. Strength and Power in Sport. Boston: Blackwell Scientific Publications, 1992:249–265.
19. Fleck SJ. Cardiovascular adaptations to resistance training. Med Sci Sports Exerc 1988;20:S146–S151.
20. Baechle TR, Earle RW, Wathen D. Resistance training. In: Baechle TR, Earle RW, eds. Essentials of Strength Training and Conditioning. Champaign, IL: Human Kinetics, 2000:395–425.
21. Rutherford OM, Jones DA. The role of learning and coordination in strength training. Eur J Appl Physiol 1986;55:100–105.
22. Ploutz LL, Tesch PA, Biro RL, Dudley GA. Effect of resistance training on muscle use during exercise. J Appl Physiol 1994;76:1675–1681.
23. Berger RA. Optimum repetitions for the development of strength. Res Q 1962;33:334–338.
24. Weiss LW, Coney HD, Clark FC. Differential

functional adaptations to short-term low-, moderate-, and high-repetition weight training. J Strength Cond Res 1999;13:236–241.

25. MacDougall JD, Ward GR, Sale DG, Sutton JR. Biochemical adaptation of human skeletal muscle to heavy resistance training and immobilization. J Appl Physiol 1977;43:700–703.

26. Staron RS, Karapondo DL, Kraemer WJ, et al. Skeletal muscle adaptations during early phase of heavy-resistance training in men and women. J Appl Physiol 1994;76:1247–1255.

27. Kraemer WJ. A series of studies—the physiological basis for strength training in American football: fact over philosophy. J Strength Cond Res 1997;11:131–142.

28. Anderson T, Kearney JT. Effects of three resistance training programs on muscular strength and absolute and relative endurance. Res Q Exerc Sport 1982;53:1–7.

29. Fleck SJ. Periodized strength training: a critical review. J Strength Cond Res 1999;13:82–89.

30. Häkkinen K, Pakarinen A, Alen M, et al. Relationships between training volume, physical performance capacity, and serum hormone concentrations during prolonged training in elite weight lifters. Int J Sports Med 1987;8(suppl):61–65.

31. Tesch PA, Komi PV, Häkkinen K. Enzymatic adaptations consequent to long-term strength training. Int J Sports Med 1987;8(suppl):66–69.

32. Kraemer WJ, Fleck SJ, Dziados JE, et al. Changes in hormonal concentrations after different heavy-resistance exercise protocols in women. J Appl Physiol 1993;75:594–604.

33. Dudley GA, Djamil R. Incompatibility of endurance- and strength-training modes of exercise. J Appl Physiol 1985;59:1446–1451.

34. Housh DJ, Housh TJ, Johnson GO, Chu WK. Hypertrophic response to unilateral concentric isokinetic resistance training. J Appl Physiol 1992;73:65–70.

35. Sale DG, Jacobs I, MacDougall JD, Garner S. Comparisons of two regimens of concurrent strength and endurance training. Med Sci Sports Exerc 1990;22:348–356.

36. Capen EK. Study of four programs of heavy resistance exercises for development of muscular strength. Res Q 1956;27:132–142.

37. Ostrowski KJ, Wilson GJ, Weatherby R, et al. The effect of weight training volume on hormonal output and muscular size and function. J Strength Cond Res 1997;11:148–154.

38. Berger RA. Comparison of the effect of various weight training loads on strength. Res Q 1963; 36:141–146.

39. Jacobson BH. A comparison of two progressive weight training techniques on knee extensor strength. Athl Train 1986;21:315–319.

40. Silvester LJ, Stiggins C, McGown C, Bryce GR. The effect of variable resistance and free-weight training programs on strength and vertical jump. NSCA J 1982;3:30–33.

41. Starkey DB, Pollock ML, Ishida Y, et al. Effect of resistance training volume on strength and muscle thickness. Med Sci Sports Exerc 1996;28:1311–1320.

42. Stone MH, Johnson RL, Carter DR. A short term comparison of two different methods of resistance training on leg strength and power. Athl Train 1979;158–161.

43. Stowers T, McMillan J, Scala D, et al. The short-term effects of three different strength-power training modes. NSCA J 1983;5:24–27.

44. Sanborn K, Boros R, Hruby J, et al. Short-term performance effects of weight training with multiple sets not to failure vs a single set to failure in women. J Strength Cond Res 2000;14:328–331.

45. Schlumberger A, Stec J, Schmidtbleicher D. Single- vs. multiple-set strength training in women. J Strength Cond Res 2001;15:284–289.

46. Kramer JB, Stone MH, O'Bryant HS, et al. Effects of single vs. multiple sets of weight training: impact of volume, intensity, and variation. J Strength Cond Res 1997;11:143–147.

47. Kraemer WJ, Ratamess N, Fry AC, et al. Influence of resistance training volume and periodization on physiological and performance adaptations in college women tennis players. Am J Sports Med 2000;28:626–633.

48. McGee D, Jessee TC, Stone MH, Blessing D. Leg and hip endurance adaptations to three weight training programs. J Appl Sports Sci Res 1992;6:92–95.

49. Marx JO, Ratamess NA, Nindl BC, et al. Low-volume circuit versus high-volume periodized resistance training in women. Med Sci Sports Exerc 2001;33:635–643.

50. Colliander EB, Tesch PA. Effects of eccentric and concentric muscle actions in resistance training. Acta Physiol Scand 1990;140:31–39.

51. Stone MH, O'Bryant H, Garhammer J. A hypothetical model for strength training. J Sports Med 1981;21:342–351.

52. Häkkinen K, Pakarinen A, Alen M, et al. Daily hormonal and neuromuscular responses to intensive strength training in 1 week. Int J Sports Med 1988;9:422–428.

53. Häkkinen K, Pakarinen A, Alen M, et al. Neuromuscular and hormonal responses in elite athletes

to two successive strength training sessions in one day. Eur J Appl Physiol 1988;57:133–139.

54. Häkkinen K, Pakarinen A, Alen M, et al. Neuromuscular and hormonal adaptations in athletes to strength training in two years. J Appl Physiol 1988;65:2406–2412.

55. Stone MH, Plisk SS, Stone ME, et al. Athletic performance development: volume load—1 set vs multiple sets, training velocity and training variation. Strength Cond 1998;20:22–31.

56. Sforzo GA, Touey PR. Manipulating exercise order affects muscular performance during a resistance exercise training session. J Strength Cond Res 1996;10:20–24.

57. Kraemer WJ, Noble BJ, Clark MJ, Culver BW. Physiologic responses to heavy-resistance exercise with very short rest periods. Int J Sports Med 1987;8:247–252.

58. Robinson JM, Stone MH, Johnson RL, et al. Effects of different weight training exercise/rest intervals on strength, power, and high intensity exercise endurance. J Strength Cond Res 1995;9:216–221.

59. Pincivero DM, Lephart SM, Karunakara RG. Effects of rest interval on isokinetic strength and functional performance after short term high intensity training. Br J Sports Med 1997;31:229–234.

60. Coyle EF, Feiring DC, Rotkis TC, et al. Specificity of power improvements through slow and fast isokinetic training. J Appl Physiol 1981;51:1437–1442.

61. Ballor DL, Becque MD, Katch VL. Metabolic responses during hydraulic resistance exercise. Med Sci Sports Exerc 1987;19:363–367.

62. Kanehisa H, Miyashita M. Specificity of velocity in strength training. Eur J Appl Physiol 1983;52:104–106.

63. Mookerjee S, Ratamess NA. Comparison of strength differences and joint action durations between full and partial range-of-motion bench press exercise. J Strength Cond Res 1999;13:76–81.

64. Keogh JWL, Wilson GJ, Weatherby RP. A cross-sectional comparison of different resistance training techniques in the bench press. J Strength Cond Res 1999;13:247–258.

65. Keeler LK, Finkelstein LH, Miller W, Fernhall B. Early-phase adaptations to traditional-speed vs. superslow resistance training on strength and aerobic capacity in sedentary individuals. J Strength Cond Res 2001;15:309–314.

66. LaChance PF, Hortobagyi T. Influence of cadence on muscular performance during push-up and pull-up exercises. J Strength Cond Res 1994;8:76–79.

67. Hay JG, Andrews JG, Vaughan CL. Effects of lifting rate on elbow torques exerted during arm curl exercises. Med Sci Sports Exerc 1983;15:63–71.

68. Jones K, Hunter G, Fleisig G, et al. The effects of compensatory acceleration on upper-body strength and power in collegiate football players. J Strength Cond Res 1999;13:99–105.

69. Moss BM, Refsnes PE, Abildgaard A, et al. Effects of maximal effort strength training with different loads on dynamic strength, cross-sectional area, load-power and load-velocity relationships. Eur J Appl Physiol 1997;75:193–199.

70. Wilson GJ. Strength and power in sport. In: Bloomfield J, Ackland TR, Elliott BC, eds. Applied Anatomy and Biomechanics in Sport, Boston: Blackwell Scientific Publications, 1994:110–208.

71. Hickson RC, Hidaka K, Foster C. Skeletal muscle fiber type, resistance training, and strength-related performance. Med Sci Sports Exerc 1994;26:593–598.

72. Graves JE, Pollock ML, Jones AE, et al. Specificity of limited range of motion variable resistance training. Med Sci Sports Exerc 1989;21:84–89.

73. McLester JR, Bishop P, Guilliams ME. Comparison of 1 day and 3 days per week of equal-volume resistance training in experienced subjects. J Strength Cond Res 2000;14:273–281.

74. Hunter GR. Changes in body composition, body build and performance associated with different weight training frequencies in males and females. NSCA J 1985;7:26–28.

75. Pollock ML, Graves JE, Bamman MM, et al. Frequency and volume of resistance training: effect of cervical extension strength. Arch Phys Med Rehabil 1993;74:1080–1086.

76. Gillam GM. Effects of frequency of weight training on muscle strength enhancement. J Sports Med 1981;21:432–436.

77. Calder AW, Chilibeck PD, Webber CE, Sale DG. Comparison of whole and split weight training routines in young women. Can J Appl Physiol 1994;19:185–199.

78. Hoffman JR, Kraemer WJ, Fry AC, et al. The effects of self-selection for frequency of training in a winter conditioning program for football. J Appl Sport Sci Res 1990;4:76–82.

79. Zatsiorsky V. Science and Practice of Strength Training, Champaign, IL: Human Kinetics, 1995.

80. Häkkinen K, Kallinen M. Distribution of strength training volume into one or two daily sessions and neuromuscular adaptations in female athletes. Electromyogr Clin Neurophysiol 1994;34:117–124.

81. Huczel HA, Clarke DH. A comparison of strength and muscle endurance in strength-trained and untrained women. Eur J Appl Physiol 1992;64:467–470.

82. Mazzetti SA, Kraemer WJ, Volek JS, et al. The influence of direct supervision of resistance training on strength performance. Med Sci Sports Exerc 2000;32:1175–1184.

83. Stone WJ, Coulter SP. Strength/endurance effects from three resistance training protocols with women. J Strength Cond Res 1994;8:231–234.

84. Adeyanju K, Crews TR, Meadors WJ. Effects of two speeds of isokinetic training on muscular strength, power and endurance. J Sports Med 1983;23:352–356.

85. Moffroid M, Whipple RH. Specificity of speed of exercise. Phys Ther 1970;50:1692–1700.

86. Fleck SJ, Kraemer WJ. Resistance training: basic principles. Phys Sportsmed 1988;16:160–171.

87. Baker D, Wilson J, Carlyon B. Generality versus specificity: a comparison of dynamic and isometric measures of strength and speed-strength. Eur J Appl Physiol 1994;68:350–355.

88. Murphy AJ, Wilson GJ. Poor correlations between isometric tests and dynamic performance: relationships to muscle activation. Eur J Appl Physiol 1996;73:353–357.

89. Fry AC, Kraemer WJ, Weseman CA, et al. The effects of an off-season strength and conditioning program on starters and non-starters in women's intercollegiate volleyball. J Appl Sport Sci Res 1991;5:174–181.

90. Ploutz-Snyder L, Giamis EL. Orientation and familiarization to 1 RM strength testing in old and young women. J Strength Cond Res 2001;15:519–523.

91. Biddle SJ. Personal beliefs and mental preparation in strength and muscular endurance tasks: a review. Phys Educ Rev 1986;8:90–103.

92. Rhea MR, Landers DM, Alvar BA, Arent SM. The effects of competition and the presence of an audience on weight-lifting performance. J Strength Cond Res 2003;17:303–306.

93. Ikai M, Steinhaus AH. Some factors modifying the expression of human strength. J Appl Physiol 1961;16:157–163.

94. Shaw CE, McCully KK, Posner JD. Injuries during the one repetition maximum assessment in the elderly. J Cardiopulm Rehabil 1995;15:283–287.

95. Barnard KL, Adams KJ, Swank AM, et al. Injuries and muscle soreness during the one repetition maximum assessment in a cardiac rehabilitation population. J Cardiopulm Rehabil 1999;19:52–58.

96. Kraemer WJ, Fry AC. Strength testing: development and evaluation of methodology. In: Maud PJ, Foster C, eds. Physiological Assessment of Human Fitness, Champaign, IL: Human Kinetics, 1995:115–138.

97. Lewis CL, Spitler DL. Effect of tibial rotation on measures of strength and endurance of the knee. J Appl Sport Sci Res 1989;3:19–22.

98. Hoeger WK, Barette SL, Hale DF, Hopkins DR. Relationship between repetitions and selected percentages of one repetition maximum. J Appl Sport Sci Res 1987;1:11–13.

99. Schoffstall JE, Branch JD, Leutholtz BC, Swain DE. Effects of dehydration and rehydration on the one-repetition maximum bench press of weight-trained males. J Strength Cond Res 2001;15:102–108.

100. Behm DG, Reardon G, Fitzgerald J, Drinkwater E. The effects of 5, 10, and 20 repetition maximums on the recovery of voluntary and evoked contractile properties. J Strength Cond Res 2002;16:209–218.

101. Mayhew JL, Prinster JL, Ware JS, et al. Muscular endurance repetitions to predict bench press strength in men of different training levels. J Sports Med Phys Fitness 1995;35:108–113.

102. Rose K, Ball TE. A field test for predicting maximum bench press lift of college women. J Appl Sport Sci Res 1992;6:103–106.

103. Graves JE, James RJ. Concurrent augmented feedback and isometric force generation during familiar and unfamiliar muscle movements. Res Q 1990;61:75–79.

104. Fry AC, Powell DR, Kraemer WJ. Validity of isokinetic and isometric testing modalities for assessing short-term resistance exercise strength gains. J Sport Rehabil 1992;1:275–283.

105. Cisar CJ, Johnson GO, Fry AC, Ryan AJ. Assessment of preseason muscular strength as a basis for specific conditioning. J Appl Sport Sci Res 1987;1:60.

106. Kraemer WJ, Ratamess NA, French DN. Resistance training for health and performance. Curr Sports Med Rep 2002;1:165–171.

RELATED WEB SITES

National Strength and Conditioning Association
www.nsca-lift.org

American College of Sports Medicine
www.acsm.org

4

Differences Between Men and Women for Exercise Testing and Exercise Prescription[a]

Jack H. Wilmore

The decade of the 1970s and the first half of the 1980s produced considerable interest in the physical abilities and limitations of women, both in the workplace and in the athletic arena. In the United States, passage of the Civil Rights Act of 1964 prohibited job discrimination on the basis of sex. The Women's Equal Rights Amendment of 1972, although never ratified, increased the awareness of women's rights under the law. Finally, the passage in 1972 of the U.S. Education Amendment (Title IX) forbade sex discrimination in any institution receiving federal funds. The first two legislative acts opened many employment opportunities for women that were previously unavailable. Women are now found in such occupations as commercial airline pilots, law enforcement officers, telephone linemen, construction workers, and heavy equipment operators, and hold combat assignments in the military. The U.S. Education Amendment (Title IX) has also had a major impact on athletic programs in public and private schools at all grade

levels. In the past, compared with programs for boys and men, girls and women were denied the opportunity for high quality athletic experiences. Title IX accomplished much in a relatively short period of time, creating more athletic opportunities for girls and women.

The sudden changes brought about by this federal legislation caused considerable confusion and raised many questions. Are girls and women physically capable of assuming new roles as they take advantage of these opportunities? Can girls and women physically cope with the rigors of high-level athletic competition? Can women perform physically demanding jobs, jobs previously restricted to men? Can girls and women obtain the traditional benefits of exercise and sport that boys and men have enjoyed for centuries? Finally, can girls and women be trained for sport or conditioned for fitness by using a format identical to that for boys and men, or are there special considerations that dictate a unique training or conditioning format? The intent of this chapter is to investigate similarities and differences between the sexes with respect to body size and composition, physiologic responses to a short-term bout of exercise, and physiologic adaptations to periods of exercise training to

[a]This chapter was adapted from Wilmore JH, Costill DL. Physiology of Sport and Exercise. 3rd ed. Champaign, IL: Human Kinetics, 2003, with permission of the publisher.

determine how exercise testing and exercise prescription might need to be modified to accommodate any differences.

Body Size and Composition

From the data of McCammon, which summarizes the Child Research Council's longitudinal growth study in Denver, it appears that differences in height, weight, circumferences, diameters, and skinfold thicknesses between the sexes do not appear until the age of 12 to 14 years, i.e., approximately at the time of puberty (1). Before puberty, there is a striking similarity between boys and girls of the same socioeconomic background for all indices of size and maturity. Forbes estimated fat-free mass (FFM) from ^{40}K assessment in 609 normal boys and girls 7.5 to 20.5 years of age and found no sex differences prior to puberty in FFM expressed per unit height (2). At 12 to 13 years of age, the FFM-to-height ratio began to plateau in girls but continued to increase in boys until the age of 20 years. The FFM tended to peak in males at 18 to 20 years of age and was approximately 1.4 times greater than the peak value attained by females at 15 to 16 years of age.

Body density data from hydrostatic weighings are somewhat inconsistent with the preceding data, as girls typically demonstrate lower body density values at all ages, including the preadolescent period. Lohman, however, has shown that lower body density values in girls do not indicate a higher relative body fat content (3).

At puberty, rather major differences in size and body composition begin to develop between the sexes, due largely to the associated endocrine changes. Testosterone secretion by the testes, which stops at birth, is reinstituted in the male at puberty, producing increased deposition of protein in muscle, bone, skin, and other parts of the body. The ultimate result is that the male adolescent is larger and more muscular than the female adolescent, characteristics that carry over into adulthood. Before puberty, the anterior pituitary gland is unable to secrete any gonadotrophic hormones. Thus, in girls, at the time when a sufficient quantity of follicle-stimulating hormone begins to be secreted, the ovaries develop, and estrogen secretion

begins. Estrogen has a significant influence on body growth, broadening the pelvis, increasing the size of the breasts, and proliferating the deposition of fat, particularly in the thighs and hips. Additionally, estrogen increases the growth rate of bone, allowing the ultimate bone length to be reached within 2 or 4 years after the onset of puberty. As a result, the female adolescent grows rapidly for the first few years after puberty and then ceases to grow. Boys have a much longer growth phase, allowing a greater height to be attained.

As a result of these endocrine changes at puberty, the average man at full maturity is nearly 13 cm (5 in.) taller, 14 to 18 kg (30–40 lb) heavier in total weight, 18 to 22 kg (40–50 lb) heavier in FFM, 3 to 6 kg (7–13 lb) lighter in fat weight, and 8 to 10 percentage units less in relative body fat, e.g., 15 versus 23 to 25% fat.

There are rather substantial gender differences in anthropometric measurements at maturity (4–7). Men have broader shoulders, narrower hips, and a greater chest girth relative to total body size. Men also tend to carry body fat in the abdominal and upper regions of the body, whereas women pattern their fat in the hips, buttocks, and thighs.

With aging, both men and women tend to accumulate fat and decrease FFM. In one of the few longitudinal studies conducted, Forbes found an average decrease in FFM of approximately 3 kg (6.6 lb) per decade or 0.3 kg (~0.7 lb) per year (8). These data confirm previous cross-sectional data indicating a loss in FFM of about 0.2 kg per year (0.44 lb per year). This decline is associated with lower levels of physical activity and testosterone. Apparently, the concomitant increase in total body fat with aging is also associated with the general decline in physical activity, without an equivalent decrease in caloric intake. Table 4–1 outlines the changes in relative body fat with aging for both sexes.

These normative data on relative body fat can be misleading. As an example, the average difference in relative body fat between young men and women, 20 to 29 years of age, is 7 to 10 percentage units, i.e., 15 to 20% for men versus 22 to 25% for women. This difference was thought to result from sex-specific differences in fat depots, e.g., breast tissue and hips. Subsequent research with female athletes, however, particularly women distance runners, indicated that these women were

TABLE 4-1   RELATIVE BODY FAT VALUES FOR MEN AND WOMEN OF VARIOUS AGES AND IN VARIOUS SPORTS

	% Fat	
Group or Sport	Men	Women
Baseball/softball	8–14	12–18
Basketball	6–12	10–16
Bodybuilding	5–8	6–12
Canoeing/kayaking	6–12	10–16
Cycling	5–11	8–15
Fencing	8–12	10–16
Football	6–18	—
Golf	10–16	12–20
Gymnastics	5–12	8–16
Horse racing (jockey)	6–12	10–16
Ice/field hockey	8–16	12–18
Orienteering	5–12	8–16
Pentathlon	—	8–15
Racquetball	6–14	10–18
Rowing	6–14	8–16
Rugby	6–16	—
Skating	5–12	8–16
Skiing (alpine and Nordic)	7–15	10–18
Ski jumping	7–15	10–18
Soccer	6–14	10–18
Swimming	6–12	10–18
Synchronized swimming	—	10–18
Tennis	6–14	10–20
Track and field, field events	8–18	12–20
Track and field, running events	5–12	8–15
Triathlon	5–12	8–15
Volleyball	7–15	10–18
Weightlifting	5–12	10–18
Wrestling	5–16	—
Age Group (Years)		
15–19	13–16	20–24
20–29	15–20	22–25
30–39	18–26	24–30
40–49	23–29	27–33
50–59	26–33	30–36
60–69	29–33	30–36

Adapted from Wilmore JH, Costill DL. Physiology of Sport and Exercise. 3rd ed. Champaign, IL: Human Kinetics, 2004:463, 572.

exceptionally lean, well below the average woman, and even below the average for young men (9). Many of the better runners were below 10% body fat (10). These low values can result from either a genetic predisposition toward leanness or the high training mileage run by these women each week, which in some cases exceeded 100 miles per week. In any event, obviously, women can reduce their fat stores to levels well below those considered normal for women of this age.

Differences between the sexes have also been noted for body fluids. In the newborn, total body water (TBW) is approximately 77% of total body weight, with the extracellular water (ECW) and intracellular water (ICW) contributing 44 and 33%, respectively. By 1 year of age, the infant has achieved the adult fraction of TBW (~61%), composed of approximately 25% ECW and 36% ICW. Sex differences are evident by the age of 18 years, with the TBW of girls dropping to approximately 47 to 54% of total body weight. This difference comes almost totally from the ICW, which is only 23 to 29%. It is quite possible that the lower percentages for TBW and ICW in women are due to the increased levels of body fat, because adipose tissue contains only a small fraction of water and because both TBW and ICW are expressed relative to total body weight. Fluid levels are also altered considerably consequent to menstruation. Weight gains of 2 to 3 kg caused by fluid retention are common.

Physiologic Responses to Acute Exercise

When men and women are exposed to a short-term bout of exercise, whether it be an all-out run to exhaustion on the treadmill or a one-time attempt to lift the heaviest weight possible, there are characteristic responses that differentiate the sexes.

NEUROMUSCULAR RESPONSES—STRENGTH

Women have typically been regarded as the weaker sex. In previous studies, women have been found to be 43 to 63% weaker than men in upper body strength, but only 25 to 30% weaker in lower body strength. Because there is a considerable size difference between the sexes, as noted above, several studies have expressed strength relative to body weight (absolute strength/body weight) or relative to FFM as a reflection of the muscle mass (absolute strength/FFM). When lower body strength is expressed relative to body weight, there is still a

5 to 15% difference between the sexes. When expressed relative to FFM, however, the difference between the sexes disappears, which indicates that the histologic and biochemical qualities of muscle and its motor control properties are similar for the two sexes (11). In fact, studies using computed tomography (CT) scans to identify the cross-sectional area of the primary muscles involved in a specific movement have clearly demonstrated a very high correlation between muscle strength and muscle cross-sectional area, totally independent of sex (12).

Although the differences in upper body strength are reduced somewhat when expressed relative to body weight and FFM, substantial differences remain (11). There are at least two possible explanations for the different findings in upper and lower body strength. First, a woman has a higher percentage of her muscle mass in the lower body. Second, and probably related, she uses the muscle mass in her lower body to a greater extent than she uses her upper body muscle mass, particularly when compared to patterns of use in men. Some women of normal body size have phenomenal strength, exceeding even that of the average man. This fact points to the importance of neuromuscular recruitment and synchronization of motor unit firing in determining ultimate levels of strength.

Recently, there has been a great deal of interest in muscle-fiber typing. In the 1960s, researchers started using the muscle biopsy technique to investigate several aspects of muscle physiology. Through various staining techniques, it was possible to identify the different muscle fiber types, which led to an interest in how athletes might differ in various sports. Over the years, biopsies have become more common among female athletes. This has led to a natural interest in the differences and similarities between male and female athletes participating in the same sport or event. The classification system most commonly used identifies three basic fiber types: slow-twitch oxidative (type I), fast-twitch oxidative (type II_a), and fast-twitch glycolytic (type II_b). Other fiber types or classifications have also been identified but are not considered in this discussion. Athletes who participate in events or activities requiring a high degree of aerobic activity (e.g., distance runners and cross-country skiers) have a high proportion of type I fibers (typically 60% or higher). Athletes who participate in speed or anaerobic-type activities (e.g., sprinters) have a predominance of type II fibers (again, usually 60% or higher). Interestingly, weight event athletes have a nearly equal distribution of type I and type II fibers, even though these sports are generally considered to be short-burst, power activities. Male and female athletes in the same sport or event have similar distributions of fiber types, although the men appear to reach greater extremes (i.e., >90% type I or >90% type II) as well as have larger fiber areas (13).

CARDIOVASCULAR RESPONSES

When placed on a cycle ergometer whose power output can be precisely controlled independent of body weight, men generally have a lower heart rate (HR) response at each absolute submaximal power output. Maximal heart rate (HR_{max}), however, does not differ between sexes of the same age. Because cardiac output ($\dot{Q}$) is nearly identical for the same absolute submaximal power output, the lower HR response in men is associated with a higher stroke volume (SV). The enhanced SV is primarily the result of at least three factors. First, men have a larger heart and therefore a larger left ventricle, both advantages of a larger body size. Second, and also related to body size, men have a greater blood volume. Finally, on average, men are typically less sedentary and therefore exhibit the classic alterations (discussed in the next section) that are associated with physical training. When the power output is controlled to provide the same relative intensity of exercise, which is usually expressed as a fixed percentage of the maximal oxygen uptake ($\dot{V}O_{2max}$), e.g., 60% $\dot{V}O_{2max}$, $\dot{Q}$, SV, and $\dot{V}O_{2submax}$ are generally lower and HR is slightly higher in women (14). At maximal rates of work, women have lower values for SV_{max} and $\dot{Q}_{max}$, largely due to their smaller body size, heart, and blood volume.

There are also differences in the arterial-mixed venous oxygen difference ($AVD-O_2$), with women having lower values at both the same submaximal power outputs and at maximal rates of work. These differences are largely the result of a lower hemoglobin content in women, resulting in a lower arterial oxygen content.

RESPIRATORY RESPONSES

The differences between men and women in the respiratory responses to exercise largely result from differences in body size. There appears to be little difference in breathing frequency when working at the same relative power output, although women tend to breathe at a higher frequency for the same absolute power output. This latter response is probably due to the fact that women would be working at a higher percentage of their $\dot{V}O_{2max}$ at the same absolute power output. Tidal volume and ventilation volume are generally smaller in the female at both the same relative and absolute power outputs, up to and including maximal rates of work. Highly trained male athletes have maximal ventilation volumes of 150 L·min^{-1}, with some exceeding 250 L· min^{-1}; most female athletes have maximal values below 125 L·min^{-1}. Again, these differences in volume are closely associated with differences in body size.

METABOLIC RESPONSES

The $\dot{V}O_{2max}$ is regarded by exercise scientists as the single best index of an individual's cardiorespiratory endurance capacity. For this reason, numerous studies have been conducted to compare $\dot{V}O_{2max}$ values of men and women, both untrained and trained. Åstrand conducted the first study and compared a large population of males and females, from 4 years of age up to adulthood (15). Subsequently, additional data have been published confirming the original work of Åstrand and adding considerably to the data pool.

Before puberty, there are no significant differences in $\dot{V}O_{2max}$ values for boys and girls when $\dot{V}O_{2max}$ is expressed relative to body weight, i.e., mL·kg^{-1}·min^{-1}. Girls tend to reach their peak $\dot{V}O_{2max}$ between the ages of 13 and 15 years, whereas boys do not reach their peak until 18 to 22 years of age. Beyond puberty, the $\dot{V}O_{2max}$ of untrained women is only 70 to 75% of that found in untrained men (16).

Differences in $\dot{V}O_{2max}$ between men and women must be interpreted carefully. In 1965, Hermansen and Andersen published data indicating that there is considerable variability within each sex and that there is considerable overlapping of values between sexes (17). Taking a group of men and women, 20 to 30 years of age, they compared the physiologic responses to submaximal and maximal exercise of four subgroups: male athletes, male nonathletes,

female athletes, and female nonathletes. First, for the same absolute level of work, they found that there was a tendency for athletes to have slightly higher $\dot{V}O_{2max}$ values at submaximal levels and for men to have slightly higher values than women. With respect to $\dot{V}O_{2max}$ expressed relative to body weight, average values for the male athletes were 61% higher than those of male nonathletes, whereas those of the female athletes were 45% higher than those of female nonathletes. Values of male athletes were 29% higher than those of the female athletes, but the mean $\dot{V}O_{2max}$ of female athletes was 25% higher than the mean value for the male nonathletes. From this study, Drinkwater calculated that 76% of the female nonathletes overlapped 47% of the male nonathletes, and that 22% of the female athletes overlapped 7% of the male athletes (18). These data demonstrate the importance of considering both the level of physical conditioning of the population studied and of looking beyond mean values to the extent of overlap between samples that are being compared.

Because $\dot{V}O_2$ is the product of $\dot{Q}$ and AVD-O$_2$, $\dot{V}O_{2max}$ represents that point during exhaustive exercise at which the subject has maximized oxygen delivery and use capabilities. Typical values range from less than 20 mL·kg^{-1}·min^{-1} in highly deconditioned, aging individuals to values in excess of 85 mL·kg^{-1}·min^{-1} in superbly conditioned endurance athletes. The highest recorded value (94 mL·kg^{-1}·min^{-1}) for a man was found in a champion Norwegian cross-country skier; the highest recorded value for a woman was 77 mL·kg^{-1}·min^{-1} for a Russian cross-country skier.

Although $\dot{V}O_{2max}$ values of boys and girls are similar until puberty, there is a question as to the validity of comparing male and female subjects beyond the age of 12 years. The data might reflect an unfair comparison of relatively sedentary females with relatively more active male subjects. Thus, the differences would reflect the level of conditioning, as well as possible sex differences. To overcome this potential problem, investigators began to look at highly trained male and female athletes, with the assumption that the level of training would be similar for the sexes. Saltin and Åstrand compared $\dot{V}O_{2max}$ values of male and female athletes who participated on Swedish national teams (19). In comparable events, the men had 15 to 30% higher values. Wilmore and Brown,

TABLE 4-2 $\dot{V}O_{2max}$ VALUES FOR MALE AND FEMALE POPULATIONS OF DIFFERENT AGES AND IN VARIOUS SPORTS

Group or Sport	Age	Males	Females
Nonathletes	10–19	47–56	38–46
	20–29	43–52	33–42
	30–39	39–48	30–38
	40–49	36–44	26–35
	50–59	34–41	24–33
	60–69	31–38	22–30
	70–79	28–35	20–27
Baseball/softball	18–32	48–56	52–57
Basketball	18–30	40–60	43–60
Bicycling	18–26	62–74	47–57
Canoeing	22–28	55–67	48–52
Football	20–36	42–60	—
Gymnastics	18–22	52–58	36–50
Ice hockey	10–30	50–63	—
Jockey	20–40	50–60	—
Orienteering	20–60	47–53	46–60
Racquetball	20–35	55–62	50–60
Rowing	20–35	60–72	58–65
Skiing, alpine	18–30	57–68	50–55
Skiing, nordic	20–28	65–94	60–75
Ski jumping	18–24	58–63	—
Soccer	22–28	54–64	50–60
Speed skating	18–24	56–73	44–55
Swimming	10–25	50–70	40–60
Track and field, discus	22–30	42–55	—
Track and field, running	18–39	60–85	50–75
	40–75	40–60	35–60
Track and field, shot put	22–30	40–46	—
Volleyball	18–22	—	40–56
Weightlifting	20–30	38–52	—
Wrestling	20–30	52–65	—

Adapted from Wilmore JH, Costill DL. Physiology of Sport and Exercise. 3rd ed. Champaign, IL: Human Kinetics, 2004:295.

in their study of 11 women long-distance runners of national and international caliber, reported $\dot{V}O_{2max}$ values (mean, 59.1 mL·kg^{-1}·min^{-1}) that were considerably higher than those of the average woman or man of similar age (9). Still, compared with equally trained men distance runners, the women had values 15.9% lower when expressed relative to body weight and 8.6% lower when expressed relative to FFM. The three best runners from this study had an average $\dot{V}O_{2max}$ value of 67.4 mL·kg^{-1}·min^{-1}, which is similar to the average value of 70.3 mL·kg^{-1}·min^{-1} reported for nationally ranked marathon runners of similar age.

Table 4-2 details $\dot{V}O_{2max}$ values for male and female athletes of different ages and in different sports.

A number of investigators have attempted to scale $\dot{V}O_{2max}$ values relative to height, weight, FFM (as described in the previous paragraph), leg muscle mass, or leg limb volume in an attempt to compare men and women more objectively. Several studies have yielded results demonstrating that differences between the sexes disappear when $\dot{V}O_{2max}$ is expressed relative to FFM or active muscle mass, but there are also studies that continue to demonstrate differences, even when accounting for differences in total body fat mass. A study by Cureton and Sparling used a novel approach to investigate this problem (20). They studied the submaximal and maximal responses to treadmill runs under various conditions in 10 men and 10 women who regularly engaged in distance running. The men were studied both at normal weight and under an artificial condition in which they had to run with external weight added to the trunk so that the total percentage of excess plus fat weight was equal to the percentage fat of matched women. The women exercised only under normal weight conditions. Equating the men and women for excess weight resulted in a reduction of 32% in the original mean sex differences in treadmill run time, of 38% in the oxygen required per unit fat-free weight to run at various submaximal speeds, and of 65% in $\dot{V}O_{2max}$. They concluded that the greater sex-specific, essential body fat stores of women is a major determinant of the sex differences in the metabolic responses to running (20). Finally, Davies found that when the $\dot{V}O_{2max}$ values of 116 boys and girls were expressed relative to body weight or to FFM, definite sex differences were observed (21). When expressed relative to the volume of the leg, however, these differences disappeared. Davies concluded that $\dot{V}O_{2max}$ is directly related to the volume or mass of active tissue involved in the exercise.

With respect to submaximal $\dot{V}O_2$ values, there appears to be little, if any, difference between men and women for the same absolute power output. Bunc and Heller found no significant differences in the net energy cost of treadmill running of similarly trained men and women athletes representing various sports (22). However, at the same absolute submaximal work rate, women usually are performing at a higher percentage of their $\dot{V}O_{2max}$.

Peak blood lactate values are generally higher in men than in women, both for active, but untrained, and for highly trained, men and women. There is no obvious reason to expect differences between the sexes in peak blood lactate values, so these results remain unexplained. With respect to lactate threshold, values are generally similar between equally trained men and women, providing the values are expressed in relative (%$\dot{V}O_{2max}$) and not absolute terms.

Physiologic Adaptations to Long-Term Exercise

Substantial alterations in basic physiologic function occur as a result of physical training, both at rest and during exercise. This section discusses how women adapt to long-term exercise, emphasizing the areas in which their responses differ from those of men.

BODY COMPOSITION, BONE, AND CONNECTIVE TISSUE

With exercise training, emphasizing either cardiorespiratory endurance activities or strength training, both women and men experience losses in total body weight, fat weight, and relative fat, in addition to small-to-moderate gains in FFM (23). The gains in FFM and losses in fat mass are generally lower in women, however the magnitude of change in body composition, with the exception of FFM, appears to be more related to the total energy expenditure associated with training activities than to sex (24). Increases in FFM are much larger in response to strength training than to endurance training, but again, the changes in women are generally small compared with those in men.

Alterations in bone and connective tissue with training are not as well understood. In general, results of studies with animals and limited studies with humans support an increase in the density of the weight-bearing long bones; this adaptation appears to be independent of sex, at least in young and middle-aged populations. There are exceptions to this conclusion, which are discussed in detail in the last section of this chapter. Connective tissue appears to be strengthened with endurance training, but sex-specific differences in response have not been identified. There has been some concern that women are more susceptible to injury while participating in physical activity and sport. This susceptibility has been largely attributed to sex-specific differences in joint integrity as well as to the strength of ligaments, tendons, and bones. Unfortunately, few published reports serve to confirm or deny the validity of such concerns. When differences in the rate of injury have been observed, it is highly possible that the injury was related more to the level of conditioning than to the sex of the participant. Objective data are difficult to obtain, but this area is nevertheless an important one that needs further study.

NEUROMUSCULAR ADAPTATIONS

For a number of years, it was not considered appropriate to prescribe strength training programs for women athletes. During the 1960s and 1970s, it became evident that many of the better female athletes in the United States were not doing well in international competition and that this was mainly due to the fact that they were weaker than their competitors. Slowly, research demonstrated that women could gain considerable benefit from strength training programs, and that strength gains were usually not accompanied by large increases in muscle bulk. One of the first studies compared the strength training response of 47 women and 26 men, previously untrained, who volunteered to participate in identical progressive-resistance, weight-training programs (11). The program was conducted two times per week, 40 min per day, for a total of 10 weeks. Bench press and leg press strength increased by 28.6 and 29.5%, respectively, in the women and 16.5 and 26.0%, respectively, in the men. There were only small increases in muscle girth in the women, whereas the men exhibited classic muscle hypertrophy. Thus, it is apparent that hypertrophy is neither a necessary consequence nor a prerequisite of gains in muscular strength. Many subsequent studies have confirmed these results.

From the aforementioned results, it appears that women have the potential to develop substantial levels of strength. Will women ever be able to attain the same levels of strength as men for all major regions of the body? From the similarity of leg strength to weight or muscle cross-sectional area ratios between the two sexes, it appears that the quality of muscle is the same, irrespective of sex. Because of the higher levels of testosterone in men, however, men will continue to have a larger total muscle mass. If muscle mass is the major determinant of strength, then men have a distinct advantage. If neural factors are as important, or even more important, than size, then the potential for absolute strength gains in women is considerable. Because the basic mechanisms that allow the expression of greater levels

of strength have yet to be clearly established, it is premature to draw conclusions.

CARDIOVASCULAR AND RESPIRATORY ADAPTATIONS

Major cardiovascular and respiratory adaptations result from cardiorespiratory endurance, or aerobic, training, and most do not appear to be sex specific. In a major review article, Saltin and Rowell describe the classic cardiovascular, respiratory, and metabolic adaptations to physical activity and inactivity (25). With aerobic training, there are major increases in $\dot{Q}_{max}$. Because HR_{max} generally does not change with training, this increase in $\dot{Q}_{max}$ results from a large increase in SV, which is the result of both a greater end-diastolic volume and a reduced end-systolic volume. The former is related to an increased blood volume and a more efficient venous return, and the latter is the result of a stronger myocardium (i.e., a stronger contraction) and a reduction in peripheral resistance. At submaximal power outputs, there is usually no change in $\dot{Q}$, although SV is considerably higher for the same absolute level of work. Consequently, HR for any given level of work is reduced. When $\dot{Q}$ does change with training, it is generally a reduction due to a reduction in $\dot{V}O_{2\,submax}$. The decrease in $\dot{V}O_{2\,submax}$ is the result of an increase in metabolic or mechanical efficiency. With the oxygen requirement reduced, there is a consequent reduction in the need for $\dot{Q}$ (14). Resting HR is generally reduced with aerobic training and can reach values of 50 beats·min^{-1} or less. Several women distance runners have had resting HRs below 36 beats·min^{-1} (9). These extremely low resting HRs are considered a classic training response and correspond to exceptionally high SVs.

The increases in $\dot{V}O_{2max}$ that accompany cardiorespiratory endurance training are discussed in the next section, but they are primarily the result of the large increases in $\dot{Q}_{max}$, with only small increases in AVD-O_2. Saltin and Rowell state that the major limitation to $\dot{V}O_{2max}$ resides in the transport of oxygen to the working muscles (25). Whereas $\dot{Q}$ is important in this respect, it is the position of these researchers that the increases in maximal aerobic power that accompany training can be attributed primarily to increased maximal muscle blood flow and muscle capillary density. There is no reason to suspect that women would differ in this response to training. In fact, Ingjer and Brodal demonstrated that endurance-trained women have considerably higher capillary-to-fiber ratios than do untrained women, i.e., 1.69 and 1.11, respectively (26).

With respect to respiration, women experience considerable increases in maximal ventilation, which reflect increases in both tidal volume and breathing frequency. These changes are generally assumed to be unrelated to the increase in $\dot{V}O_{2max}$.

METABOLIC ADAPTATIONS

With cardiorespiratory endurance training, women experience the same relative increase in $\dot{V}O_{2max}$ that has been observed in men. Several studies have reported that the magnitude of increase is highly related to the initial level of fitness, i.e., those with low fitness levels prior to the start of training will generally experience a greater percentage increase. However, several recent studies have not been able

to confirm this in that they have found no relationship between the initial fitness level and the magnitude of increase in $\dot{V}O_{2max}$. Each person, theoretically, has a genetically established upper limit of $\dot{V}O_{2max}$ that they cannot exceed, irrespective of the duration or intensity of training. Consequently, the closer one is to this upper limit, the more difficult it is to obtain large improvements with subsequent training. Thus, it would be expected that most women would experience rather substantial improvements in $\dot{V}O_{2max}$ with endurance training, because they have relatively low initial values, and most have been relatively inactive. On the basis of findings in the research literature, women can improve their $\dot{V}O_{2max}$ by up to 50% with aerobic training, the magnitude of change being dependent on the intensity and duration of the individual exercise sessions, the frequency of sessions per week, and the length of the study. Figure 4-1 illustrates the wide variation in response to exercise training (i.e., percentage increase in $\dot{V}O_{2max}$) in men and women ages 17 to 71 years of age (27,28). Further, it

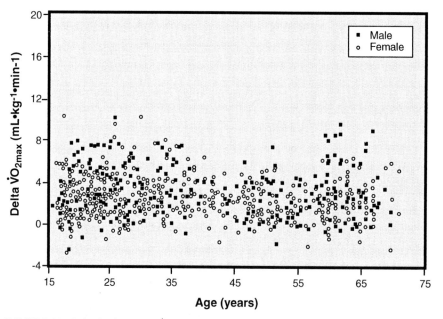

FIGURE 4-1 Variation in changes in $\dot{V}O_{2max}$ (percentage change) with endurance exercise training in men and women ages 17 to 71 years. (Adapted from Skinner JS, Jaskólski A, Jaskólska A, et al. Age, sex, race, initial fitness and response to training: The HERITAGE Family Study. J Appl Physiol 2001;90:1770–1776 and Kohrt WM, Malley MT, Coggan AR, et al. Effects of gender, age and fitness level on response of VO2max to training in 60–71 yr olds. J Appl Physiol 1991;71: 2004–2011.)

illustrates that irrespective of age, women have the same range of improvement as men.

Oxygen uptake at the same absolute submaximal power output either does not change or is reduced slightly as mentioned in the section above. Blood lactate levels are reduced for the same absolute submaximal power output, and peak lactate levels are generally increased. Thus, the anaerobic or lactate threshold increases with training, and this increase seems to be independent of sex (29). Finally, endurance training also improves the ability to use free fatty acids, an adaptation that is important for glycogen sparing.

Therefore, it appears that women respond to physical training in exactly the same manner as men. Whereas the adaptations to training may differ somewhat in magnitude (e.g., FFM), the trends do appear to be identical. This consideration is extremely important when prescribing exercise for women.

Special Considerations

Although men and women respond to short-term exercise and adapt to long-term exercise in much the same manner, there are several areas that must be considered when prescribing exercise for women. Although there is a possibility of some overlap with other chapters in this book, replication is minimized.

AGING

Once full maturity is reached, there is generally a gradual decline in $\dot{V}O_{2max}$. This fact was first noted in men by Robinson in 1938 (30). I. Åstrand conducted a similar study on women in 1960 and noted the same decline (31). The decrease with age is linear, and although the slopes detailing this decline are nearly identical for men and women, the intercept for the women's curve is approximately 9 mL·kg^{-1}·min^{-1} lower than that for men (32). In addition, men and women tend to both increase the amount of total body fat and decrease FFM as they age. Thus, women are fatter and have less FFM at any given age. These differences in endurance capacity and body composition definitely influence both exercise testing and exercise prescription.

Are the changes in endurance capacity and body composition a necessary consequence of aging or are other factors involved? With respect to body composition, there is accumulating evidence that the increases in body fat and decreases in FFM primarily result from physical inactivity, and overeating to a lesser extent. Likewise, the $\dot{V}O_{2max}$ values of trained individuals is considerably higher than values for untrained individuals of similar age at all ages. Maintaining an active lifestyle will not, however, prevent the decrease in $\dot{V}O_{2max}$ with age, for the slope of the regression line is similar for trained and untrained individuals. Vaccaro et al. compared trained women swimmers and untrained women from ages 20 to 69 years and found that although the trained swimmers had significantly higher $\dot{V}O_{2max}$ values, they demonstrated a 7% decrease per decade in $\dot{V}O_{2max}$ (33). The untrained group demonstrated a similar 8% decrease per decade. Therefore, maintaining an active lifestyle will promote a healthier and more attractive physique and body composition and may also allow the individual to have the endurance capacity equal to that of a sedentary person of the same sex who is 30 to 40 years younger.

OSTEOPOROSIS

There is evidence that maintaining a healthy lifestyle may also retard one of the detrimental aging processes that is a major health concern of women— osteoporosis. Osteoporosis is characterized as an increase in bone porosity, a decrease in bone mineral content, and an increase in the risk of fractures that typically begins in the late thirties and is accelerated two to five times that rate at the onset of menopause. Although there is still a good deal to discover concerning the etiology of osteoporosis, there are three major contributing factors in postmenopausal women: an overall reduction in calcium intake, an estrogen deficiency, and a reduction in physical activity.

In addition to postmenopausal women, women with amenorrhea and those with anorexia also suffer from osteoporosis, the results of either decreased calcium intake or reduced serum estrogen levels, or possibly both. Rigotti et al. assessed the skeletal mass of 18 women who were known anorexics and 28 normal controls by direct photon absorptiometry and found that the patients with anorexia had significantly lower bone densities than the control subjects (34). Drinkwater et al. compared radial and vertebral bone densities of 14 amenorrheic women endurance athletes with those of 14 eumenorrheic women endurance athletes and discovered that amenorrheic group had substantially lower bone density values (35). When bone density values of the amenorrheic endurance athletes were compared with the age-related regression equation of Riggs et al. (36), the amenorrheic endurance athletes' values (mean age 24.9 years) were equivalent to values of normal, untrained women of 51.2 years of age. Eumenorrheic endurance athletes tend to exhibit higher bone mineral content values than eumenorrheic sedentary women. Drinkwater et al. found a reversal of this bone mineral loss in amenorrheic endurance athletes who resumed normal menses, but subsequently reported that bone mineral density may not be fully recovered, that is, the ability to regain bone mineral may be limited (37).

To date, there are insufficient data to draw any firm conclusions concerning the effects of exercise and amenorrhea on osteoporosis. It does seem logical, however, that regular physical activity, normal estrogen levels, and adequate calcium intake combined with an adequate caloric intake is a sensible approach to maintaining the integrity of the skeletal system at any age.

MENSTRUATION

Two questions foremost in the minds of many women, particularly women athletes, relate to the influence of their menstrual cycle on athletic performance and the influence of their physical activity and competition on menstruation, pregnancy, and childbirth. The question of pregnancy and childbirth is addressed in Chapter 25. With respect to alterations in athletic performance during different phases of the menstrual cycle, there appears to be considerable individual variability. Some women have absolutely no noticeable change in their ability to perform at any one time in their monthly cycle, whereas other women have considerable difficulty in the preflow and initial flow phases. The limited research that has been conducted tends to suggest that performance ability is best in the immediate postflow period up to the fifteenth day of the cycle, with the first day of the cycle corresponding to the initiation of the flow or menstrual phase, and ovulation occurring on about day 14. The number of women who report impaired performance during the flow phase is approximately the same as those who experienced no difficulty. In fact, some women athletes have reportedly set world records during the flow phase.

With respect to the question concerning the influence of various training programs and intense competition on the menstrual cycle, athletes who have trained and competed intensely in such sports as figure skating, ballet dancing, gymnastics, diving, cycling, and distance running have reported the absence of menses for months or even years. The prevalence of secondary amenorrhea, as well as oligomenorrhea (abnormally infrequent or scanty menses), among women athletes is not well documented, but its occurrence is estimated to be as high as 5 to 40% or higher in certain sports or events, which is considerably higher than the estimated prevalence of 2 to 3% for secondary amenorrhea and 10 to 12% for oligomenorrhea in the general population. The prevalence appears to be higher in women who train for many hours each day and in those who work at high intensities.

Identifying the cause of secondary amenorrhea and oligomenorrhea has proven difficult. Over the years, the following have been proposed as potential causal mechanisms:

- Acute effects of stress
- High quantity and/or intensity of training
- Hormonal alterations
- Low total body weight or low body fat mass
- Inadequate nutrition (caloric deficit) and disordered eating

During the past 10 years, it has become increasingly clear that a chronic caloric deficit, in which caloric intake does not match caloric expenditure for an extended period of time, is likely the precipitating factor. A series of well-designed studies by Loucks has demonstrated that simply inducing a caloric or energy deficit is sufficient to induce significant hormonal alterations associated with amenorrhea (38). This response appears to be totally independent of the quality or quantity of training. Eating disorders, such as anorexia nervosa, are generally characterized by a chronic caloric deficit, and menstrual dysfunction typically occurs.

The long-term consequences of secondary amenorrhea or oligomenorrhea are not totally understood. Some women have become pregnant while amenorrheic, which indicates that fertility is possibly not influenced in the absence of menstruation. This latter point is an important one, for many women assume that they have a simple but effective form of birth control while amenorrheic. As discussed above, there can be significant loss of bone during periods of amenorrhea. In fact, a triad of disorders has been identified that are closely related. This has been termed the *female athlete triad* and consists of disordered eating, menstrual dysfunction, and bone mineral loss (39). It appears that when women are in a sustained period of energy deficit, there are subtle hormonal changes that eventually can lead to secondary amenorrhea, and sustained secondary amenorrhea can lead to bone mineral loss.

ENVIRONMENTAL FACTORS

Exercise in the heat, in the cold, or at altitude provides an additional stress or challenge to the body's adaptive abilities. Results of many early studies indicated that women are less tolerant to heat than men, particularly when physical work is involved. Much of this difference, however, is the result of lower levels of fitness in those women who were tested, because the men and women were tested at the same absolute level of work. When work load is adjusted relative to the individual's capacity ($\dot{V}O_{2max}$), women respond in an almost identical manner. Women generally have lower sweat rates for the same exercise and heat stress, although they do possess a larger number of active sweat glands. When exposed to repeated bouts of heat stress, the body undergoes considerable adaptation (acclimatization), which enables it to survive future heat stress more efficiently. Evidence suggests that men and women undergo similar reductions in the internal temperature thresholds for sweating and vasodilation, and the sensitivity of the sweating response per unit of internal temperature increases after both physical training and heat acclimation (40). Any differences noted between the sexes were attributed to the initial differences in physical conditioning and not to sex. With respect to cold exposure, women do have a slight advantage as a result of their higher levels of subcutaneous body fat. Their smaller muscle mass, however, is a disadvantage in exposure to extreme cold, because shivering is the major adaptation for generating body heat. The greater the active muscle mass, the greater the subsequent generation of heat. An excellent review on this subject was published in 1984 by Drinkwater (41).

Several investigators have reported differences between the sexes in response to hypoxia, both at rest and during submaximal exercise. Although there is a decrease in $\dot{V}O_{2max}$ during hypoxic work, with the decrement in direct proportion to the decrement in barometric pressure, the differences between men and women are small and do not seem to have an adverse effect on the ability of women to work at high altitude. Studies of maximal exercise at high altitude demonstrate no difference in response between men and women.

EXERCISE TESTING AND THE PRESCRIPTION OF EXERCISE

In reviewing the acute responses and chronic adaptations to exercise, it is apparent that few differences exist between men and women. Consequently, few adjustments need to be made when testing or prescribing exercise for women. The most important point to consider is discussed in the section on aging. When compared with men of the same age, the average woman is fatter, has less FFM, and has a lower endurance capacity. This difference is probably related more to physical inactivity than to sex, although sex differences must still be considered. When selecting a protocol for exercise testing, women may require a protocol that has a lower ramp, i.e., the step increments should progress more slowly. Also, when using the same test protocol, different regression equations should be applied when test duration is used to estimate $\dot{V}O_{2max}$. With respect to the interpretation of the exercise electrocardiogram, one must recognize that women exhibit a higher percentage of false-positive test results. In several studies, as many as one-half (50%) of a sample of asymptomatic women were found to have S-T segment changes indicating myocardial ischemia.

In the prescription of exercise, one must match the intensity of the exercise to the capacity of the individual. When exercise testing precedes the exercise prescription, it is relatively easy to prescribe intensity on the basis of a training HR range or perceived exertion range that has been determined from the results of the exercise test. When exercise testing is not conducted prior to prescribing exercise, it is best to be conservative in the prescription of exercise intensity. Because women are fatter and have less FFM to support their total body weight, in addition to their lower endurance capacity, they must have their exercise intensity adjusted accordingly. It might also be appropriate to reduce exercise duration and frequency during the first few months, because the exercise program will probably constitute a considerable physical stress, with a potentially greater risk of injury. Consideration should be given to walking or swimming programs, in which the potential for injury is minimized, and success is a more likely outcome. Another excellent activity that is popular with women of all ages is aerobic dance. Aerobic dance classes, however, must be graded according to endurance capacity, as well as dancing ability.

Do not misconstrue the aforementioned statements to imply that women should be pampered or coddled. Women who have the same body composition and endurance capacity as men of similar age should be given a similar exercise prescription. The preceding advice simply recognizes that most women are not similar to their male counterparts when they initiate their program, and these precautions are taken to provide the participant with the best conditions in which to be successful.

REFERENCES

1. McCammon RW. Human Growth and Development. Springfield, IL: Charles C Thomas, 1970.
2. Forbes GB. Relation of lean body mass to height in children and adolescents. Pediatr Res 1972;6: 32–37.
3. Lohman TG. Applicability of body composition techniques and constants for children and youths. Exerc Sport Sci Rev 1986;14:325–357.
4. Pollock ML, Hickman T, Kendrick Z, et al. Prediction of body density in young and middle-aged men. J Appl Physiol 1976;40:300–304.
5. Pollock ML, Laughridge EE, Coleman B, et al. Prediction of body density in young and middle-aged women. J Appl Physiol 1975;38:745–749.
6. Wilmore JH, Behnke AR. An anthropometric estimation of body density and lean body weight in young men. J Appl Physiol 1969;27:25–31.
7. Wilmore JH, Behnke AR. An anthropometric estimation of body density and lean body weight in young women. Am J Clin Nutr 1970;23:267–274.
8. Forbes GB. The adult decline in lean body mass. Hum Biol 1976;48:161–173.
9. Wilmore JH, Brown CH. Physiological profiles of women distance runners. Med. Sci. Sports 1974;6:178–181.
10. Wilmore JH, Brown CH, Davis JA. Body physique and composition of the female distance runner. NY Acad Sci 1977;301:764–776.
11. Wilmore JH. Alterations in strength, body composition, and anthropometric measurements consequent to a 10-week weight training program. Med Sci Sports 1974;6:133–138.
12. Schantz P, Randall-Fox E, Hutchison W, et al. Muscle fibre type distribution, muscle cross-sectional area and maximal voluntary strength in humans. Acta Physiol Scand 1983;117:219–226.
13. Wilmore JH. The application of science to sport: physiological profiles of male and female athletes. Can J Appl Sport Sci 1979;4:103–115.
14. Wilmore JH, Stanforth PR, Gagnon J, et al. Cardiac output and stroke volume changes with endurance training: The HERITAGE Family Study. Med Sci Sports Exerc 2001;33:99–106.
15. Åstrand P-O. Experimental Studies of Physical Working Capacity in Relation to Age and Sex. Copenhagen: Munksgaard, 1952.
16. Shvartz E, Reibold RC. Aerobic fitness norms for males and females aged 6 to 75 years: a review. Aviat Space Environ Med 1990;61:271–276.
17. Hermansen L, Andersen KL. Aerobic work capacity in young Norwegian men and women. J Appl Physiol 1965;20:425–431.
18. Drinkwater BL. Physiological responses of women to exercise. Exerc Sport Sci Rev 1973;1:125–153.
19. Saltin B, Åstrand P-O. Maximal oxygen uptake in athletes. J Appl Physiol 1967;23:353–358.
20. Cureton KJ, Sparling PB. Distance running performance and metabolic responses to running in men and women with excess weight experimentally equated. Med Sci Sports Exerc 1980;12:288–294.
21. Davies CTM. Body composition in children: a reference standard for maximum aerobic power output on a stationary ergometer. Acta Paediatr Scand 1971;217(suppl):136–137.
22. Bunc V, Heller J. Energy cost of running in similarly trained men and women. Eur J Appl Physiol, 1989;59:178–183.
23. Wilmore JH. Body composition in sport and exercise: directions for future research. Med Sci Sports Exerc 1983;15:21–31.
24. Wilmore JH, Després J-P, Stanforth PR, et al. Alterations in body weight and composition consequent to

20 wk of endurance training: the HERITAGE Family Study. Am J Clin Nutr 1999;70:346–352.

25. Saltin B, Rowell LB. Functional adaptations to physical activity and inactivity. Fed Proc 1980;39:1506–1513.

26. Ingjer F, Brodal P: Capillary supply of skeletal muscle fibers in untrained and endurance-trained women. Eur J Appl Physiol 1978;38:291–299.

27. Skinner JS, Jaskólski A, Jaskólska A, et al. Age, sex, race, initial fitness and response to training: The HERITAGE Family Study. J Appl Physiol 2001;90:1770–1776.

28. Kohrt WM, Malley MT, Coggan AR, et al. Effects of gender, age and fitness level on response of VO_{2max} to training in 60–71 yr olds. J Appl Physiol 1991;71:2004–2011.

29. Gaskill SE, Walker AJ, Serfass RA, et al. Changes in ventilatory threshold with exercise training in a sedentary population: The Heritage Family Study. Int J Sports Med 2001;22:586–592.

30. Robinson S. Experimental studies of physical fitness in relation to age. Arbeitsphysiol 1938;10:251–323.

31. Åstrand I. Aerobic work capacity in men and women with special reference to age. Acta Physiol Scand 1960;49(suppl):169.

32. Wilmore JH. Inferiority of female athletes: myth and reality. J Sports Med 1975;3:1–6.

33. Vaccaro P, Ostrove SM, Vandervelden L, et al. Body composition and physiological responses of masters female swimmers 20 to 70 years of age. Res Q Exerc Sport 1984;55:278–284.

34. Rigotti NA, Nussbaum SR, Herzog DB, et al. Osteoporosis in women with anorexia nervosa. N Engl J Med 1984;311:1601–1606.

35. Drinkwater BL, Nilson K, Chesnut CH, et al. Bone mineral content of amenorrheic and eumenorrheic athletes. N Engl J Med 1984;311:277–281.

36. Riggs BL, Wahner HW, Seeman E, et al. Changes in bone mineral density of the proximal femur and spine with aging: differences between the postmenopausal and senile osteoporosis syndromes. J Clin Invest 1982;70:716–723.

37. Drinkwater BL, Bruemner B, Chesnut CH. Menstrual history as a determinant of current bone density in young athletes. JAMA 1990;263:545–548.

38. Loucks AB, Verdun M, Heath EM. Low energy availability, not stress of exercise, alters LH-pulsatility in exercising women. J Appl Physiol 1998;84:37–46.

39. Otis CL, Drinkwater B, Johnson M, et al. The female athlete triad. Med Sci Sports Exerc, 1997;29(5):i–ix.

40. Nadel ER, Roberts MF, Wenger CB. Thermoregulatory adaptation to heat and exercise: comparative responses of men and women. In: Folinsbee LJ, et al., eds. Environmental Stress. New York: Academic Press, 1978.

41. Drinkwater BL. Women and exercise: physiological aspects. Exerc Sport Sci Rev 1984;12:21–51.

5

Differences Between Children and Adults for Exercise Testing and Exercise Prescription

Helge U. Hebestreit and Oded Bar-Or

Most knowledge of the physiologic responses of humans to exercise is based on studies with adults. Fewer data are available on the effects of short- or long-term exercise on children and adolescents. Although some of our considerations regarding exercise testing and prescription for children can be borrowed from those available for adults, specific characteristics of the child require a special approach. First, a child's metabolic, cardiopulmonary, neuromuscular, thermoregulatory, and perceptual responses to exercise differ somewhat from those of mature individuals. Secondly, methods and protocols used for testing adults are not always applicable to children, whether owing to differences in size, mental ability, attention span, and emotional maturity or to ethical constraints. Additional differences are clinical, i.e., the major pediatric diseases differ from those prevalent in young or middle-aged adults. The questions, guidelines, and precautions relevant for exercise testing or rehabilitation of an adult with coronary heart disease are not applicable to most pediatric patients. Inversely, the rationale for exercise provocation in such conditions as congenital heart defects, growth hormone deficiency, bronchial asthma, cystic fibrosis, or progressive muscular dystrophy is of little relevance to adults.

The purpose of this chapter is to highlight the main differences in exercise testing and prescription between children and adults. Readers interested in exercise testing or physical training of healthy children or those with a chronic health condition may find further information in recent textbooks on this topic (1–6).

Developmental Aspects of Exercise Physiology

BODY SIZE

One obvious difference between children and adults is body stature and body weight. Furthermore, children are growing individuals. Especially during the first year of life and the growth spurt at puberty, height may change by more than 10 cm per year. Differences and changes in body size may interfere with the interpretation of performance when comparing individuals of different ages and/or stature or when evaluating longitudinal data. Furthermore, growth poses an increased risk of injuries to bone at the growth plates. Body proportions are also subject to change during childhood and adolescence. Young children are characterized by a relatively larger head and trunk, while older individuals have relatively longer extremities. In consequence, biomechanical properties change, and the neuromotor control must adapt.

MUSCLE SIZE AND PROPERTIES

Absolute muscle mass increases considerably during growth. Relative to total body weight, muscle mass remains more or less constant at 40 to 46% between the ages of 5 years and 29 years in females (7). In males, relative muscle mass increases during childhood and adolescence from about 42 to 53% (7).

Although muscle biopsy data are scarce in children for ethical reasons, muscle fiber composition and muscle metabolic properties change during childhood and adolescence. Some studies found a larger proportion of slow oxidative type I fibers and fewer type II fibers in younger individuals (8,9).

Several studies suggest that the concentrations of creatine phosphate (CP), adenosine triphosphate (ATP), and glycogen in the resting muscle of children are the same as, or only slightly lower than, those of young adults (10,11). Although there is no age-related difference in the utilization rate of ATP or CP, the utilization rate of glycogen is greatly diminished in the child. This difference is reflected in the rate of lactate production, e.g., 13- to 15-year-old boys may reach only 65 to 70% of lactate concentration in muscle observed in adults during maximal exercise (12). Younger children reach even lower levels. Likewise, maximal exercise results in a smaller decrease in muscle pH and a smaller increase in the ratio of inorganic phosphate to CP in children (13). These differences may be explained by a lower activity of phosphofructokinase (a rate-limiting enzyme of glycolysis) in children (12,14). Scant data suggest that oxidative capacity in children's muscles is similar to that of sedentary adults (15).

In addition to metabolic differences in muscles, there is some evidence that functional properties of the muscle also change during childhood. Lin et al. measured half-relaxation time of the soleus muscle after a single Achilles tendon tap in 3- to 10-year-old children (16). Half-relaxation time was negatively correlated with age. At age 10, half-relaxation time was about 40 ms, which is close to the values found in adults (males, 35.6 ms; females, 41.1 ms).

NEUROMOTOR CONTROL

During childhood and adolescence, performance in tasks requiring fast movements that are not limited by muscle power (e.g., finger or ankle tapping) improves considerably with age (17). This is most likely due to an improvement in motor control during the first two decades of life. The reasons for this development are only partly understood. Branching of neurons with increasing density of interneuron contacts, which is stimulated by motor learning, probably plays a significant role. In healthy children, a mature movement pattern in such fundamental motor tasks as running, throwing, hopping, etc. is usually achieved by the age of 5 to 8 years (18). Other skills may mature somewhat later.

NEUROPSYCHOLOGIC DEVELOPMENT

There is fast development of attention, memory, language, and learning skills, as well as executive, sensorimotor and visuospatial functions, during childhood. The effects of age are more significant in the 5- to 8-year age range than in the 9- to 12- year age range (19). At least some neuropsychologic skills improve further during adolescence (20). Low attention span and language skills may interfere with exercise testing and prescription, especially in young children or those with developmental disorders.

RATING OF PERCEIVED EXERTION (RPE)

Like adults, children can discriminate among several exercise intensities and use the RPE scale (21). For cognitive and semantic reasons, the classical 6–20 or 0–10 Borg scales may not be appropriate for children younger than 8 to 9 years, and several illustrated scales have been proposed (22). The children's OMNI scale of perceived exertion (Fig. 5-1) has been validated for walking/running and cycling exercise (23,24).

An interesting feature of a child's RPE is that for a given heart (HR) or percentage HR_{max}, children

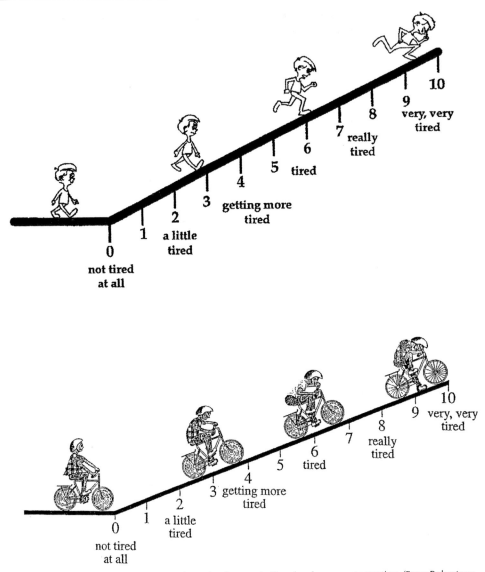

FIGURE 5-1 The OMNI scale of perceived exertion for treadmill and cycle ergometer testing. (From Robertson RJ, Goss FL, Boer NF, et al. Children's OMNI scale of perceived exertion: mixed gender and race validation. Med Sci Sports Exerc 2000;32:452–458 and Utter AC, Robertson RJ, Nieman DC, et al. Children's ONMI scale of perceived exertion: walking/running evaluation. Med Sci Sports Exerc 2002;34:139–144.)

rate the exertion level lower than adolescents, who rate it lower than adults (21). An exception in this study of some 1300 individuals ranging in age from 7 to 68 years were children in the 7- to 9-year-old group who rated RPE on the 6–20 Borg scale higher than did the 10- to 12-year-olds.

Children who are first subjected to an incremental cycling task to determine their individual power–RPE relationship and who are later asked to reproduce a power corresponding to a given RPE value may be less able to do so than adults (25,26). However, if adequate practice is offered, RPE may be used in children to prescribe exercise intensity. In a study of 20 healthy boys and girls aged 7 to 10 years to produce three different power levels using RPE, there was a large bias and intraindividual variation of power between the first two trials (27). In contrast, there was better agreement between the third and the fourth trial. Using the children's OMNI scale of perceived exertion, Robertson et al. showed that 8- to 12-year-old boys and girls may even be able to reproduce a prescribed cycling intensity without several practice trials (28).

THERMOREGULATION

The major task of the thermoregulatory system during exercise is to dissipate metabolic heat (MH) produced in proportion to exercise intensity and duration. The rate of MH production per kilogram of body mass during activities such as running and walking is greater in children. Thus, a greater thermal load is imposed upon their thermoregulatory apparatus. The major avenue for heat dissipation during exercise is sweat evaporation, especially on a hot day, when other avenues become less effective. Sweating rate of children is much lower than that in adults, even when corrected for body surface area (29). Even though children have a greater density of active sweat glands, each gland produces less sweat. Whether at rest or during exercise, the gland of an adult produces 2.5 times as much sweat (30). Furthermore, the threshold for perspiration (i.e., core temperature at which sweating starts) is higher in children (31).

Additional avenues for heat exchange with the environment are conduction, convection, and radiation, all of which depend on the surface area of the skin and on the temperature gradient between the skin and the environment. The surface area of a child relative to body mass is greater than that of an adult. Heat exchange to and from the environment is therefore greater in children. Although this is an advantage for the child in neutral or warm climates, it can become a major handicap when the body is exposed to a hot or cold environment. These geometric and functional differences make the child an inefficient thermoregulator during exercise.

Heat Tolerance
Children cannot sustain activity for as long as adults whenever the ambient temperature exceeds 40°C

(32–34). Their tolerance to swimming in cool water is also deficient (35).

Acclimatization to Exercise in the Heat
Children acclimatize to hot climates somewhat less efficiently than adults (29,34), primarily because of their slower rate of acclimatization (30). Thus, if children pursue intense athletic activities before reaching acclimatization, they are at a potential risk of a heat-related illness.

Hypohydration
Clinical reports indicate that hypohydrated children are at risk of heatstroke and other heat-related illnesses during heat waves. The core temperature of progressively dehydrating 10- to 12-year-old boys who exercise intermittently in a hot climate was found to rise in proportion to the level of fluid deficit (36). The rate of rise in core temperature was greater in these children than in young adults. One way to prevent hypohydration in a child who exercises for prolonged periods is to ensure fluid replenishment every 15 to 20 min. Otherwise, "involuntary dehydration" takes place. Another approach is to add flavor and NaCl to a drink. In one study, the addition of flavor to tap water increased voluntary drinking by 45%. Further addition of 18.8 mmol·L^{-1} NaCl and 6% carbohydrate increased voluntary drinking by an additional 45% (37).

Only scant information is available on the effect of hypohydration on the performance of the exercising child. In one study, mild dehydration (loss of as little as 1% of body weight) significantly decreased endurance time during cycling at 90% of peak oxygen intake (V̇O$_2$ peak) in 10- to 12-year-old boys (38).

Children at Special Risk of Heat-Related Illness
Some juvenile populations are at a special risk when exerting in a hot climate. These include healthy children who are hypohydrated or who are wearing protective clothing (e.g., American football) (39). Children with such diseases as anorexia nervosa (due to low insulative protection, inadequate peripheral circulation, and vomiting); cystic fibrosis (excessive salt loss, reduced thirst sensation leading to hypohydration); type I diabetes (hypohydration); febrile states; gastroenteritis (fast

TABLE 5-1   HEMODYNAMIC AND RESPIRATORY CHARACTERISTICS OF CHILDREN'S RESPONSES TO EXERCISE

Function	Typical for Children (compared with adults)
Hemodynamic	
HR at submaximal intensity	Higher, especially at first decade
HR max	Higher
$SV_{submax\ and\ max}$	Lower
Q at given $\dot{V}O_2$	Somewhat lower
AV-difference for O_2 at given $\dot{V}O_2$	Somewhat higher
Blood flow to active muscle	Higher
SBP, $DBP_{submax\ and\ max}$	Lower
Respiratory	
$\dot{V}_E$ at given $\dot{V}O_2$	Higher
$\dot{V}_E$ "breaking point"	Similar
Respiratory rate	Higher
Vt/VC	Lower

dehydration); hypocaloric malnutrition (low insulative protection); mental retardation (insufficient drinking); and obesity are also at risk of heat-related illness (for details, see Bar-Or [40]).

CARDIORESPIRATORY RESPONSES TO EXERCISE

Qualitatively, hemodynamic and respiratory adjustments to exercise are similar in children and adults. There are quantitative differences, however, as summarized in Table 5-1.

Hemodynamic Aspects

A distinct hemodynamic characteristic of the child is a low stroke volume (SV) at rest and during submaximal and maximal exercise (41). Although HR is higher, cardiac output ($\dot{Q}$, or HR × SV) is 1 to 3 $L\cdot min^{-1}$ lower than in adults at any given $\dot{V}O_2$. This "hypokinetic" response seems to be more pronounced in younger children (42). Based on the Fick principle, the calculated arteriovenous difference in O_2 content (AVD-O_2) is higher in children at submaximal, but apparently not at maximal, exercise (43,44). Blood flow (BF) to the exercising muscle is greater in children, and they have a greater

reserve for BF increase beyond the metabolic needs of maximal exercise, i.e., when ischemic changes are superimposed (45,46). Such better peripheral BF adjustment compensates for the lower $\dot{Q}$ and explains their higher AVD-O_2. Yet it is premature to infer that such a peripheral advantage is an end result of a "hypokinetic" central mechanism or vice versa. During exercise, arterial blood pressure (BP), especially the systolic BP (SBP), is lower in children (47–49). Such low BP values seem neither beneficial nor detrimental to the working capacity of the child.

Respiratory Aspects

The ventilatory apparatus of exercising children is less efficient, mainly because of a greater minute ventilation ($\dot{V}_E$) at any given level of $\dot{V}O_2$ (50,51) or $\dot{V}CO_2$ (52). This is more pronounced in younger children and represents lower use of O_2 from the inspired air. One reason for this inefficient respiration could be the shorter time period of each respiratory cycle, caused by a higher respiratory frequency. Indeed, a child's breathing pattern is relatively shallow, as reflected by a low ratio of tidal volume to vital capacity (V_t/VC) during maximal exercise (50). In spite of this breathing pattern, the dead space to tidal volume ratio is similar in exercising children and adults, and the child's alveolar ventilation is adequate (53). The major disadvantage of excessive $\dot{V}_E$ in children is the greater O_2 cost of respiration, which could contribute in part to their overall higher $\dot{V}O_2$ during exercise. When defined per percentage $\dot{V}O_2$ peak, the ventilatory threshold is somewhat higher in children than in adolescents and adults (54).

EXERCISE CAPACITY

In physical activities that require sustained or intense energy turnover, children can seldom compete at par with adolescents or young adults. Such is the case in tasks that comprise long or short distance running, jumping, cycling, rowing, or skiing. A basic question is whether this handicap of children is primarily due to a deficiency in their maximal aerobic power or their anaerobic capacity.

Maximal Aerobic Power

Taking $\dot{V}O_{2peak}$ as a criterion, one might conclude that maximal aerobic power is distinctly lower in children. An 8-year-old boy, for example, may have a $\dot{V}O_{2peak}$ of 1.3 to 1.5 L·min^{-1}, while that of an 18-year-old boy is 3.0 to 3.5 L·min.$^{-1}$. However, because many tasks require the translocation of the whole body, a child whose body weight is low may not need as high a $\dot{V}O_{2peak}$ as is needed by a heavier adolescent. It has been customary, therefore, to describe $\dot{V}O_2$ per kilogram of body weight, rather than in absolute values, whenever individuals who differ in body weight are to be compared. When expressed per kilogram of body weight, the $\dot{V}O_{2peak}$ of young boys is similar to that of male adolescents and young men. $\dot{V}O_{2peak}$ per kilogram is even higher in prepubescent girls than in older girls and women (55,56). However, the per kilogram standardization may not be correct either. When using a ratio of $\dot{V}O_{2peak}$ divided by body mass$^{0.67}$, there is a considerable increase in normalized $\dot{V}O_{2peak}$ during childhood and adolescence (57). If more complex allometric equations are used to correct $\dot{V}O_{2peak}$ for the influences of body size, adiposity, and gender, there is still an increase in $\dot{V}O_{2peak}$ with age (58).

Short-Term Exercise and Anaerobic Capacity

Unlike maximal aerobic power, anaerobic performance of children, even when expressed per kilogram of body weight, is distinctly lower than that of older age groups. When such short-term, all-out power output tasks as isokinetic dynamometry or the Wingate and the force–velocity cycling tests are undertaken, performance rises continuously with age (43,59–61). As found in the authors' laboratories, an 8-year-old boy produces only 45 to 50% of the mechanical power produced by a 14-year-old boy. When normalized for body weight, the figure is still 65 to 70%. With girls, the same trend exists, although the performance per kilogram of body weight does not increase beyond 11 to 12 years. Even when allometric scaling techniques are applied to longitudinal data, a dependency of short-term exercise performance on age is observed (62).

It is unclear why children have a lower short-term exercise capacity than adults. It has been suggested that the lower glycolytic capacity of children (as evidenced from lower peak lactate levels and higher pH at peak exercise in the muscle) may limit anaerobic energy turnover and thereby impair performance at very high exercise intensities. However, the lower maximal power output in children

during brief exercise tasks such as the vertical jump test or the Wingate anaerobic test may also be attributed to several other factors such as relatively fewer type II muscle fibers (8,9), poor motor coordination during fast movements (17), and a relatively long relaxation time of muscle fibers (16). In the latter cases, the low peak lactate levels and high pH in children reflect a lesser drive for glycolysis and not a basic problem in energy production. Since it does not make physiologic sense that only one body system is limiting performance in everyday tasks in which multiple systems are required in an integrated fashion, it is most likely that more than one of the above factors play a role.

Metabolic Cost of Locomotion/ Mechanical Efficiency

The metabolic cost of walking and running (and possibly other activities) at a given speed is distinctly higher in children than in older individuals (51,63). This difference cannot be explained by the higher resting metabolic rate in children but probably reflects a mechanically "wasteful" running or walking style in smaller children. Whatever its cause, the end result of greater O_2 cost of locomotion leaves the child with a lower energy "reserve" between a submaximal task and maximal aerobic power during walking and running (43). Interestingly, gross mechanical efficiency determined during cycling exercise seems to be similar in children and young adults (64).

Kinetics of $\dot{V}O_2$

Children rarely engage in activities with a constantly high intensity. In contrast, their play consists of short bursts of high-intensity activities separated by intervals of low-intensity activities (65). In consequence, various techniques have been developed to study acute cardiorespiratory adaptations to changes in exercise intensity. Most investigations in children have focused on the responses of $\dot{V}O_2$ to changes in exercise intensities. While some studies indicate that $\dot{V}O_2$ kinetics are faster in children than in adults (66), others do not (67,68).

Recovery

Children recover faster than adults from strenuous exercise. This observation is supported by a set of studies in which recovery was determined following a 30-sec, all-out exercise task in prepubertal boys and young men (69,70). It was found that the boys had a faster recovery of performance, $\dot{V}O_2$, HR, VE, and electrolyte changes than the men.

Trainability of Children

Training of sufficient frequency, duration, and intensity may significantly improve endurance performance in children and adolescents. However, some studies suggest that the aerobic trainability of children in the first decade of life is lower than would be expected from improvement in their athletic performance. A case in point is a study in which 91 children, ages 9 to 10 years, underwent various training regimens for 9 weeks (71). Even strenuous interval runs of 145 m, undertaken four times a week, did not increase their $\dot{V}O_{2peak}$, although running performance improved. Similar results were obtained by other researchers (72–74). Improved performance in the reported studies can possibly be due to an increase in anaerobic threshold, which might be more responsive to endurance training than $\dot{V}O_{2peak}$ (75). A more efficient running style or a better anaerobic capacity may also play a role. Other studies found that $\dot{V}O_{2peak}$ of children increased with aerobic training, as reviewed lately by Pate and Ward (76) and Mahon (77). Apparently, when the training regimen complies with principles established for adults, the aerobic system of prepubescents is trainable, although trainability may be lower than in adults.

Specific (78–80) and nonspecific (79) exercise training has been shown to improve short-term exercise performance in children aged 10 years and older by 3 to 20%. However, these findings were not always conclusive in that one but not other indices of performance improved with high-intensity, short-duration training (79,80). Possible mechanisms for an improved performance during high-intensity exercise tasks in children could include better neuromotor control and a higher glycolytic capacity (14,81,82).

Most (83–85) but not all (86) studies using resistance training in pre- and postpubertal children found significant improvements in muscle strength. Trainability of strength appears to be independent of age or maturity during childhood and adolescence (87,88). However, the mechanisms with which strength is improved might be different across ages. In prepubertal children, only minor increases in muscle bulk have been observed with strength training (83,84), suggesting that the improvement might partially reflect an improved neural drive (83). In contrast, strength gain during training in adults is related to both muscle hypertrophy and improved neural activation.

Is there a specific developmental age at which trainability is especially high (or low)? Trainability will depend on the training stimulus in relation to the baseline physical activity or baseline fitness. Because children are generally more active than adults, a sufficient stimulus may be harder to achieve. In addition, not chronological age but maturation might be important. A mixed longitudinal and cross-sectional study on Japanese boys showed no regularity regarding the chronological age at which aerobic training was most effective but a greater effectiveness of training around peak height velocity than at any earlier age (89). However, this has not been shown in other studies.

Exercise Testing in Children

Formal exercise tests have been performed in children as early as age 3 years (90). However, due to their short attention span and fast local muscle fatigue, routine testing is usually done at age 6 years and older.

REASONS TO PERFORM AN EXERCISE TEST

Exercise testing in children is usually conducted for the following reasons:

1. To determine physical working capacity as an index of fitness or physical activity in healthy individuals, or to describe the level of impairment in those with a chronic health condition. Exercise capacity may also allow one to predict prognosis in some diseases, e.g., patients with cystic fibrosis (91).
2. Adverse reactions to exercise may indicate the need for further evaluation (e.g., dysrhythmia, exercise-induced bronchial obstruction, exercise-induced hypoxia).
3. The effects of a specific intervention on exercise capacity or adverse responses to exercise are evaluated (e.g., physical training, drug therapy, surgery, bracing, oxygen supplementation).

4. The child, parents, or a physician are concerned about exercise safety, and exercise testing is indicated to reassure them.

REASONS NOT TO PERFORM AN EXERCISE TEST

Because exercise testing may be harmful, a careful analysis of the possible gain in information expected versus the potential harm induced is mandatory before a test is scheduled. A reevaluation should take place before the test is conducted.

In individuals in whom increased risks from exercise testing are suspected (Table 5-2), other, less risky means of obtaining the desired information should be used first. In suspected heart disease, for example, echocardiography and Holter monitoring may be sufficient to diagnose and treat. If the exercise-related risks are only temporarily increased (i.e., during acute infections or asthma attacks), exercise testing may have to be postponed until a more stable condition is reached.

SAFETY ISSUES AND MONITORING DURING THE EXERCISE TEST

The exercise test should be conducted by experienced staff. When patients are tested, a physician

TABLE 5-2 CONTRAINDICATIONS FOR EXERCISE TESTING

- Acute febrile infections
- Acute exacerbation of bronchial asthma
- Acute metabolic crisis (diabetes mellitus)
- Acute myocarditis
- Active rheumatic fever with carditis
- Uncontrolled severe hypertension
- Hypertrophic cardiomyopathy with a history of syncope
- Severe pulmonary hypertension
- Poorly compensated congestive heart failure
- Severe aortic or mitral stenosis
- Unstable dysrhythmia
- Marfan syndrome with suspected aortic dissection
- Severe pulmonary vascular disease

Modified from Washington RL, Bricker JT, Alpert BS, et al. Guidelines for exercise testing in the pediatric age group. Circulation 1994;90: 2166–2179 and Hebestreit H. Ergometrie in der Pädiatrie. In: Löllgen H, Erdmann E, eds. Ergometrie. Belastungsuntersuchungen in Klinik und Praxis. 2nd ed. Berlin: Springer Verlag, 2000:285–300.

should be available in the exercise laboratory or nearby. The laboratory should be equipped with well-maintained emergency equipment.

In healthy children, an HR monitor may be all that is needed, along with an ergometer and one or two exercise physiologists. In patients, additional equipment and personnel may be necessary to monitor for adverse reactions during exercise. Depending on the disease and the purpose of the test, ECG, pulse-oximetry, BP monitoring, blood gas analysis, spirometry, and monitoring of ventilation and respiration during exercise may be necessary.

Before an exercise test is conducted, a medical history and physical examination should be performed to identify possible contraindications. The testing protocol and risks and benefits of the test are explained to the child and the parent, and consent should be obtained.

The child should not have eaten a large meal for at least 2 hours prior to testing. Familiarization of the child with the testing equipment and procedures is highly recommended to obtain optimal test results.

The exercise test should be terminated if the child does not want to continue, if (severe) adverse effects of exercise occur, or if the monitoring equipment fails.

CHOICE OF AN ERGOMETER

Treadmills and cycle ergometers are used for exercise testing of children, especially for medical purposes (92). Only in rare cases, such as arm ergometry in spina bifida or muscular dystrophy patients, is other equipment used. For small children or those with advanced disease, walk tests on a (hospital) floor are also useful.

Both treadmill and cycle ergometer have advantages and disadvantages. However, the ergometer of choice for children younger than 6 to 8 years is the treadmill, especially when an all-out test is attempted. A young child who is tested on a cycle ergometer often can no longer pedal even though the HR is only 170 to 180 beats·min^{-1}. The same child, if tested on a treadmill, may reach a heart rate of 200 to 210 beats·min^{-1} and a measured $\dot{V}O_{2peak}$ that is 20 to 30% higher than the peak value obtained on the cycle ergometer. The apparent cause of this discrepancy is the undeveloped muscle mass in the thigh (especially the knee extensors) in the young child, which results in early local muscle fatigue during cycling. Further advantages of the treadmill are that walking and running are much more common in children than cycling and that a larger muscle mass is involved in running, putting a higher stress on the cardiorespiratory system. With small children, a treadmill should allow for slow speed settings of the belt and small increments of speed and slope.

For aerobic exercise tests, cycle ergometers should have a constant power mode that allows the child to accelerate and decelerate during the test without changes in power output (PO). Most electronically braked ergometers have this option. If only a constant torque mode is available (e.g., mechanically braked ergometers), testing may be difficult or impossible with young children or with older ones of a low mental age. Most anaerobic exercise tests (e.g., Wingate test and the force–velocity test) require a constant-torque ergometer. Most cycle ergometers have to be modified for (smaller) children. The horizontal and vertical position of the seat should be adjustable, and the crank arm length of the pedals should vary between 9 and 17 cm (93).

CHOICE OF A PROTOCOL

Many protocols have been used to test children. In a survey of 30 pediatric cardiac exercise testing facilities, a treadmill (17 laboratories) was used more often than a cycle ergometer (13 laboratories) (92). Most laboratories used the Bruce treadmill protocol or modified versions thereof. The Godfrey, James, and McMaster protocols were used for cycle ergometry.

The choice of protocol depends on the age, body size, and attention span of the child, the question asked, and the equipment available. Sometimes, more than one exercise test is necessary to address all questions about an individual. In general, total exercise duration for an aerobic test should be kept between 6 and 10 min to avoid premature muscle fatigue and/or boredom. Protocols with shorter stage duration are preferred if the test is conducted to measure peak exercise capacity. If BP measurements or blood gas analyses are scheduled during exercise, a stage duration of 3 to 5 min is best.

The following protocols for exercise testing are commonly used to determine aerobic working capacity and detrimental effects of exercise in children.

Bruce Protocol

The Bruce treadmill protocol can be used for individuals of all ages, although exercise time may be very short in small children and quite long in fit adults. Some laboratories use 2-min instead of 3-min stages. Normal values for children aged 4 to 14 have been established by Cumming et al. (94).

James Protocol

This cycle ergometer protocol is often used for cardiac exercise testing. We use a modified protocol for testing patients with suspected pulmonary fibrosis. The initial PO is 200 kp·m·min^{-1} ($\approx$33 W). This is then increased every 3 min by: 100 kp·m·min^{-1} ($\approx$16 W) if body surface area (BSA) is <1 m^2; 200 kp·m·min^{-1} ($\approx$33 W) for BSA 1 to 1.2 m^2; or 300 kp·m·min^{-1} ($\approx$50 W) for BSA >1.2 m^2. After the third stage, PO is increased by 100 to 200 kp·m·min^{-1} (16–33 W) every minute. Normative data for children have been published by James et al. (95) and Washington et al. (96).

Godfrey Protocol

This protocol for cycle ergometry has been widely used for the exercise evaluation of patients with cystic fibrosis (91). Stage duration is 1 min. PO increases depend on the height of the person tested. Children shorter than 120 cm start at 10 W, with increases of 10 W each minute until they cannot maintain a cycling cadence of 60 rpm. Initial PO and PO increments in children 120 to 150 cm tall are 15 W. In children with a height > 150 cm, the respective value is 20 W. Reference values for maximal PO and peak $\dot{V}O_2$ can be estimated from equations reported by Godfrey (97) and Orenstein (98), respectively.

In some situations, none of the above protocols is suitable to address the question to be solved. The following testing protocols may be helpful in such cases.

Wingate Anaerobic Test

The Wingate test (WAnT) is a 30-sec all-out cycle ergometer test to measure short-term muscle power (see [60] for details). The test is mainly used with healthy subjects and those with a neuromuscular disease but has also been applied to patients with cystic fibrosis. Briefly, following a warm-up, the child is instructed to pedal as fast as possible against a constant and high resistance. Test–retest reliability of peak power and mean power generated during the test are high, and the correlation of these parameters with performance in sprint running, sprint swimming, and high-jumping is also high (60). In children with cerebral palsy, mean power in the WAnT correlates well with performance in such everyday activities as standing, walking, and running (99). Performance data of healthy children have been reported by Bar-Or (43) and Inbar et al. (60).

Force–Velocity Test

The force–velocity test consists of several 5- to 8-sec, all-out sprints on a cycle ergometer against various braking forces. Peak cycling cadence and the corresponding PO are plotted over braking force, and optimal force and cadence are determined. If flywheel inertia is taken into account, PO is constant across a large range of applied forces. So far, the test has mainly been used to study the performance of healthy children (59,100).

Test for Exercise-Induced Bronchoconstriction

If exercise-induced bronchoconstriction is suspected, an exercise provocation test may help to establish this diagnosis (see [101] for details). The test procedures and interpretation are identical for children and adults. Sensitivity of this test is about 60 to 70%.

6-Min Walk Test

The 6-min walk test has been used to assess performance in severely sick patients with cardiac or pulmonary disease. In some hospitals, the test is also used to determine when a patient should be listed for transplantation (102). In patients with cystic fibrosis, a distance < 400 m walked in 6 min is taken as indicator for a poor prognosis. Test–retest reliability is good ($r = 0.90$) (103).

Test for Growth Hormone (GH) Deficiency

In short-statured children, an exercise provocation can be used to assess GH release (104). Various protocols using cycle or treadmill exercise of 10- to 30-min duration and a submaximal intensity have been used successfully. A 20-min exercise at about 70% of peak $\dot{V}O_2$ seems to be practical and effective in suggesting or rejecting the diagnosis of GH deficiency (104).

OUTCOME VARIABLES: MEASURES OF AEROBIC PERFORMANCE

For the indicators of aerobic performance commonly used in children, an exercise test to exhaustion is required. If the child does not give a maximal effort, performance should not be reported or should be commented on in the summary. In adults, a plateau of $\dot{V}O_2$ despite an increase in PO has been accepted as an indicator for all-out efforts. However, a plateau is observed in only about half of all children (105). Children who do reach a plateau achieve similar scores to those who do not (51,106–108). Therefore, several other criteria for a maximal effort have been suggested. Rowland (92) recommends an average target HR of 195 beats $\cdot$min^{-1} during cycle ergometry and 200 beats$\cdot$min^{-1} during treadmill exercise, but acknowledges the large interindividual differences in maximal HR. A mean respiratory exchange ratio >1.00 (treadmill) or >1.05 (cycle ergometer) has also been used. Armstrong and Welsman recommend the appearance of the subject at peak exercise as an indicator for a maximal effort (55).

Ventilatory Threshold, Lactate Threshold

For children who will not perform with an all-out effort or for whom a maximal effort is not warranted, the ventilatory threshold (VAT) or lactate threshold (LT) can be used. Some studies suggest that VAT may be more sensitive than $\dot{V}O_{2peak}$ to physical training (75).

Two problems limit the practical use of VAT: (*a*) VAT cannot be determined from a single exercise test in about 5 to 10% of children, and (*b*) two investigators may determine different VAT values from the same data set. However, if more than one criterion is used to determine VAT in children, intra- and interobserver reliability is high (intraclass correlation coefficients >0.90) (109).

LT is determined from a series of blood lactate measurements during an incremental exercise task. While a definite cutoff threshold for lactate concentration has been used in the past (e.g., 2 mmol$\cdot$L^{-1}, 3 mmol$\cdot$L^{-1}, or 4 mmol$\cdot$L^{-1}), most investigators now determine an individual LT as the first definite increase in lactate concentration above baseline with increasing exercise intensity.

Test–retest reliability of VAT and LT in children is high. VAT correlates closely with $\dot{V}O_{2peak}$ (109). Some normal values for VAT in children are available (110).

MONITORING FOR ADVERSE EFFECTS OF EXERCISE

ECG

Typical indications for exercise ECG in children are thoracic pain with exercise, dysrhythmia (benign arrhythmias tend to cease with increasing exercise intensity), heart surgery in the past (dysrhythmia?), and Kawasaki's disease with aneurysms of the coronary arteries. A 12-lead ECG is usually recorded during an incremental exercise test. The extremity leads are placed in the subclavicular fossae and on the abdomen, the precordial leads in the same locations as during a resting ECG.

In general, the pattern of physiologic and pathologic ECG changes is similar in children and adults. However, arrhythmias are much more common than ST-changes in children. In some patients, a long-QT syndrome can be evident only during exercise. Therefore, at different levels of exercise intensity, a proper correction of QT interval for the influence of heart rate is mandatory whenever a long-QT syndrome is suspected. At least in children, the Bazet equation seems to be less suitable for this correction than the equation suggested by Karjalainen et al. (111,112).

Blood Pressure (BP)

SBP at maximal exercise depends on body size and race (113). In children, peak SBP rarely exceeds 200 mm Hg, a peak exercise SBP up to 220 mm Hg is considered normal in adults. There is no proof that an SBP of up to 250 mm Hg is harmful in a healthy child (48).

Pulse Oximetry

In patients with pulmonary fibrosis, oxygen saturation (SaO_2) during exercise may help to establish the diagnosis and is valuable for follow-up. A drop in SaO_2 of more than 4% is considered pathologic, although a decrease of up to 10% has been observed in healthy, highly trained adults. In patients with cystic fibrosis, an exercise-induced fall in SaO_2 below 90% may indicate that intense exercise over a prolonged period of time without oxygen supplementation may lead to stress on the right heart.

The easiest way to measure SaO_2 is by means of pulse oximetry. A sensor on the forehead (e.g., Nelcor RS10 forehead sensor) has been shown to provide accurate readings with only few artifacts; finger sensors are less suitable for exercise testing (114).

Spirometry

Spirometry before and after exercise is used to identify patients with exercise-induced bronchoconstriction. Spirometry before exercise may also help to explain reduced exercise capacity in patients with cystic fibrosis. The value of flow-volume loops obtained during exercise has yet to be established.

Blood Gas Analysis

Blood gas analysis during exercise can be helpful to calculate the alveolar–arterial difference in oxygen partial pressure. This difference is widened in patients with pulmonary fibrosis. Blood gas analysis may also be used to detect an excessive increase in PCO_2 during exercise, although monitoring of end-tidal PCO_2 is a less invasive measure that can be obtained online.

Tidal Volume

Tidal volume (V_T) usually increases with increasing exercise intensity. A failure to increase V_T sufficiently during exercise results in a relatively high respiratory frequency at moderate exercise intensities and limits performance. Patients with cystic fibrosis may experience increased air trapping during exercise, leading to an impaired rise in V_T. Patients with pulmonary fibrosis and reduced vital capacity may also show low V_T during exercise.

Exercise Prescription

As a rule, a healthy child does not require an exercise prescription. Children are generally more active than adults or adolescents, and their spontaneous activity seems sufficient to maintain a fair level of fitness. However, demands by adults that the child be quiet and excessive television and computer access may suppress a child's normal desire to be physically active. Space and time to play outdoors with friends is often all that is needed to have as much activity as necessary. In healthy adolescents, especially in girls, some recommendations toward physical activity (e.g., "do the activity you like, but do it nearly every day") may be necessary. The two subgroups of children who do require guidance and planned regimens of activity are some sick (or disabled) children and those aspiring to athletic excellence. The latter group is not discussed.

A major difference to recognize while planning activity programs for adults and children is that the latter group does not require special motivation. Sedentary adults recruited to an activity program must first undergo a "campaign" to modify their awareness and attitude toward physical activity. Children do not need motivational tactics. Most healthy children (and many sick ones) have a built-in urge to stay active whenever they are not inhibited or distracted by their environment. Physical activity is a way to express and is an integral part of play. The games they select often include such elements as running, jumping, and climbing. However, children will rarely comply with "boring" exercise programs. It cannot be overemphasized that physical activities should be fun, especially at younger ages.

A child will seldom voluntarily pursue such prolonged, monotonous activities as distance walking, running, or swimming. More typically, children select intermittent-type exercise, during which bouts of intense exertion are interspersed with short rest periods or less strenuous activities (65). Their fast rate of recovery after a strenuous task (69) enables children to sustain such intermittent activities for many hours.

One segment of the pediatric population that merits special attention is children with real or presumed physical or mental handicaps. Such children may benefit from an exercise prescription beyond the positive effects every child may experience (Table 5-3). However, these children are often hypoactive. A summary of causes of hypoactivity in the sick child is given in Table 5-4. The main message to be derived from these data is that conditions in which there is a definite, objective cause for hypoactivity are outnumbered by those in which hypoactivity is imposed by fear, shame, overprotection, or sheer ignorance. In addition, a given disease can

TABLE 5-3 BENEFITS OF EXERCISE IN CHILDREN WITH CHRONIC HEALTH CONDITIONS

Disease	Potential Benefits of Exercise
Diabetes mellitus type I	• Increased physical fitness • Increased sensitivity to insulin • Possibly, fewer long-term complications
Bronchial asthma	• Increased physical fitness • Improved self-esteem, body image, and social development • Fewer hospital visits and days absent from school
Cystic fibrosis	• Increased physical fitness • Improved self-concept • Possibly, decreased morbidity and mortality
Juvenile idiopathic arthritis	• Increased physical fitness • Increased strength in muscles and ligaments • Improved joint protection • Increased bone mineral content
Epilepsy	• Increased physical fitness • Improved self-esteem • Improved overall health
Obesity	• Increased physical fitness • Decreased adiposity • Preserved muscle mass during diet • Improved self-esteem • Improved overall risk profile
Muscular dystrophy	• Preserved range of motion of the joints • Possibly, slowed decrease in strength • Improved self-esteem
Hemophilia	• Improved physical fitness • Increase in levels of clotting factors • Increased strength of muscles and ligaments • Improved joint protection

TABLE 5-4   CAUSES OF HYPOACTIVITY IN SICK CHILDREN

Cause	Related Condition
Handicap causes motor limitation	Paralysis, muscle dystrophy or atrophy, advanced arthritis, extreme obesity, amputation, and cerebral palsy
Handicap causes cardiopulmonary or metabolic limitation	Advanced cyanotic heart disease, cystic fibrosis or kyphoscoliosis, and extreme obesity or undernutrition (anorexia)
Child is ashamed and is afraid of being active	Obesity, kyphoscoliosis, cerebral palsy, blindness, hemophilia, bronchial asthma, diabetes mellitus, epilepsy, Down syndrome, and other types of mental retardation
Overprotection by parents and educators	Any "heart disease" (also benign murmur), cystic fibrosis, bronchial asthma, diabetes mellitus, epilepsy, and hemophilia
"Take-it-easy" approach by uninitiated physicians and school nurses	Dysrhythmia, congenital heart disease, diabetes mellitus, bronchial asthma, cystic fibrosis, epilepsy, and hemophilia

be accompanied by hypoactivity of more than one cause.

To prescribe an activity regimen for the sick child, one should first identify the specific reason for the hypoactivity. For example, it is only logical that an obese child who is inhibited by shame and peer rejection not be forced to join a team sport at school, but rather be able to join special programs with other obese children. Such programs can be carried out at school (115) or elsewhere. Children with a rare disorder or those who require an individual training program may have to exercise at or near their home (e.g., patients with CF, children after transplantation). Children with asthma who are simply detrained due to hypoactivity can be given a variety of activities to increase their general fitness level. One patient with hemophilia may choose to be inactive due to fear of bleeding; another is habitually active but has undergone recent muscle atrophy due to knee hemarthrosis. The approach to these two patients should obviously be individualized. A diabetic youth can perform any kind of activity, but proper education is necessary to adapt diet and/or insulin dose to prevent hypoglycemia.

Unlike healthy children, a child with a disease must often be motivated to assume an active way of life. More important, however, and often more difficult to accomplish is the modification of parental attitude, involvement and action. Parents must first be convinced of the need for increased physical activity, as well as of its benefits and lack of hazard to their child. Otherwise, chances are slim that the child will assume an adequate activity pattern. Parents are often reluctant to allow their children to

be active because of sheer ignorance of the health consequences of exertion. Such ignorance may stem from prejudice, but also from a misinterpretation of the physician's instructions or even from wrong medical advice. It has been shown, for example, that 53% of parents who curtailed the activity of their child with a *benign* cardiac murmur did so because a physician mentioned the heart murmur (116). Seventy percent of these parents expressed doubt and confusion about their child's health status. Thus, for success in instituting adequate activity patterns among sick (or presumed sick) children, the physician and physical educator must first and foremost obtain parental cooperation. The parents' fear should be alleviated, and their level of uncertainty about the benefits and hazards of physical exertion should be reduced.

As with adults, exercise prescription for children should be well defined in terms of the intensity, duration, frequency, and content of each element. A major challenge is to describe to the child the notion of "intensity." An attempt has been made to use an RPE scale to prescribe intensity. This seems to be feasible with obese children (25). Because of the greater spontaneity of children and their shorter attention span, one can assume a priori that adherence to a preset program may not be as expected. Nevertheless, good adherence can be achieved when activities are administered by an instructor who can communicate to the child that activity is fun rather than boring. Fitting an exercise program to the child with motor disability must be based on residual functional capacity rather than merely on classification of pathologic findings.

REFERENCES

1. Docherty D, ed. Measurement in Pediatric Exercise Science. Champaign, IL: Human Kinetics, 1996.
2. Rowland TW, ed. Pediatric Laboratory Exercise Testing. Clinical Guidelines. Champaign, IL: Human Kinetics, 1993.
3. Bar-Or O, ed. The Child and Adolescent Athlete. Oxford: Blackwell Science, 1996.
4. Sullivan JA, Anderson SJ, eds. Care of the Young Athlete. Chicago, IL: American Academy of Orthopaedic Surgeons & American Academy of Pediatrics, 2000.
5. Armstrong N, van Mechelen W, eds. Paediatric Exercise Science and Medicine. Oxford: Oxford University Press, 2000.
6. Goldberg B, ed. Sports and Exercise for Children with Chronic Health Conditions. Champaign, IL: Human Kinetics, 1995.
7. Malina RM. Quantification of fat, muscle and bone in man. Clin Orthop 1969;65:9–38.
8. Lexell J, Sjöström M, Nordlund A-S, et al. Growth and development of human muscle: a quantitative morphological study of whole vastus lateralis from childhood to adult age. Muscle Nerve 1992;15:404–409.
9. Elder GCB, Kakulas BA. Histochemical and contractile property changes during human muscle development. Muscle Nerve 1993;16:1246–1253.
10. Eriksson BO. Muscle metabolism in children—a review. Acta Pediatr Scand 1980;283(suppl):20–27.
11. Eriksson BO, Saltin B. Muscle metabolism during exercise in boys aged 11 to 16 years compared to adults. Acta Paediatr Belg 1974;28:257–265.
12. Eriksson BO, Karlsson J, Saltin B. Muscle metabolites during exercise in pubertal boys. Acta Paediatr Scand 1971;217(suppl):154–157.
13. Zanconato S, Buchthal S, Barstow TJ, et al. ^{31}P–Magnetic resonance spectroscopy of leg muscle metabolism during exercise in children and adults. J Appl Physiol 1993;74:2214–2218.
14. Fournier M, Ricci J, Taylor AW, et al. Skeletal muscle adaptation in adolescent boys: sprint and endurance training and detraining. Med Sci Sports Exerc 1982;14:453–456.
15. Bell RD, MacDougall JD, Billeter R, et al. Muscle fiber types and morphometric analysis of skeletal muscle in six-year-old children. Med Sci Sports Exerc 1980;12:28–31.
16. Lin JP, Brown JK, Walsh EG. Physiological maturation of muscles in childhood. Lancet 1994;343:1386–1389.
17. Lin JP, Brown JK, Walsh EG. The maturation of motor dexterity or why Johnny can't go any faster. Dev Med Child Neurol 1996;38:244–254.
18. Seefeldt V, Haubenstricker J. Patterns, phases, or stages: an analytical model for the study of developmental movement. In: Kelso JAS, Clark JE, eds. The Development of Movement Control and Coordination. New York: Wiley, 1982:309–318.
19. Korkman M, Kemp SL, Kirk U. Effects of age on neurocognitive measures of children ages 5 to 12: a cross-sectional study on 800 children from the United States. Dev Neuropsychol 2001;20:331–354.
20. Anderson VA, Anderson P, Northam E, et al.. Development of executive functions through late childhood and adolescence in an Australian sample. Dev Neuropsychol 2001;20:385–406.
21. Bar-Or O. Age-related changes in exercise perception. In: Borg G, ed. Physical Work and Effort. Oxford: Pergamon Press, 1977:255–266.
22. Eston R, Lamb KL. Effort perception. In: Armstrong N, van Mechelen W, eds. Paediatric Exercise Science and Medicine. Oxford: Oxford University Press, 2000:85–91.
23. Robertson RJ, Goss FL, Boer NF, et al. Children's OMNI scale of perceived exertion: mixed gender and race validation. Med Sci Sports Exerc 2000;32:452–458.
24. Utter AC, Robertson RJ, Nieman DC, et al. Children's OMNI scale of perceived exertion: walking/running evaluation. Med Sci Sports Exerc 2002;34:139–144.
25. Ward DS, Bar-Or O. Use of the Borg Scale in exercise prescription for overweight youth. Can J Sport Sci 1990;15:120–125.
26. Ward DS, Jackman JD, Galiano FD. Exercise intensity reproduction: children versus adults. Pediatr Exerc Sci 1991;3:209–218.
27. Eston RG, Parfitt G, Campbell L, et al. Reliability of effort perception for regulating exercise intensity in children using the Cart and Load Effort Rating (CALER) scale. Pediatr Exerc Sci 2000;12:388–397.
28. Robertson RJ, Goss FL, Bell JA, et al. Self-regulated cycling using children's OMNI scale of perceived exertion. Med Sci Sports Exerc 2002;34:1168–1175.
29. Inbar O. Acclimatization to dry and hot environment in young adults and children 8–10 years old. Ed.D. dissertation, Columbia University, 1978.
30. Bar-Or O. Climate and the exercising child—a review. Int J Sports Med 1980;1:53–65.
31. Araki T, Tsujita J, Matsushita K, et al. Thermoregulatory responses of prepubertal boys to heat and cold in relation to physical training. J Hum Ergol 1980;9:69–80.
32. Drinkwater BL, Kupprat IC, Denton JE, et al. Response of prepubertal girls and college women to

work in the heat. J Appl Physiol 1977;43:1046–1053.

33. Haymes EM, Buskirk ER, Hodgson JL, et al. Heat tolerance of exercising lean and heavy prepubertal girls. J Appl Physiol 1974;36:566–571.

34. Wagner JA, Robinson S, Tzankoff SP, et al. Heat tolerance and acclimatization to work in the heat in relation to age. J Appl Physiol 1972;33:616–622.

35. Sloan REG, Keatinge WR. Cooling rates of young people swimming in cold water. J Appl Physiol 1973;35:371–375.

36. Bar-Or O, Dotan R, Inbar O, et al. Voluntary hypohydration in 10- to 12-year-old boys. J Appl Physiol 1980;48:104–108.

37. Wilk B, Bar-Or O. Effect of drink flavor and NaCl on voluntary drinking and rehydration in boys exercising in the heat. J Appl Physiol 1996;80:1112–1117.

38. Wilk B, Yuxiu H, Bar-Or O. Effect of body hypohydration on aerobic performance of boys who exercise in the heat. Med Sci Sports Exerc 2002;34(suppl):S48.

39. Fox EL, Mathews DK, Kaufman WS, et al. Effects of football equipment on thermal balance and energy cost during exercise. Res Q Am Assoc Health Phys Educ 1966;37:332–339.

40. Bar-Or O. Temperature regulation during exercise in children and adolescents. In: Gisolfi CV, Lamb DR, eds. Perspectives in Exercise Science and Sports Medicine, vol 2. Indianapolis: Benchmark Press, 1989:335–367.

41. Turley KR, Wilmore JH. Cardiovascular responses to treadmill and cycle ergometer exercise in children and adults. J Appl Physiol 1997;83:948–957.

42. Mocellin R, Sebening W, Buhlmeyer K. Cardiac output and oxygen uptake at rest and during submaximal loads in 8 to 14 year-old boys. Z Kinderheilkd 1973;114:323–339.

43. Bar-Or O. Pediatric Sports Medicine for the Practitioner. From Physiological Principles to Clinical Applications. Berlin: Springer-Verlag, 1983.

44. Eriksson BO. Cardiac output during exercise in pubertal boys. Acta Pediatr Scand 1971;217:53–55.

45. Koch G. Muscle blood flow after ischemic work and during bicycle ergometer work in boys aged 12 years. Acta Paediatr Belg 1974;28:29–39.

46. Koch G. Muscle blood flow in prepubertal boys—effect of growth combined with intensive physical training. In: Borms J, Hebbelinck M, eds. Pediatric Work Physiology. Basel: Karger, 1978:39–46.

47. Strong WB, Miller MD, Striplin M, et al. Blood pressure response to isometric and dynamic exercise in healthy black children. Am J Dis Child 1978;132:587–591.

48. Alpert BS, Fox ME. Blood pressure response to dynamic exercise. In: Rowland TW, ed. Pediatric Laboratory Exercise Testing. Champaign, IL: Human Kinetics, 1993:67–90.

49. Riopel DA, Taylor AB, Hohn AR. Blood pressure, heart rate, pressure rate product and electrocardiographic changes in healthy children during treadmill exercise. Am J Cardiol 1979;44:697–704.

50. Robinson S. Experimental studies of physical fitness in relation to age. Int Z angew Physiol 1938;10:251–323.

51. Åstrand PO. Experimental Studies of Physical Working Capacity in Relation to Sex and Age. Copenhagen: Munksgaard, 1952.

52. Cooper DM, Kaplan MR, Baumgarten L, et al. Coupling of ventilation and CO_2 production during exercise in children. Pediatr Res 1987;21:568–572.

53. Shephard RJ, Bar-Or O. Alveolar ventilation in near maximum exercise. Data on pre-adolescent children and young adults. Med Sci Sports 1970;2:83–92.

54. Reybrouck TM. The use of the anaerobic threshold in pediatric exercise testing. In: Bar-Or O, ed. Advances in Pediatric Sport Sciences. Vol 3. Biological Issues. Champaign, IL: Human Kinetics, 1989:131–149.

55. Armstrong N, Welsman JR. Assessment and interpretation of aerobic fitness in children and adolescents. Exerc Sport Sci Rev 1994;22:435–476.

56. Krahenbuhl GS, Skinner JS, Kohrt WM. Developmental aspects of maximal aerobic power in children. Exerc Sport Sci Rev 1985;13:503–538.

57. Léger L. Aerobic performance. In: Docherty D, ed. Measurement in Pediatric Exercise Science. Champaign, IL: Human Kinetics, 1996:183–223.

58. Armstrong N, Welsman JR, Nevill AM, et al. Modeling growth and maturation changes in peak oxygen uptake in 11–13 yr olds. J Appl Physiol 1999;87:2230–2236.

59. Falgairette G, Bédu M, Fellmann N, et al. Bioenergetic profile in 144 boys aged from 6 to 15 years with special reference to sexual maturation. Eur J Appl Physiol 1991;62:151–156.

60. Inbar O, Bar-Or O, Skinner JS. The Wingate Anaerobic Test. Champaign, IL: Human Kinetics, 1996.

61. Martin JC, Malina RM. Developmental variations in anaerobic performance associated with age and sex. In: van Praagh E, ed. Pediatric Anaerobic Performance. Champaign, IL: Human Kinetics, 1998:45–64.

62. Armstrong N, Welsman JR, Chia MY. Short term power output in relation to growth and maturation. Br J Sports Med 2001;35:118–124.

63. Daniels J, Oldridge N, Nagle F, et al. Differences and changes in $\dot{V}O_2$ among young runners 10 to 18 years of age. Med Sci Sports 1978;10:200–203.

64. Rowland TW, Staab JS, Unnithan VB, et al. Mechanical efficiency during cycling in prepubertal and adult males. Int J Sports Med 1990;11:452–455.

65. Bailey RC, Olson J, Pepper SL, et al. The level and tempo of children's physical activities: an observational study. Med Sci Sports Exerc 1995;27:1033–1041.

66. Fawkner SG, Armstrong N, Pooter CR, et al. Oxygen uptake kinetics in children and adults after the onset of moderate-intensity exercise. J Sports Sci 2002;20:319–326.

67. Cooper DM, Berry C, Lamarra N, et al. Kinetics of oxygen uptake and heart rate at onset of exercise in children. J Appl Physiol 1985;59:211–217.

68. Hebestreit H, Kriemler S, Hughson RL, et al. Kinetics of oxygen uptake at the onset of exercise comparing boys and men. J Appl Physiol 1998;85:1833–1842.

69. Hebestreit H, Mimura K, Bar-Or O. Recovery of muscle power after high-intensity short-term exercise: comparing boys and men. J Appl Physiol 1993;21:1–6.

70. Hebestreit H, Meyer F, Htay-Htay, et al. Plasma metabolites, volume and electrolytes following 30-s high-intensity exercise in boys and men. Eur J Appl Physiol 1996;72:563–569.

71. Bar-Or O, Zwiren LD. Physiological effects of increased frequency of physical education classes and of endurance conditioning on 9- to 10-year-old girls and boys. In: Bar-Or O, ed. Pediatric Work Physiology. Natanya: Wingate Institute, 1973:183–198.

72. Daniels J, Oldridge N. Changes in oxygen consumption of young boys during growth and running training. Med Sci Sports 1971;3:161–165.

73. Mocellin R, Wasmund U. Investigations on the influence of a running-training programme on the cardiovascular and motor performance capacity in 53 boys and girls of a second and third primary school class. In: Bar-Or O, ed. Pediatric Work Physiology. Natanya:Wingate Institute, 1973:279–285.

74. Stewart KJ, Gutin B. Effects of physical training on cardiorespiratory fitness in children. Res Q Am Assoc Health Phys Educ 1976;47:110–120.

75. Becker DM, Vaccaro P. Anaerobic threshold alterations caused by endurance training in young children. J Sports Med 1983;23:445–449.

76. Pate RR, Ward DS. Endurance trainability of children and youth. In: Bar-Or O, ed. The Child and Adolescent Athlete. Oxford: Blackwell Science, 1996:130–137.

77. Mahon AD. Exercise training. In: Armstrong N, van Mechelen W, eds. Paediatric Exercise Science and Medicine. Oxford: Oxford University Press, 2000:201–222.

78. Grodjinovsky A, Bar-Or O, Dotan R, et al. Training effect on the anaerobic performance of children as measured by the Wingate anaerobic test. In: Borg K, Eriksson BO, eds. Children and Exercise IX. Baltimore: University Park Press, 1980:139–145.

79. McManus A, Armstrong N, Williams CA. Effect of training on the aerobic and anaerobic performance of prepubertal girls. Acta Paediatr 1997;86:456–459.

80. Sargeant AJ, Dolan P, Thorne A. Effect of supplemental physical activity on body composition, aerobic and anaerobic power in 13-year old boys. In: Binkhorst RA, Kemper HCG, Saris WHM, eds. Children and Exercise XI. Champaign, IL: Human Kinetics, 1985:135–139.

81. Eriksson BO, Gollnick PD, Saltin B. Muscle metabolism and enzyme activities after training in boys 11–13 years old. Acta Physiol Scand 1973;87:485–497.

82. Cadefau J, Casademont J, Grau JM, et al. Biochemical and histochemical adaptation to sprint training in young athletes. Acta Physiol Scand 1990;140:341–351.

83. Ozmun JC, Mikelsky AE, Surburg PR. Neuromuscular adaptations following prepubescent strength training. Med Sci Sports Exerc 1994;26:510–514.

84. Weltman A, Janney C, Rians CB, et al. The effects of hydraulic resistance strength training in pre-pubertal males. Med Sci Sports Exerc 1986;18:629–638.

85. Komi PV, Viitasalo JHT, Rauramaa R, et al. Effect of isometric strength training on mechanical, electrical and metabolic aspects of muscle function. Eur J Appl Physiol 1978;40:45–55.

86. Docherty D, Wenger HA, Collis ML, et al. The effects of variable speed resistance training in strength development in prepubertal boys. J Hum Move Stud 1987;13:377–382.

87. Sailors M, Berg K. Comparison of responses to weight training in pubescent boys and men. J Sports Med 1987;27:30–37.

88. Pfeiffer RD, Francis RS. Effects of strength training on muscle development in prepubescent, pubescent, and postpubescent males. Phys Sportsmed 1986;14:134–143.

89. Kobayashi K, Kitamura K, Miura M, et al. Aerobic power as related to body growth and training in Japanese boys: a longitudinal study. J Appl Physiol 1978;44:666–672.

90. Shuleva KM, Hunter GR, Hester DJ, et al. Exercise oxygen uptake in 3- through 6-year-old children. Pediatr Exerc Sci 1990;2:130–139.

91. Nixon PA, Orenstein DM, Kelsey SF, et al. The prognostic value of exercise testing in patients with cystic fibrosis. N Engl J Med 1992;327:1785–1788.

92. Rowland TW. Aerobic exercise testing protocols. In: Rowland TW, ed. Pediatric Laboratory Exercise Testing. Champaign, IL: Human Kinetics, 1993:19–41.

93. Hebestreit H, Lawrenz W, Zelger O, et al. Ergometrie im Kindes- und Jugendalter. Monatsschr Kinderheilkd 1997;145:1326–1336.

94. Cumming GR, Everatt D, Hastman L. Bruce treadmill test in children: normal values in a clinic population. Am J Cardiol 1978;4:69–75.

95. James FW, Kaplan S, Glueck CJ, et al. Responses of normal children and young adults to controlled bicycle exercise. Circulation 1980;61:902–912.

96. Washington RL, van Gundy JC, Cohen C, et al. Normal aerobic and anaerobic exercise data for North American school-age children. J Pediatr 1988;112:223–233.

97. Godfrey S, Davies CTM, Wozniak E, et al. Cardiorespiratory response to exercise in normal children. Clin Sci 1971;40:419–431.

98. Orenstein DM. Assessment of exercise pulmonary function. In: Rowland TW, ed. Pediatric Laboratory Exercise Testing. Clinical Guidelines. Champaign, IL: Human Kinetics, 1993:141–163.

99. Parker DF, Carriere L, Hebestreit H, et al. Muscle performance and gross motor function in children with spastic cerebral palsy. Develop Med Child Neurol 1993;35:17–23.

100. Doré E, Bédu M, Franca NM, et al. Anaerobic cycling performance characteristics in prepubescent, adolescent and young adult females. Eur J Appl Physiol 2001;84:476–481.

101. Hebestreit H. Exercise and physical activity in the child with asthma. In: Armstrong N, van Mechelen W, eds. Paediatric Exercise Science and Medicine. Oxford: Oxford University Press, 2000:323–330.

102. Kadikar A, Maurer J, Kesten S. The six-minute walk test: a guide to assessment for lung transplantation. J Heart Lung Transplant 1997;16:313–319.

103. Gulmans VA, van Veldhoven NH, de Meer K, et al. The six-minute walking test in children with cystic fibrosis: reliability and validity. Pediatr Pulmonol 1996;22:85–89.

104. Saggese G, Meossi C, Cesaretti G, et al. Physiological assessment of growth hormone secretion in the diagnosis of children with short stature. Pediatrician 1987;14:121–137.

105. Rowland TW, Cunningham LN. Oxygen uptake plateau during maximal treadmill exercise in children. Chest 1992;101:485–489.

106. Cooper DM, Weiler-Ravell D, Whipp BJ, et al. Aerobic parameters of exercise as a function of body size during growth in children. J Appl Physiol 1984;56:628–634.

107. Rivera-Brown AM, Rivera MA, Frontera WR. Applicability of criteria for $\dot{V}O_2$ max in active adolescents. Pediatr Exerc Sci 1992;4:331–339.

108. Mahon AD, Marsh ML. Ventilatory threshold and $\dot{V}O_2$ plateau at maximal exercise in 8 to 11 year old children. Pediatr Exerc Sci 1993;5:332–338.

109. Hebestreit H, Staschen B, Hebestreit A. Ventilatory threshold: a useful method to determine aerobic fitness in children? Med Sci Sports Exerc 2000;32:1964–1969.

110. Reybrouck T, Weymans M, Stijns H, et al. Ventilatory anaerobic threshold in healthy children. Age and sex differences. Eur J Appl Physiol 1985;54:278–284.

111. Karjalainen J, Viitasalo M, Manttari M, et al. Relation between QT intervals and heart rates from 40 to 120 beats/min in rest electrocardiograms of men and a simple method to adjust QT interval values. J Am Coll Cardiol 1994;23:1547–1553.

112. Bhatia NG, Heise CT, Barber G. Exercise and QT interval corrections. Pediatr Exerc Sci 1995;8:94.

113. Alpert BS, Flood NL, Strong WB. Responses to ergometer exercise in healthy biracial population of children. J Pediatr 1982;101:538–545.

114. Yamaya Y, Bogaard HJ, Wagner PD, et al. Validity of pulse oximetry during maximal exercise in normoxia, hypoxia, and hyperoxia. J Appl Physiol 2002;92:162–168.

115. Ward DS, Bar-Or O. Role of the physician and physical education teacher in the treatment of obesity at school. Pediatrician 1986;13:44–51.

116. Bergmann AB, Stamm SJ. The morbidity of cardiac nondisease in schoolchildren. N Engl J Med 1967;276:1008–1013.

117. Washington RL, Bricker JT, Alpert BS, et al. Guidelines for exercise testing in the pediatric age group. Circulation 1994;90:2166–2179.

118. Hebestreit H. Ergometrie in der Pädiatrie. In: Löllgen H, Erdmann E, eds. Ergometrie. Belastungsuntersuchungen in Klinik und Praxis. 2nd ed. Berlin: Springer Verlag, 2000:285–300.

6

Aging for Exercise Testing and Exercise Prescription

James S. Skinner

The population of older persons is expanding rapidly in the United States; this is especially so with persons over the age of 65 years (1). More importantly, those over 65 years have the highest proportion of chronic diseases and disabilities and use the health care system most often (2). Equally important, persons over the age of 50 years are the most inactive group of adults; this is especially so for those over 75 years of age (3). Therefore, increasing the level of activity among the older members of our society should be a priority because regular activity has potential functional, health, economic, and psychosocial benefits.

General Effects of Aging

Functional and structural changes occur in most cells of the body throughout life. Although the aging process actually begins before birth, its effects are generally counterbalanced by growth. Once maturity is reached at age 20 to 25 years and growth stops, however, the effects become noticeable, usually around the age of 30 years. The rate with which the age-related changes occur varies from one person to another and from one body system to another within the same person (4), but the changes seem to be inevitable and irreversible.

With aging, there is a loss in size or number, or both, of functional units within every system of

the body, as well as a loss in function of those units that remain. As a result, aging can be characterized by a decreased ability to adapt to, and recover from, physiologic displacing stimuli. It seems that the greater the intensity of the stimulus and the larger the number of physiologic mechanisms involved in adjusting to that stimulus, the greater will be the loss of function with age (5).

Because exercise is a form of physiologic stimulation requiring complex forms of regulation and interaction among many systems, it is not surprising that the performance of certain types of exercise diminishes with age; this is particularly the case with high-intensity exercise that requires more adaptations. Similarly, because training is a form of adaptation to repeated exercise stimulation, one might assume that adaptation to training will be less or that older persons might need more time to adapt (6). Therefore, those who test and prescribe exercise for middle-aged and older persons should be aware of the effects of aging on the various systems and on the ability to exercise and train, as well as the general characteristics and specific needs of older persons. For more detailed descriptions of age-related changes in different systems, the reader is referred to published reviews (4,5,7–10).

There are many changes in body composition with age. For example, body weight and fat mass increase in middle-aged persons, after which there is a reduction in height, weight, fat-free mass (bone, protein, and muscle), and body cell mass (11). With age, there is a gradual loss of bone mass in almost all humans, beginning at age 30 to 35 years and accelerating after menopause in women and at age 50 to 55 years in men. These weaker bones are more susceptible to fracture spontaneously or after mild trauma (please refer to Chapter 11 for more details). Along with a decrease in bone mass, the amount of body fat tends to increase. and muscle mass (size and number of muscle cells) decreases. Although the loss of muscle mass is more profound than is the overall loss of body weight, this difference is partially masked by an increased amount of body fat.

The increase in body fat appears to be more related to lifestyle than to age per se. Skrobak-Kaczynski and Andersen found that Norwegian lumberjacks had mean values of about 13% body fat from age 20 to 70 years (12). It is not known how much exercise was needed to maintain these "younger" levels, but it is clearly more than most people do in our technological society. With age, the pattern of fat distribution changes, such that more fat is deposited internally and on the torso than under the skin and on the limbs (11,13). Shimokata et al. (14) found that men had progressive increases in central adiposity with age but that this trend was not apparent in women until the age of 54 years, suggesting that menopause might affect their fat distribution. Add to this the fact that skinfolds may be more compressible in the elderly (13), and it becomes obvious that estimates of body fat based on skinfolds should be age, gender, and population specific. Although some equations of this type have been developed (15,16), there is still a debate as to whether population-specific equations are better than general ones (17). Using quadratic regression analysis, general equations independent of age and body composition have been developed for men (18) and for women (19). Unfortunately, the upper age in these two studies was 61 years for the men and 55 years for the women, suggesting the need to develop the same type of equations specific to elderly men and women. There are also problems determining body composition by hydrostatic weighing in old age. For example, there are age-related and variable decreases in bone density among men and women, as well as a rise in the amount of connective tissue within the body and a higher residual volume with increasing age.

Early studies found a greater reduction in the number and size of fast-twitch, glycolytic muscle fibers used for strength and speed than in slow-twitch, oxidative, endurance muscle fibers (20). However, Rogers and Evans (10) reviewed more recent findings and state that both muscle types are equally affected when there is a loss of muscle mass with age. Along with the loss of functional units in muscle cells, there are smaller stores of adenosine triphosphate (ATP), CP, and glycogen and less effective enzymes for all three mechanisms of energy production, i.e., use of stored energy (ATP and CP), anaerobic glycolysis, and the aerobic metabolism of fats and carbohydrates.

Within the nervous system, there is a decrease in the number and size of neurons, nerve conduction velocity, and maximal conduction frequency, as well as an increase in the amount of connective tissue in the neurons and in the excitability threshold of muscle. As a result, the control of movement is less precise, less harmonious and more hesitant and seems to require more attention (5,21,22).

Cartilage, tendons, and ligaments become stiffer and more rigid with age. As a result, adults become significantly less flexible with increasing age, but less so in the upper extremities (23). The loss of flexibility is less pronounced in those areas of the body that are used on a regular basis, suggesting that disuse and aging both play a role.

Changes in the respiratory system have little effect on the function of healthy lungs at rest, but do make it more difficult for the lungs to supply adequate levels of oxygen to the body during intense exercise. As stated by Reddan (24), the older person has less reserve and has less room for error in the systems that control ventilation.

Because of increasing amounts of connective tissue, decreased elasticity, higher total peripheral resistance (TPR), and higher blood pressure (BP), the heart has to work harder to pump the same amount of blood. The higher BP and TPR and somewhat lower cardiac output ($\dot{Q}$) at rest are of little consequence, however, unless disease is present.

With increasing amounts of exercise, the aging cardiovascular and respiratory systems are less capable of adapting (9). At the same moderate submaximal power output, aging is characterized by (*a*) little change in oxygen intake ($\dot{V}O_2$) and heart rate (HR); (*b*) higher values for ventilation ($\dot{V}_E$), BP, arteriovenous difference for oxygen (AVD-O_2), blood lactic acid concentration (LA), and oxygen debt; (*c*) lower values for Q̇ and stroke volume (SV); and (*d*) a lower *rate* of adaptation to, and recovery from, exercise. The effects of age are most evident at maximal levels of exercise. With the exception of increased BP and TPR, there are reductions in maximal values of $\dot{V}O_2$, $\dot{V}_E$, Q̇, HR, SV, AVD-O_2, and LA. With the decrease in $\dot{V}O_{2max}$, a given amount of submaximal exercise becomes relatively more strenuous, i.e., a higher percentage of $\dot{V}O_{2max}$.

From this brief review, it is clear that the aged are weaker, slower, and less powerful and that there is a reduction in those performances requiring the regulating and coordinating functions of the nervous system, e.g., balance, reaction time, agility, and coordination. It is also easy to understand why older people cannot perform as well in almost any type of activity, except for low-intensity activities in which energy demands are easily met (25).

Age, Deconditioning, and Disease

When a middle-aged or older person comes for assistance, the physician or exercise leader must determine the relative effects of age, deconditioning, and disease. For example, dyspnea with moderate exercise may be due to age, poor fitness, or pulmonary disease. The structural and functional changes that occur with age and deconditioning tend to be more "normal," whereas those associated with disease are not.

Although aging and deconditioning are not diseases, all three factors are often treated in the same manner (26). Not only can the aged, the deconditioned, and the sick have similar physiologic traits, they are often similar psychologically. While deconditioning and aging are not synonymous, they do have common attributes. In fact, Smith states that deconditioning and aging each account for about one-half the "normal" functional decline (i.e., without the presence of disease) occurring from age 30 to 70 years (27).

Different diseases affect people at different ages, and age can have a modifying effect on various disease processes. Therefore, the ability to distinguish deconditioning and age-related changes from disease processes is a major challenge for physicians. This distinction is important, however, because it

will influence the type of exercise test that is given and the exercise programs that are prescribed.

Certain diseases, as well as the presence of factors associated with a higher risk of developing them, are found more frequently with advancing age. Some examples of these are arthritis, cardiovascular diseases, chronic obstructive pulmonary diseases, diabetes mellitus, hypertension, osteoporosis and renal disease. For more detailed descriptions of these disorders and their effects on exercise testing and exercise prescription, the reader is referred to the specific chapters in this book.

Exercise Testing of the Elderly

Whether an exercise tolerance test is needed depends on the patient's health status, present level of habitual activity, and the level of activity desired. In other words, low-risk, nonsymptomatic patients with no evidence of cardiovascular disease may not need to be tested if walking or mild calisthenics will be their main form of exercise. On the other hand, high-risk patients with a history of clinical problems that might be aggravated by exercise or persons who want to do more vigorous exercise should be tested for their personal safety.

The main purposes of exercise testing are the same for the elderly as they are for all adults, i.e., to define the degree of risk associated with varying levels and amounts of exercise and to establish the appropriate intensities for the exercise prescription. Although the contraindications to exercise testing are no different for older and younger persons (28), the fact that age is a risk factor and that certain diseases might be more prevalent in older people makes safety a major issue.

Assuming that the physician (*a*) is familiar with the patient's prior and current status in terms of health and physical activity and (*b*) understands the contraindications for exercise testing (28), the Council on Scientific Affairs of the American Medical Association recommends exercise tests for the elderly "when appropriate" (29). Thus, not all older people can or should be given exercise tests to determine their fitness. For example, Sidney and Shephard found that medical screening eliminated 21% of elderly volunteers for a training program (30). Because older persons are at greater risk (even those who are apparently healthy), a physician should be in visual contact or in close proximity at all times. Interpretation of exercise test results also can be a problem. Schlenker reported that 77% of older adults take at least one prescription medication on a regular basis, whereas 65% take one to three, and 20% take four to nine (31). The interactions of these medications with each other, as well as their possible interaction with exercise, may affect test results and any subsequent exercise prescription.

Except for research purposes, there is little reason to do maximal exercise tests with older adults. Thomas et al. found test–retest reliability coefficients of 0.67, 0.87, and 0.90 for three treadmill protocols with 224 men aged 55 to 68 years (32). Although higher peak values for $\dot{V}O_2$ were found when tests were repeated, only one third of the men reached a plateau in $\dot{V}O_2$; this raises more doubts about the value of and need for maximal tests. A better approach would be to estimate fitness from submaximal tests so that more persons can be evaluated with less risk.

Two practical questions arise, however. Most submaximal tests determine HR at several levels of $\dot{V}O_2$ or power output (PO). By extrapolating the linear relationship between HR and either of these two variables to that individual's known or estimated maximal HR, the maximal $\dot{V}O_2$ or PO can be predicted. However, because of the large variation in maximal HR (30) and the concern about approaching or going to maximum, how does one select the correct maximal HR to which one should extrapolate? In addition, a recent study has shown that the often-used equation of 220 minus age underestimates the true maximal HR in older persons (33) Similarly, if older subjects are limited by muscular weakness and cannot push themselves to maximal levels of $\dot{V}O_2$ (or are not motivated to do so), of what practical significance are these "maximal" values to their health, well-being, and independence? Submaximal tests of progressively increasing intensity to some fixed end-point (e.g., to a known HR or to the onset of predetermined signs and symptoms) may be more useful.

Many normative values are based on data on young men and may not be directly applicable to an older population, especially one with more women. Thus, more information on typical values in the young-old (65–75 years), the old-old (75+ years), and the athletic old are needed. Perhaps more important would be information on (*a*) how much and what types of physical activity are needed to increase and maintain functional ability in the older person and (*b*) which fitness tests best measure these abilities.

FACTORS INFLUENCING EXERCISE TESTING

As mentioned above, age is a risk factor in the development of various diseases. The effects of each of these diseases should therefore be considered when a suitable exercise test is selected. Nevertheless, common characteristics of the elderly can modify the type of test given (Table 6-1).

With age, there is a reduction in the average values of $\dot{V}O_{2max}$ of about 10% per decade in healthy sedentary men and women (8). Starting at about 12 to 13 metabolic equivalents (METs; [42–46 mL·kg^{-1}·min^{-1}]) at age 25 years, there is a drop of approximately 1 MET each 7 years or a $\dot{V}O_2$ of 0.5 mL·kg^{-1}·min^{-1} each year. Men tend to have average values about 1 MET higher than women. Thus, the average 60-year-old has a $\dot{V}O_{2max}$ of 7 to 8 METs; this value drops to 5 to 6 METs in the average healthy 75-year-old. Smith reports average values of 5 to 7 METs in the young-old (65 to 75 years) living in the community, 2 to 4 METs in the old-old (75+ years) living in nursing homes, and about 10 METs in the athletic old (27). Given the low values in all but the athletic old, the initial PO of any exercise test should have a fairly low energy requirement. Thus, the Bruce test is not the test of choice because the second stage (2.5 mph, 12% grade) requires 7 METs and is at or near the $\dot{V}O_{2max}$ of most elderly persons (28).

Older persons require more time to reach a relative steady state in $\dot{V}_E$, $\dot{V}O_2$, and HR. An ideal test therefore incorporates a long period of warm-up, i.e., the intensity of the initial PO is low (2–3 METs) and is continued for at least 3 min or longer until the steady state is attained. Increases in exercise intensity should be small (0.5–1.0 MET), and the time at each PO should not be too brief (at least 2–3 min). Again, the big increase in intensity found from one stage to the next in the Bruce test argues against its use with older subjects. Even the modified Balke test, which starts at 3 mph, 0% grade (3.2 METs) and increases by 2.5% grade

TABLE 6-1   EXERCISE TESTING FOR THE ELDERLY

Characteristic	Suggested Test Modification
Low $\dot{V}O_{2max}$	Start at low intensity (2–3 METs)
More time required to reach a steady state	Long warm-up (3+ min). Small rise in power outut (0.5–1 MET) and/or 2–3 min at each stage
Increased fatiguability	Reduce total test time to 12–15 min or use an intermittent protocol
Increased need to monitor ECG, BP, and HR	Bike > treadmill > step test
Poor balance	Bike > treadmill > step test. Use treadmill built into floor
Poor strength (especially upper thighs)	Treadmill > bike or step test
Less ambulatory ability	Increase treadmill grade rather than speed (maximum of 3–3.5 mph)
Poor neuromuscular coordination	Increase amount of practice. May require more than one test
Difficulty holding mouthpiece with dentures	Add support or use face mask to measure $\dot{V}O_2$
Impaired vision	Bike > treadmill or step test
Impaired hearing	Treadmill > bike or step test, if person needs to follow a cadence. Difficulty understanding and responding in a noisy environment (use electronic bike)
Senile gait patterns and foot problems (e.g., bunions and calluses)	Bike > treadmill or step test

(1 MET) every 2 min, may not always be the test of choice because of the insufficient time at each stage to reach a steady state. Smith and Gilligan recommend another modification of the Balke test starting at 2 mph, 2% grade (2 METs) and increasing by 2% (0.55 MET) each 2 min (34). For nursing home patients with a very low maximum, they suggest a four-stage chair step test that allows patients to sit while raising their legs to various heights (33). This test begins at 2.3 METs, and intensity increases by about 0.5 MET after 2 to 5 min at each stage, to a maximum of 3.9 METs.

Because fatigability increases with age, total test time should not be too long. Of course, duration will depend on the objectives of the test, the ability to estimate an individual's fitness before testing, and the ability to modify a protocol depending on the test results.

With advancing age, medical problems are more likely, suggesting that the need for monitoring is greater. Although it is easier to monitor BP with the use of the bicycle ergometer than with the treadmill and step test, there is no problem recording HR with the electrocardiographic systems available today.

Poor balance and poor muscular strength are characteristics of the older, sedentary person. In terms of balance, weight-supported exercise on a bicycle ergometer is easier than exercise on the treadmill or step test. Nevertheless, the treadmill is preferred for those persons with poor muscle strength, especially those with weakness in the upper thigh. Individuals with poor balance probably feel more comfortable walking on a treadmill that is not too high off the ground. Although many persons are allowed to hold the treadmill railing, the energy cost of a particular PO can be greatly altered. Whereas this effect may not be a problem if $\dot{V}O_2$ is measured, it can cause significant errors when HR is used to predict maximal working capacity or maximal $\dot{V}O_2$ (35).

Associated with the lack of balance is a decrease in ambulatory ability and neuromuscular coordination with age. Increasing treadmill grade rather than speed should therefore be easier. Older persons may require more practice before they feel comfortable keeping the proper cadence during a bicycle ergometer or step test and while walking on the treadmill. As a result, more than one testing session may be required before the tester is confident that the results indicate the older person's responses to that amount and type of exercise.

Other characteristics of the elderly should be considered when deciding on the need for exercise testing and the type of test to be given. Persons with dentures may have difficulty holding a mouthpiece, so that added support or use of a face mask will be needed for the direct determination of $\dot{V}O_2$. Impaired vision may reduce the ability to perform treadmill and step tests adequately and safely. Persons with hearing loss may not be able to follow the proper cadence in bicycle ergometer and step tests or to respond as well to questions during a test, especially in a noisy environment. Persons with senile gait patterns and such foot problems as bunions and calluses may have difficulty walking on a treadmill or performing a step test.

It would appear, therefore, that there is much heterogeneity among the elderly, and that no one exercise test protocol or apparatus is optimal. Nevertheless, if one considers the factors discussed above, as well as the reasons why exercise testing is done with each person, suitable alternatives may be found.

More emphasis should be placed on evaluating factors important to health and well-being, such as flexibility, endurance, strength, balance, and body fat. In other words, fitness testing for the older adult should relate more to health and independent living than to performance. As well, their results should not be compared with "average" values. Given that "average" is not always satisfactory and that performance per se is less important to most older people, evaluations should use such terms as "desirable," "acceptable," "minimal," and "undesirable" to inform the aged about the possible interrelationships among certain aspects of fitness, health, and independence.

Exercise Prescription for the Elderly

The general principles of exercise prescription for the aged are not much different from those used with younger people, except that the principles may have to be modified because of restrictions caused by the normal effects of aging. Smith has found that the "young-old" have few problems, while the "old-old" are hindered by a variety of age-related disorders (27). Additional modifications should be made when clinical problems or disabilities common to the elderly are present (e.g., atherosclerosis, hypertension, emphysema, arthritis, and neuromuscular incoordination). Thus, there is a wide spectrum of ability and need among the elderly. Generally speaking, the longer individuals have been sedentary and the more restrictions or limitations they have, the higher will be the number of modifications that should be made in their exercise prescription.

Aging of the cardiovascular system is almost always associated with atherosclerosis (5,36). In addition, aging and cardiovascular disease have similar effects on exercise capacity (37). As a result, patients with coronary disease could be considered to have advanced aging of the arterial system. Given these similarities, most principles of exercise prescription for these heart disease patients would also apply to older persons; programs for both groups require a more systematic and cautious approach. Thus, some supervision may be needed, especially at the beginning of an exercise program or when there is a significant increase in the intensity of the exercise performed.

OBJECTIVES OF EXERCISE PROGRAMS

Depending on the health status and level of habitual activity, which can vary greatly, the goals of the elderly can be quite different. Whereas performance and appearance are more important for young people, health, independence, and general well-being become more important with age. In fact, Paterson et al. found that the desire to remain independent is paramount in older adults (38). Thus, the primary goal of exercise programs for the elderly (Table 6-2) should be to improve general well-being, to increase their ability to take care of themselves, and to feel better during the later years of life.

Because a loss in cardiovascular endurance, strength, balance, or flexibility is associated with a loss of independence and a diminished ability to adjust to the requirements of daily living, improvement of these factors should be emphasized. Unless programs also attempt to increase socialization and enjoyment, however, it is unlikely that older people will continue to participate in what should be a regular part of their lifestyle. Although the other

TABLE 6-2   OBJECTIVES OF EXERCISE PROGRAMS FOR THE ELDERLY

Improve self-care capabilities and general well-being
Improve cardiovascular condition and general endurance
Increase muscular strength and endurance
Maintain or improve flexibility, coordination, and balance
Maximize social contact and enjoyment of life
Improve weight control and nutrition
Aid digestion and reduce constipation
Promote relaxation
Relieve anxiety, insomnia, and depression
Sustain sexual vigor

objectives listed in Table 6-2 may be secondary for program planning, they are still associated with self-care and general well-being.

A good exercise prescription is one that sets realistic goals for persons of all ages. As with younger people, the elderly want success. This can be accomplished by setting many small and attainable short-term goals and by selecting goals with a high probability of success (e.g., improved performance of such basic motor skills as walking, instead of better performance of complex movements that require practice and are difficult to master). Because the elderly have a desire to be wanted and to have their advice sought and valued, the prescription should involve setting goals; this should improve the chances that the elderly person will adhere to the prescribed program.

CONSIDERATIONS IN PRESCRIBING EXERCISE

There are factors to consider when prescribing exercise for the aged (Table 6-3). Because the same amount of exercise requires the same amount of energy, and because there is a marked drop in $\dot{V}O_{2max}$ with age, a given submaximal PO becomes more intense relative to the maximum. With high-intensity exercise, older persons have a slower rate of increase in $\dot{V}O_2$, $\dot{V}_E$, and HR; they must provide more energy via the anaerobic mechanism, and they cannot exercise for as long a time (5,37). Aging appears to have a minimal effect on the ability to work at or below 50% $\dot{V}O_{2max}$, however. People can work at these lower intensities for as many as 8 hours with little problem (25). Thus, the elderly have more

difficulty if the intensity is high and if the pace is imposed; less difficulty can be expected when they can select their own work rate.

Given that the functional ability of many sedentary elderly people is so low, such simple activities as walking, housework, and gardening may be intense enough to stimulate improvements. Thus, even a small increment in habitual activity may improve their functional ability, independence, and quality of life.

An exercise prescription should include the frequency, duration, intensity, and types of activity that the older person can do. It should also include instructions on what to do if the patient develops such effort-related symptoms as marked dyspnea with moderate exercise, chest pain, dizziness, claudication, or extreme fatigue.

Intensity

The risks of cardiovascular and musculoskeletal problems are much greater with intense exercise, especially in older people with bone, joint, and neuromuscular problems (39). The elderly also are more easily fatigued and are more susceptible to

TABLE 6-3   CONSIDERATIONS IN PRESCRIBING EXERCISE FOR THE ELDERLY

Medical-physiologic factors
    Reduced cardiorespiratory capacity
    Less ability to perform moderate and high intensity exercise
    Decreased ability to adapt to and to recover from exogenous physiologic stimuli (e.g., exercise, heat, and cold)
    Reduced adaptability to physical training (degree and/or rate of improvement)
    Muscle weakness and increased fatiguability
    Degenerative bone, joint, and tendon problems
    Increased susceptibility to soreness and injury
    Impaired balance and neuromuscular coordination
    Impaired vision and hearing
    Senile gait disorders and foot problems
Psychologic factors
    Lack of encouragement to be active
    Inaccurate perception by young and old of how active the elderly are, can be, or should be
    Increased inhibitions and depression
    Negative attitudes toward physical activity
    Distorted self-image

injury. Therefore, training programs should start with exercise at a low intensity to allow a more gradual increase in activity. Because it seems that older adults prefer moderate exercise, keeping the intensity at a comfortable level should improve program compliance and maintenance (40).

The longer individuals have been sedentary and the more restrictions or limitations they have, the lower should be the starting intensity, e.g., 30 to 40% $\dot{V}O_{2max}$. Because average 65-year-old persons have a maximum of 7 to 8 METs, they should begin at 2 to 3 METs (walking 2–3 mph). To put this in context, daily activities of independent living for healthy sedentary men and women aged 55 to 65 years require a VO_2 of about 15 mL·kg^{-1}·min^{-1} ($\sim$ 4 METs) (38). Thus, walking is or should be within the capabilities of most older persons and would be a good intensity for them.

After an interval that is longer than that usually required for younger people, intensity can be gradually raised to 50 to 70% $\dot{V}O_{2max}$ (3.5–5.5 METs). This slower progression should allow sufficient time for the older person to adapt to the training stimulus.

If one decides not to do a maximal test with an older person, how can exercise intensity be estimated for a prescription? The key is to have measurements of HR at several POs on a treadmill or during such standardized activities as walking at known speeds. Using the Borg scale, ratings of perceived exertion (RPE) at the various POs and HRs also would be useful. An RPE of 12 to 13 (somewhat hard) is associated with moderate-intensity exercise (6). Knowing the HR obtained at this RPE would allow older persons to have some idea of the exercise intensity.

Skinner et al. trained a large sample of healthy, sedentary adults from the age of 17 to 65 years for 20 weeks (41). When subjects were grouped by age and their data before and after training were analyzed, it was found that subjects in all three age groups had significantly lower HRs (P <.01) at the same absolute POs after training (Fig. 6-1). As expected, the youngest subjects had a higher maximal HR (P <.01) and higher HRs at any given % $\dot{V}O_{2max}$ (P <.01) than the other two age groups. The middle group also had a higher maximal HR (P <.01) and higher HRs at any given % $\dot{V}O_{2max}$ (P <.01) than those in the oldest age group. However, there was no difference in HR at the same %

$\dot{V}O_{2max}$ after training in any age group. The same was found for men and women (Fig. 6-1). Because a given HR in a given person is associated with the same relative intensity (% $\dot{V}O_{2max}$) for that person, when adults aged 17 to 65 years exercise at the same HR and/or RPE over several months, they are working at the same intensity, even though their $\dot{V}O_{2max}$ might change; there is little reason to expect that this will be different in those over 65 years.

Duration

Because the older person is less able to adapt to, and recover from, physiologic stimuli, any major increase in activity should be preceded and followed by prolonged periods of mild, gradually increasing (or decreasing) exercise. The older and more sedentary the individual, the longer should be the warm-up and cool-down periods. Avoiding rapid or major changes (up or down) in intensity, gives the older person more time to adapt to, and recover from, activities of higher intensity.

With prolonged periods of lower-intensity exercise, the total duration of each session will have to be longer to produce a significant total energy turnover. Balke suggests that the amount of energy expended during an exercise session be at least 10% of the person's daily caloric intake (42). For most older persons, this amount would be 10% of 1800 to 2200 kcal, or about 200 kcal per day of exercise, and would require approximately 1 hour of walking by persons with a low $\dot{V}O_{2max}$. Less time is needed with correspondingly greater speeds or work rates. Once an individual is exercising regularly, the minimal duration of each session should be 30 min. If the exercise sessions go much longer than 30 min, the older person should consider doing two shorter sessions rather than one long session. One study that might apply in this situation is that of DeBusk et al. (43). They found that three 10-min sessions per day were as effective as one 30-min session for improving the $\dot{V}O_{2max}$ of middle-aged men. There is probably no reason why the same would not apply to older persons. Also, if they can find times throughout the day when they can walk (even for 10 to 15 min), then walking could become a part of their lifestyle.

Frequency

As with individuals of any age who wish to improve cardiovascular endurance and have better control

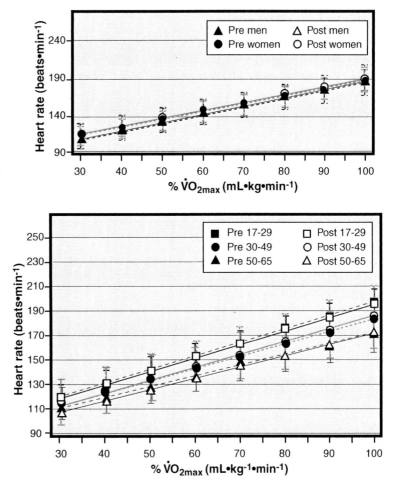

FIGURE 6-1 Heart rates at fixed relative intensities (% $\dot{V}O_{2max}$) for 293 men and 360 women *(top)* and for 295 young (17–29 years), 229 middle-aged (30–49 years), and 129 older (50–65 years) subjects *(bottom)* pre- and posttraining in the HERITAGE Family Study (see ref. 41).

of the composition of their body weight, the elderly should exercise at least three times per week. Because the aged are also trying to improve general well-being and the ability to take care of themselves, however, they need to be mentally and physically active every day. By finding ways to be active and by incorporating these activities into a given lifestyle, significant amounts of exercise can be performed. As well, it will be possible to improve such important aspects as flexibility, strength, and balance and to avoid or reduce the loss of function usually associated with disuse.

Type of Activity

In programs for the elderly, rhythmic, continuous exercise involving the use of large muscle groups should be emphasized. Activities of low-to-moderate intensity, such as walking, jogging, cycling, and swimming, are excellent for weight control and to improve general muscular and cardiovascular endurance. Games of low organization are an excellent means to improve hand–eye coordination, balance, and flexibility while having fun.

The keys to maintaining adequate joint function are movement to the joint's range of motion and adequate levels of strength. Therefore, exercise programs should include rhythmic stretching of all joints (especially during warm-up and cool-down phases) to improve flexibility; this stretching will help to maintain the ability to stoop, bend, and reach. Rhythmic calisthenics are ideal to increase strength and muscle tone, especially in those areas (thighs, back, abdomen, and arms) in which muscle weakness is common in the older adult. This type of exercise with light-to-moderate resistance is also potentially less dangerous. As with coronary disease patients, lifting heavy weights, isometric exercise, and arm exercises should be avoided or carefully controlled because they cause marked increases in HR and BP (28).

In general, the activities selected for the elderly will depend on the number and type(s) of limitations they possess. For example, if an older person has a problem with balance, exercise can be performed with some sort of support (sitting, lying on the floor, standing while holding a chair, or in warm water). The usual limitations of the aged generally preclude activities involving bodily contact, rapid or complicated movements, sharp turns, excessive competition, and environmental extremes (heat, cold, or altitude). Table 6-4 describes different types of exercise suitable for the elderly and gives examples of how programs can be modified in relation to characteristics of many older persons.

Progression

Because the older adult is generally less adaptable, more time should be spent at each level of exercise to allow more complete adaptation before increasing frequency, duration, or intensity. Because

of the potential problems associated with high-intensity exercise, it is usually better to exercise longer, more often, or both. Nevertheless, increases in any of these three important components of training should be made gradually and without major changes in the total amount of work done.

Other Considerations

As stated in the introduction to this chapter, persons over the age of 50 years are the most inactive group of adults; this is especially so for those over 75 years of age (3). Thus, people tend to become less active with advancing age. Cunningham et al. studied the activity patterns of 1695 men, aged 20 to 70 years, and found that their frequency of participation in active leisure-time activities decreased with age (44). More importantly, the average and peak energy expenditures also declined. Although part of these reductions in activity might be associated with the effects of aging on the ability to exercise, there are also sociopsychologic factors to consider.

The general stereotype of the older person in North America is not one of an active individual. Young people are taught that a reduction in habitual activity is an inevitable process of aging (45). The

TABLE 6-4   MEDICAL-PHYSIOLOGIC CONSIDERATIONS IN PRESCRIBING EXERCISE FOR THE ELDERLY AND EXAMPLES OF POSSIBLE MODIFICATIONS

Characteristic	Example of a Possible Modification
Greater chance of diseases that put patients at high risk	Increased monitoring for safety; changes depend on limitations (e.g., avoid intense isometrics and Valsalva maneuver in patients with hypertension)
Lower cardiovascular ability	Start at lower work loads
Less ability to perform moderate- to high-intensity exercise	Decrease intensity and allow patients to select their own pace
Less able to adapt to and recover from exercise	Longer warm-up and cool-down periods
Reduced adaptability to training (degree and/or rate of improvement)	More gradual progression in frequency, duration, and intensity of exercise
Muscle weakness	Moderate strength training
Increased fatiguability	Short intervals with more rest periods
Degenerative bone, joint, and tendon problems	No activities with bodily contact
Increased susceptibility to injury and soreness	No fast turns or movements
Poorer flexibility	Emphasize stretching
Poorer coordination and balance	Hold on to chair and exercise while seated or supine; exercise in warm water
Impaired vision and hearing	Exercise on a stationary bicycle
Senile gait disorder and foot problems	Use supportive, shock-absorbing shoes with good traction

general population also believes that older persons are less active than the older persons say they are (46). Thus, inactivity among the aged is perceived to be "natural."

There is also a problem in perception among the elderly themselves. Older persons perceive that chronic disorders are part of normal aging, and that they cannot do anything about it (47). Sedentary persons over the age of 50 years tend to have a distorted image of their bodies, i.e., they feel broader and heavier than they actually are (36). Sidney and Shephard asked Canadians over age 65 years if they felt that they got enough physical activity (46). Although most individuals said that they had more than enough and were more active than other persons in their age group, most respondents were below average in their level of fitness when tested on the treadmill. Thus, older persons appear to believe that their activity levels are adequate and do not perceive the need to do more (i.e., that they are just as active as their friends). Unfortunately, they are probably correct. Some of this perception problem may be due to the fact that results from most fitness tests are compared with "average" values. Even though an average rating may not reflect an acceptable or desirable level, a person might feel that "average" is adequate and see no reason to take corrective action. Because persons tend to overestimate what they do and to underestimate what they eat, this inaccurate self-perception is probably not limited to the elderly.

Coupled with the stereotype that one is not supposed to be active and the lack of encouragement to become active, the attitudes and perceptions mentioned above promote a sedentary lifestyle for the aging adult. As a result, the distorted stereotype is reinforced, and a vicious circle is created. Unfortunately, many older persons feel that they have little or no control over the aging process and therefore do not try to prevent or delay many of the functional losses that occur (5,27). Increasing the habitual activity of the elderly might reinforce the idea that they are capable of doing more. If they then attempt to do more, the downward spiral of the vicious circle might be reversed.

Perhaps by emphasizing the possible relationships between desirable fitness levels and independence, by giving fitness tests that evaluate those factors important to health and well-being, and by showing the elderly the types and amounts of activity needed to maintain functional ability, these perceptions can be changed, and the overall health of the older population improved. In this regard, cardiorespiratory fitness and leg strength are critical for maintaining physical function at a level compatible with independent living by older adults (48).

Several sociocultural factors can influence how well the elderly will accept and participate in exercise programs. The experiences, lifestyle, beliefs, and attitudes of young persons today are not the same as those of older persons. In other words, older individuals have different values and norms and may not easily accept those of a young exercise leader or physician. As an example, an older woman may feel uncomfortable exercising in a class and wearing shorts, leotards, or even slacks. Older persons also tend to be more inhibited. Therefore, these feelings and inhibitions should be considered when planning exercise programs.

Just exposing older persons to activity in a caring environment might affect their willingness to exercise. In a study on the effects of exercise on older adults with rheumatoid arthritis and osteoarthritis, some participants were originally assigned to a control group that did only mild activities to increase their range of motion (49). The researchers noted an increase in physical activity in this group after the study was over. They hypothesized that the exercise content was less important than the positive exercise experience for motivating some of the older adults to become more active.

Related to this positive experience, remember that exercise is a form of social activity for persons of all ages; this is especially so for the elderly who have more time. Therefore, exercise sessions should emphasize fun, enjoyment, social contact, and regular participation more than fitness, performance, or health, even though these important benefits might and should result.

Strength Training in the Elderly

Data from cross-sectional and longitudinal studies report a drop in muscle strength of about 15% per decade from 50 to 70 years, followed thereafter by a decrease of about 30% (7). Although a loss of muscle mass and the subsequent drop in muscle strength are considered normal aspects of aging, there are serious health consequences such as a higher incidence of falls and a loss of independence (50).

Little is known about the longitudinal or cross-sectional changes in the strength of various muscle groups with age, especially in active and inactive persons. Thus, age- and gender-specific norms for strength and muscular endurance are needed. It would be useful if these norms could be related to minimal and acceptable levels needed for independence, because this would give the older adult some idea of what is needed to remain functional.

Until the late 1980s, exercise programs for the elderly emphasized aerobic activities. Since that time, an increasing number of studies and position stands have stressed the need for, and the desirability of, including programs to improve strength at all ages, but especially in the elderly (6,7,51). When elderly persons become stronger, they tend to increase their level of spontaneous physical activity; this has been shown in healthy, free-living older adults and in very old and frail adults (7). Thus, improving strength seems to allow and encourage the elderly to become more active. This positive effect on their lifestyle is often accompanied by improved cardiovascular and metabolic functions, as well as increases in insulin action, bone mineral density, flexibility, and functional status (7,52).

The general principles of strength training for the elderly are essentially the same as those for younger persons. The reader is referred to Chapter 3 in this book for more details. As with younger persons, older persons have only modest gains when the intensity of the resistance is low (7). Similarly, if there is an adequate training stimulus, older adults also can have marked increases in strength (53). Even persons over the age of 90 years have had significant increases in strength with resistance training (54). As is the case with aerobic exercise programs, a major difference between young and old adults is that older persons may need to start at lower intensities and amounts of resistance and progress more slowly.

Trainability of the Elderly

Because aging is characterized by a loss in number, size, and performance of functional units within the body and by a reduced adaptability to physiologic stimuli, adaptability to training may also be impaired with age. In fact, studies done 20 to 30 years ago found that older humans and animals required more time to improve and that less improvement occurred in such variables as strength, $\dot{V}O_{2max}$, mitochondrial volume in muscle, and activity of oxidative enzymes (37,55). Even though researchers differed concerning whether trainability is affected by age, the consensus today is that the trainability of the elderly is similar to that of younger adults (6,7).

Part of the problem in the controversy over age and trainability was that most training programs for the elderly were less strenuous. Because researchers did not know how much exercise the elderly could or should do, they were more conservative in their approaches to training. As a result, their exercise programs did not require either the same absolute (e.g., running at 6 mph) or relative (75% $\dot{V}O_{2max}$) intensities or amounts of exercise as those in programs used with younger persons. Unless similar programs are given to young and old alike and a direct comparison is then made, it is difficult to discuss this problem.

Although the HERITAGE Family Study was primarily a study on the influence of genetic factors, it has provided information on age and adaptation to endurance training because it gave the same standardized, 20-week exercise program to 633 subjects from ages 17 to 65 years (56). Figure 6-2 shows the change in $\dot{V}O_{2max}$ (mL·kg^{-1}·min^{-1}) of the men and women of various ages in this study (57). Included in this figure are the results from the study by Kohrt et al., who gave a similar exercise program to 110 subjects aged 60 to 71 years (58). As can be seen in Figure 6-2, there was a wide variation in response (i.e., there were high, medium and low responders at all ages), but there was no difference between men and women or among subjects of different ages. Thus, it appears that older adults respond in a manner similar to that seen in the young and middle-aged subjects.

One comment made in the position stand of the American College of Sports Medicine was that older participants may need more time to adapt to endurance training (6). Because the subjects in both studies were tested only at the beginning and end of the training program, it was not possible to test this hypothesis. Nevertheless, it appears from these two studies that the trainability of $\dot{V}O_{2max}$ in older subjects does not differ significantly from that in

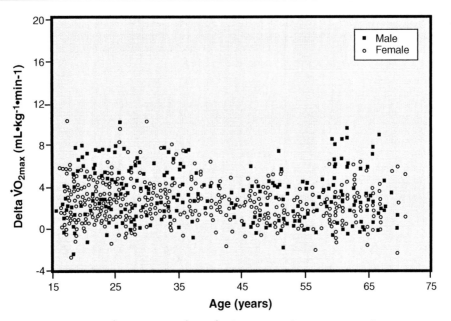

FIGURE 6-2 Change in $\dot{V}O_{2max}$ (mL·kg^{-1}·min^{-1}) of 287 men and 346 women aged 17 to 65 years in the HERITAGE Family Study (57) and of 53 men and 57 women aged 60 to 71 years in the study by Kohrt, et al. (58).

younger subjects when they are given 20 or more weeks to adapt.

Summary

- The main goal of an exercise program is not to train the elderly to become athletes.
- Improved psychologic and physiologic functioning are the usual results of systematic, progressive programs of increased exercise.
- Although some of these changes may not be as great or come as rapidly, especially in older persons who have been sedentary for many years, self-sufficiency and the ability to move with relative ease are attainable and are probably more important for daily living and independence than the high $\dot{V}O_{2max}$ often seen in those who train intensely to improve their fitness.
- Those involved with older patients should emphasize that the *process* of being active is more important than the *product* of being fit. That is, some persons can train regularly and intensely but not improve their strength or endurance very much,

whereas others (*a*) may train irregularly and get marked improvements or (*b*) do not train at all and are still fitter and can perform better.
- The important thing to remember is that it is possible to improve the ability to exercise at any age.

REFERENCES

1. Bureau of the Census. Current population reports: population projections of the United States by age, sex, race, and Hispanic origin: 1995–2050. Washington, DC: U.S. Department of Commerce, Economics and Statistics Administration, Bureau of the Census, 1996.
2. Berg RI, Casells JS, eds. The second fifty years: promoting health and preventing disability. Washington, DC: National Academy Press, 1990.
3. U.S. Department of Health and Human Services. Physical activity and health: a report of the Surgeon General. Atlanta, GA: U.S. Department of Health and Human Services, Centers for Disease Control and Prevention, National Center for Chronic Disease Prevention and Health Promotion, 1996.
4. Shock NW, Greulich RC, Andres R, et al. Normal Human Aging: The Baltimore Longitudinal Study

of Aging. NIH Publ no. 84-2450. Washington, DC: U.S. Department of Health and Human Services, 1984.

5. Skinner JS, Tipton CM, Vailas AC. Exercise, physical training and the aging process. In: Viidik A, ed. Lectures on Gerontology. Vol 1B. London: Academic Press, 1982:407–440.

6. American College of Sports Medicine Position Stand. The recommended quantity and quality of exercise for developing and maintaining cardiorespiratory and muscular fitness, and flexibility in healthy adults. Med Sci Sports Exerc 1998;30:975–991.

7. American College of Sports Medicine, Position stand. Exercise and physical activity for older adults. Med Sci Sports Exerc 1998;30:992–1008.

8. Holloszy JO, Kohrt WM. Exercise. In: Masoro EJ, ed. Handbook of Physiological Aging. New York: Oxford University Press, 1995:633–666.

9. Spina RJ. Cardiovascular adaptations to endurance exercise training in older men and women. Exerc Sport Sci Rev 1999;27:317–332.

10. Rogers MA, Evans WJ. Changes in skeletal muscle with aging: effects of exercise training. Exerc Sport Sci Rev 1993;21:65–102.

11. Going S, Williams DP, Lohman TG. Aging and body composition: biological changes and methodological issues. Exerc Sport Sci Rev 1995;23:411–458.

12. Skrobak-Kaczynski J, Andersen KL. The effect of a high level of habitual physical activity in the regulation of fatness during aging. Int Arch Occup Environ Health 1975;36:41–46.

13. Stevens J, Cai J, Pamuk ER, et al. The effect of age on the association between body-mass index and mortality. N Engl J Med 1998;338:1–7.

14. Shimokata H, Tobin JD, Muller DC, et al. Studies in the distribution of body fat: I. Effects of age, sex, and obesity. J Gerontol 1989;44:M66–M73.

15. Jackson AS, Pollock ML. Steps toward the development of generalized equations for predicting body composition in adults. Can J Appl Sports Sci 1982;7:189–196.

16. Pollock ML, Hickman T, Kendrick Z, et al. Prediction of body density in young and middle-aged men. J Appl Physiol 1976;40:300–304.

17. Pollock ML, Jackson AS. Research progress in validation of clinical methods of assessing body composition. Med Sci Sport Exerc 1984;6:606–615.

18. Jackson AS, Pollock ML. Generalized equations for predicting body density of men. Br J Nutr 1978;40:497–504.

19. Jackson AS, Pollock ML, Ward A. Generalized equations for predicting body density of women. Med Sci Sport Exerc 1980;12:175–181.

20. Larsson L. Morphological and functional characteristics of the aging skeletal muscle in man. Acta Physiol Scand Suppl 1978;457:1–36.

21. Fitts RH. Aging and skeletal muscle. In: Smith EL, Serfass RC, eds. Exercise and Aging: The Scientific Basis. Hillside, NJ: Enslow Publishing, 1981:31–44.

22. Grabiner MD, Enoka RM. Changes in movement capabilities with aging. Exerc Sport Sci Rev 1995;23:65–104.

23. Bell RD, Hoshizaki TB. Relationships of age and sex with range of motion of seventeen joint actions in humans. Can J Appl Sport Sci 1981;6:202–206.

24. Reddan W. Respiratory system and aging. In: Smith EL, Serfass RC, eds. Exercise and Aging: The Scientific Basis. Hillside, NJ: Enslow Publishing, 1981:89–107.

25. Åstrand I. Degree of strain during building work as related to individual work capacity. Ergonomics 1967;10:293–303.

26. Bortz WM II. Disuse and aging. JAMA 1982;248:1203–1208.

27. Smith EL. Age: the interaction between nature and nurture. In: Smith EL, Serfass RC, eds. Exercise and Aging: The Scientific Basis. Hillside, NJ: Enslow Publishing, 1981:11–17.

28. American College of Sports Medicine. Guidelines for Exercise Testing and Exercise Prescription. 6th ed. Philadelphia: Lippincott Williams & Wilkins, 2000.

29. American Medical Association Council on Scientific Affairs. Indications and contraindications for exercise testing. JAMA 1981;246:1015–1018.

30. Sidney KH, Shephard RJ. Maximum and submaximum exercise tests in men and women in the seventh, eighth, and ninth decades of life. J Appl Physiol 1977;43:280–287.

31. Schlenker E. Nutrition in Aging. St. Louis: Mosby College Publishing, 1984.

32. Thomas S, Cunningham DA, Rechnitzer P, et al. Protocols and reliability of maximal oxygen uptake in the elderly. Can J Sport Sci 1987;12:144–151.

33. Tanaka H, Monahan KD, Seals DR. Age-predicted maximal heart rate revisited. J Am Coll Cardiol 2001;37:153–156.

34. Smith EL, Gilligan C. Physical activity prescription for the older adult. Physician Sportsmed 1983;11:91–101.

35. Haskell WL. Factors influencing estimated oxygen uptake during exercise testing soon after myocardial infarction. Am J Cardiol 1982;50:299–304.

36. Skinner JS. The cardiovascular system with aging and exercise. In: Brunner D, Jokl E, eds. Physical Activity and Aging. Basel: Karger, 1970:100–109.

37. Skinner JS. Aging and performance. In: Keul J, ed. Limiting Factors of Physical Performance. Stuttgart: Thieme Verlag, 1973:271–282.

38. Paterson DH, Cunningham DA, Koval JJ, et al. Aerobic fitness in a population of independently living men and women aged 55–65 years. Med Sci Sports Exerc 1999;31:1813–1820.

39. Mazzeo RS, Tanaka H. Exercise prescription for the elderly: current recommendations. Sports Med 2001;31:809–818.

40. King AC, Haskell WL, Taylor CB, et al. Group- vs. home-based exercise training in healthy older men and women: a community-based clinical trial. JAMA 1991;266:1535–1542.

41. Skinner JS, Gaskill SE, Rankinen T, et al. Heart rate vs % VO_{2max}: Age, sex, race, initial fitness & training response—HERITAGE. Med Sci Sports Exerc 2003; 35:1908–1913.

42. Balke B. Prescribing physical activity. In: Ryan AJ, Allman FL, eds. Sports Medicine. New York: Academic Press, 1974:505–523.

43. DeBusk RF, Stenestrand U, Sheehan M, et al. Training effects of long versus short bouts of exercise in healthy subjects. Am J Cardiol 1990;65:1010–1013.

44. Cunningham DA, Montoye HJ, Metzner HL, et al. Active leisure time activities as related to age among males in a total population. J Gerontol 1968;23:551–556.

45. Ostrow C, Jones DC, Spiker DD. Age role expectations and sex role expectations for selected sport activities. Res Q Exerc Sport 1981;52:216.

46. Sidney KH, Shephard RJ. Activity patterns of elderly men and women. J Gerontol 1977;32:25–32.

47. Petrella RJ. Exercise for older patients with chronic disease. Physician Sportsmed 1999;27:79.

48. Paterson DH, Stathokostas L. Physical activity, fitness, and gender in relation to morbidity, survival, quality of life, and independence in older age. In: Shephard RJ, ed. Gender, Physical Activity, and Aging. Boca Raton, FL: CRC Press, 2002:99–119.

49. Minor MA, Hewett JE, Webel RR, et al. Efficacy of physical conditioning exercise in patients with rheumatoid arthritis and osteoarthritis. Arthritis Rheum 1989;32:1396–1405.

50. Young A, Skelton D. Applied physiology of strength and power in old age. Int J Sports Med 1994;15:149–151.

51. American College of Sports Medicine. Position stand. The recommended quantity and quality of exercise for developing and maintaining cardiorespiratory and muscular fitness in healthy adults. Med Sci Sports Exerc 1990;22:265–274.

52. Hurley BF, Roth SM. Strength training in the elderly: effects on risk factors for age-related diseases. Sports Med 2000;30:249–268.

53. Frontera WR, Meredith CN, O'Reilly KP, et al. Strength conditioning in older men: skeletal muscle hypertrophy and improved function. J Appl Physiol 1988;64:1038–1044.

54. Fiatarone MA, Marks EC, Ryan ND, et al. High-intensity strength training in nonagenarians: effects on skeletal muscle. JAMA 1990;263:3029–3034.

55. Orlander J, Aniansson A. Effects of physical training on skeletal muscle metabolism and ultrastructure in 70 to 75-year-old men. Acta Physiol Scand 1980;19:149–154.

56. Skinner JS, Wilmore KM, Jaskólska A, et al. Adaptation to a standardized training program and changes in fitness in a large, heterogeneous population: the HERITAGE Family Study. Med Sci Sports Exerc 2000;32:157–161.

57. Skinner JS, Krasnoff J, Jaskólski A, et al. Age, sex, race, initial fitness and response to training: the HERITAGE Family Study. J Appl Physiol 2001;90:1770–1776.

58. Kohrt WM, Malley MT, Coggan AR, et al. Effects of gender, age and fitness level on response of VO_2 max to training in 60–71 years olds. J Appl Physiol 1991;2004–2011.

RELATED WEB SITES

The National Blueprint: Increasing Physical Activity Among Adults Age 50 and Older
www.agingblueprint.org

The Blueprint Steering committee of this organization consists of members from the following organizations:

American Association of Retired Persons (AARP)
www.aarp.org

American College of Sports Medicine
www.acsm.org

American Geriatrics Society
www.americangeriatrics.org

Centers for Disease Control and Prevention
www.cdc.gov/netinfo.htm

National Council on the Aging
www.ncoa.org

National Institute on Aging
www.nia.nih.gov

Robert Wood Johnson Foundation
www.rwjf.org

Also on this web site are *Aging and Physical Activity Links,* which give information about aging and physical activity on 23 different links.

7

Environmental Factors for Exercise Testing and Exercise Prescription

Samuel N. Cheuvront, Michael N. Sawka, and Kent B. Pandolf

The clinical use of exercise testing to evaluate an individual's cardiorespiratory reserve and to enable the appropriate prescription of aerobic activity has attained wide medical acceptance. The physiologic stress from the metabolic intensity imposed by exercise, however, is only one consideration in testing and prescription. An equally important stress is that imposed by the environment (heat, cold, altitude, and air quality). Both exercise and environment alter the physiologic responses of the cardiorespiratory system. These environmental factors, either singly or in combination with exercise, can result in potentially hazardous health conditions.

Temperature Regulation and Energy Balance

The control mechanisms of temperature regulation for dealing with overcooling (cold stress) are not as effective as those for regulation against overheating (heat stress). Consequently, humans are thought of as tropical animals. Such behavioral modifications as increased food intake and adequate clothing are typical human reactions to overcooling. In contrast, control mechanisms for thermoregulation are primarily structured to protect the body against overheating. This fact becomes readily apparent when one considers that greater variations in core tem-

perature (T_c) than $\pm4°C$ are associated with reduced physiologic and psychologic performance, whereas deviations of about $+6°C$ or $-12°C$ from $37°C$ (normal T_c) are usually lethal. Combined exercise and heat stress can result in greater strain on the thermoregulatory system than either stress alone, whereas exercise stress may counteract cold stress and result in less overcooling. Fortunately, the human thermoregulatory system has a remarkable ability to maintain physiologic control through appropriate adjustments over an extremely wide range of different heat productions, heat losses, and environmental temperatures.

Physical exercise dramatically alters the rate of metabolic energy (heat) production (M), with resultant physiologic adjustments for heat loss. During exercise, T_c initially increases rapidly and then increases at a reduced rate until heat loss equals heat production and essentially steady-state values are achieved (1). The T_c increase represents storage of metabolic heat produced as a byproduct of muscle contraction. At the onset of exercise, metabolic rate increases immediately, while thermoregulatory responses for heat loss respond more slowly. The classic energy balance equation for evaluating heat gain or heat loss from the body is $S = M - (\pm W) + Q_s \pm K \pm (R + C) - E$, in which S = rate of body heat storage; M = rate of metabolic energy (heat) production estimated from measured oxygen uptake ($\dot{V}O_2$); W = mechanical work, either

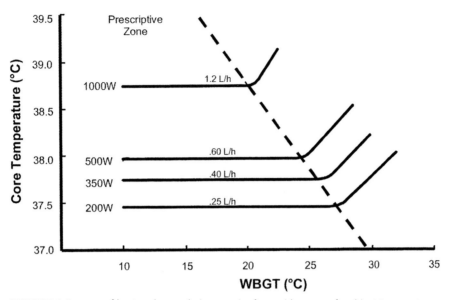

FIGURE 7-1 Avenues of heat exchange during exercise for a wide range of ambient temperatures. (Modified from Sawka MN, Wenger CB, Pandolf KB. Thermoregulatory responses to acute exercise-heat stress and heat acclimation. In: Fregly MJ, Blatteis CM, eds. Handbook of Physiology, section 4, environmental physiology. New York, Oxford University Press, 1996:157–185.)

concentric (positive) or eccentric (negative) exercise; Q_s = rate of solar radiative energy absorbed (differentiates between heat loss in sunlight and that lost from skin in an environment without solar flux); K = rate of conduction (important only when in direct contact with an object, e.g., clothing, or a substance, e.g., water); R + C = rate of radiant and convective energy exchanges; and E = rate of evaporative loss. The three major physical avenues of heat loss are radiation, convection, and evaporation. The thermoregulatory effector responses that enable dry (radiative and convective) and evaporative heat loss increase in proportion to the rate of heat production. Eventually, these mechanisms increase heat loss sufficiently to balance metabolic heat production, allowing a steady-state T_c to be achieved, so long as the environment allows.

Steady-state T_c increases in proportion to metabolic rate during exercise (2–5). Although this relationship between metabolic rate and T_c is adequate for a given person, it does not always hold for comparisons among different people. The use of relative intensity ($\%\dot{V}O_{2max}$), rather than absolute metabolic rate (absolute intensity), removes most of the intersubject variability for the T_c elevation during exercise (6,7). Therefore, relative exercise intensity is an important factor when prescribing exercise. Figure 7-1 illustrates that the magnitude of T_c increase during steady-state exercise at low (200 W) to very high (1000 W) metabolic rates is often independent of a wide range of environments (with low humidity) (1,2). This is true, however, only within a climatic "prescriptive zone" (2) that narrows as metabolic rate increases.

Ultimately, the combination of the level of exercise and the particular environmental conditions determines the rate of sweat production and dictates the required rate of evaporative cooling (E_{req}). The maximal evaporative capacity of the environment (E_{max}), however, determines the maximal possible evaporative loss. Figure 7-2 illustrates heat exchange data during exercise ($\sim$650 W) in a broad range of climatic conditions (5 to 36°C dry bulb temperatures with low relative humidity, % rh) (1,8). The difference between metabolic rate and total heat loss represents the energy used for mechanical work and heat storage. The relative contributions of dry and evaporative heat exchange to total heat loss, however, vary with climatic conditions.

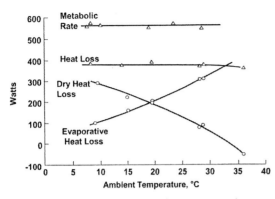

FIGURE 7-2 T_c response and required sweating rates for exercise in relation to metabolic rate and environment (Modified from Sawka MN, Wenger CB, Pandolf KB. Thermoregulatory responses to acute exercise-heat stress and heat acclimation. In: Fregly MJ, Blatteis CM, eds. Handbook of Physiology, section 4, environmental physiology. New York, Oxford University Press, 1996:157–185.)

As ambient temperature increases, the gradient for dry heat exchange is less and evaporative heat exchange is more important. When ambient temperature equals mean skin temperature ($\overline{T}_{sk}$), evaporative heat exchange accounts for virtually all heat loss. For individuals exercising outdoors, the solar radiant load becomes an important consideration.

It is beyond the scope of this chapter to present a detailed essay on temperature regulation and exercise. The reader is directed to other reviews and books (9–13).

Exposure to High Environmental Temperatures

HUMAN PHYSIOLOGIC RESPONSES TO HEAT

The two physiologic responses primarily concerned with dynamic regulation against overheating are skin blood flow and sweating. The main function of the former is to transport heat from the deep body to the surface. Sweat glands produce and secrete sweat required for evaporative cooling at the skin surface. During exercise, regulation by these systems is increasingly challenged when air temperature (T_a) rises from temperate (~22°C) to hotter conditions.

Metabolic (exercise-induced) and environmental heat stress can result in normal or expected physiologic responses to the particular stress, but may also produce a variety of abnormal heat disorders. Although the primary purpose of this section is not to detail the pathologic manifestations of excessive heat exposure, a few comments on how to prevent these heat disorders are warranted. Exercise-induced heat exhaustion can be minimized by providing proper heat acclimation, by grading the exercise to consider hot climate extremes, and by avoiding sudden postural changes or maintenance of upright static exercise. Heat cramps and salt-depletion heat exhaustion can occur when fluid and electrolyte losses are profound. These disorders are most prevalent in chronically hot climates, particularly when food and water intakes are limited or restricted. Avoid drinking in excess of sweat losses to avoid hyponatremia (14). Fluid needs rarely exceed 8 to 12 L·day^{-1}, even in very hot climates (15,16). Salt tablets should not be used and, if necessary, supplemental sodium can be easily obtained by salting foods (16). Anhidrotic heat exhaustion, which is related to reduced functional sweating, has been linked to such skin disorders as heat rash and sunburn; both disorders have been associated with exercise-heat intolerance, as depicted by elevations in T_c and reductions in performance time (1,17). Heat intolerance was seen with as little as 20% of the body surface involved and persisted up to 3 weeks after the clinical rash had resolved. Pandolf et al. (18) also showed that both sweating sensitivity and sweating rate were reduced by mild sunburn during exercise in a hot/dry environment (49°C, 20% rh). Thus, both of these common hot-weather ailments can significantly impair thermoregulation. Heat rash is prevented by drying the skin when possible and by wearing clean, dry clothing that allows unimpeded evaporation. Sunburn is reduced by wearing proper clothing, by exercising during hours of minimal solar load (before 10 AM or after 4 PM), or by using an appropriate sunscreen. Heat hyperpyrexia and exertional heat injury/heat stroke present dramatic elevations of T_c, usually in the range of 41 to 42°C. The former disorder is usually characterized by lower T_cs in this range, with the individual still capable of sweating. The latter condition presents higher T_cs and generalized anhidrosis. Elevations in T_c, however, may not be causally related to these disorders, because both competitive distance runners and patients with passively induced hyperthermia tolerate T_cs of 41 to 42°C with minimal side effects (19,20). Both heat hyperpyrexia and heat stroke can be prevented by adapting exercise to the climate, by ensuring proper heat acclimation, and most importantly by screening for a past history of heat illness.

THERMOREGULATORY AND CARDIOVASCULAR ADJUSTMENTS TO EXERCISE IN DRY AND HUMID HEAT

Effects of Solar Heat Load

The importance of quantifying the physiologic effects of solar radiation becomes apparent when considering exercise prescriptions for outdoor environments. The effect of simulated solar heat load in hot/dry (40°C, 32% rh) and hot/wet (35°C, 75% rh) environments has been reported for heat-acclimated men while walking at 1.34 m·sec^{-1} (0 and 5% grade) (21). Evaluation of solar load by copper manikin predicted the delivery of an effective 300 W (seminude) and 120 W (clothed) of radiant heat load to the skin. Individuals were evaluated with or without this solar load while wearing shorts, socks, and running shoes (seminude) or a slightly heavier clothing ensemble. After 100 min of exercise, physiologic responses were greater while exercising with solar load (range of mean differences; heart rate (HR), 22–42 beats·min^{-1}; rectal temperature (ΔT_{re}), 0.45–1.48°C; sweat rate ($\dot{m}_{sw}$), 145–314 g·m^{-2}·h^{-1}. Nielsen et al. (22) measured net solar heat gain (short- and long-wave radiation gains − long wave radiation losses) during 2 hours of light (92 W) cycle ergometer exercise performed outdoors between July and September during maximal solar zenith angle hours (10 AM to 4 PM). With temperate climates (21–25°C), direct solar heat amounted to ~22% of the total heat load (22). Taken together, these studies suggest the need for altering exercise prescriptions during outdoor activity, especially on hot, clear days.

Role of Cardiorespiratory Training and Fitness

The importance of training and cardiorespiratory fitness on physiologic responses to exercise in the heat and on the rate of heat acclimation is controversial, but there are several detailed reviews (23–25). Although most authors agree that training in a cool environment improves exercise-heat tolerance, the degree of improvement is controversial. To achieve optimal gains, researchers suggest using intensive interval or continuous training at an intensity >50% $\dot{V}O_{2max}$ (26–29). Improvement in heat tolerance produced by mild-to-moderate training at <50% $\dot{V}O_{2max}$ is questionable (30). It seems that training must exceed 1 week, but the best improvement reportedly occurs after 8 to 12 weeks (26,27). It seems that training should increase $\dot{V}O_{2max}$ by 15 to 20% to improve tolerance. Improvement in exercise-heat tolerance after appropriate training appears to apply to both dry and wet heat. Persons with high $\dot{V}O_{2max}$ values and such athletes as marathoners (whose endurance training causes high levels of body hyperthermia and regulatory sweating) seem to be at an advantage.

Another debatable issue is whether $\dot{V}O_{2max}$ is related to improved exercise-heat tolerance or to a faster rate of heat acclimation. Two authors using different climates independently report that an individual's $\dot{V}O_{2max}$ accounts for 42 to 46% of the variability that determines T_c level during 3 hours of exercise in the heat of the acclimation day for a plateau in T_c (31,32). Other authors report insignificant relationships (33–35). Most studies in which a lack of relationship was shown, however, evaluated relatively few subjects or homogeneously fit subjects. The $\dot{V}O_{2max}$, per se, may not be important, but the physiologic adaptations associated with various fitness levels may play a vital role in determining exercise-heat tolerance. Therefore, improved aerobic fitness by endurance training is associated with significant elevations in T_c during training to improve exercise-heat tolerance (23). Athletes training in cold water have lower heat tolerance than other athletes of similar fitness (27) or experience no thermoregulatory improvement during exercise-heat stress despite significant (15%) training improvement in $\dot{V}O_{2max}$ (36). Thus, training that improves fitness without substantial elevations in T_c and sweating may not improve heat tolerance.

Advantages of Heat Acclimation

Repeated exercise-heat exposure results in a gradual acclimation with improved exercise-heat tolerance (37). The physiologic improvements seen during the first 4 days are dramatic, and acclimation is virtually complete after about 10 days. During acclimation, the major physiologic changes are an earlier onset and increased rate of sweating, lowered HR, and lowered internal body temperature during exercise in the heat (38). These changes result from many potential mechanisms, including improved sweating, more total body water and plasma volume, higher venous tone from cutaneous and noncutaneous beds, increased activity of the adrenopituitary system, and lowered metabolic demands from repeated exposures (38). No single cause explains the adaptive process, as acclimation probably results from the interplay of many mechanisms.

The full development of exercise-heat acclimation need not involve daily 24-hour exposure. A continuous, daily 100-min exposure can produce an optimal response (1,38). The acclimation response is somewhat specific to the particular climatic condition and exercise intensity. It appears to be well retained for 2 weeks after the last heat exposure but is rapidly lost during the next 2 weeks (1,38). Some authors report greater retention of acclimation benefits in physically trained persons than in sedentary individuals (31,38).

Clothing Interaction

During exercise in the heat, black clothing and possibly other dark colors are usually associated with a greater solar radiative absorption than white or lighter colors. Generally, clothing serves as a physical barrier that reduces heat exchange by radiation and convection and simultaneously lowers the maximal evaporative exchange to the environment. The more impermeable the clothing (e.g., a sweat suit or rubberized suit), the greater the reduction in evaporative heat loss and the associated rise in cardiovascular and thermoregulatory strain. For comfort, cotton clothing is generally more effective than polyester during exercise in the heat. In hot/wet environments, when T_a is less than $\overline{T}_{sk}$, exercising individuals should wear the least amount of clothing possible. When T_a exceeds $\overline{T}_{sk}$, additional clothing may protect from the ambient heat load but will interfere more with body heat loss. It is advisable to wear loose-fitting clothing that allows greater airflow between skin and the environment, with resultant greater evaporative cooling. In hot/wet or hot/dry environments, a thin layer of white cloth-

ing markedly reduces the solar heat load and should be worn when exercising under the sun. Associated concepts have been recently reviewed in detail elsewhere (39).

IMPACT OF HEAT ON EXERCISE TESTING AND EXERCISE PRESCRIPTION

Sports and occupational medicine communities commonly use wet bulb globe temperature (WBGT) as an empirical index to quantify climatic heat stress (40–42). It was originally developed for light-intensity exercise (45). Outdoor WBGT = 0.7 natural wet bulb + 0.2 black globe + 0.1 dry bulb; indoor WBGT = 0.7 natural wet bulb + 0.3 black globe. WBGT is used to decide the permitted physical activity level and strategies to minimize risk of heat injury. High WBGT values can be achieved by high humidity (43), as reflected in high wet bulb temperature, or through high air (dry bulb) temperature and solar load (44), as reflected in black globe temperature.

The American College of Sports Medicine (ACSM) position stand on preventing thermal injuries during distance running is based in part on the WBGT, which may also be adaptable for exercise testing and prescription (46). With a WBGT >28°C (82°F), the ACSM suggests that prolonged exercise be curtailed or rescheduled until a lower WBGT is prevalent. The ACSM proposes posting large signs to alert individuals of the existing risk of thermal stress using four categories. Very high risk is associated with a WBGT >28°C (82°F), high risk is 23 to 28°C (73 to 82°F), moderate risk is 18 to 20°C (65 to 73°F), and low risk is <18°C (65°F) (46). These WBGT values are representative for persons in running shorts, shoes, and a T-shirt. However, because WBGT does not consider clothing or exercise intensity (metabolic rate), it cannot predict heat exchange with the environment (40). Therefore, different clothing systems necessitate further adjustments in the WBGT values associated with each level of risk. Finally, the ACSM recommends that when environmental heat stress is prevalent, all exercise should begin in the early morning (before 8 AM) or in the evening (after 6 PM) to lessen the effects of solar load and high temperatures.

Exercise Performance

The exercise prescription often uses a target HR that is within "safe" limits to provide a beneficial training stimulus. Heat stress increases HR independently as a result of increased skin blood flow and volume, reduced cardiac filling (lower end-diastolic volume), and temperature effects on pacemaker cells (38). During submaximal exercise in the heat, cardiac output ($\dot{Q}$) can be higher, the same, or lower than in temperate conditions. At very low exercise intensities (<20% aerobic power), $\dot{Q}$ is elevated to increase skin blood flow. With high-intensity (>70% aerobic power) or prolonged exercise, $\dot{Q}$ cannot typically be sustained, despite significant tachycardia, because blood is displaced to the skin, with a resultant drop in venous return (12). However, $\dot{Q}$ may increase under the same circumstances in highly fit athletes who can maintain stroke volume at an increased HR (47).

In young male subjects after 30 min of moderate exercise (40% $\dot{V}O_{2max}$), HR increases predictably ~1 beat·min^{-1} for each 1°C increase in T_a (dry heat) above temperate levels (24 vs. 44, 55°C) (48). Recently, more quantitative predictions of equilibrium exercise HR response were made for typical hot/dry (40°C, 20% rh) and hot/humid (35°C, 75% rh) environments in contrast to a temperate (21°C, 50% rh) environment (49–51). It was assumed that the subject weighed 70 kg, wore shorts and a T-shirt, exercised at a high metabolic rate (700 W), and was not heat acclimated. Compared with values in a temperate climate, HR was 30 beats·min^{-1} higher (~1.5 beats·min^{-1} per 1°C rise in T_a) in the hot/dry and 50 beats·min^{-1} higher (~3.5 beats·min^{-1} per 1°C rise in T_a) in the hot/wet climate. Thus, whereas adjustments are needed in dry climates, particular concern should be given to the target HR in humid climates. These prediction equations should be used to *individually* adjust the exercise prescription target HR when considering the particular environmental conditions, exercise intensity, and clothing interactions (49,50). A mathematical model based on the above prediction equations has been developed to prognosticate human performance in the heat and may be useful to establish exercise prescrip-

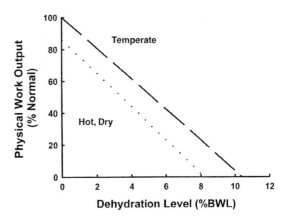

FIGURE 7-3 Effects of air temperature and dehydration on submaximal work performance. (Modified from Sawka MN, Young AJ. Physical exercise in hot and cold climates. In: Garrett WE, Kirkendall DT, eds. Exercise and Sport Science. Philadelphia: Lippincott Williams & Wilkins, 2000:385–400.)

tions (52). This prediction model calculates sustainable exercise–rest cycles, maximal single exercise time (if appropriate), and associated water requirements. Target HR responses should be adjusted and reevaluated periodically to consider seasonal effects.

Figure 7-3 provides a literature compilation regarding the effects of climatic heat stress (moderate-to-high risk categories) and dehydration on aerobic exercise capabilities (13). This analysis is based on highly motivated and heat-acclimated persons. Note that heat stress reduces physical exercise (submaximal) capabilities by ~20% of that under temperate environmental conditions. The combination of heat stress and moderate (4% body weight) dehydration can reduce work capabilities by ~50% of what is expected for fully hydrated individuals in temperate conditions (13). Mechanisms that explain this observation include increased cardiovascular strain and psychologic factors that independently or in combination diminish the will to exercise (13). When physical activity is expected in the heat, especially on a clear day (solar load) or under humid conditions, reduced exercise intensity and target HR are essential. The impact of dehydration alone on exercise testing and prescription is discussed below, along with recommendations for fluid replacement.

Special Populations

Heat tolerance is generally reduced in older individuals, and cardiovascular strain is greater because of reduced fitness and the inability to partition and regulate blood flow effectively (53). While hot environments predictably increase cardiovascular strain, as measured by changes in HR, these changes are not necessarily associated with pathologic outcomes in persons with compromised cardiovascular health. Physiologic responses to 30 min of static–dynamic work (shoveling) were compared in 10 men with stable ischemic heart disease in warm (29°C), temperate (24°C) and cold (−8°C) environments (54). While HR was higher during warm weather, no subject reported angina, and no abnormal ST-segment changes were observed during any trial. Similarly, Sheldahl et al. (55) reported higher HR without myocardial ischemia or reduced ejection fraction in coronary heart disease (CHD) patients (≥6 weeks post-cardiac event) after 60 min of cycling exercise in warm (30°C) conditions than in temperate (22°C) conditions. While these observations provide valuable insight for exercise prescription, when the level of environmental stress necessitates precaution during exercise for healthy populations, exercise for special populations should also be curtailed.

Exposure to Low Environmental Temperatures

HUMAN PHYSIOLOGIC RESPONSES TO COLD

Humans generally rely on behavioral strategies (e.g., clothing, shelter) for protection from cold. When behavioral thermoregulation provides inadequate protection, physiologic defenses to combat cold are elicited in the form of alterations in peripheral circulation that reduce heat loss and increase heat production (56). The initial response to cold stress is peripheral vasoconstriction to reduce heat loss from the deep body to the periphery. The next major response involves greater skeletal muscle activity, or shivering, which increases metabolic heat production (3–4 times the resting level) (13). These physiologic responses may influence or be influenced by the physiologic responses to exercise (13,57), which easily results in a 10-fold increase in heat production and can effectively counteract moderate cold stress.

A variety of factors can alter cold tolerance (56). Body size and shape alter heat loss to the environment. For a given cold stress, smaller persons (children and women) need a relatively greater heat production to maintain thermal equilibrium because of their larger surface area-to-mass ratios (58). Similarly, shorter persons who weigh the same as taller persons lose less heat, principally because they have less exposed surface area (shorter arms, legs, and trunk). Thickness of subcutaneous fat deposits is also important. Generally, subcutaneous fat is an effective insulator, with greater amounts being negatively related to the fall in T_{sk} or T_c (56). The advantages of increased subcutaneous fat are apparent for all types of cold exposure, but particularly cold water immersion (58). Skeletal muscle mass is another important factor because it can generate heat via voluntary (exercise) or involuntary (shivering) contraction. Respiratory heat and water loss can be substantial during exercise in the cold. Most of the loss occurs as evaporation to humidify the very dry cold air that is inhaled. Upper-airway temperatures may fall substantially during exercise if extremely cold air is breathed, but the lower respiratory tract and deep body temperatures are unaffected (59).

Most body heat loss in cold environments occurs via conductive (K) and convective (C) mechanisms. When ambient temperature is colder than body temperature, the resulting thermal gradient favors body heat loss. While the pathophysiology of cold injury is not a major consideration of this chapter, a few comments on preventing cold disorders during exercise are warranted. Cold disorders can be categorized by nonfreezing (muscle cramps, chilblains, and immersion/trench hand or foot) or freezing (frostnip and frostbite) cold injuries and whole body hypothermia. A major consideration in prevention is an adequate definition of the cold stress (i.e., the particular ambient temperature and wind velocity), as well as the presence of sweat on the skin or in the clothing. For maximal protection, clothing should be layered and thick and *must* be kept dry. To prevent cold injuries, heat supply to the periphery must be enhanced. Auxiliary heating of the extremities through battery-charged gloves and socks should help maintain safe temperatures. Alcoholic drinks produce peripheral vasodilation and therefore promote heat loss, enhancing the risk of hypothermia (60). Gradual acclimation to cold over 2 to 3 weeks may induce peripheral changes that help the individual to resist local cold injury (56). Because exercisers seldom spend much time outdoors and because exercise increases heat production, the risk of whole body hypothermia is minimal, provided the individual does not stay in the cold in a sweat-soaked or rain-soaked state.

CARDIOVASCULAR AND THERMOREGULATORY RESPONSES TO EXERCISE IN THE COLD

Cooling the body can result in marked systemic alterations (56). The most apparent alteration is perhaps peripheral vasoconstriction, which leads to a reduction in local circulation and reduced perfusion of various vascular beds, producing vascular stasis and local tissue anoxia. There is an initial paradoxical increase in HR, pulmonary ventilation, and mean arterial pressure. As deep body temperature drops, however, HR, ventilation, and blood pressure (BP) fall. Neurohumoral activation leads to release of the anterior pituitary hormones and catecholamines to conserve body heat. Other than physical exercise, however, the major reflex response for increased heat production involves higher muscle tone and shivering. In certain circumstances, periodic oscillations in $\overline{T}_{sk}$ occur reflecting transient changes in blood flow to superficial capillaries of the limbs (cold-induced vasodilation) (61). This nervous reflex appears to act as a primary mechanism to protect peripheral tissue from freezing injury or to maintain dexterity.

Mild-to-moderate cold stress of a less prolonged nature (~1 hour) is more likely to be encountered by the exerciser than is prolonged severe cold stress. Even less severe cold stress alters cardiovascular performance and produces circulatory changes that augment myocardial oxygen requirements, thus placing some individuals at added risk. For instance, mild cold stress (15°C) during rest and light exercise causes a consistently higher total peripheral resistance (TPR), higher systemic arterial pressure, and greater left ventricular work in individuals with and without CHD (62). This higher TPR occurs in the absence of reflex bradycardia and $\dot{Q}$ is not altered by the cold. Exposure of the face to a moderate cold stress (4°C) has been associ-

ated with bradycardia, resulting from a vagal reflex through trigeminal nerve stimulation (63). Sympathetic nervous system stimulation produces a rise in systolic (SBP) and diastolic BP (DBP). Thus, facial exposure to cold winds and whole body exposure might precipitate angina in an individual with CHD. Exercise would only accentuate this risk by demanding further increases in left ventricular work and myocardial oxygen demand.

COLD ACCLIMATION AND ADAPTIVE HABITUATION

Compared with chronic heat stress, physiologic adjustments to chronic cold exposure are less pronounced, slower to develop, and less practical in terms of relieving thermal strain and preventing cold injury. Cold acclimatization or acclimation must be differentiated from adaptation or habituation. Acclimatization and acclimation are functional alterations established over days or weeks in response, respectively, to either complex, natural environmental factors or artificially controlled, usually simple environmental factors (64). In contrast, adaptation suggests physiologic changes that develop over generations and are genetically transmitted to help promote survival in hostile environments (64). Habituation to cold stress seems to be associated more with nervous system regulation. Physiologic adjustments during human adaptation or acclimation to cold have been reviewed elsewhere (56).

Human Acclimation and Adaptive Habituation to Cold

Human thermoregulatory adaptations to chronic cold exposure are more modest and less understood than adaptations to chronic heat (56). Where chronic heat exposure induces a fairly uniform pattern of adjustments, chronic cold exposure induces three different patterns of adaptation. Habituation is characterized by blunted physiologic responses during cold exposure. Metabolic adaptations are characterized by enhanced thermogenic responses, and insulative adaptations are characterized by enhanced body heat conservation (56).

Brief, intermittent cold exposures can induce habituation of shivering and vasoconstrictor responses to cold, even when very limited body surface areas

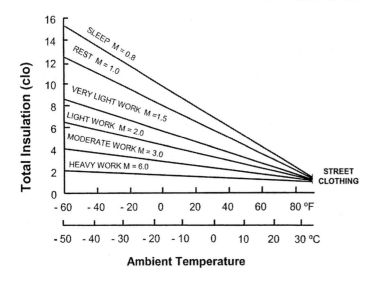

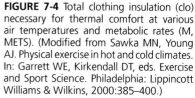

FIGURE 7-4 Total clothing insulation (clo) necessary for thermal comfort at various air temperatures and metabolic rates (M, METS). (Modified from Sawka MN, Young AJ. Physical exercise in hot and cold climates. In: Garrett WE, Kirkendall DT, eds. Exercise and Sport Science. Philadelphia: Lippincott Williams & Wilkins, 2000:385–400.)

are exposed and whole body heat losses are probably negligible (56). More pronounced physiologic adjustments are observed only when repeated cold exposure causes significant body heat loss, such as insulative adjustments in response to repeated cold exposure that are too severe to be offset by increased metabolic heat production (i.e., when cold causes a significant drop in T_c) (56). The possibility that an enhanced thermogenic capability can develop in humans in response to chronic cold cannot be dismissed. It is tempting to speculate that the stimulus for this metabolic pattern of cold adaptation is prolonged periods in which significant body heat loss is experienced, but under conditions in which body heat production increased sufficiently to prevent a significant decline in deep body temperature. This speculation is not unjustified, since the metabolic pattern of cold adjustments has only been reported in studies in which acclimatization or acclimation was induced by exposure to such conditions, i.e., prolonged exposure to moderately cold air (56).

Clothing Interaction

Using proper clothing should be stressed when prescribing exercise in cold air. Clothing should be thick and multilayered, while providing adequate ventilation to keep it dry. All areas of the body (particularly face, ears, neck, hands, and feet) should be covered adequately and kept warm. However, many outdoor winter sports and recreational activities require participants to disregard heavy insulative garments in favor of less restrictive clothing for freedom of motion. Clothing insulation needed for warmth and comfort in cold environments is much higher during rest and light activity than during strenuous activity (Fig. 7-4) (13). The solution is to dress in multiple clothing layers that allow insulation to be adjusted according to activity level, such that heat storage and sweating can be minimized. When exercise is stopped, any accumulation of sweat in clothing will compromise its insulative value and facilitate heat loss by conduction, convection, and evaporation. By the same token, rain or accidental immersion will drastically magnify these effects via disproportional moisture absorption and greater body surface area contact with wet clothing. Proper cold weather clothing should be wind resistant, but must provide adequate ventilation to reduce sweat accumulation. Proper protection of the face and extremities may be of greater concern.

IMPACT OF COLD ON EXERCISE TESTING AND EXERCISE PRESCRIPTION

Although exercise increases metabolic heat production, it also facilitates heat loss by convective heat transfer from the body core to the skin. When low ambient temperatures are combined with considerable wind speeds, convective heat losses become magnified, especially when exercise intensity is reduced because of fatigue, and the risk of hypothermia can occur in environmental temperatures of 10 to 12°C WBGT (50–54°F) (9,46). In fact, it is more common to see exhaustive collapse in distance runners suffering from hypothermia than from hyperthermia (65). The ACSM recommends canceling outdoor distance running events when air temperature is below −20°C (−4°F) (46).

While no single cold stress index integrates all the effects of environment on heat loss, the wind chill index (WCI) is widely accepted and used (66). The WCI estimates the environmental cooling rate from the combined effects of the wind and air temperature and is useful for guiding decisions about conducting or canceling outdoor activities, although some limitations exist (see ref. 67 for review). Water has a much higher thermal capacity than air, and the cooling power of the ambient environment is greatly enhanced under cold/wet conditions. Thus, even with relatively mild water temperatures, swimmers and outdoorsmen who wade streams can lose considerable body heat. Special precautions should therefore be used for those at risk, especially those who use swimming as a form of exercise. Swimming in unheated or improperly heated pools and in the ocean (50% of which is <20°C) should be approached with extreme caution.

Exercise Performance and Special Populations

Although extremely cold temperatures can affect muscle function and reduce work performance (57), sustained exercise generally results in adequate heat production and maintenance of muscle temperature. Cutaneous cold receptor stimulation can, however, lead to increased TPR, arterial pressure, myocardial contractility, and cardiac work during rest or exercise (62,68,69). These altered responses were observed even during very mild cold stress (~15°C) (62). Even localized facial exposure to moderate cold (4°C) has been associated with vagally mediated reflex bradycardia and sympathetically increased SBP and DBP (63). Thus, localized and more total body cold strain could lower the threshold and provoke an attack of angina pectoris in individuals with CHD because of an increase in TPR and arterial pressure and the consequent augmentation of myocardial oxygen demands. There is no evidence that coronary vasoconstriction per se contributes to developing myocardial hypoxia

during cold stress. During cold exposure, exercise could further increase the work of the heart through added myocardial oxygen requirements. Thus, an individual with CHD is at even greater risk because of far less functional myocardial reserve capacity. The importance of these observations for cold weather exercise prescription is only precautionary for compromised, but low-risk populations. While information is limited, one study of low-risk patients with stable ischemic heart disease reported higher SBP and DBP responses to 30 min of static–dynamic exercise in a cold environment (−8°C) than to the same activity in warmer (24–29°C) environments (54). This finding is consistent with greater TPR and potentially greater left ventricular work, but no adverse ST-segment changes (or any other ECG symptomatology) were observed.

A screening test for individual cold sensitivity may become necessary if it is suspected that a high-risk individual will be exposed to even mild cold stress (~15°C or less). The cold pressor test, which was designed to detect persons who were potentially hypertensive, might be used effectively to classify individuals in terms of reactivity to a cold stimulus (70,71). During immersion of the hand in cold water, sympathetic activity can be graded by the rise in SBP and DBP, elevation of HR, and degree of systemic vasoconstriction, as implied by the reduction in $\bar{T}_{sk}$ of the immersed hand. Extreme reactivity would contraindicate exercising in the cold for those with signs of CHD. As an additional caveat, long-term breathing of cold air can also increase respiratory passage secretions and decrease mucociliary clearance (72), potentially producing airway congestion, impairing pulmonary mechanics, and increasing the difficulty of any given exercise bout.

Exposure to Terrestrial Altitude

SHORT- AND LONG-TERM PHYSIOLOGIC ADAPTATIONS TO ALTITUDE EXPOSURE

Acute and Subacute Exposure to High Altitude

The most prominent adaptation to acute altitude exposure is an increased pulmonary ventilation ($\dot{V}_E$) at any given exercise $\dot{V}O_2$ (73,74). Hyperpnea results in an elevated respiratory exchange ratio (R), reflecting increased CO_2 elimination from the lungs, and an associated rise in blood pH (73). In contrast to long-term altitude exposure, increased $\dot{Q}$ is noted during the first few days at altitude and is attributed mainly to a higher HR (74–76). These cardiopulmonary alterations are, in part, an attempt to enhance oxygen transport and delivery and thus help compensate for the lower oxygen pressure. These compensatory mechanisms are not adequate, however, and exercise performance is usually severely limited relative to the other two adaptive stages. Other factors related to performance alterations are uncompensated alkalosis, altered endocrine function, body fluid changes, and disturbed metabolic function (73). During short-term exposure, mountain sickness can develop with such symptoms as headache, lethargy, drowsiness, fatigue, sleep disturbances, loss of appetite, digestive disorders, and, less frequently, nausea and vomiting (75,77). A more serious but rare disorder is high altitude pulmonary edema, associated with fluid accumulation in the lungs (75,77).

The functional changes observed during subacute altitude exposure are also transient (74). The subacute stage is associated with adaptations that increase the oxygen-carrying capacity of the blood. Arterial oxygen content is restored (increased hematocrit) to near sea level values secondary to a decreased plasma volume (73–76,78,79). Although this hemoconcentration may increase blood oxygen content, these alterations are also associated with small decreases in convective blood flow secondary to increased blood viscosity (73,75,76). The second major change seen involves decreased submaximal and maximal $\dot{Q}$, attributable to a reduction in SV (74), probably as a result of decreased plasma volume and compromised ventricular filling (80). A further transient increase in $\dot{V}_E$ (particularly at heavier exercise intensities) is seen during this adaptive stage and is referred to as *ventilatory acclimatization* (73,76,79). At a constant $\dot{V}O_2$, $\dot{V}_E$ at altitude may increase by nearly 100%.

Long-Term Exposure to High Altitude

Although the functional alterations seen during long-term exposure (2–3 weeks) are similar to those seen during subacute adaptation, Hannon and Vogel state that these functional alterations differ in four major respects (74). Long-term adaptations

to altitude develop more slowly, are not transient, are probably associated with all system components, and produce functional system capabilities that exceed those seen with subacute adaptation (74).

Although initiated during the acute adaptive stage, the effects of increased erythropoiesis become most pronounced during the chronic stage (78). While increasing hemoglobin content, the greater number of circulating red blood cells further decreases blood flow and increases blood viscosity. Thus, cardiac work may be increased at any given $\dot{Q}$ (73). Biochemical and histologic changes become more apparent after long-term exposure, which may facilitate the increase of either oxygen conductance or transport or both. For example, compared with the other two adaptive stages, there is a more pronounced capillary density, an increased myoglobin content in the skeletal muscles, and other modifications of enzymatic activity that may facilitate oxygen transport after long-term exposure to hypoxia (81). These functional alterations require different time periods for complete long-term adaptation and may necessitate significantly longer time periods when exercise responses are considered (74).

IMPACT OF ALTITUDE ON EXERCISE TESTING AND EXERCISE PRESCRIPTION

Maximal Exercise Performance

Many studies show a progressive reduction in $\dot{V}O_{2max}$ with increasing altitude. Fulco et al. (82) reported this relationship for altitudes from 580 to 8848 m; a slightly modified version is illustrated in Figure 7-5. The regression line in Figure 7-5 predicts a 5 to 10% decline in $\dot{V}O_{2max}$ for every 1000 m of ascent (76), although wide variability exists due to multiple factors, and disproportionately larger decrements may be observed above 6300 m (82). Smaller (1–7%) reductions in $\dot{V}O_{2max}$ are reported for well-conditioned athletes beginning at 350 to 580 m (82,83). The decrement in $\dot{V}O_{2max}$ is larger for highly fit men than for less fit men, presumably due to inherent pulmonary gas exchange limitations ($\dot{V}_A/\dot{Q}$ mismatch; $\dot{V}_A$-alveolar ventilation) exacerbated by hypoxia (82). This hypothesis is consistent with the $\dot{V}_A/\dot{Q}$ mismatch and reduced arterial oxygen saturation ($\%SaO_2$) observed for athletes with

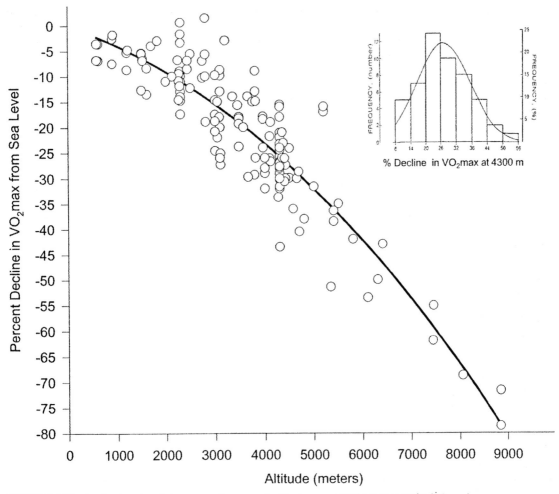

FIGURE 7-5 Effects of reduced partial pressure of oxygen at altitude on maximal oxygen uptake ($\dot{V}O_{2max}$) when expressed as a percentage of $\dot{V}O_{2max}$ at sea level. (Modified from Fulco CS, Rock PB, Cymerman A. Maximal and submaximal exercise performance at altitude. Aviat Space Environ Med 1998;69:793–801.) *Inset:* Distribution of decrement in percentage $\dot{V}O_{2max}$ at 4300 m (Modified from Young AJ, Cymerman A, Burse RL. The influence of cardiorespiratory fitness on the decrement in maximal aerobic power at high altitude. Eur J Appl Physiol 1985;54:12–15.)

elite $\dot{V}O_{2max}$ values (84,85). Although reportedly (86) sea level $\dot{V}O_{2max}$ is a poor predictor of $\dot{V}O_{2max}$ decline at altitude (4300 m), this is probably explained by the fact that only subjects with subelite $\dot{V}O_{2max}$ values were studied. These data illustrate that the decline in $\dot{V}O_{2max}$ at 4300 m is normally distributed for a range of fitness abilities usually encountered in an exercise testing arena (36–60 mL·kg^{-1}·min^{-1}) (86). Any decrease in $\dot{V}O_{2max}$

will persist at a given altitude, provided the level of cardiorespiratory physical fitness is not altered. Upon return from higher altitude, $\dot{V}O_{2max}$ returns to the sea level value so long as muscle mass is maintained (87).

The greatest reduction in $\dot{V}O_{2max}$ usually occurs during the first few days of altitude exposure, with a small but significant increase seen with persistent residence (76,81). The early reduction is generally attributed to the lowered arterial oxygen content and the persistent decrease to a reduction in $\dot{Q}_{max}$ (81,88). Reduced $\dot{Q}_{max}$ results from a decrease in SV combined with a lower maximal HR (89). Maintenance of plasma volume at altitude may maintain ventricular filling pressure and prevent a decrease in SV (90,91). Increased vagal tone (90,92) and reduced cardiac β-receptor responsiveness (81,93) have been implicated in the lower maximal HR. The reductions in $\dot{V}O_{2max}$ and $\dot{Q}_{max}$ at 4300 m are not equal (94), suggesting the involvement of such factors as ventilatory, hemodynamic, and metabolic changes that together decrease $\dot{V}O_{2max}$. Reviews of the cardiovascular and peripheral adaptations to exercise at high altitude are found elsewhere (76, 81).

Submaximal Exercise Performance

For any given power output (PO) at sea level, $\dot{V}O_2$ is similar at altitude (95). But because submaximal exercise performance is closely tied to $\dot{V}O_{2max}$, any PO corresponds to a greater relative exercise intensity at altitude. Therefore, at the same absolute sea level PO, submaximal exercise performance is reduced at high altitude. For events lasting 20 to 30 min and 2 to 3 hours at sea level, Fulco et al. (82) report that absolute performances at 2000 m altitude would be impaired by 5% and 10 to 15%, respectively, i.e., performance decrements are proportional to altitude and exercise duration (82). Limitations are more profound for short- than long-term altitude exposure (96). Whereas the limitations imposed by the cardiovascular system primarily alter maximal exercise responses at altitude, differences in the use rate of glycogen stores and anaerobic metabolism influence submaximal exercise responses during short- and long-term altitude exposure (81). The physiologic alterations at altitude that help to improve tissue oxygen delivery when oxygen availability is reduced may be classified into three separate stages: acute, subacute, and chronic adaptation. Acute adaptation occurs during the first 72 hours of exposure; subacute adaptations are seen over the next 10 to 11 days; and chronic adaptations are observed after 2 weeks of exposure. Although the adaptations are presented as three distinct stages, they really represent a continuum of change with considerable individual overlap and variability.

Submaximal and maximal exercise performance is reduced at altitude (2000–5000 m) and an exercise prescription should be adjusted accordingly.

Absolute exercise levels should be reduced 5 to 10% for each 1000 m ascent above sea level if exercise is to be performed at the same relative intensity (81). Using the information in Figure 7-5, many individuals can adjust exercise appropriately when the prescription is based on relative exercise intensity.

Special Populations

Grover implies that as long as persons with cardiovascular disease recognize their limitations and maintain exercise intensity within these limits, cardiac performance will not be compromised (75). According to Levine et al. (97), >5 million people over the age of 60 visit high altitudes annually. Because an aged population is at increased risk for cardiovascular disease, interest in the response of the elderly to hypobaric hypoxia has grown. The clinical responses of 97 older men and women (59–83 years) were studied over 5 days at moderate altitude (2500 m). Although CHD was present in 20% of subjects, no adverse signs or symptoms were observed during casual activity (98). Therefore, persons with asymptomatic cardiovascular disease can safely visit moderate altitudes. Levine et al. (97) studied the response to exercise in 20 veterans (mean age, 68 years) at sea level, 2500 m (acute), and 2500 m (chronic, 5 days). The double product (HR × SBP) that produced 1 mm of ST-segment depression was 5% lower at 2500 m (vs. sea level), but stabilized after 5 days at altitude (97). They concluded that (*a*) performance at altitude was predictable on the basis of sea level performance and (*b*) those with CHD should initially limit activity and allow several days to acclimatize to altitude (97). A study of the effects of moderate altitude on patients with CHD and impaired left ventricular function found that exercise at 2500 m was terminated more often because of dyspnea than at sea level but was otherwise tolerated well and without any adverse events (99).

In contrast, exposure to high altitude places greater demands on the right ventricle of the heart, resulting in increased total cardiac work (i.e., greater coronary blood flow), particularly during exercise (100). Some authors report such ECG disturbances during exercise as atrial and ventricular ectopic beats and prolonged QT interval, as well as diphasic, inverted, or flat T wave and lowered ST segment in nonadapted individuals at altitudes of 3000 to 5000 m (101). These results may have been confounded by the addition of cold stress.

Whether these responses are particularly important and potentially dangerous for persons with CHD may depend on the altitude studied, as well as on the seriousness and stability of the cardiovascular condition. At the very least, persons with advanced or unstable disease should (*a*) limit sojourns to low-moderate altitude near adequate facilities for cardiovascular care, (*b*) ascend to altitude slowly, and (*c*) limit activity to below symptom-limiting sea level intensities (102).

Exposure to Atmospheric Pollutants

Little is known about the effects of single agents or combinations of atmospheric air pollutants on ei-

ther submaximal or maximal exercise performance. Even less is known about the particular concentration levels and critical exposure durations of air pollutants necessary for decrements in exercise performance. Of the air pollutants, only carbon monoxide (CO) has been evaluated with any thoroughness regarding cardiovascular responses to exercise. In healthy individuals, CO does not alter submaximal exercise responses, but slightly reduces maximal exercise performance. Individuals with cardiovascular impairments show marked decreases in submaximal exercise time to angina onset while breathing CO (Table 7-1).

Among the remaining air pollutants evaluated, the photochemical oxidants ozone (O_3), nitrogen dioxide (NO_2), and peroxyacetylnitrate (PAN) and the sulfur oxides, represented by sulfur dioxide

TABLE 7-1 EFFECTS OF AIR POLLUTANTS ON EXERCISE PERFORMANCE OF NORMAL AND CARDIOVASCULAR/PULMONARY-IMPAIRED INDIVIDUALS

Subject Group Air Pollutant •Exercise Intensity	Performance Decrement	No Effect	Selected References
Normal population			
CO			
• Submaximal		X	106, 107
• Maximal	X		109, 110
O_3			
• Submaximal		X	111, 112
• Maximal	?		114, 115
NO_2			
• Submaximal		X	103, 117
• Maximal	?		103
PAN			
• Submaximal		X	106, 116
• Maximal	?		103, 108
PANCO			
• Submaximal		X	106, 116
• Maximal	?		103, 108
SO_2			
• Submaximal	?		103
• Maximal	?		103
Cardiovascular/pulmonary-impaired population[a]			
CO	X		120, 122
O_3	X[b]		103, 123, 124, 125
NO_2	?		103
PAN	?		103, 108
PANCO	?		103, 108
SO_2	?		103

[a]Denotes submaximal exercise effects only.
[b]Applies to pulmonary-impaired (COPD and asthma) populations only.

(SO_2) and PANCO, have no demonstrable cardiovascular effects during submaximal exercise in healthy individuals. There are questionable effects, however, in healthy individuals during maximal exercise and in CHD patients during submaximal exercise. Table 7-1 summarizes the effects of air pollutants on exercise performance for healthy and cardiovascularly impaired individuals. The reader is directed for further information to reviews by Raven (103), Gong and Krishnareddy (104), and Carlisle and Sharp (105).

IMPACT OF ADVERSE AIR QUALITY ON EXERCISE TESTING AND EXERCISE PRESCRIPTION

Healthy Individuals

CO impairs cardiovascular function during exercise by binding with hemoglobin (COHb) to impede oxygen transport. Minimal impairment of cardiorespiratory function and no major performance decrements were observed in healthy individuals at COHb levels below 15% at submaximal exercise intensities of 35 to 60% $\dot{V}O_{2max}$ of short or prolonged duration. HR, however, increased significantly, and added respiratory distress was noted at ~70% $\dot{V}O_{2max}$ (106,107). In contrast, $\dot{V}O_{2max}$ was inversely related to CO concentration (107–110). The critical level at which COHb significantly influences $\dot{V}O_{2max}$ is reportedly 4.3%, but even lower levels (2.7%) have been associated with significant decrements in maximal exercise time (108–110).

The photochemical oxidants seem to cause lung and respiratory tract dysfunction, with questionable effects on the cardiovascular system during exercise (103). Of these, O_3 has been studied most thoroughly. During submaximal exercise (40–70% $\dot{V}O_{2max}$) after or during exposure to 0.37, 0.50, or 0.75 ppm O_3, no significant alterations in submaximal $\dot{V}O_2$, HR, or $\dot{V}_E$ were reported (111,112). Other measurements of pulmonary function, however, were somewhat disturbed (112). No significant differences in pulmonary function were reported between continuous and intermittent submaximal exercise (0.30 ppm O_3)when the total effective dose was the same (113). The limited observations concerning a true decrement in $\dot{V}O_{2max}$ with O_3 exposure are debatable. Some authors report no change in exercise capacity or

$\dot{V}O_{2max}$ while breathing filtered air (FA) or 0.15 or 0.30 ppm O_3 and others show an 11% lower $\dot{V}O_{2max}$ while exposed to 0.75 ppm O_3 than while exposed to FA (114,115). Thus, the critical concentration level for reduced performance is questionable, particularly during maximal exercise. Raven suggests that exercise performance decrements can be predicted as a function of V_E and exposure time (103).

Of the other oxidants, PAN and PANCO have been evaluated during exercise stress (106,108, 116). During submaximal exercise (35% $\dot{V}O_{2max}$) lasting 3 hours while breathing 0.24 ppm PAN or PANCO (50 ppm; COHb, 4–6%), no remarkable changes in cardiorespiratory function were observed in younger (18–30 years) or older (40–55 years) subjects (106,116). Forced vital capacity was reduced 4 to 7% in the younger subjects with PAN, but the significance is questionable. No significant reductions in $\dot{V}O_{2max}$ were reported while breathing these same concentrations of PAN or PANCO (108,110). It seems premature to conclude that PAN or PANCO have no adverse effects on exercise performance, particularly at maximal levels. The concentration of PAN (0.24 ppm) in these few experiments may be at or slightly below the threshold level needed for demonstrable physiologic effects.

Even less is known about exercise-related effects of another oxidant (NO_2) and the sulfur oxides as represented by SO_2. Concentration levels of 0.62 ppm of NO_2 were evaluated after 2 hours of exposure at 40% $\dot{V}O_{2max}$ with no significant alterations in cardiorespiratory function (117). No significant changes were found in pulmonary function of male athletes at 50% $\dot{V}O_{2max}$ during 30 min of exercise (0.18 and 0.30 ppm of NO_2) (118). At low submaximal exercise intensity (only double the resting $\dot{V}_E$), exposure to 0.37 ppm of pure SO_2 did not change ventilatory function after 2 hours of intermittent exercise exposure (119). Maximal exercise responses to these two pollutants have not been reported. A synergistic effect between SO_2 and O_3 has been described in terms of a greater reduction in ventilatory function during exercise, raising the question of possible synergism among other pollutants (119). There is little information concerning the responses to long-term or prolonged exposure (>4 hours) to these pollutants at various concentrations during exercise.

Special Populations

Of the pollutants, only CO has been directly evaluated during exercise in cardiovascularly impaired individuals. It has been suggested that there is a relationship between CO and advanced development of CHD and that CO in the presence of significant CHD hastens myocardial infarction, angina pectoris, or sudden death. In a study of 10 CHD patients, exposure to heavy freeway traffic for 90 min increased COHb to an average of 5.08%, causing a decrease in exercise time to angina onset and significant reductions in SBP and HR at the onset of angina (120). Ischemic ST-segment depressions were noted in 3 of 10 patients while breathing freeway air, in contrast to no abnormalities during freeway driving while breathing compressed, purified air. In two studies, each involving 10 patients with documented angina, exercise angina onset time was determined while breathing 50 ppm of CO (COHb, 2.7%) for 2 hours or 50 ppm of CO (COHb, 2.9%) and 100 ppm of CO (COHb, 4.5%) for 4 hours (121,122). During both studies at either CO concentration, the average exercise times to onset of angina were lower than the values while breathing compressed, purified air. Duration of angina was significantly prolonged after breathing 100 ppm of CO, but not after breathing 50 ppm of CO (121). Generally, deeper and more prolonged ST-segment depressions were noted after breathing CO (121). Thus, CHD patients are at significant risk during exercise at low levels of COHb (2.5–3.0%). Raven concludes that "the cardiac-impaired exercising patient will be placed at increased risk of incurring additional coronary events if ambient levels of CO in the inspired air are capable of causing a rise of blood COHb levels above 1.5 to 2.0%" (103).

One might expect that individuals with cardiovascular or pulmonary disorders would be at risk during exercise while exposed to oxidants and sulfur oxides because of their limited cardiovascular or pulmonary reserve capacities. However, patients with documented CHD exposed to 0.20 or 0.30 ppm of O_3 during 40 min of treadmill exercise were no more susceptible to ozone toxicity than clinically normal persons (123). In contrast, persons performing light exercise with documented chronic obstructive pulmonary disease (COPD) exposed to 0.24 ppm of O_3 or documented asthma at 0.16 ppm

of O_3 demonstrated significant lung dysfunction (124,125).

Submaximal exercise performance of persons without cardiovascular disorders does not appear to be compromised within the limits of the particular concentration levels evaluated for the different air pollutants. At near-maximal or maximal exercise, performance does appear limited for these same people when exposed to the same pollutants. In contrast, individuals with impaired cardiovascular systems are at even greater risk during submaximal exercise and exposure to CO; tissue hypoxia and myocardial ischemia may result from the binding of CO to hemoglobin. Evidence is limited concerning the adverse effects of the oxidants and sulfur oxides on the cardiovascular system of these compromised individuals during exercise. The oxidants (O_3, NO_2, and PAN) and sulfur oxides, which increase airway resistance because of reflex bronchoconstriction, place individuals with lung and respiratory tract disorders such as COPD and asthma at particular risk during exercise. Obviously, individuals with disorders of both the cardiovascular and respiratory systems are at even greater risk during exercise when exposed to these pollutants.

Most studies on exercise performance and air pollutants involve short-term exposure to particular pollutant(s). Little is known about long-term exposure to adverse air quality and the impact on exercise performance. For many air pollutants (e.g., CO), it takes 8 to 12 hours or longer to reach an equilibrium state between the inspired concentration and the level within the body (121). Thus, the cardiovascular or pulmonary burden should be even greater during exercise after prolonged exposure to adverse air quality. The possible synergism between various pollutants (in terms of added cardiorespiratory distress for acute or prolonged exposure) has not been evaluated during exercise and may further tax the cardiac or pulmonary reserves. Given the many unanswered questions concerning adverse air quality and those specifically at risk during exercise, supervising professionals who prescribe/lead exercise programs should act conservatively when this environmental stress is considered (103).

The current primary U.S. government concentration standards for these common atmospheric air pollutants are 9 ppm/8 h and 35 ppm/1 h of CO exposure; 0.12 ppm/1 h of O_3 exposure; 0.05 ppm/

1 year of NO_2 exposure; 0.14 ppm/24 h of SO_2 exposure, and 150 $\mu g/m^3$/24 h of particulate matter exposure (104). Exercise should not be done outdoors by those with cardiovascular or respiratory disorders when these first-alert levels of adverse air quality are reported (103). As a general precaution for greatly industrialized or densely populated urban areas, exercise prescriptions for impaired individuals should focus on indoor exercise.

Exposure to Various Interstressors

Of the various environmental stressors discussed in this chapter, only the physiologic responses during exercise to the combined effects of environmental heat and adverse air quality, the combined effects of hypoxia (high altitude) and adverse air quality, and the combined effects of environmental cold and high altitude have been reported. The combined effects of heat stress and air pollutants (specifically CO, O_3, PAN, and PANCO) have been evaluated. Only O_3, however, has been systematically studied at a variety of ambient temperatures. All pollutants (except for one series of experiments in which maximal exercise responses to CO, PAN, and PANCO were evaluated) have been studied at only low exercise intensities (35–40% $\dot{V}O_{2max}$) in the heat. The combined effects of high altitude and CO were reported in cardiovascularly impaired individuals, and the combined effects of O_3 on adult hikers at Mt. Washington were studied. Much of the information on cold temperatures and altitude results from the prevalence of these colder temperatures in the high mountains rather than by specific experimental design per se. Generally, the physiologic responses during exercise to cold and altitude have been evaluated from brief exposures to the extremes for these two conditions. To date, few studies have assessed the effects of any of these interstressors on individuals with specific cardiovascular or respiratory disorders.

ENVIRONMENTAL HEAT, HYPOXIA (HIGH ALTITUDE), AND ADVERSE AIR QUALITY

Because the level of many air pollutants is high during periods of air stagnation and is often ac-

companied by elevated T_a, individuals with an impaired cardiovascular or respiratory system are at even greater risk. Submaximal exercise performance (40% $\dot{V}O_{2max}$) during O_3 exposure (0.50 ppm) was evaluated at different environmental conditions (25°C, 45% rh; 31°C, 85% rh; 35°C, 40% rh; and 40°C, 50% rh). There was a trend toward greater impairment in pulmonary function during combined exposure to O_3 and heat stress (111). Decrements in pulmonary function after exposure to ozone and heat were greatest immediately after exercise. Reductions in vital capacity and maximal voluntary ventilation were significant during the most extreme heat exposure (40°C, 50% rh); exercise $\dot{V}_E$ was highest at this T_a (plus ozone). Because heat and O_3 exposure were not related to additional reductions in any flow variables compared with O_3 alone, other unknown mechanism(s) besides bronchoconstriction probably are related to the decrements in pulmonary function during exposure to the combined stresses.

Although other air pollutants (CO, PAN, and PANCO) have been evaluated during exercise-heat stress, the environmental conditions were limited to 30% rh at 25°C and 35°C (106,108,110,116) during maximal and submaximal (35% $\dot{V}O_{2max}$) exercise intensities. $\dot{V}O_{2max}$ was not altered during exposure to CO, PAN, or PANCO at 35°C. While breathing filtered air, exposure to 35°C lowered $\dot{V}O_{2max}$ (~4%) more than exposure to either single pollutant or the two in combination at 25°C. Although no significant changes in physiologic responses were reported while breathing CO, PAN, or PANCO at 35°C during submaximal exercise, subjective complaints were greater, particularly for PAN and PANCO. Drinkwater et al. speculate that the combination of CO and heat stress is important in the more pronounced respiratory disturbances seen at this elevated temperature (108).

Because these two environmental stressors (heat and pollution) pose additional risks when presented separately to the exercising individual with an impaired cardiovascular or respiratory system, it is not surprising that the risk is potentiated when they are combined. Information available suggests that individuals with limited cardiac or pulmonary reserve capacities are at greater risk during combined exposure to environmental heat plus either CO or O_3. Because evidence is limited, it is premature to conclude that other pollutants do not adversely affect exercise performance at elevated T_a, particularly in those at risk. Therefore, outdoor physical exercise should not be prescribed for individuals at risk when heat stress levels necessitate caution for healthy individuals or when the current primary federal standards for air pollutants are exceeded (103).

Recently, men with CHD performed exercise stress tests at a simulated 2.1-km altitude while exposed to CO (COHb = 4.2%). The time to onset of angina was reduced by 18%, and there was greater susceptibility to ventricular ectopy than at sea level (126,127). Hikers aged 18 to 64 years climbed Mt. Washington while exposed to low levels of O_3, fine particulate matter, and strong aerosol acidity (128). Those with asthma or wheeze had significantly greater changes in pulmonary dysfunction.

ENVIRONMENTAL COLD AND HIGH ALTITUDE

As one ascends mountainous terrain, both T_a and humidity decrease, with corresponding increases in wind velocity and solar radiation. Although there is considerable variation, T_a decreases $\sim 1°C$ for every 150 m of ascent (129). The low humidity seen at high altitude promotes increased heat loss through more effective evaporative cooling. Low humidity combined with high pulmonary ventilation can markedly increase heat loss, with serious performance consequences (130). The increased wind velocity decreases the effective temperature at the skin surface. The effects of this wind-chill factor are of particular consequence for preventing peripheral freezing cold injuries due to cooling of exposed surface areas. Increased wind velocity may hamper locomotion, elevate $\dot{V}O_2$, and contribute to fatigue or exhaustion (129). In addition, wind penetration of clothing disturbs the trapped dead air layer and decreases insulation. Although precautions must be taken to prevent sunburn damage, solar radiation provides a necessary source of heat. In contrast to hot environments, it seems important to wear dark colors at altitude, because black clothing absorbs 88% of the solar radiation, khaki 57%, and white only 20% (129).

In addition to selecting dark clothing at altitude, three basic principles for clothing design are suggested to help reduce heat loss (130). They are (*a*) trapping air within clothing and using its in-sulative properties plus that of the fabric to reduce heat loss, (*b*) using multiple-layered clothing that helps to maximize the use of the entrapped air layer and allows removal or addition of clothing layers as needed, and (*c*) layering heavier and less permeable clothing over more coarsely woven clothing to reduce dampness and heat transfer. The clothing must be kept as dry as possible because wet clothing (from either sweat production or environmental moisture) reduces its insulative properties and results in increased heat loss.

The interactive effects of cold and hypoxic stresses on exercise performance are not well understood, principally because of a lack of experimental information. Ward suggests a number of factors that may decrease exercise performance (129). Cold and hypoxic stresses combined may decrease mental function and could alter exercise performance. Because $\dot{V}O_{2max}$ is reduced at altitude, heat production during exercise is limited at altitude and therefore is associated with a greater risk of cold injury. The increased $\dot{V}_E$ at altitude increases heat and water loss, both of which are an obvious disadvantage. Both cold and hypoxic stress are associated with hemoconcentration and a possible additive increase in blood viscosity, leading to decreased blood flow. Severe peripheral vasoconstriction (cold stress) and high blood viscosity (enhanced by dehydration at altitude) can lead to impaired tissue perfusion and possible tissue necrosis. Because skin blood flow is reduced by hypoxic vasoconstriction at altitude in thermoneutral temperatures, this response may magnify the reduction during cold exposure. Cold and hypoxic stresses may increase lactic acid production for a given exercise intensity, possibly complicating exercise performance. Finally, because the combined stress can produce a life-threatening situation for the normal, healthy individual during exercise, the added risks to those with disorders of the cardiovascular or pulmonary systems are obvious.

HYDRATION IN HOT, COLD, AND HIGH-ALTITUDE ENVIRONMENTS

Hot Environments

Water deficits develop because of fluid nonavailability or a mismatch between thirst and sweat loss. Hypohydration increases T_c responses during exercise in both temperate and hot climates (16,131); fluid deficits as small as 1% of body weight can elevate T_c and HR during exercise (16,131,132). The T_c rises 0.1 to 0.23°C, and HR increases ~6 beats·min^{-1} per 1% body weight lost (131,133,134). As the water deficit increases, there is a concomitant graded increase in physiologic strain during exercise-heat stress (131,133), and heat tolerance is reduced (131). When exercise is expected to cause fluid losses >2% body weight, target HR prescriptions should be modified. Besides elevating T_c and HR responses, hypohydration negates the thermoregulatory advantages conferred by high aerobic fitness and heat acclimation (135,136). Because thirst does not develop until modest dehydration (1–2%) is present, exercise prescriptions for hot climates should include recommendations to drink early and often and to replace fluids at a rate that approximates sweat loss (137). Intake should not exceed 1.5 L·h^{-1} for extended durations of heavy sweating (14,15).

Cold and High-Altitude Environments

As air temperature decreases, saturation vapor pressure also declines. Thus, cold air has less water content than warmer air, even if the relative humidity is the same. Breathing cold air may increase body fluid loss during exercise because more respiratory water is required to humidify the inspired air as it passes into the lungs. This fact becomes especially important during exercise when $\dot{V}_E$ is increased and at altitude during both rest and exercise (relative to sea level), since hypohydration is a hallmark of successful altitude acclimatization (138). Standard calculations (139) show that respiratory water loss can be ~50% greater during exercise ($\dot{V}O_2 = 3$ L·min^{-1}) when breathing cold (0°C) rather than hot (35°C) air of similar relative humidity (50%). Although short-term respiratory water losses in cold environments can range widely (10–100 mL·h^{-1}, depending on $\dot{V}_E$), these losses can add considerably to total fluid requirements if extrapolated over a prolonged outdoor exposure. In addition, thirst is blunted in cold weather (140), and fluid may be voluntarily restricted to avoid the need to urinate outdoors in freezing temperatures. Because sweating rates can exceed 1 L·h^{-1} during work in cold environments, especially when heavy clothing is worn (140), dehydration can be a problem in cold, high-altitude environments. It is also suspected that peripheral cold injury may be exacerbated by dehydration (141), possibly through an impaired vasoconstrictor response to cold (142). Exercise prescriptions for cold, high-altitude environments must also consider the importance of proper fluid replacement strategies.

Acknowledgment

The authors gratefully acknowledge Terry Hovagimian for her technical assistance in manuscript preparation. The views, opinions, and/or findings contained in this report are those of the authors and should not be construed as an official Department of the Army position, policy, or decision, unless so designated by other official documentation.

REFERENCES

1. Sawka MN, Wenger CB, Pandolf KB. Thermoregulatory responses to acute exercise-heat stress and heat acclimation. In: Fregly MJ, Blatteis CM, eds. Handbook of Physiology, section 4, environmental physiology. New York: Oxford University Press, 1996:157–185.
2. Lind AR. A physiological criterion for setting thermal environmental limits for everyday work. J Appl Physiol 1963;18:51–56.
3. Nielsen B, Nielsen M. Body temperature during work at different environmental temperatures. Acta Physiol Scand 1962;56:120–129.
4. Nielsen M. Heat production and body temperature during rest and work. In: Hardy JD, Gagge AP, Stolwijk JAJ. Physiological and Behavioral Temperature Regulation. Springfield, IL: Charles C Thomas, 1970:205–214.
5. Saltin B, Hermansen L. Esophageal, rectal, and muscle temperature during exercise. J Appl Physiol 1966; 21:1757–1762.
6. Åstrand I. Aerobic work capacity in men and women. Acta Physiol Scand 1960;49:64–73.
7. Davies CTM. Influence of skin temperature on sweating and aerobic performance during severe work. J Appl Physiol 1979;47:770–777.
8. Nielsen M. Die Regulation der Körpertemperatur bei Muskelarbeit. Skand Arch Physiol 1938;79: 193–230.
9. Cheuvront SN, Haymes EM. Thermoregulation and marathon running: biological and environmental influences. Sports Med 2001;31:743–762.
10. Gisolfi CV, Lamb DR, Nadel ER. Perspectives in Exercise Science and Sports Medicine. Vol 6, Exercise, Heat, and Thermoregulation. Traverse City, MI: Cooper Publishing, 1993.

11. Gisolfi CW, Wenger CB. Temperature regulation during exercise: old concepts, new ideas. Exerc Sport Sci Rev 1984;12:339–372.
12. Rowell LB. Human cardiovascular adjustments to exercise and thermal stress. Physiol Rev 1974;54:75–159.
13. Sawka MN, Young AJ. Physical exercise in hot and cold climates. In: Garrett WE, Kirkendall DT, eds. Exercise and Sport Science. Philadelphia: Lippincott Williams & Wilkins, 2000:385–400.
14. Montain SJ, Sawka MN, Wenger CB. Hyponatremia associated with exercise: risk factors and pathogenesis. Exerc Sport Sci Rev 2001;29:113–117.
15. Montain SJ, Latzka WA, Sawka MN. Fluid replacement recommendations for training in hot weather. Mil Med 1999;164:502–508.
16. Sawka MN, Montain SJ. Fluid and electrolyte balance: effects on thermoregulation and exercise in the heat. In: Bowman BA, Russell RM, eds. Present Knowledge in Nutrition. Washington, DC: ILSI Press, 2001:115–126.
17. Pandolf KB, Griffin TB, Munro EH, et al. Persistence of impaired heat tolerance from artificially induced miliaria rubra. Am J Physiol 1980;239:R226–232.
18. Pandolf KB, Gange RW, Latzka WA, et al. Human thermoregulatory responses during heat exposure after artificially induced sunburn. Am J Physiol 1992;262:R610–616.
19. Bynum GD, Pandolf KB, Schuette WH, et al. Induced hyperthermia in sedated humans and the concept of critical thermal maximum. Am J Physiol 1978;235:R228–236.
20. Cheuvront SN, Sawka MN. Physical exercise and exhaustion from heat strain. J Korean Soc Living Environ Syst 2001;8:134–145.
21. Pandolf KB, Shapiro Y, Breckenridge JR, et al. Effects of solar heat load on physiological performance at rest and work in the heat. Fed Proc 1979;38:1052 (abstr).
22. Nielsen B, Kassow K, Aschengreen FE. Heat balance during exercise in the sun. Eur J Appl Physiol 1988;58:189–196.
23. Armstrong LE, Pandolf KB. Physical training, cardiorespiratory physical fitness and exercise-heat tolerance. In: Pandolf KB, Sawka MN, Gonzalez RR, eds. Human Performance Physiology and Environmental Medicine at Terrestrial Extremes. Indianapolis, IN: Benchmark Press, 1988:199–226.
24. Gisolfi CV, Cohen JS. Relationships among training, heat acclimation, and heat tolerance in men and women: the controversy revisited. Med Sci Sports 1979;11:56–59.
25. Pandolf KB. Effects of physical training and cardiorespiratory physical fitness on exercise-heat tolerance. recent observations. Med Sci Sports 1979;11:60–65.
26. Gisolfi CV. Work-heat tolerance derived from interval training. J Appl Physiol 1973;35:349–354.
27. Henane R, Flandrois R, Charbonnier JP. Increase in sweating sensitivity by endurance conditioning in man. J Appl Physiol 1977;43:822–828.
28. Nadel ER, Pandolf KB, Roberts MF, et al. Mechanisms of thermal acclimation to exercise and heat. J Appl Physiol 1974;37:515–520.
29. Roberts MF, Wenger CB, Stolwijk JAJ, et al. Skin blood flow and sweating changes following exercise training and heat acclimation. J Appl Physiol 1977;43:133–137.
30. Shvartz E, Saar E, Meyerstein N, et al. A comparison of three methods of acclimatization to dry heat. J Appl Physiol 1973;34:214–219.
31. Pandolf KB, Burse RL, Goldman RF. Role of physical fitness in heat acclimatisation, decay and reinduction. Ergonomics 1977;20:399–408.
32. Shvartz E, Shapiro Y, Magazanik A, et al. Heat acclimation, physical fitness, and responses to exercise in temperate and hot environments. J Appl Physiol 1977;43:678–683.
33. Drinkwater BL, Denton JE, Kupprat IC, et al. Aerobic power as a factor in women's response to work in hot environments. J Appl Physiol 1976;41:815–821.
34. Greenleaf JE, Castle BL, Ruff WK. Maximal oxygen uptake, sweating and tolerance to exercise in the heat. Int J Biometeorol 1972;16:375–387.
35. Wyndham CH, Strydom NB, Williams CG, et al. An examination of certain individual factors affecting the heat tolerance of mine workers. J S Afr Inst Mining Metallurgy 1967;68:79–91.
36. Avellini BA, Shapiro Y, Fortney SM, et al. Effects on heat tolerance of physical training in water and on land. J Appl Physiol, 1982;53:1291–1298.
37. Wenger CB. Human heat acclimatization. In: Pandolf KB, Sawka MN, Gonzalez RR, eds. Human Performance Physiology and Environmental Medicine at Terrestrial Extremes. Indianapolis, IN: Benchmark Press, 1988:153–197.
38. Sawka MN, Cheuvront SN, Kolka MA. Human adaptations to heat stress. In: Nose H, Mack GW, Imaizumi K, eds. Exercise, Nutrition, and Environmental Stress, Vol 3. Traverse City, MI: Cooper Publishing Group, 2003:129–153.
39. Gonzalez RR. Biophysical and physiological integration of proper clothing for exercise. Exerc Sport Sci Rev 1987;15:261–295.

40. Gonzalez RR. Biophysics of heat exchange and clothing: applications to sports physiology. Med Exerc Nutr Health 1995;4:290–305.

41. Kark JA, Burr PQ, Wenger CB, et al. Exertional heat illness in Marine Corps recruit training. Aviat Space Environ Med 1996;67:354–360.

42. National Institute of Occupational Safety and Health. Occupational exposure to hot environments. Washington, DC: U.S. Department of Health and Human Services, 1986.

43. Ladell WSS. Terrestrial animals in humid heat: man. In: Dill DB, Adolf EF, Wilber CG. Handbook of Physiology, section 4, Adaptation to the environment. Washington, DC: American Physiological Society, 1964:625–659.

44. Lee DHK. Terrestrial animals in dry heat; man in the desert. In: Dill DB, Adolf EF, Wilber CG. Handbook of Physiology, section 4, Adaptation to the environment. Washington, DC: American Physiological Society, 1964:551–582.

45. Yaglou CP, Minard D. Control of heat casualties at military training centers. AMA Arch Ind Health 1957;16:302–316.

46. American College of Sports Medicine. Heat and cold illnesses during distance running. Med Sci Sports Exerc 1996;28:i–x.

47. Gonzalez-Alonso J, Mora-Rodriguez R, Coyle EF. Stroke volume during exercise: interaction of environment and hydration. Am J Physiol Heart Circ Physiol 2000;278:H321–H330.

48. Pandolf KB, Cafarelli E, Noble BJ, et al. Hyperthermia: effect on exercise prescription. Arch. Phys Med Rehabil 1975;56:524–526.

49. Givoni B, Goldman RF. Predicting effects of heat acclimatization on heart rate and rectal temperature. J Appl Physiol 1973;35:875–879.

50. Givoni B, Goldman RF. Predicting heart rate response to work, environment, and clothing. J Appl Physiol 1973;34:201–204.

51. Givoni B, Goldman RF. Predicting rectal temperature response to work, environment, and clothing. J Appl Physiol 1972;32:812–822.

52. Pandolf KB, Stroschein LA, Drolet LL, et al. Prediction modeling of physiological responses and human performance in the heat. Comput Biol Med 1986;16:319–325.

53. Kenney WL. Thermoregulation at rest and during exercise in healthy older adults. Exerc Sport Sci Rev 1997;25:41–76.

54. Dougherty SM, Sheldahl LM, Wilke NA, et al. Physiological responses to shoveling and thermal stress in men with cardiac disease. Med Sci Sports Exerc 1993;25:790–795.

55. Sheldahl LM, Wilke NA, Dougherty S, et al. Cardiac responses to combined moderate heat and exercise in men with coronary artery disease. Am J Cardiol 1992;15:186–191.

56. Young AJ. Homeostatic responses to prolonged cold exposure: human cold acclimatization. In: Fregly MJ, Blatteis CM, eds. Handbook of Physiology, section 4, Environmental physiology. New York: Oxford University Press, 1996:419–438.

57. Horvath SM. Exercise in a cold environment. Exerc Sport Sci Rev 1981;9:221–263.

58. Toner MM, McArdle WD. Human thermoregulatory responses to acute cold stress with special reference to water immersion. In: Fregly MJ, Blatteis CM, ed. Handbook of Physiology, section 4, Environmental physiology. New York: Oxford University Press, 1996:379–418.

59. Jaeger JJ, Deal EC, Roberts DE, et al. Cold air inhalation and esophageal temperature in exercising humans. Med Sci Sports Exerc 1980;12:365–369.

60. Freund BJ, O'Brien C, Young AJ. Alcohol ingestion and temperature regulation during cold exposure. J Wilderness Med 1994;5:88–98.

61. Ducharme MB, VanHelder WP, Radomski MW. Cyclic intramuscular temperature fluctuations in the human forearm during cold-water immersion. Eur J Appl Physiol 1991;63:188–193.

62. Epstein SE, Stampfer M, Beiser GD, et al. Effects of a reduction in environmental temperature on the circulatory response to exercise in man. N Engl J Med 1969;280:7–11.

63. LeBlanc J. Man in the Cold. Springfield, IL: Charles C Thomas, 1975.

64. Glossary of Terms for Thermal Physiology. 2nd ed. Revised by the Commission for Thermal Physiology of the International Union of Physiological Sciences. Pflugers Arch 1987;410:567–587.

65. Roberts WO. A 12-yr profile of medical injury and illness for the Twin Cities Marathon. Med Sci Sports Exerc 2000;32:1549–1555.

66. National Weather Service, Office of Climate, Water, and Weather Services. Wind Chill Temperature Index, November 1, 2001, at http://www.nws.noaa.gov/om/notif.htm. Accessed June 5, 2002.

67. Danielsson U. Windchill and the risk of tissue freezing. J Appl Physiol 1996;81:2666–2673.

68. Leon DF, Amidi M, Leonard JJ. Left heart work and temperature responses to cold exposure in man. Am J Cardiol 1970;26:38–45.

69. Neill WA, Duncan DA, Kloster F, et al. Response of coronary circulation to cutaneous cold. Am J Med 1974;56:471–476.

70. Dubois-Rande JL, Dupouy P, Aptecar E, et al. Comparison of the effects of exercise and cold pressor test on the vasomotor response of normal and atherosclerotic coronary arteries and their relation

to the flow-mediated mechanism. Am J Cardiol 1995;76:467–473.

71. Malacoff RF, Mudge GH, Holman BL, et al. Effect of the cold pressor test on regional myocardial blood flow in patients with coronary artery disease. Am Heart J 1983;106:78–84.

72. Giesbrecht GG. The respiratory system in a cold environment. Aviat Space Environ Med 1995; 66:890–902.

73. Åstrand PO, Rodahl K. Textbook of Work Physiology. 3rd ed. New York: McGraw-Hill, 1986.

74. Hannon JP, Vogel JA. Oxygen transport during early altitude acclimatization: a perspective study. Eur J Appl Physiol 1977;36:285–297.

75. Grover RF. Performance at altitude. In: Strauss RH, ed. Sports Medicine and Physiology. Philadelphia: WB Saunders, 1979:327–343.

76. Grover RF, Weil JV, Reeves JT. Cardiovascular adaptation to exercise at high altitude. Exerc Sport Sci Rev 1986;14:269–302.

77. Hultgren HN. High Altitude Medicine. Palo Alto, CA: Hultgren Publications, 1997.

78. Sawka MN, Convertino VA, Eichner ER, et al. Blood volume: importance and adaptations to exercise training, environmental stresses, and trauma/sickness. Med Sci Sports Exerc 2000;32:332–348.

79. Young AJ, Young PM. Human acclimatization to high terrestrial altitude. In: Pandolf KB, Sawka MN, Gonzalez, RR, eds. Human Performance Physiology and Environmental Medicine at Terrestrial Extremes. Carmel, CA: Cooper Publishing Group, 1988:497–544.

80. Kollias J, Buskirk ER. Exercise and altitude. In: Johnson WR, Buskirk ER. Structural and Physiological Aspects of Exercise and Sport. Princeton, NJ: Princeton Book Company, 1980:211–227.

81. Saltin B. Exercise and the environment: focus on altitude. Res Q Exerc Sport 1996;67:1–10.

82. Fulco CS, Rock PB, Cymerman A. Maximal and submaximal exercise performance at altitude. Aviat Space Environ Med 1998;69:793–801.

83. Jackson CG, Sharkey BJ. Altitude, training and human performance. Sports Med 1988;6:279–284.

84. Dempsey JA, Hanson PG, Henderson KS. Exercise-induced arterial hypoxaemia in healthy human subjects at sea level. J Physiol 1984;355:161–175.

85. Powers SK, Lawler J, Dempsey JA, et al. Effects of incomplete pulmonary gas exchange on $\dot{V}_{O_2 max}$. J Appl Physiol 1989;66:2491–2495.

86. Young AJ, Cymerman A, Burse RL. The influence of cardiorespiratory fitness on the decrement in maximal aerobic power at high altitude. Eur J Appl Physiol 1985;54:12–15.

87. Ferretti G, Hauser H, di Prampero PE. Maximal muscular power before and after exposure to chronic hypoxia. Int J Sports Med 1990;(suppl 1):S31–34.

88. Stenberg J, Ekblom B, Messin R. Hemodynamic response to work at simulated altitude, 4,000 m. J Appl Physiol 1966;21:1589–1594.

89. Alexander JK, Hartley LH, Modelski M, et al. Reduction of stroke volume during exercise in man following ascent to 3,100 m altitude. J Appl Physiol 1967;23:849–858.

90. Grover RF. Future studies in adaptations to altitude. In: Horvath S, Yousef MK, eds. Environmental Physiology. Aging, Heat and Altitude. New York: Elsevier-North Holland, 1981:281–290.

91. Grover RF, Reeves JT, Maher JT, et al. Maintained stroke volume but impaired arterial oxygenation in man at high altitude with supplemental CO_2. Circ Res 1976;38:391–396.

92. Hartley LH, Vogel JA, Cruz JC. Reduction of maximal exercise heart rate at altitude and its reversal with atropine. J Appl Physiol 1974;36:362–365.

93. Richalet JP, Larmignat P, Rathat C, et al. Decreased cardiac response to isoproterenol infusion in acute and chronic hypoxia. J Appl Physiol 1988;65:1957–1961.

94. Saltin B, Grover RF, Blomqvist CG, et al. Maximal oxygen uptake and $\dot{Q}$ after 2 weeks at 4,300 m. J Appl Physiol 1968;25:400–409.

95. Levine BD, Stray-Gundersen J. Living high-training low: effect of moderate-altitude acclimatization with low-altitude training on performance. J Appl Physiol 1997;83:102–112.

96. Pandolf KB, Young AJ, Sawka MN, et al. Does erythrocyte infusion improve 3.2-km run performance at high altitude? Eur J Appl Physiol 1998;79:1–6.

97. Levine BD, Zuckerman JH, deFilippi CR. Effect of high-altitude exposure in the elderly: the Tenth Mountain Division Study. Circulation 1997;96:1224–1232.

98. Roach RC, Houston CS, Honigman B, et al. How well do older persons tolerate moderate altitude? West J Med 1995;162:32–36.

99. Erdmann J, Sun KT, Masar P, et al. Effects of exposure to altitude on men with coronary artery disease and impaired left ventricular function. Am J Physiol 1998;81:266–270.

100. Balke B. Cardiac performance in relation to altitude. Am J Cardiol 1964;14:796–810.

101. Politte LL, Almond CH, Logue JT. Dynamic electrocardiography with strenuous exertion at high altitudes. Am Heart J 1968;75:570–572.

102. Alexander JK. Coronary problems associated with altitude and air travel. Cardiol Clin 1995;13:271–278.

103. Raven PB. Heat and air pollution: the cardiac patient. In: Pollock ML, Schmidt DH, eds. Heart

Disease and Rehabilitation. Boston: Houghton Mifflin, 1979:563–586.

104. Gong H, Krishnareddy S. How pollution and airborne allergens affect exercise. Physician Sportsmed 1995;23:35–43.

105. Carlisle AJ, Sharp NCC. Exercise and outdoor ambient air pollution. Br J Sports Med 2001;35:214–222.

106. Gliner JA, Raven PB, Horvath SM, et al. Man's physiologic response to long-term work during thermal and pollutant stress. J Appl Physiol 1975;39:628–632.

107. Vogel JA, Gleser MA. Effect of carbon monoxide on oxygen transport during exercise. J Appl Physiol 1972; 32:234–239.

108. Drinkwater BL, Raven PB, Horvath SM, et al. Air pollution, exercise, and heat stress. Arch. Environ Health 1974;28:177–181.

109. Horvath SM, Raven PB, Dahms TE, et al. Maximal aerobic capacity at different levels of carboxyhemoglobin. J Appl Physiol 1975;38:300–303.

110. Raven PB, Drinkwater BL, Ruhling RO, et al. Effect of carbon monoxide and peroxyacetyl nitrate on man's maximal aerobic capacity. J Appl Physiol 1974;36:288–293.

111. Folinsbee LJ, Horvath SM, Raven PB, et al. Influence of exercise and heat stress on pulmonary function during ozone exposure. J Appl Physiol 1977;43:409–413.

112. Folinsbee LJ, Silverman F, Shephard RJ. Exercise responses following ozone exposure. J Appl Physiol 1975;38:996–1001.

113. McKittrick T, Adams WC. Pulmonary function response to equivalent doses of ozone consequent to intermittent and continuous exercise. Arch Environ Health 1995;50:153–158.

114. Folinsbee LJ, Silverman F, Shephard RJ. Decrease of maximum oxygen uptake following exposure to ozone. Physiologist 1975;18:215 (abstr).

115. Savin WM, Adams WC. Effects of ozone inhalation on work performance and $\dot{V}_{O_2\,max}$. J Appl Physiol 1979;46:309–314.

116. Raven PB, Gliner JA, Sutton JC. Dynamic lung function changes following longterm work in polluted environments. Environ Res 1976;12:18–25.

117. Horvath SM, Folinsbee LJ. The effect of nitrogen dioxide on lung function in normal subjects. Washington, DC: U.S. Department of Commerce, National Technical Information Service PB-277 671, 1978.

118. Kim SU, Koenig JQ, Pierson WE, et al. Acute pulmonary effects of nitrogen dioxide exposure during exercise in competitive athletes. Chest 1991;99:815–819.

119. Hazucha M, Bates DV. Combined effect of ozone and sulphur dioxide on human pulmonary function. Nature 1975;257:50–51.

120. Aronow WS, Harris CN, Isbell MW, et al. Effect of freeway travel on angina pectoris. Ann. Intern Med 1972;77:669–676.

121. Anderson EW, Strauch JM, Fortuin NJ, et al. Effect of low-level carbon monoxide exposure on onset and duration of angina pectoris: a study in ten patients with ischemic heart disease. Ann Intern Med 1973;79:46–50.

122. Aronow WS, Isbell MW. Carbon monoxide effect on exercise-induced angina pectoris. Ann Intern Med 1973;79:392–395.

123. Superko HR, Adams WC, Webb-Daly P. Effects of ozone inhalation during exercise in selected patients with heart disease. Am J Med 1984;77:463–470.

124. Gong H, Shamoo DA, Anderson KR, et al. Responses of older men with and without chronic obstructive pulmonary disease to prolonged ozone exposure. Arch Environ Health 1997;52:18–25.

125. Horstman DH, Ball BA, Brown J, et al. Comparison of pulmonary responses of asthmatic and nonasthmatic subjects performing light exercise while exposed to a low level of ozone. Toxicol Ind Health 1995;11:369–385.

126. Kleinman MT, Leaf DA, Kelly E, et al. Urban angina in the mountains: effects of carbon monoxide and mild hypoxemia on subjects with chronic stable angina. Arch Environ Health 1998;53:388–397.

127. Leaf DA, Kleinman MT. Urban ectopy in the mountains: carbon monoxide exposure at high altitude. Arch Environ Health 1996;51:283–290.

128. Korrick SA, Neas LM, Dockery DW, et al. Effects of ozone and other pollutants on the pulmonary function of adult hikers. Environ Health Perspect 1998;106:93–99.

129. Ward M. Mountain Medicine: A Clinical Study of Cold and High Altitude. London: Crosby Lockwood Staples, 1975.

130. Baker PT. The Biology of High-Altitude Peoples. Cambridge: Cambridge University Press, 1978.

131. Sawka MN, Montain SJ, Latzka WA. Body fluid balance during exercise-heat exposure. In: Buskirk ER, Puhl SM, eds. Body Fluid Balance: Exercise and Sport. Boca Raton, FL: CRC Press, 1996:139–158.

132. Ekblom B, Greenleaf CJ, Greenleaf JE, et al. Temperature regulation during exercise dehydration in man. Acta Physiol Scand 1970;79:475–483.

133. Montain SJ, Coyle EF. Influence of graded dehydration on hyperthermia and cardiovascular drift during exercise. J Appl Physiol 1992;73:1340–1350.

134. Strydom NB, Holdsworth DL. The effects of different levels of water deficit on physiological responses

during exercise heat stress. Int Z angew Physiol 1968;26:95–102.

135. Buskirk ER, Iampietro PF, Bass DE. Work performance after dehydration: effects of physical conditioning and heat acclimatization. J Appl Physiol 1958;12:189–194.

136. Sawka MN, Toner MM, Francesconi RP, et al. Hypohydration and exercise: effects of heat acclimation, gender, and environment. J Appl Physiol 1983;55:1147–1153.

137. American College of Sports Medicine. Exercise and fluid replacement. Med Sci Sports Exerc 1996;28:i–vii.

138. Hoyt RW, Honig A. Environmental influences on body fluid balance during exercise: altitude. In: Buskirk ER, Puhl SM, eds. Body Fluid Balance: Exercise and Sport. Boca Raton, FL: CRC Press, 1996:183–196.

139. Mitchell JW, Nadel ER, Stolwijk JAJ. Respiratory weight losses during exercise. J Appl Physiol 1972;22:474–476.

140. Freund BJ, Young AJ. Environmental influences on body fluid balance during exercise: cold exposure. In: Buskirk ER, Puhl SM, eds. Body Fluid Balance: Exercise and Sport. Boca Raton, FL: CRC Press, 1996:159–181.

141. Roberts DE, Berberich JJ. The role of hydration on peripheral response to cold. Milit Med 1988;153:605–608.

142. O'Brien C, Young AJ, Sawka MN. Hypohydration and thermoregulation in cold air. J Appl Physiol 1998; 84:185–189.

8

Exercise Adherence and Prescription for Special Populations

John S. Raglin and Gregory S. Wilson

The need for establishing effective methods to increase participation in regular programs of physical activity in the general population has never been more critical. Estimates of the proportion of adults who engage in vigorous exercise on a regular basis range from a low of 10% (1) to a high of 22% (2). In contrast, a greater proportion of adults (~25%) are chronically inactive and do not exercise at all (1). Participation in regular physical activity decreases across the lifespan, with this trend beginning at adolescence (3). From 1991 to 1998, the percentage of adult Americans classified as medically obese has risen by 49.2% (4), and this has led to sharp increases in diseases related to excess weight, most notably type 2 diabetes. Even among persons who begin an exercise program, an average of 50% will fail to adhere, a figure that has remained essentially unchanged across the past two decades (5). Typically, the greatest rate of dropout occurs during the first 6 to 8 weeks of an exercise program (6), before most participants begin to experience obvious gains in fitness and other desirable consequences.

Simple solutions to the problem of exercise adherence are unlikely. For example, among the reasons given for quitting an exercise program, the most frequently cited is the lack of time, with as many as 40% of dropouts stating it is the chief reason they failed to adhere (7). Time-management techniques have been proposed as a solution to create sufficient leisure time for physical activity and to enhance adherence (7). Nevertheless, exercise dropout rates remain unaltered even in situations in which time constraints are glaringly absent. For example, in studies of prisoners (8) enrolled in supervised exercise programs, adherence rates (55%, 57%) were found to be no better than the average for the general population.

Educational programs have long been used to promote the benefits of physical activity, create positive attitudes toward exercise programs, and ultimately increase participation. The anticipated benefit to adherence from possessing information on the proper prescription and benefits of exercise is supported by theories of exercise behavior, including social learning theory, protection motivation theory, and the health belief model. Each of these theories emphasizes the importance of rational decision-making processes whereby an individual weighs the potential costs and benefits of exercise and alters behavior accordingly (9). Based on these theories, it follows that adherence rates would be greater for persons with an increased personal health risk (e.g., hypertension) or with a medical condition that benefits from increased physical activity (e.g., coronary artery disease), particularly given that health benefits would accrue from a relatively mild regimen often fully covered by health insurance policies.

However, in a summary of adherence studies involving several thousand adults, Franklin (10) found the dropout rate of patients enrolled in exercise programs for cardiac rehabilitation to be essentially identical to that of healthy adults enrolled in exercise programs for the purpose of general fitness and health (44 vs. 46%, respectively), an observation supported in a recent meta-analysis of the literature (11). Hence, the assumption that adherence rates would increase for persons who have the most to gain from participating in an exercise program has not consistently been borne out.

Reviewers have been undivided in calling for exercise adherence research and for application to be grounded in an appropriate theoretical framework (9,12). However, at least 10 theories have been applied to exercise behavior research (6), some of which involve as many as 20 independent variables. These variables have not been measured consistently across studies and in some cases were assessed using instruments of questionable validity. Further complicating the successful application of theory, both levels of physical activity and rates of adherence have been measured using different standards and instruments (13). Finally, inappropriate statistical modeling can inflate the association between a variable and adherence or result in spurious correlations (14). Although there is evidence that theoretically guided research can result in a greater understanding of exercise adherence and reduce dropout, particularly in the case of the transtheoretical model (14), the rigorous and appropriate use of this and other theoretical models remains vexingly difficult.

Despite these sobering findings, research has shown that various intervention techniques yield modest improvements in exercise adherence in some circumstances (11). A wide variety of techniques have been used in the attempt to reduce exercise dropout, and interventions can be targeted toward the individual, group, or entire communities. In addition, intervention techniques can be tailored for different stages of exercise under the assumption that this will enhance their effectiveness. The following section describes the major techniques used in the attempt to enhance physical activity levels while reducing the risk of dropout.

Intervention Strategies

BEHAVIOR MODIFICATION

Much of the research involving exercise intervention has used behavioral modification (15). These techniques do not involve teaching skills that would directly strengthen exercise behavior or change beliefs, attitudes, or self-perception toward exercise. Rather they are targeted toward antecedent behaviors inconsistent with exercise (e.g., smoking, sedentary recreation) or consequent behaviors to reinforce and strengthen habitual physical activity behaviors (e.g., taking the stairs rather than an elevator). Generally, behavior modification techniques are regarded as therapist centered because they are initiated and supervised by the care provider.

One of the major behavioral modification techniques is *stimulus control*, whereby cues that either weaken or strengthen the likelihood of exercise are first identified and then manipulated (11). Cues can be categorized as *physical* (e.g., fatigue after a day at work); *emotional* (e.g., feeling guilty for not exercising); *cognitive* (e.g., thinking about the benefits of exercising or not exercising); or *environmental* (e.g., a memo indicating the schedule of an exercise class). The salience of these cues is influenced by personal characteristics such as attitudes toward exercise and physical conditions that constrain the ability to exercise (e.g., obesity). Thus, they can differ considerably across individuals.

Stimulus control is applied so that positive cues are introduced and strengthened while attempting to minimize or eliminate cues that are contrary to exercise. Positive cues include the use of signs or posters encouraging physical activity or placement of exercise equipment in a conspicuous location with easy access. The use of telephone calls to prompt exercise is another example of a stimulus control cue. A study of adults enrolled in a walking program found that once-a-week phone calls either to "touch base" or provide information on skills such as goal setting enhanced exercise frequency to a similar degree, while a less frequent phone schedule was significantly less effective (16).

Another major behavioral modification strategy that has been used in exercise adherence studies is *reinforcement control*, which works to increase the frequency of the target behavior through the use of rewards. This technique can be implemented either through positive reinforcement, in which a desirable stimulus is presented after the behavior, or through negative reinforcement, whereby a negative stimulus is withdrawn following the target behavior. An example of negative reinforcement would include exercise resulting in the reduction of dysphoric feelings (e.g., guilt, anxiety) or symptoms a disease (e.g., pain, fatigue). However, it is more common to use positive reinforcement to introduce rewards during and following a physical activity session (15). Some examples include praise or an award such as a T-shirt when an exercise goal has been met. Positive and negative reinforcers can be conceptualized as either intrinsic or extrinsic. Intrinsic rewards are internally generated by the exerciser and would include feelings of satisfaction, accomplishment, or mastery. Extrinsic rewards are typically controlled by a person other than the exerciser, and examples include T-shirts, awards, or prizes.

The conditions when rewards will be presented can be determined through behavioral contracts that specify acceptable activities and their appropriate duration and intensity. Contracts may also include a penalty clause to be applied when the target activity has not been met. Penalties must not be perceived as being contrary to exercise or excessively punitive. One means of achieving this is to choose penalties that result in some incidental gain for the client, such as a donation to a charity.

A technique called treatment-matching can be useful to identify the appropriate intervention and to tailor it to the individual's present stage of exercise behavior on the basis of the transtheoretical model. Using this model, exercise and other health-related behaviors are classified according to the following discrete stages: (*a*) *precontemplation*, in which individuals have no intention to exercise; (*b*) *contemplation*, in which individuals are inactive but intend to begin exercising within 6 months, (*c*) *preparation*, in which individuals are active but have not yet met the exercise prescription, although they intend to do so; (*d*) *action*, in which individuals have been exercising at the exercise prescription for less than 6 months and, (*e*) *maintenance*, in which individuals have been exercising regularly for longer than 6 months (17). Using treatment-matching, individuals who are planning to begin an exercise program (the preparation stage) would

benefit from physical and psychosocial assessments that identify exercise barriers and reinforcements. In contrast, persons who have been exercising regularly for some time (the maintenance stage) would benefit from reevaluating exercise goals and planning for potential lapses in their exercise routine.

COGNITIVE BEHAVIORAL MODIFICATION

Cognitive behavioral modification targets stimulus control and reinforcement control techniques toward psychologic variables that are assumed to mediate the exercise behavior, rather than directly affect the exercise behavior itself (18). Skills are taught in the attempt to alter and control conditions that prompt and strengthen exercise behavior; these include goal setting, decision making, self-monitoring, and relapse prevention training. In contrast to strict behavior modification methods, the exerciser assumes the central role in applying cognitive behavior techniques. Therefore, these methods are regarded as client, rather than therapist, centered. For example, instead of simply being assigned a standard exercise prescription in the case of an exercise contract, the client would determine the appropriate level of activity as well as specify the rewards and punishments, with the assistance of an exercise professional or physician.

Goal setting is perhaps the most commonly used cognitive behavior technique and is a central feature of cognitive theories of exercise behavior. Goal setting works by directing attention and marshaling resources toward the target behavior, and providing objective markers of progress. An inherent aspect of goal setting is that the goals be realistic and within the capacity of the individual to achieve. Rewards should be structured into the goal-setting program to provide incentives and maintain persistence. While these points may seem obvious, it is not uncommon for beginning exercisers to have unrealistic goals about what a physical activity program can achieve (e.g., immediate and dramatic weight loss), which can sabotage the effectiveness of a goal-setting program. Conversely, persons with physical conditions that limit their ability to exercise (e.g., heart disease) may have physical activity goals that fall below their physical capability, or may possess inadequate levels of confidence about their ability to achieve an exercise goal within their physical capacity. Information gained from baseline exercise and health tests can be used to formulate efficacious exercise goals that are also personally relevant, as well as to provide objective information later used to map progress and improvement. Since persons who quit exercise programs typically do so within the initial few weeks, a goal-setting strategy must include short-term goals that can be achieved during a single exercise session or within a week.

Self-monitoring by means of a written record of thoughts, feelings, and environmental factors associated with successful or unsuccessful attempts to exercise can be useful for identifying both barriers and reinforcers of physical activity. This information may also aid participants to schedule exercise more effectively into a regular routine to optimize convenience (15).

Relapse prevention techniques are typically used in the attempt to reduce or eliminate undesired habitual behaviors such as smoking, particularly when the individual is in a situation or environment that increases the risk of recidivism (15). In the case of exercise, relapse prevention focuses on so-called high-risk variables that lead to inactivity or missing a scheduled exercise session. Commonly cited high-risk variables include inclement weather, smoking, social eating and drinking, and fatigue from overwork or insufficient sleep. Because these risks can differ across individuals and change over time, one must use self-monitoring or interviews to identify causes of past exercise dropout. Based on this information, the individual is provided with skills training such as the use of coping strategies and contingency plans that are targeted toward previously identified high-risk situations. For example, if rain or inclement weather is identified as a common reason for missing a scheduled exercise session, then appropriate backup plans such as indoor exercise (mall walk) or having all-weather exercise gear on hand would be implemented.

Behavior modification and cognitive behavior modification techniques have been found to provide some benefit in increasing exercise adherence. A meta-analysis of the adherence literature (11) examining the benefit of behavior intervention techniques yielded an estimated population effect corrected by sample size of 0.75, which predicts a success rate of 88%. No differences in effectiveness occurred for age, sex, or race, but larger effect sizes were found for low-intensity exercise programs, in large part because of the increased risk of injury associated with more vigorous activity. The beneficial effects of behavioral intervention techniques on adherence compare closely to the degree of improvement in adherence associated with social support found in another meta-analysis (19). In contrast, no improvements in adherence were found for interventions based on health education or health-risk appraisals. Unfortunately, there has been little systematic study of either behavioral intervention techniques or social influences on special populations, and empirical information on how to specifically prescribe behavioral techniques for special populations is generally absent (12).

OTHER VARIABLES ASSOCIATED WITH EXERCISE ADHERENCE

Various psychologic and social variables have been studied in the context of exercise behavior. The results of this work indicate that surprisingly few factors have a significant impact on adherence (20). For example, a positive personal attitude about the importance of physical activity would logically be assumed to increase exercise activity and reduce the likelihood of dropout. Attitudes about exercise are also central features to a number of theories of exercise adherence. However, research indicates that possessing a positive attitude toward physical activity often has only a marginal effect on reducing dropout (21).

Self-efficacy is another psychologic variable that has been studied extensively. Self-efficacy is a measure of the self-perception of one's capability to perform a prescribed behavior in a specific situation. High self-efficacy has been found to be associated with increases in effort expended on a task and persistence in studies of a variety of health behaviors, including exercise. Several measures of exercise self-efficacy have been developed to determine the degree of confidence an individual has in completing successively longer exercise prescriptions. Research indicates that high exercise self-efficacy is associated with adoption of physical activity programs, but its effect on the maintenance of activity is smaller (22). As noted by Dishman (14), the degree to which one's confidence in the ability to adhere successfully to an exercise program is mediated by past successes or failures and their interaction with barriers. Nonetheless, the use of techniques that can build self-efficacy is recommended (18). Self-efficacy for exercise can be enhanced by creating mastery experiences in an exercise prescription that are scheduled regularly and broken into discrete components progressing from easy to more challenging. When participants reach an exercise "milestone," they are rewarded and provided specific feedback about their accomplishment (e.g., "Congratulations, you walked 5 minutes longer than you were able to last week").

Another means by which self-efficacy can be increased is to provide information about the normal physical signs and sensations that occur with exercise, as well as how to correctly interpret this information. For example, appropriate elevations in respiration and heart rate should be perceived as normal sensations of exercise that can be used to monitor and regulate exercise effort, rather than as signs of fatigue or a lack of fitness.

Self-motivation is a stable trait that assesses "the tendency to persevere independent of situational reinforcements" (23; p. 421). Research involving a validated measure of self-motivation indicates that high scores are moderately correlated with greater adherence to physical activity in both recreational (24) and sport competition settings (25), but the strength of this relationship is insufficient for practical application. Self-motivation has high test–retest reliabilities of the magnitude associated with stable psychologic traits, and it does not change significantly following long-term exercise participation. Hence, in contrast to self-efficacy and other more labile psychologic variables, self-motivation is not amenable to intervention techniques.

SOCIAL SUPPORT

Research has shown that forms of social support can sometimes result in enhanced exercise behavior. Various forms of social support (e.g., family, friends) can increase participation in exercise programs by adult women (26). The support of one's spouse is a significant predictor of exercise adherence in men. For example, in a study of over 200 men enrolled in a medically based exercise program (27), adherence averaged 80% for participants whose spouse had a positive attitude toward the exercise program, but only 40% for men whose spouse had either a neutral or negative attitude toward the program. Other research indicates that spousal support is associated with improved adherence by men enrolled in cardiac rehabilitation programs (28,29). A study (30) of healthy men and women enrolled in a general fitness program found that married participants who attended the program with their spouse had far greater adherence 1 year following enrollment than married participants whose spouses enrolled alone (93.7 vs. 57%). The participants who exercised with their spouses enrolled together in the exercise program on their own accord; no efforts or inducements were provided to encourage married couples to join as a pair. Whether an incentive program targeted toward getting spouses to participate in an exercise program together would result in an adherence rate comparable to that observed in this study is unclear. Processes that create social support by strengthening cohesiveness among exercise participants in organized programs have been hypothesized to result in greater success (31), but studies on the effects of team-building interventions in exercise programs indicate their benefit to be only modest and equivalent to a placebo treatment (32). Given that research on other intervention techniques has also tended to yield only modest reductions in dropout, it is likely that the benefit of spouse support observed in the present study was a consequence of many variables.

EXERCISE PRESCRIPTION FOR SUCCESS IN SPECIAL POPULATIONS

The American College of Sports Medicine (ACSM) (33) recommends that the general principles of exercise prescription apply to adults of all ages, regardless of special need. In special populations such as the elderly, however, physical inactivity is more common, and additional consideration may need to be given to developing an exercise program that will promote successful adherence (34). Research indicates that the use of exercise prescriptions does not systematically enhance exercise adherence (11), but this conclusion was based on studies that largely involved healthy populations, and the impact of exercise programing on special populations is less well understood. Some evidence suggests that home-based lifestyle programs that involve accruing 30 min of daily activity through several short periods provide health benefits comparable to traditional prescriptions while also enhancing adherence (35). One must identify an activity that is both convenient and enjoyable to the individual (36). Because special populations often have conditions or symptoms that make physical activity more difficult and lower their quality of life, careful prescription of an exercise program could well make a crucial difference in ensuring long-term adherence.

The following sections discuss behavioral and social issues associated with exercise programs for special populations. Readers should refer to the specific chapter that deals with the health problem or the special population for more information on exercise prescription.

The Elderly

Although the benefits of regular participation in physical activity among special populations are widely recognized, participation and long-term adherence to exercise remains low. Currently, it is estimated that two thirds of persons over the age of 65 do not exercise on a consistent basis (37), with women over the age of 55 more likely to limit or avoid physical activity than men (38). Consistent with studies involving younger samples, among sedentary elderly who do begin an exercise program, 50% will drop out within the first 6 months of involvement (39).

Medical conditions that make exercise more difficult become increasingly common with age, but many nonmedical variables are important determinants of nonparticipation and dropout (38). To improve exercise adherence with the elderly, factors associated with reasons for not exercising must be identified and, if possible, remedied. Baseline fitness testing, interviews, and the judicious use of questionnaires can each aid toward this end, if this information is used to create achievable exercise goals that are personally meaningful and that minimize or eliminate barriers to physical activity.

BEHAVIORAL AND SOCIAL ISSUES

No single variable explains and predicts exercise behavior. As a result, specific factors must be examined in the context of personal, environmental, and behavioral factors (18). For instance, Satariano

et al. (38) found that the elderly often have more than one reason for not participating in exercise programs and that gender may influence perceived obstacles. These researchers reported that elderly women were most likely to cite the absence of an exercise companion as the primary reason for avoidance of physical activity, while a lack of interest was the leading factor for men. Hence, for women, social support may be more important in the early stages of exercise adoption to ensure successful adherence (18). Additionally, socioeconomic factors present a more significant barrier to participation in exercise programs for women than for men (38). Despite initial gender differences, with increasing age both men and women report the fear of falling as a major factor in the avoidance of physical activity. In contrast, a study of elderly African-American women found that the most frequent barrier to exercise was the accessibility and availability of fitness facilities (40).

Research has also found that self-motivation is often a clear discriminator between those elderly individuals who adhere to an exercise program and those that drop out (24). Dishman (20) has suggested that a simple lack of knowledge concerning the benefits of an exercise program often affects individual levels of motivation. Exercise leaders who focus on motivating the elderly to both participate in and maintain an exercise program can increase adherence rates. A crucial aspect of their success is to educate the elderly about the potential benefits of physical activity (37).

Pregnancy

One of the initial special population groups to be directly examined in terms of the potential harmful and beneficial effects of exercise was pregnant women (41). However, recent research suggests that the benefits of a properly prescribed program of exercise during pregnancy outweigh the potential risks (33,42).

BEHAVIORAL ISSUES

Perceived stress and social support have both been associated with exercise behavior in pregnant women. In a study of Swedish women, Rodriguez et al. (43) reported that social support had a significant effect on compliance with health professional's recommendations for exercise throughout pregnancy. The degree of understanding of the partner toward the pregnancy and social isolation all affected the motivation of the women to both participate in and adhere to a prescribed exercise program.

Obesity

Exercise has been firmly established as a vital component of an effective weight-management program. However, the long-term adherence rates of obese individuals is very low (44). Because most obese individuals are sedentary and are likely to have had poor experiences with previous exercise programs, ACSM (33) guidelines suggest that exercise professionals conduct an interview with obese participants prior to the start of an exercise regime to determine the extent of past exercise history, potential problems, and preferred locations where an exercise program may be performed.

BEHAVIORAL ISSUES

Exercise leaders and personal trainers need to be sensitized to the particular challenges facing overweight individuals. Self-consciousness and anxieties about personal physical appearance are common among overweight individuals engaging in physical activity programs, and these feelings can result in greater dropout. The exercise setting itself may exacerbate these feelings, and efforts should be made to create a nonthreatening environment. For success with the obese individual, the exercise prescription must be designed to minimize discomfort and social anxiety associated with many exercise environments. In some cases, this may require scheduling separate exercise classes.

Mental Illness

There is substantial evidence that physical exercise programs can provide considerable psychologic benefits (45). Reductions in anxiety and increased feelings of calmness have been consistently observed following single bouts of exercise, and these changes may persist for several hours (46). Long-

term participation in exercise programs is also associated with improvements in mental health, particularly for clinical populations (47). In studies on samples of clinically depressed and anxiety individuals, regular participation in supervised exercise is associated with psychologic improvements that approach (48) or equal those associated with medication (49). With individuals scoring in the normal range for these variables, the changes in depression and anxiety are generally smaller and often not statistically significant (45).

PROGRAMMATIC ISSUES

Unlike the use of exercise as a means to treat or prevent physical conditions such as hypertension or osteoporosis, relatively little information exists regarding the appropriate exercise prescription for psychologic conditions. However, some general guidelines can be provided based on the published literature. In studies of different exercise programs (e.g., aerobic vs. anaerobic), it appears that the effectiveness of exercise to improve mental health is similar for aerobic and anaerobic forms of exercise, although studies using vigorous strength training programs are scant (46). Aerobic training programs used in mental health research have been based on accepted guidelines and involve prescriptions of walking/jogging programs three times a week. It has been speculated that improvements in mental health are directly linked to increased physical capacity, but the extant evidence has found only a small correlation between these variables (47,49). Other work has found that even mild stretching programs provide psychologic benefits comparable with those from more rigorous regimens of walking/jogging (47). Hence, the initial exercise prescription can be quite mild and easily tolerated, an issue of additional significance because fatigue and lethargy are common symptoms in depression.

It has long been proposed that vigorous exercise will not provide psychologic benefits to individuals suffering from anxiety disorders, and that the exercise itself could worsen symptoms or provoke panic attacks (50). However, a comprehensive review of the literature indicates there is no empirical support for this contention (51). Recent work involving clinically diagnosed panic disorder patients indicated that most can complete bouts of high-intensity exercise without experiencing a panic attack (52). Some evidence does indicate that depressed and anxious patients are lower in fitness than age-matched individuals free from psychologic disorders. Given this and the finding that the relationship between improvements in cardiovascular fitness and psychologic symptoms is weak, a mild exercise program will likely result in meaningful improvement in clinical symptoms and greater adherence than a more vigorous regimen.

BEHAVIORAL ISSUES

Although substantial evidence indicates that physical exercise can be effective in treating mild-to-moderate mental health disorders, many patients—particularly those with anxiety disorders—avoid exercise because of widely circulated but unfounded fears that it will exacerbate their symptoms (51). Educating individuals about the psychologic benefits of exercise and research indicating that exercise does not provoke panic attacks can help alleviate these concerns. Providing information about sensations and normal discomfort that occurs with exercise (e.g., increased heart rate and ventilation, sweating) is crucial, given that many of these symptoms commonly occur in panic attacks and may be interpreted as a sign of anxiety. Attention should also be accorded to the exercise setting. Patients with phobias or other anxiety disorders may be uncomfortable exercising in the middle of a group, in an enclosed space, or far from an exit in a room. Exercise in large open spaces or outdoors can be provoke anxiety in other individuals, and in such cases, an exercise partner can help alleviate fears as can the use of well-defined exercise trails.

Psychiatric medication can be used safely by most patients who are exercising, but these medications do have side effects that can make physical activity uncomfortable, such as dry mouth and drowsiness. Chlorpromazine and tricyclic antidepressants have been found to be associated with lower blood pressure and orthostatic intolerance (53). Muscle tremor and weakness may occur with lithium usage. Fewer side effects have been reported for selective serotonin reuptake inhibitors, although one report found that the combination of fluoxetine and lithium may exacerbate exercise-induced hyperthermia (59). Although it has been speculated that the combination of exercise and medication may have a synergistic effect that could potentiate both the benefits and side effects of medication, no evidence to this effect has been observed (49,53).

Summary

Getting healthy individuals who are inactive to begin and successfully adhere to physical activity programs is a multidimensional challenge that is compounded when dealing with special populations. Research indicates that behavior-modification and cognitive–behavior-modification techniques are associated with increased adoption and maintenance of physical activity. Health education or health risk appraisals have not been found to be consistently effective (11,55). However, in the case of special populations, these procedures provide important information that can be integrated into a broad intervention strategy that includes behavioral techniques. Information on exercise prescription, while not associated with improved adherence in general (11), could be particularly valuable for special populations with conditions that result in exercise barriers not faced by the general population. Moreover, past research has often combined cognitive–behavioral interventions with other techniques, so it is difficult to evaluate the influence of a single intervention objectively on the basis of the literature (11). In the case of special populations who have conditions that would benefit from physical exercise, the need for empirical information concerning effective ways to improve participation and success in physical activity programs and research is especially needed.

REFERENCES

1. Caspersen CJ, Merritt RK. Physical activity trends among 26 states, 1986–1990. Med Sci Sports Exerc 1995;27:713–720.
2. Stephens T, Jacobs DR, White CC. A descriptive epidemiology of leisure time physical activity. Pub Health Rep 1985;100:147–151.
3. Caspersen CJ, Pereira MA, Curran KM. Changes in physical activity patterns in the United States by sex, and cross-sectional age. Med Sci Sports Exerc 2000;32:1601–1609.
4. Mokdad AH, Serdula MK, Dietz WH, et al. The spread of the obesity epidemic in the United States, 1991–1998. JAMA 1999;282:1519–1522.

5. Morgan WP. Prescription of physical activity: a paradigm shift. Quest 2000;53:366–382.

6. Dishman RK. Advances in Exercise Adherence. Champaign, IL: Human Kinetics, 1994.

7. Gettman LR. Management skills required for exercise programs. In: Blair SN, et al., ed. Resource Manual for Guidelines for Exercise Testing and Prescription. Philadelphia: Lea & Febiger, 1988:377–389.

8. Morgan WP. Involvement in vigorous physical activity with special reference to adherence. Proceedings of the NCPEAM/NAPECW national conference 1977:235–246.

9. Godin G, Shephard RJ. Use of attitude-behavior models in exercise promotion. Sports Med 1990;10:103–121.

10. Franklin BA. Program factors that influence exercise adherence: practical adherence skills for the clinical staff. In: Dishman RK, ed. Exercise Adherence: Its Impact on Public Health. Champaign, IL: Human Kinetics, 1988:237–258.

11. Dishman RK, Buckworth J. Increasing physical activity: a quantitative synthesis. Med Sci Sports Exerc 1996;28:706–719.

12. Kosma M, Cardinal BJ, Kintala P. Motivating individuals with disabilities to be physically active. Quest 2002;54:116–132.

13. Dishman RK, Buckworth J. Adherence to physical activity. In: Morgan WP, ed. Physical Activity and Mental Health. Washington, DC: Taylor & Francis, 1997:163–180.

14. Dishman RK. The problem of exercise adherence: fighting sloth in nations with marketing economies. Quest 2000;53:279–294.

15. Buckworth, J. Exercise determinants and interventions. Int J Sport Psychol 2000;31:305–320.

16. Lombard DN, Lombard TN, Winett RA. Walking to meet health guidelines: the effect of prompting frequency and prompt structure. Health Psychol 1995;14:164–170.

17. Prochaska, JO, Marcus BH. The transtheoretical model: applications to exercise. In: Dishman RK, ed. Advances in Exercise Adherence. Champaign, IL: Human Kinetics, 1994:161–180.

18. Buckworth J, Dishman R. Exercise Psychology. Champaign, IL: Human Kinetics, 2002.

19. Carron, AV, Hausenblas, HA, Mack D. Social influence and exercise: a meta-analysis. J Sport Exerc Psychol 1996;18:1–16.

20. Dishman RK. Motivating older adults to exercise. South Med J 1994;87:79–82.

21. Sonstroem RJ. Psychological models. In: Dishman RK, ed. Exercise Adherence: Its Impact on Public Health. Champaign, IL: Human Kinetics, 1988: 125–153.

22. McAuley E, Blissmer B. Self-efficacy determinants and consequences of physical activity. Exerc Sport Sci Rev 2000;28:85–88.

23. Dishman RK, Ikes W. Self-motivation and the adherence to therapeutic exercise. J Behav Med 1981;4: 421–438.

24. Dishman R, Ickes W, Morgan W. Self-motivation and adherence to habitual physical activity. J Appl Psychol 1980;10:115–132.

25. Raglin JS, Morgan WP, Luchsinger AL. Mood and self-motivation in successful and unsuccessful rowers. Med Sci Sports Exerc 1990;22:849–853.

26. Lee C. Factors related to the adoption of exercise among older women. J Behav Med 1993;16:323–334.

27. Heinzelmann F, Bagley RW. Response to physical activity programs and their effects on health behavior. Public Health Rep 1970;85:905–911.

28. Erling J, Oldridge NB. Effect of a spousal-support program on compliance with cardiac rehabilitation. Med Sci Sports Exerc 1985;17:284.

29. Knapp D, Gutmann M, Squires R, et al. Exercise adherence among coronary artery bypass surgery (CABS) patients. Med Sci Sports Exerc 1983;15:120.

30. Wallace JP, Raglin JS, Jastremski C. Twelve month adherence of adults who joined a fitness program with a spouse vs. without a spouse. J Sports Med Phys Fitness 1995;35:206–213.

31. Estabrooks PA. Sustaining exercise participation through group cohesion. Exerc Sport Sci Rev 2000;28:63–67.

32. Estabrooks PA, Carron AV. Group cohesion in older adult exercisers: prediction and intervention effects. J Behav Med 1999;22:575–588.

33. American College of Sports Medicine. Guidelines for Exercise Testing and Prescription. 6th ed. Philadelphia: Lippincott Williams & Wilkins, 2000.

34. McArdle WM, Katch FI, Katch VL. Essentials of Exercise Physiology. 2nd ed. Philadelphia: Lippincott Williams & Wilkins, 2000.

35. Jakicic JM, Winters C, Lang W, Wing RR. Effects of intermittent exercise and use of home exercise equipment on adherence, weight loss, and fitness in overweight women. JAMA 1999;282:1554–1660.

36. Brennan FH. Exercise prescriptions for active seniors. Physician Sports Med 2002;30(2):19–27.

37. Grove N, Speir B. Motivating the well elderly to exercise. J Community Health Nurs 1999;16:179–180.

38. Satariano WA, Thaddeus J, Haight MA, et al. Reasons given by older people for limitation or avoidance of leisure time physical activity. J Am Geriatr Soc 2000;48:502–512.

39. Resnick B. Prescribing an exercise program and motivating older adults to comply. Educ Gerontol 2001;27:209–227.

40. Jones M, Neis MA. The relationship of perceived benefits of and barriers to reported exercise in older African-American women. Public Health Nurs 1996;13:151–158.

41. Durak E. Special populations and exercise. Total Health 1983;15:23–28.

42. Clapp JF. The effect of continuing regular endurance exercise on the physiologic adaptations to pregnancy outcome. Am J Sports Med 1996;24:28–29.

43. Rodriguez A, Bohlin G, Lindmark G. Psychosocial predictors of smoking and exercise during pregnancy. J Reprod Infant Psychol 2000;18:203–226.

44. Goodrick GK, Malek JN, Foreyt JP. Exercise adherence in the obese: self-regulated intensity. Med Exerc Nutr Health 1994;3:335–338.

45. Morgan WP. Physical Activity and Mental Health. Washington, DC: Taylor & Francis, 1997:107–126.

46. Raglin JS. Anxiolytic effects of exercise. In: Morgan WP, ed. Physical Activity and Mental Health. Washington, DC: Taylor & Francis, 1997:107–126.

47. Martinsen EG, Morgan WP. Antidepressant effects of physical activity. In: Morgan WP, ed. Physical Activity & Mental Health. Washington: Taylor & Francis, 1997:93–106.

48. Broocks A, Bandelow B, Pekrun G, et al. Comparison of aerobic exercise, clomipramine, and placebo in the treatment of panic disorder. Am J Psychol 1998;55:603–609.

49. Blumenthal JA, Babyak MA, Moore KA, et al. Effects of exercise training on older patients with major depression. Arch Int Med 1990;159:2349–2356.

50. Pitts JW, McClure JN. Lactate metabolism in anxiety neurotics. N Engl J Med 1967;227:1329–1336.

51. O'Connor PJ, Smith JC, Morgan WP. Physical activity does not provoke panic attacks in patients with panic disorders. Anxiety Stress Coping 2000;13:333–353.

52. Martinsen EG, Raglin JS, Hoffart A, et al. Tolerance to intensive exercise and high levels of lactate in panic disorder. J Anxiety Disord 1998;12:333–342.

53. Martinsen EG, Stanghelle JK. Drug therapy and physical activity. In: Morgan WP, ed. Physical Activity & Mental Health. Washington, DC: Taylor & Francis, 1997:81–90.

54. Epstein Y, Albukrek D, Kalmovitz B, et al. Heat intolerance induced by antidepressant. Ann NY Acad Sci 1997;813:553–558.

55. Dishman RK, Buckworth J. Exercise determinants and interventions. Int J Sport Psychol 2000;31:305–320.

9

Economic Evaluation: Comprehensive Cardiac Rehabilitation as an Example

Neil B. Oldridge

The rapidly growing burden of chronic illnesses on the health care system has created increased interest in the economic impact of strategies to treat chronic diseases such as coronary artery disease (CAD). In 1995, first-year costs of treatment for the estimated 616,900 incident cases of CAD in the United States amounted to a total of $5.54 billion, with the 5- and 10-year cumulative costs an estimated $71.5 billion and $126.6 billion, respectively (1). Extrapolating from a study of nearly 10,000 patients with acute myocardial infarction (MI) or angina following catheterization discharged to the 1993 U.S. population of patients with catheterization, the mean 10-year costs amounted to an estimated $63.3 billion (2).

These data reinforce the enormous cost burden of treating chronic disease and the associated risk factors, and identifying the most efficient use of limited and finite resources available for health care has become a major challenge. With demographic shifts and improved life-expectancy, escalating demands for more and higher-quality health care and the increased availability of expensive technologic advances each play a significant part in the increasing cost of health care seen in most countries. Economic evaluations, de-

fined as "the comparative analysis of alternative courses of action in terms of both costs and consequences," provide a framework for a systematic evaluation of both the benefits and costs of alternative health care services (3). There are two key questions in the economic evaluation of health care services:

- Is health care service A more cost-effective than the alternative service B, which most frequently is usual care?
- What is the cost impact for the health care system if service A is substituted for service B?

As evidence for effectiveness is often of poor quality and, in many cases, entirely lacking, making decisions about which alternative to choose from among the many current and emerging medical practices is often problematic (4). Additionally, we know little about the cost-effectiveness of many of our current interventions (5).

The purpose of this chapter is to provide a brief description of the types of economic evaluations commonly used in health care and to summarize the available economic evaluation data for comprehensive cardiac rehabilitation.

Economic Evaluation in Health Care

The claim that a specified medical practice is cost-effective frequently is not supported with appropriate documentation of associated costs and benefits. With the increased awareness of having to stay within a given budget, economic evaluation is one strategy to help decision makers make rational choices about effective and efficient health care. The different perspectives at each level result in attitudes toward economic evaluations that differ considerably (6). Decision making takes place at the macro level, where politicians and regulators make decisions about health care reimbursement; at an intermediate level, where organizations make formulary and guideline decisions; and at the micro level, where health care practitioners and patients make treatment decisions. Additional concerns about economic evaluations include (*a*) methodological issues in analytic strategies, for example, costing challenges, which often result in contradictory results and create confusion; (*b*) results that are often counterintuitive; and (*c*) other arguments of a psychologic and philosophic nature, such as from whose perspective—the social perspective using community-based preference data or the patient perspective using individual patient data—should the economic evaluation be carried out (6). Economic evaluations provide a balance sheet of the effects, either benefits (i.e., advantages) or harms (i.e., disadvantages), and costs for making choices between alternative health care services. Ultimately, the question comes down to "Who should do what to whom, with what health resources, and with what relation to other health services?" (3).

Standardization of economic evaluation methodology is needed if comparisons of the cost-effectiveness of various treatments are to be made by clinicians, payers, and policy makers. A standard set of cost-effectiveness analysis methods, the "reference case" analysis, has been recommended by the Panel on Cost-Effectiveness in Health and Medicine (7) and is summarized in a series of 3 articles in JAMA (5,8,9).

PERSPECTIVE

The panel recommends that the "reference case" analysis be conducted from the societal perspective using community-based preference data, as this represents the public interest rather than that of any group and allows comparisons across conditions and interventions when assessing the relative value or merit of alternative health care services (7). This approach to the economic evaluation of health care services gives consideration to the costs of all resources used and to all the health effects, even in individuals not directly affected by the intervention. The societal perspective approach directly acknowledges the value of our limited resources for competing uses, such as education, welfare, and justice. As decisions about the relative value or merit of alternative health care services are made in the light of the increasing societal demands for scarce and finite resources, "no perspective has a stronger claim to be the basis for comparability across studies."

However, although patient preferences should not be seen as equivalent to community preferences, there may be good reasons for using patient preference data under certain circumstances. For example, when a study is designed to compare the impact of alternative treatments for the same condition, e.g., clinic-based and home-based cardiac rehabilitation, the use of patient preferences would be preferable to use of community preferences (7). This is because the focus of this kind of analysis is to examine the most efficient way of treating patients for a specific condition, given that there are alternative treatment choices, and is not intended for resource allocation decisions over a wide range of conditions. Patient perspective preference measures better capture the small but important differences often seen with treatments and so can better capture the effects of a given treatment (7).

HEALTH CARE COSTS AND EFFECTS

Cost (inputs) and effect (outcomes) data collected on two or more alternatives provide the basis for economic evaluations and calculating a cost-effectiveness (C/E) ratio (7). The numerator term in the C/E ratio is the "net incremental" cost of treatment A, which is the difference between the resources used or the costs of the treatment under investigation and the costs of the comparison treatment, typically "routine care." The health effect is the denominator term in the C/E ratio and is the "net incremental" improvement, which captures the change in health or the outcomes. The cost-effectiveness analysis is therefore always comparative, and the incremental C/E ratio for treatment A versus routine care is calculated as the additional cost of treatment A compared with the cost of routine care as described below.

$$\text{Incremental Cost-effectiveness}_A = \frac{\text{Cost}_A - \text{Cost}_{\text{routine care}}}{\text{Effect}_A - \text{Effect}_{\text{routine care}}}$$

Costs of a health care service, the numerator term in the C/E ratio, reflect the resources used. Direct costs can be medical (activities of the hospital and health professionals, patients' own costs) or nonmedical (food, transportation, lodging, family care) and are usually based on the price of the factors involved. Indirect costs reflect the impact of the resources lost because of either mortality or morbidity (reflecting premature death and the time lost from production and/or consumption activities). Intangible costs, those associated with pain and suffering, grief, and other nonmonetary outcomes of illness and health care, are difficult to estimate.

The health effect or outcome can be measured either in natural units (e.g., years of life gained [LYG]; years of life saved [YOLS]; laboratory measures such as blood pressure, blood lipids, or health-related quality of life [HRQL]) or derived units (e.g., quality-adjusted life-years [QALYs]). Preference-based scales are designed to provide preference scores for health states and are used to assess HRQL and estimate QALYs (3,7). Preference scores may be measured either indirectly using community-based multi-attribute health classification systems such as the Quality of Well-Being (QWB) (10) and the Health Utilities Index (11,12) or direct patient preferences using techniques such as the time-tradeoff (TTO) (13) and the standard gamble (14).

With the QWB multi-attribute health classification system, patients are asked to report on their own health status using standardized interviewer-administered questionnaires. The QWB is designed to elicit a patient's perspective of his or her limitations and problems with health including symptoms, mobility, physical activity, and social activity. Using the QWB linear additive preference function, an indirect community preference score is calculated for each patient. With the TTO methodology, patients provide a preference score for their own subjectively defined comprehensive current health state, whose content is implicit and personal. Both the indirect and direct preference approaches are based on a scale in which dead = 0.00 and perfect health = 1.00.

Theory and experience have shown that patient-level preference scores, such as estimated with the TTO, are generally higher than community-level preference scores, such as estimated with the QWB (15). These differences in approaches to preference measurement have led to questions such as "Do we know how similar the estimated QALYs are when using both community QWB and patient TTO preference scores generated by the same group of patients?"

TYPES OF ECONOMIC EVALUATION

The form of the economic evaluation is determined basically by the response to two sets of questions (Fig. 9-1). Two sets of questions can be asked and answered: (*a*) Were both costs and effects of the health care service considered? (*b*) Were alternative health care services compared? According to Drummond et al. (3), only when the answer to both questions is "yes" is there a full economic evaluation, otherwise the analyses provide only partial economic evaluations. A further determinant of the type of economic evaluation is the way that the health effect or outcome, the denominator term in the C/E ratio, is calculated (7).

The following answers to the two sets of questions distinguish the types of cost studies.

Partial Economic Evaluation
a. Cost description: the information presented pertains only to one service and only cost information is provided.
b. Cost–outcome description: the information presented pertains only to one service and both cost and effect information is provided.
c. Cost analysis: the information presented pertains to two or more services and only cost, not effect, information is provided.

	Are both costs and consequences examined?	
	NO	**YES**
	Partial evaluations	
	Costs only	
NO	Cost description	Cost-outcome description
Are alternatives compared?		**FULL EVALUATIONS**
YES	Cost analysis	Cost minimization Cost-benefit Cost-effectiveness Cost-utility

FIGURE 9-1 Spectrum of health care economic evaluation.

Full Economic Evaluation

The answer here to the questions posed above is that if there are two or more alternative courses of action and both costs and consequences of each alternative course of action are available, then the analysis is a full economic evaluation. The following characteristics distinguish between the different types of full economic evaluations.

a. Cost minimization: if the effectiveness of alternative interventions is similar or the same and their outcomes are similar or the same, the less expensive intervention will be preferred as it is considered the more efficient.

b. Cost–benefit: both costs and health effects are given a monetary value, which permits comparison across different health care services, and the service with the highest ratio of benefit to cost is the service of choice. However, as it is difficult to put a monetary value on the complex outcomes of health care, such as on a LYG or YOLS, cost–benefit analysis is used infrequently for health care research and decision making.

c. Cost-effectiveness: The effectiveness of an intervention and its costs are incorporated into a C/E analysis ensuring that both are considered in clinical decision-making. Two forms of cost-effectiveness analyses have been identified.

(i) Cost-effectiveness analysis is used when the outcomes, or denominator term in the C/E ratio, are measured in natural units and are expressed in a single dimension, most commonly LYG or YOLS, and when the outcomes of alternative health care services are expected to differ. Incremental costs are determined per unit effect, and the lower the C/E ratio, the greater the cost-effectiveness.

(ii) Cost-utility analysis is a form of C/E analysis in which the outcome, or denominator term, is based on the desirability of a specific health state or treatment outcome. This typically is measured as a preference score that is anchored at 0.00 (death) and 1.00 (full health), with the score used to adjust the value of the time spent in a given health state (14). Most commonly, this is calculated as a QALY, but similar measures such as the healthy years equivalent also can be estimated. If intervention A improves the preference measure more than intervention B, then more QALYs will be gained with intervention A than with B. The net incremental cost per unit of effect, in this case QALYs, then can be compared across diseases, conditions, and treatments, and the lower the C/U ratio, the greater the cost utility. Cost-utility analysis, conducted from the societal perspective with community-based preferences, is recommended for making health care policy decisions in Canada (16), in Australia (17), and increasingly in the United States (7). However, although patient preferences are not equivalent to community preferences, when a study is designed to compare the impact of alternative treatments for the same condition (e.g., clinic-based and home-based cardiac rehabilitation), the use of patient preferences is preferable to use of community preferences (7).

DATA SOURCES

Valid effectiveness data for an intervention, relative to an alternative such as usual care, should be established before an economic evaluation is attempted (3). Valuable sources of effectiveness data include the randomized controlled trial (RCT), although there is some controversy over carrying out economic evaluations alongside RCTs (18,19). RCTs meet the criteria for best experimental scientific evidence and hypothesis testing, i.e., high internal validity with replication, verification, falsification, and assessment of uncertainty. On the other hand, from the policymakers' perspective, there are problems with the level of generalizability of RCT evidence, including the choice of alternative intervention, protocol-driven costs, an artificial environment, choice of outcomes, inadequate patient follow-up, and patient or provider selection bias (20). The use of decision theory modeling is a legitimate and complementary alternative to RCT-generated data for economic evaluations and can enrich and broaden the results of experimental research and substitute for experimental data when it is not available. In this approach, retrospective clinical study effectiveness evidence is combined with cost data from secondary sources in a decision analysis model (20,21).

OTHER ECONOMIC EVALUATION ISSUES

The validity of the assumptions determines the usefulness of an economic evaluation. For example, assuming a reinfarction rate of 2% per year may be inaccurate, as the actual rate may turn out to be 4%. Therefore, sensitivity analyses should be carried out with a range of possible assumptions to examine the robustness of the initial assumption (7). Time preference is another important consideration as we tend to value present costs and benefits more than we value future costs and benefits. The diminished value of future costs and benefits is handled by discounting both present costs and benefits (7). For example, preventive strategies such as medical treatment of hypertension have high initial costs but delayed benefits; medical treatment of angina has relatively uniform costs and benefits over the long term; bypass surgery has high present costs but produces immediate benefits.

While there is a need to know what society deems acceptable in terms of costs and outcomes, guidelines for determining whether a treatment is or is not cost-effective have not been universally agreed on. Interventions with incremental costs (updated by medical care consumer price index to US$ in 2001) below $25,000 are considered highly attractive, between $25,000 and $50,000 per year of life saved or per QALY are attractive, and more than $50,000, increasingly unattractive (22,23).

Economic Evaluation of Comprehensive Cardiac Rehabilitation

The essence of an economic evaluation is that it provides a balance sheet of the benefits (advantages) or harms (disadvantages) and the costs of each option, allowing comparisons to assist in choosing among the available alternatives. Drummond et al. have suggested that economic evaluations are most helpful when proceeded by demonstration of efficacy, effectiveness, and availability (3).

Cigarette smoking, hyperlipidemia, and lack of physical activity are three major modifiable risk factors for both primary and secondary prevention of heart disease, with considerable evidence that modification of these factors, either singly or in combination, is beneficial (24). Unfortunately, and despite the available evidence of their efficacy, secondary preventive strategies are frequently underused (25), with as few as 11% of patients with an acute coronary event referred to cardiac rehabilitation in routine clinical practice (26), and as many as 38% of U.S. and 32% of Canadian patients referred at tertiary medical centers in the GUSTO Trial (27). Further, patient adherence with secondary prevention strategies is often low and a major concern (28).

As an example, the evidence that smoking cessation as part of secondary prevention decreases the risk for cardiovascular disease end-points is considered proven (24). There are limited experimental data on smoking cessation after MI, but in one study, the 61% cessation rate in patients randomized to a nurse-managed intervention was nearly double the 32% rate observed in the usual care group (29). A recent meta-analysis of smoking cessation after MI included 12 cohort studies with data on

5878 patients from 6 countries between 1949 and 1988, with a follow-up duration ranging from 2 to 10 years (30). All 12 studies showed a mortality benefit associated with smoking cessation, with an aggregate odds ratio of 0.54 (95% confidence interval, 0.46–0.62) for death after MI in those who quit smoking, and the estimated number needed to quit smoking to save one life is 13, assuming a mortality rate of 20% in continuing smokers (30). Decision-theory modeling has been used (31) to examine the cost-effectiveness of the nurse-managed smoking cessation program reported above in patients with MI (29). The cost was estimated by considering the resources necessary to implement the program, and years of life saved were estimated by modeling life expectancy using a single declining exponential approximation of life expectancy based on data from published reports. The cost-effectiveness of the nurse-managed smoking cessation program was estimated to be $220/year of life saved (about $340 in 2001 US$) and remained below $20,000/year of life saved even if the cessation rate was 3% or if it cost as much as $8,840/smoker (29).

CARDIAC REHABILITATION

Clinical practice guidelines for cardiac rehabilitation services, based on 334 studies of efficacy and effectiveness, were established in 1995 for comprehensive cardiac rehabilitation in the United States (26). Key cardiac rehabilitation services are exercise, education, and risk factor management counseling, and the most substantial benefits, as documented in the guidelines (26) and supported by systematic review and meta-analysis (32), include the following:

- Increased exercise tolerance
- Improved symptoms
- Improved blood lipid levels
- Improved well-being
- Decreased cigarette smoking
- Reduced stress
- Reduced mortality

There are only a limited number of economic evaluations of cardiac rehabilitation (33,34) and even fewer that meet the following criteria:

1. A full economic evaluation or a cost-analysis
2. Adults with CAD

3. Cardiac rehabilitation with an exercise component
4. Primary outcomes providing costs in dollars or an incremental cost-effectiveness or cost-utility ratio

Three of the six studies that meet the eligibility criteria are cost-analysis studies (35–37), and three are full economic evaluations (38–40). An additional full economic evaluation of exercise-based cardiac rehabilitation in patients with heart failure (41), which meets each of the inclusion criteria other than the diagnostic criterion, is described below.

This small number of rigorous economic evaluations clearly demonstrates both the paucity of, and the need for more, economic evaluations of cardiac rehabilitation services. However, the limited data are encouraging and suggest that cardiac rehabilitation probably is an efficient use of health care resources that can be economically justified. Two of the full economic evaluations were carried out in Canada (38,40) and one each in the United States (39) and Italy (41); of the three cost analyses, two were carried out in Sweden (35,37) and one in the United States (36). With no universal approach to the delivery of cardiac rehabilitation services in the same country, let alone between different countries, the generalizability of the data on the cost-effectiveness of comprehensive cardiac rehabilitation to different health care systems is uncertain.

PARTIAL ECONOMIC EVALUATION

Cost Analysis

1. The purpose of this prospective, nonrandomized 5-year follow-up study (Sweden, published in 1991) was to compare 5-year costs associated with comprehensive cardiac rehabilitation services with standard care following MI in patients <65 years of age from the perspective of the Swedish National Health Insurance System (35). Following MI, 147 patients (124 males, 23 females) from one hospital district were invited to participate in a medically supervised physical training program for 3 months, with encouragement to continue home training. Controls (134 males, 24 females) were recruited from the adjacent hospital district and received

standard care consisting of 1 post-MI clinic visit, followed by referral to primary health care.

A cost analysis was carried out with 5-year direct costs estimated for the program participation, rehospitalization, clinic visits procedures, medications, and travel. The difference in direct costs per patient was 3,910 Swedish Kronor (SEK) per patient in favor of rehabilitation. Indirect costs accounted for most of the total cost and were associated primarily with lost productivity. The overall rate of active employment at 5 years was significantly higher ($P < .01$) among the rehabilitation patients (51.8%) than the control patients (27.4%), giving a total indirect cost of SEK 69,600 in favor of the rehabilitation patients. The rehabilitation program, therefore, resulted in savings of SEK 73,510 per patient over the 5-year follow-up, with positive clinical results favoring rehabilitation patients (42). According to the authors of the study, "The outstanding winner of the rehabilitation programme was the Swedish National Health Insurance System. It must be concluded that the comprehensive cardiac rehabilitation programme is a major strategy that leads to both lowered costs and positive health effects. The cardiac rehabilitation programme therefore is highly cost-effective" (35). Even though the data were not generated in a randomized study design, the controlled nature of the study, the comparison of two real-life clinical situations, and the prospective nature of the data collection each strengthens the usefulness of the information about the cost-effectiveness of cardiac rehabilitation.

2. A computerized retrospective review of billing data (United States, published in 1992) was carried out using the hospital perspective to determine total hospitalization charges for cardiac admissions after MI or for bypass surgery over a 3-year period for 580 patients (36). Of these 580 patients, 230 were referred to a 12-week cardiac rehabilitation program with cardiac risk factor management education, while 350 patients were not referred. Rehabilitation entrants and nonentrants had similar left ventricular function but entrants were more likely to have had an MI, to be younger, male, nonsmokers, and white collar workers and less likely to have had bypass surgery or other medical complications.

A cost-analysis was carried out and, before correction for clinical differences at baseline, rehabilitation entrants had significantly lower ($P = .022$) cardiac hospitalization charges of $1,197 ($\pm$$3,911$) per patient over the 3-year follow-up period, compared with nonentrants $1,936 ($\pm$$5,359$). This difference remained significant after stepwise analysis of covariance to adjust for the baseline differences between the two groups. The authors point out that since physician charges were not included in the cost-analysis, the cost differential was underestimated, and they conclude that the "results of this study show an association between participation in comprehensive cardiac rehabilitation and lowered cardiac rehospitalization costs in the years after an acute coronary event" (36). However, the retrospective study design and the differences in baseline characteristics of the patients limit the usefulness of these data.

3. Bondestam et al. (37) examined the effects of early rehabilitation on the use of medical care following MI in patients 65 years of age and older, using the perspective of the primary health care provider. The study design was similar to that used by Levin et al. (35), with patients in one hospital primary care clinic serving as the rehabilitation group ($n = 91$) and those in a nearby hospital, without rehabilitation services, serving as controls ($n = 99$). Patients were followed for 1 year with registration of deaths from the national registry and documentation of rehospitalization or unplanned visits to the emergency department.

The intervention consisted of low-intensity exercise for 4 to 8 weeks, followed by a group discussion on risk factor management. Rehabilitation patients had a total of 70 emergency visits and rehospitalizations compared with 149 among the control patients ($P < .001$), resulting in significantly ($P < .05$) fewer days of hospitalization. The authors conclude that "an uncomplicated rehabilitation model characterized by very early intervention and performed within the primary health care system can significantly reduce the consumption of health care 1 year after myocardial infarction in patients ≥ 65 years old" (37). This is the only study that has examined the use of health care in older patients with MI and as such provides useful information about the effectiveness of cardiac rehabilitation in reducing health care use for at least the first year following MI.

FULL ECONOMIC EVALUATION

Two different approaches to economic evaluation, *(a)* RCTs with an a priori economic evaluation and *(b)* decision-theory modeling, are available and should be considered as complementary rather than competitive sources of information (21). As stated above, RCTs meet the criteria for best experimental scientific evidence and hypothesis testing, while decision-theory modeling combines retrospective clinical study effectiveness evidence with cost data from secondary sources in a decision analysis model, broadening the results of experimental research (20,21). There are two decision-theory modeling studies with full economic evaluations in cardiac rehabilitation, one (39) in patients who survived the MI and one (40) in patients with symptomatic cardiovascular disease. There are two full economic evaluations using RCT-derived data, one in patients surviving the MI (38) and one in patients with heart failure (41).

Decision-Theory Modeling: Cost-Effectiveness

1. Ades et al. (39) carried out a decision-theory cost-effectiveness analysis of cardiac rehabilitation after MI from the perspective of the patient or insurance payer, using data from published results of RCTs on mortality, epidemiologic studies of long-term survival, and published studies of patient charges for rehabilitation services and averted medical expenses. The data source for the clinical effectiveness information (i.e., all-cause mortality) was a meta-analysis of cardiac rehabilitation, with controls randomized to either no or light exercise in the first 3 post-MI years (43), with rates similar to those reported earlier by Oldridge et al. (44). Longer-term survival data were generated from the Duke University Cardiovascular Disease database (45). An annual discount rate of 5% was used to reduce YOLS to their 1995 value. Cost data were derived from survey data obtained from 626 operating cardiac rehabilitation centers, 78% of which were hospital based (46).

These investigators estimated an incremental life expectancy of 0.202 years during the 15 years following rehabilitation with a 1985 estimated net cost of $430 (direct costs, $1,280; savings, $850) for rehabilitation and exercise testing. Using inflationary factors and changes in post-MI mortality, the cost-effectiveness ratio for 1995 was $4,950/YOLS. Sensitivity analyses, considering survival, efficacy, and averted expenses were carried out, supporting the study results. The authors conclude by stating that "cardiac rehabilitation is more cost-effective than thrombolytic therapy, coronary bypass surgery, and cholesterol lowering drugs, though less cost-effective than smoking cessation … and should stand alongside these therapies as standard of care in the post-MI setting" (39).

2. Lowensteyn et al. (40) carried out the second decision-theory modeling economic evaluation study (perspective not stated) in patients with cardiovascular disease. Risk factor data were derived from the Canadian Heart Health Survey (47); these were then applied to the Cardiovascular Disease Life Expectancy Model (48) to estimate YOLS with exercise-training cardiac rehabilitation. Canadian costs associated with fatal and nonfatal events, surgical procedures, and medical follow-up were estimated from previously published research (49), and costs were estimated for unsupervised and supervised exercise training rehabilitation assuming 50% adherence in year 1 and 30% in all other years. The cost-effectiveness per YOLS (in 1996 US dollars) of secondary prevention of cardiovascular disease was estimated for both unsupervised and supervised settings and for men and women by age (35–54, 55–64, and 65–75 years) (40).

The cost-effectiveness ratios, as expected, were always worse for supervised exercise training than for unsupervised exercise training, and unsupervised exercise training was actually cost saving in women 55 to 64 years of age (Table 9-1). With unsupervised exercise training, the ratios were worse in women than in men in the youngest age group but worse for men than women in the oldest age group. With supervised exercise training, the ratios were worse for women than men at each age group. The authors conclude that unsupervised exercise-training cardiac rehabilitation "appears to be an

TABLE 9-1 DECISION-THEORY MODELING COST-EFFECTIVENESS OF EXERCISE-TRAINING CARDIAC REHABILITATION FOR PERSONS WITH CARDIOVASCULAR DISEASE

	Unsupervised Cost/YOLS[a]		Supervised Cost/YOLS	
Age	Women	Men	Women	Men
35–54 years	$6,765	$1,734	$42,367	$13,719
55–64 years	($634)[b]	$341	$12,015	$8,562
65–74 years	$965	$1,723	$20,307	$14,464

[a]Cost per year of life saved in 1996 US dollars.
[b]Cost saving per YOLS.

extremely efficient use of resources" at all ages in both men and women; they further state "supervised exercise is highly cost-effective for all men with cardiovascular disease and women with cardiovascular disease between 55 and 64 years of age ... and relatively cost-effective for older women with cardiovascular disease" (40).

Randomized Controlled Trials: Cost-effectiveness and Cost Utility

1. There is only one randomized controlled trial of early cardiac rehabilitation after MI which included an a priori economic evaluation with both cost-effectiveness and cost-utility analyses (38). The RCT was carried out in Canada and included patients ($n = 201$) with a documented MI who were moderately anxious or depressed and were identified while in hospital. They were then stratified and randomized to either 8 weeks of exercise and group behavioral and risk factor management counseling ($n = 99$) or usual community care (control, $n = 101$) within 6 weeks of the MI (50).

The smaller number of cardiac rehabilitation visits ($P < .001$) among early rehabilitation patients ($N = 2.1$) than in control patients ($N = 8.4$) during the 10 months of follow-up after the experimental 8-week intervention amounted to a direct cost savings of $310 per rehabilitation patient. With total direct costs of $790, the net direct costs amounted to $480 per rehabilitation patient, which is the numerator for each of the calculations that follow. Two denominator terms were generated. The first was estimated QALYs using the direct TTO preference instru-

ment (13,51,52) which was administered to all patients at five assessment points: on entry into the RCT and at the end of the intervention at 2 months, 4 months, 8 months, and 12 months. The TTO approach resulted in an incremental aggregate mean of 0.052 QALYs gained per rehabilitation patient. The second approach was to estimate the number of LYGs using data from meta-analyses of cardiac rehabilitation (43,44), which demonstrated a 25% lower mortality rate with rehabilitation than with usual care, amounting to an incremental 0.022 LYG per rehabilitation patient.

Using these data and 1991 US dollars, the best-estimate cost-effectiveness ratio in the original analysis (38) was $21,800 per LYG and the best estimate cost-utility ratio was $9,200 per QALY gained with cardiac rehabilitation. Combining the differences in QALYs and the reduction in mortality from the meta-analyses, a mean of 0.071 QALYs attributable to the rehabilitation program was gained per patient, and the best estimate comprehensive cost-utility ratio for cardiac rehabilitation was estimated at $6,800 per QALY gained per rehabilitation patient. The investigators in this study concluded that "the data provide evidence that brief cardiac rehabilitation initiated soon after MI for patients with mild to moderate anxiety or depression, or both, is an efficient use of health care resources and can be economically justified" (38).

The data collected in that study have been reanalyzed recently using more up-to-date measurement, and analytic strategies provide some tantalizing information (53). These strategies include the following:

a. In addition to using the direct TTO utility measure in the RCT, we also administered the indirect, multi-attribute, community-based QWB to all patients.

b. We used linear-regression modeling to impute all missing preference and cost data.

c. We estimated individual-level preference scores (estimating the QALYs experienced by each patient over the 12-month follow-up using each of the five imputed preference score data sets) rather than group-level preference scores.

d. We used contemporary methods to estimate the confidence interval (CI) around a ratio.

With QWB preference scores at the group-level, rehabilitation was associated with 0.011 more QALYs than the control group, whereas the difference with TTO preference scores was 0.040 QALYs. As we imputed all missing data, we were able to estimate the 95% CI around the mean change at the individual level. We observed an individual-level mean difference of 0.011 QALYs (95% CI, –0.030 to 0.052) with QWB preference scores and QALYs 0.040 (95% CI, –0.029 to 0.103) with TTO preference scores, both in favor of rehabilitation. There was no significant difference between the two (Table 9-2).

Incremental costs over and above the usual care costs and the results of all subsequent calculations are inflated from the published figure of 1991 US$ to 2001 US dollars (54) with estimated net incremental costs of $ 702 (lower 95% CI, –$200; upper 95% CI, $1605).

The mean cost-utility ratio for the group-level and individual-level QWB-derived QALYs was $63,818/QALY; with TTO-derived QALYs, the mean cost-utility ratio for the group-level and individual-level was $17,550/QALY. The lower and upper 95% CIs for the individual-level QWB- and TTO-derived cost-utility ratios were estimated using the normal approximation method (Table 9-2).

The key finding in this secondary analysis of data is that community preference and patient preference scores give different results (53). This was true for baseline scores, for the change over the 12-month follow-up, for the estimation of QALYs, and for the cost-utility ratios. As we were able to estimate the 95% confidence limits with the individual-level data, we were able to document that there was no statistically significant difference in the estimated individual-level QWB and TTO cost-utility ratios. However, the individual-level cost-utility ratio with the community-level QWB preference scores was qualitatively unattractive, while the individual-level cost-utility ratio with the patient-level TTO preference scores was attractive and highly cost-effective.

2. There is one randomized controlled trial of early cardiac rehabilitation in patients with heart failure that included an a priori economic evaluation with a cost-effectiveness evaluation (41). The RCT was carried out in Italy, and eligible patients between the ages of 54 and 65 years with class II and III heart failure ($n = 99$) were randomized to either a 14-month exercise

---

TABLE 9-2   QUALITY-ADJUSTED LIFE-YEARS (QALYs) AND COST-UTILITY RATIOS (CURs)

| | QALYs and Cost-Utility Ratios[a] | | | | | |
| | Quality of Well-being | | | Time Tradeoff | | |
	Lower 95% CI	Mean	Upper 95% CI	Lower 95% CI	Mean	Upper 95% CI
Individual-level QALYs	−0.030	0.011	0.052	−0.029	0.040	0.103
Individual-level CUR ($)		63,818			17,550	
95% CI - Normality ($)	−180,424		304,475	−19,286		54,321

[a]Incremental with lower and upper 95% confidence intervals (CI) in 2001 US$ and individual-level and incremental net rehabilitation program costs (mean, $702; lower 95% CI, – $200; upper 95% CI, $1605.

training program ($n = 50$) or usual community care (control, $n = 49$) (55).

The hospitalization rate during the follow-up was 29% in the usual care group (14 of 49 patients) compared with 10% among the rehabilitation patients (5 of 50 patients), which resulted in an estimated savings of $1,336/patient using a 3% discount rate, 1999 US dollars, and New York City cost figures. As the cost of the rehabilitation program amounted to $5,282, the incremental costs of the program were $3,227. The incremental life expectancy was estimated over a 10-year period with survival rates of 42% in the rehabilitation group and 30% in the usual care group. When discounted at 3%, the incremental life expectancy was 1.82 years/patient. The cost-effectiveness ratio is expressed as the incremental cost of cardiac rehabilitation as the numerator and the incremental years of live saved as the denominator. With an incremental cost of $3,227 and 1.82 incremental years of life saved, the cost-effectiveness ratio is $1,773/life-year saved with upper and lower limits of $8,274 to $1,012 per life-year saved. The authors suggest that the cost-utility ratio per QALY would possibly be lower as the significant improvements in health-related quality of life observed in the RCT (55) suggest that "quality adjustment would result in a cost-effectiveness ratio that would more heavily favor exercise training" (41).

Discussion

Economic evaluation provides data on alternative courses of action and should be helpful when developing clinical practice guidelines and health policies to improve clinical practice. The characteristics of the patients treated and the assumptions underlying the effectiveness of the intervention affect the cost-effectiveness of an intervention. In addition, questions that need to be addressed when evaluating the cost-effectiveness of alternative secondary prevention interventions for CAD include

- What is the expected impact on mortality and health-related quality-of-life?
- How do the costs of the strategy compare with those of the alternatives?

- Will the costs be offset by economic savings due to delays or prevention of adverse events?
- What is the time frame in which costs and benefits are expected to occur?
- How likely is the patient to adhere to the recommended therapy?

With certain limitations, economic evaluations of comprehensive cardiac rehabilitation suggest that it is a cost-effective intervention in patients with CAD. The limitations include the following. First, there are only limited data on which to base any estimate of the cost-effectiveness of cardiac rehabilitation. Second, in the only randomized controlled trials in which an economic evaluation of cardiac rehabilitation was carried out, cardiac rehabilitation was associated with increased costs (38,41), whereas the studies with less rigorous designs showed actual savings or a decrease in health care use. This reinforces the need for more research on the cost-effectiveness of cardiac rehabilitation before any definitive statement is made about reimbursement.

While both community and patient preferences have been used in cost-effectiveness studies to calculate QALYs, the Panel on Cost-Effectiveness has pointed out that in 1996 there were no studies comparing the impact of using one or the other preference in the same analysis in the same patients undergoing the same interventions (5,7) (and to our knowledge this is still true). Although there was a large interindividual variability in both preference measures in the secondary analysis of the data originally published by our group (38), all but one of the 15 comparisons (three comparisons at each of the five assessment points) were significantly different, always with higher TTO patient-preference than QWB community-preference scores. The mean cost-utility ratio with individual-level QWB-derived QALYs was $63,818/QALY and was $17,550/QALY with individual-level TTO-derived QALYs. This suggests that the cost-effectiveness of a particular intervention, in this case cardiac rehabilitation, differs substantially depending upon whether community preferences or patient preferences are used to estimate QALYs. The results of this secondary analysis would suggest that the Panel was right to be concerned about the measurement approach taken to estimate QALYs and that every study should carefully consider whether or not to add an analysis from both the community and the patients' perspective. Further, and importantly for cardiac rehabilitation, the incremental cost-utility ratios derived with either QWB- or TTO-derived QALYs suggest that for a unit of effectiveness (i.e., improved HRQL), there is evidence that patient-level preferences result in considerably more attractive cost-effectiveness ratios than with community-level preferences. The wide and overlapping confidence limits preclude a conclusion of significant differences, and although these observations cannot be generalized to other studies, they are a cause for concern.

Economic evaluation is only one component of the evaluation of health care services and permits the comparison of alternative courses of action in monetary terms per unit of consequence. Cardiac rehabilitation services are undergoing considerable reexamination (56–59). These new approaches to service delivery have not been subjected to extensive economic evaluation, although the limited evidence on the more traditional approach to delivering cardiac rehabilitation suggests that it can be economically justified as a cost-effective intervention. Further, cardiac rehabilitation appears to be at least as cost-effective as many of the other secondary prevention strategies except smoking cessation, which has an estimated cost-effectiveness ratio (2001 US$) of approximately $340/LYG (31). However, at the end of this discussion on the cost-effectiveness of comprehensive cardiac rehabilitation, we still do not have definitive answers to the following two critical questions:

1. "If exercise is a key component of comprehensive cardiac rehabilitation, what is the incremental value of exercise when added to other cost-effective secondary prevention interventions such as smoking?"
2. "Does cardiac rehabilitation actually reduce costs and save scarce health care resources?"

Summary

- Economic evaluation is defined as the comparative analysis of alternative courses of action in terms of both costs and effects and provides a framework for systematic evaluation of both the costs and effects of alternative health care services.

- The incremental cost-effectiveness ratio is calculated as the difference in costs between the alternatives divided by the differences in health effects between the alternatives.
- Economic evaluations of comprehensive cardiac rehabilitation suggest that it is a cost-effective intervention in patients with CAD.
- The cost-effectiveness of cardiac rehabilitation appears to differ substantially depending upon whether community preferences or patient preferences are used to estimate QALYs.
- The cost-effectiveness of cardiac rehabilitation is particularly attractive in patients with heart failure.
- These conclusions are based on limited information, and considerably more research is needed.

REFERENCES

1. Russell MW, Huse DM, Drowns S, et al. Direct medical costs of coronary artery disease in the United States. Am J Cardiol 1998;81:1110–1115.
2. Eisenstein EL, Shaw LK, Anstrom KJ, et al. Assessing the clinical and economic burden of coronary artery disease: 1986–1998. Med Care 2001;39:824–835.
3. Drummond MF, O'Brien BJ, Stoddart GL, Torrance GW. Methods for the Economic Evaluation of Health Care Programmes. Oxford: Oxford University Press, 1997.
4. Eddy DM, Billings J. The quality of medical evidence: implications for quality of care. Health Affairs 1988;7:19–32.
5. Russell LB, Gold MR, Siegel JE, et al. for the Panel on Cost-Effectiveness in Health and Medicine. The role of cost-effectiveness analysis in health and medicine. JAMA 1996;276:1172–1177.
6. Zwart-van Rijkom JE, Leufkens HG, Busschbach JJ, et al. Differences in attitudes, knowledge and use of economic evaluations in decision-making in The Netherlands. The Dutch results from the EUROMET Project. Pharmacoeconomics 2000;18: 149–160.
7. Gold MR, Siegel JE, Russell L, Weinstein M, eds. Cost-Effectiveness in Health and Medicine. New York: Oxford University Press, 1996.
8. Weinstein MC, Siegel JE, Gold MR, et al., for the Panel on Cost-Effectiveness in Health and Medicine. Recommendations of the Panel on Cost-Effectiveness in Health and Medicine. JAMA 1996;276:1253–1258.
9. Siegel JE, Weinstein MC, Russell LB, Gold MR, for the Panel on Cost-Effectiveness in Health and Medicine. Recommendations for reporting

cost-effectiveness analyses. JAMA 1996;276:1339–1341.

10. Kaplan R, Bush J. Health-related quality of life measurement for evaluation research and policy analysis. Health Psychol 1982;1:61–80.

11. Feeny D, Furlong W, Barr RD. Multiattribute approach to the assessment of health-related quality of life: Health Utilities Index. Med Pediatr Oncol 1998;(suppl):54–59.

12. Furlong WJ, Feeny DH, Torrance GW, Barr RD. The Health Utilities Index (HUI) system for assessing health-related quality of life in clinical studies. Ann Med 2001;33:375–384.

13. Torrance GW, Thomas WH, Sackett DL. A utility maximization model for evaluation of health care programs. Health Serv Res 1972;7:118–113.

14. Torrance GW, Feeny D. Utilities and quality-adjusted life years. Int J Technol Assess Health Care 1989;5:559–575.

15. Torrance GW, Furlong W, Feeny D. Health utility estimation. Expert Rev Pharmacoecon Outcomes Res 2002;2:99–108.

16. Canadian Coordinating Office for Health Technology Assessment. Guidelines for the Economic Evaluation of Pharmaceuticals: Canada. 1st ed. Ottawa: 1994.

17. Commonwealth of Australia. Background document on the use of economic evaluation as a basis for the inclusion of pharmaceutical products on the Pharmaceutical Benefits Scheme. Canberra: Australian Government Publishing Service, 1993.

18. O'Brien BJ, Drummond MF, Labelle RJ, Willan A. In search of power and significance: issues in the design and analysis of stochastic cost-effectiveness studies in health care. Med Care 1994;32:150–163.

19. Coyle D, Davies L, Drummond MF. Trials and tribulations. Emerging issues in designing economic evaluations alongside clinical trials. Int J Technol Assess Health Care 1998;14:135–144.

20. Rittenhouse B. Uses of Models in Economic Evaluations of Medicines and Other Health Technologies. London: Office of Health Economics, 1996.

21. Brennan A, Akehurst R. Modelling in health economic evaluation. What is its place? What is its value? Pharmacoeconomics 2000;17:445–459.

22. Mark DB, Hlatky MA. Medical economics and the assessment of value in cardiovascular medicine: Part I. Circulation 2002;106:516–520.

23. Goldman L, Garber AM, Grover SA, Hlatky MA. Cost effectiveness of assessment and management of risk factors. J Am Coll Cardiol 1996;27:1020–1030.

24. 27th Bethesda Conference. Matching the intensity of risk factor management with the hazard for coronary disease events. J Am Coll Cardiol 1996;27:957–1047.

25. Meyers DG. Relative survival benefits of risk factor modifications. Am J Cardiol 1996;77:298–299.

26. Wenger NK, Froelicher ES, Smith LK, et al. Cardiac Rehabilitation. Clinical Practice Guideline #17. AHCPR #96-0672. Rockville, MD: U.S. Dept of Health & Human Services, Public Health Service, Agency for Health Care Policy & Research, and the National Heart, Blood & Lung Institute; 1995.

27. Mark DB, Naylor CD, Hlatky MA, et al. Use of medical resources and quality of life after acute myocardial infarction in Canada and the United States. N Engl J Med 1994;331:1130–1135.

28. Oldridge NB, Pashkow FJ. Adherence and motivation in cardiac rehabilitation. In: Pashkow FJ, Dafoe WA, eds. Clinical Cardiac Rehabilitation. A Cardiologist's Guide. Baltimore: Williams & Wilkins; 1999:487–503.

29. Taylor CB, Houston-Miller N, Killen JD, DeBusk RF. Smoking cessation after acute myocardial infarction: Effects of a nurse-managed intervention. Ann Intern Med 1990;113:118–123.

30. Wilson K, Gibson N, Willan A, Cook D. Effect of smoking cessation on mortality after myocardial infarction: meta-analysis of cohort studies. Arch Intern Med 2000;160:939–944.

31. Krumholz HM, Cohen BJ, Tsevat J, et al. Cost-effectiveness of a smoking cessation program after myocardial infarction. J Am Coll Cardiol 1993;22:1697–1702.

32. Taylor R, Brown A, Ebrahim A, et al. Exercise-based rehabilitation for patients with coronary heart disease: systematic review & meta-analysis of randomized controlled trials. Am J Med 2004;116:682–692.

33. Oldridge NB. Comprehensive cardiac rehabilitation: Is it cost-effective? Eur Heart J 1998;19(suppl O):O42–O49.

34. Taylor R, Kirby B. The evidence base for the cost effectiveness of cardiac rehabilitation. Heart 1997;78:5–6.

35. Levin L-A, Perk J, Hedback B. Cardiac rehabilitation—cost analysis. J Intern Med 1991;230:427–434.

36. Ades PA, Huang D, Weaver SO. Cardiac rehabilitation participation predicts lower rehospitalization costs. Am Heart J 1992;123:916–921.

37. Bondestam E, Breikks A, Hartford M. Effects of early rehabilitation on consumption of medical care during the first year after acute myocardial infarction in patients >65 years of age. Am J Cardiol 1995;75:767–771.

38. Oldridge N, Furlong W, Feeny D, et al. Economic evaluation of cardiac rehabilitation soon after acute myocardial infarction. Am J Cardiol 1993;72:154–161.

39. Ades PA, Pashkow FJ, Nestor JR. Cost-effectiveness of cardiac rehabilitation after myocardial infarction. J Cardiopulm Rehabil 1997;17:222–231.

40. Lowensteyn I, Coupal L, Zowall H, Grover SA. The cost-effectiveness of exercise training for the primary and secondary prevention of cardiovascular disease. J Cardiopulm Rehabil 2000;20:147–155.

41. Georgiou D, Chen Y, Appadoo S, et al. Cost-effectiveness analysis of long-term moderate exercise training in chronic heart failure. Am J Cardiol 2001;87:984–988.

42. Hedback B, Perk J. Five-year results of a comprehensive rehabilitation programme on mortality, morbidity and risk factors. Eur Heart J 1987;8:234–242.

43. O'Connor GT, Buring JE, Yusuf S, et al. An overview of randomized trials of rehabilitation with exercise after myocardial infarction. Circulation 1989;80:234–244.

44. Oldridge NB, Guyatt GH, Fischer M, Rimm AR. Cardiac rehabilitation after myocardial infarction: combining data from randomized clinical trials. JAMA 1988;260:945–980.

45. Mark DB, Hlatky MA, Califf RM, et al. Cost effectiveness of thrombolytic therapy with tissue plasminogen activator as compared with streptokinase for acute myocardial infarction. N Engl J Med 1995;332:1418–1424.

46. Byl N, Reed P, Franklin BA, Gordon S. Cost of phase II cardiac rehabilitation: implications regarding ECG monitoring practices. Circulation, 1988;78(suppl II):II-136 (abstr)

47. The Canadian Heart Health Database 1986–92. Canadian Heart Health Database Centre, Memorial University of Newfoundland. St. John's, 1998.

48. Grover SA, Paquet S, Levinton C, et al. Estimating the benefits of modifying risk factors of cardiovascular disease: a comparison of primary vs secondary prevention. Arch Intern Med 1998;158:655–662.

49. Grover SA, Coupal L, Paquet S, Zowall H. Cost-effectiveness of 3-hydroxy-3-methylglutaryl-coenzyme A reductase inhibitors in the secondary prevention of cardiovascular disease: forecasting the incremental benefits of preventing coronary and cerebrovascular events. Arch Intern Med 1999;159:593–600.

50. Oldridge N, Guyatt G, Jones N, et al. Effects on quality of life with comprehensive rehabilitation after acute myocardial infarction. Am J Cardiol 1991;67:1084–1089.

51. Torrance GW. Measurement of health state utilities for economic appraisal. A review. J Health Econ 1986;5:1–30.

52. Bennett KJ, Torrance GW. Measuring health state preferences and utilities: rating scale, time trade-off, and standard gamble techniques. In: Spilker B, ed. Quality of Life and Pharmacoeconomics in Clinical Trials. Philadelphia: Lippincott-Raven; 1996:253–265.

53. Furlong W, Oldridge N, Perkins A, et al. Community or patient preferences for cost-utility analyses: does it matter? Value in Health 2003;6:298.

54. Economic Report of the President. Washington, DC: United States Government Printing Office; 2002.

55. Belardinelli R, Georgiou D, Cianci G, Purcaro A. Randomized, controlled trial of long-term moderate exercise training in chronic heart failure: effects on functional capacity, quality of life, and clinical outcome. Circulation 1999;99:1173–1182.

56. Dafoe W, Huston P. Current trends in cardiac rehabilitation. Can Med Assoc J 1997;156:527–532.

57. Franklin BA, Hall L, Timmis GC. Contemporary cardiac rehabilitation services. Am J Cardiol 1997;79:1075–1077.

58. Gordon NF, Haskell WL. Comprehensive cardiovascular disease risk reduction in a cardiac rehabilitation setting. Am J Cardiol 1997;80:69H–73H.

59. Ades PA, Balady GJ, Berra K. Transforming exercise-based cardiac rehabilitation programs into secondary prevention centers: a national imperative. J Cardiopulm Rehabil 2001;21:263–272.

RELATED WEB SITES

Cochrane Library
www.cochrane.org

McMaster University Centre for Health Economics and Policy Analysis, Ontario, Canada
www.chepa.org

The University of York, United Kingdom
www.york.ac.uk/inst/che

Neuromuscular and Skeletal Conditions

10

Arthritis

Ilkka M. Vuori

Arthritis is a chronic degenerative condition of joints. Two distinctive forms of arthritis can be discerned: osteoarthritis (OA) and rheumatoid arthritis (RA). OA is much more common, and its pathophysiology is more related to physical activity than those features of RA. Therefore, this chapter focuses mainly on OA. However, there is a need for more information on how to do exercise testing, how to prescribe exercise, and what to expect with RA.

OA is a heterogeneous condition that can affect any diarthrodial joint. It is not clear if OA is a single disease or many disorders with a similar common pathway (1). One classification of OA is into primary and secondary forms (2). Primary OA is the more common form. Its cause is not known, but it is commonly related to aging and heredity. Secondary OA may occur in any joint as a result of articular injury (e.g., repetitive joint use, fracture, or metabolic disease) and may occur at any age.

Clinically, OA can be defined as a disease that combines the pathology of disease with pain that occurs when the joint is used (1). The pathology of OA involves the whole joint and also adjacent tissues and their functions. The primary problem is in the joint cartilage, which gets softer and less resilient, and there is focal and progressive hyaline cartilage loss. The cartilage gets thinner, and its cushioning function to reduce the mechanical forces in the joint, as well as its covering of the bone ends, are decreased. Consequently, the bone underneath the cartilage grows thicker (osteosclerosis), marginal outgrowths (osteophytes) develop as compensatory changes, and the joint space gets narrower (3–5).

Soft tissue structures in and around the joint are also affected. These changes include progressive inflammatory infiltrates in, and thickening of, the synovium; laxity of the ligaments; and weakness of the bridging muscles. During the arthritic process, friction in the joint increases, shock absorption decreases, and impact loading increases. These changes tend to facilitate structural and functional degeneration of the joint (3,6).

The signs of OA include localized tenderness, crepitation on motion, mild joint enlargement, synovitis, and possibly deformities in later stages. Radiologic changes include narrowing of joint space, osteophytes, and bone remodeling around the joints. A large proportion of subjects with radiologic findings of OA have no symptoms (1). Usual symptoms are pain on motion in the early stages and also at rest in the more advanced stages, aggravation of pain by prolonged or intensive activity, and localized stiffness, especially in the morning and after periods of inactivity during the day. In severe cases, patients have limited range of motion of the affected joint as a result of incongruous joint surfaces, muscle or capsular contracture, or mechanical block (usually temporary) caused by loose bodies in the joint space or by osteophytes (4,7). Especially older patients with knee OA also have increased body sway and impaired balance (8,9). Individuals with OA may also report symptoms of joint instability, periarticular muscle weakness, and fatigue (10). Together with decreased proprioception and flexibility, these functional deteriorations increase the risk of patient falls (11).

The onset of OA symptoms is almost invariably insidious. The signs and symptoms of the disease usually manifest only after there is significant damage to the cartilage. Lack of symptoms in the early stage of OA is due to the lack of nerve endings in the cartilage. Although the exact cause of pain in OA is not known (12), there are several possible sources such as periostal irritation as a result of remodeling, denuded bone due to cartilage damage, compression of soft tissue by osteophytes, synovitis, effusion, stress on ligaments, spasm of surrounding tissues, and microfractures of subchondral bone (13).

OA affects most commonly knee and hip joints, especially in old age (14) (Fig. 10-1), and they represent two of the most significant causes of pain and disability in adult individuals (6). Therefore, this chapter concentrates on OA of the knee and hip.

Estimates of the prevalence and incidence of OA show wide variation, depending on the criteria of diagnosis and the population. Figure 10-1 depicts the higher incidence of OA in women than in men and its steep increase with age. In the U.S. population 30 years of age and older, 6% are estimated to have symptomatic knee OA, and 3% symptomatic hip OA (15). In subjects older than 60 years, the prevalence of clinically significant disease is 10 to 20%, and knee OA is about twice as prevalent as hip disease (about 10 vs. 5 %) (16,17).

Especially in its advanced form, OA leads to serious individual and social consequences. In the Western countries, OA ranks fourth in health impact among women and eighth among men (18). OA causes more trouble with climbing stairs and walking than any other disease (19). Older individuals with OA are more likely to need help with personal care activities and instrumental activities of daily living than individuals without OA. These patients make twice as many visits to a health care provider as those without the disease (20). OA leads frequently to decreased quality of life and social isolation (21). OA is the most common reason for total hip and knee replacements and causes considerable burden to the economy in terms of lost time at work and early retirement (22). Total costs of arthritis, including OA, may exceed 2% of the gross

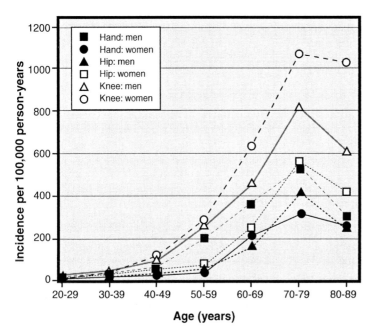

FIGURE 10-1 Incidence of osteoarthritis of the hand, hip, and knee in members of the Fallon Community Health Plan, 1991–1992, by age and sex. (Reproduced with permission from Oliveria SA, Felson DT, Reed JI, et al. Incidence of symptomatic hand, hip, and knee osteoarthritis among patients in a health maintenance organization. Arthritis Rheum 1995;38:1134–1141.)

domestic product (22). In the United States OA is the second and globally the eighth most common cause of disability (6).

Risk Factors for the Development and Progression of OA

Several systemic factors increase the risk of development and progression of OA (1) (Fig. 10-2). The role of increasing age and female sex as risk factors has already been mentioned. Evidence for the role of ethnicity is conflicting, and the role of biology, lifestyle, and socioeconomic factors as possible confounders is unclear (1). All forms of OA appear to be strongly genetically determined, as genetic factors account for at least 50% of OA in the hips and a smaller percentage in the knees (1). Several possible candidate genes have been identified (1,7). Low levels of estrogen seem to increase the risk, as evidenced by a higher incidence of OA after menopause. However, the evidence of a protective value of estrogen replacement therapy is only suggestive because of conflicting observations (1,7). Bone density is in complex relationship to OA. High bone density increases the risk of developing OA, but it may protect against progression of already existing disease. High bone loss in OA patients may accelerate progression of the disease (1). Some nutritional factors may be related to risk of OA. Continuous exposure to oxidants may increase the risk, but vitamins C and D seem to be protective (1).

Local factors that influence the risk of OA include overweight and obesity, mechanical environment of the joint, acute joint injury, joint deformity, muscle weakness, occupational factors, and sports participation. Overweight and obesity increase the risk of developing OA and its radiographic progression (23–27) in most but not all studies, more in women than in men. On the other hand, even a modest (~10 lb) weight loss decreases the risk of knee OA by about 50% (28). Weight loss can also slow down the progression and decrease the symptoms of already existing knee OA (6,29). The relationship of overweight with hip OA is weaker than its association with knee OA (1,4). The increased risk of OA associated with overweight is mainly explained by overloading of the joints, but systemic factors also may be involved (1).

The long-term mechanical environment of the joint is determined by its stability, alignment, and

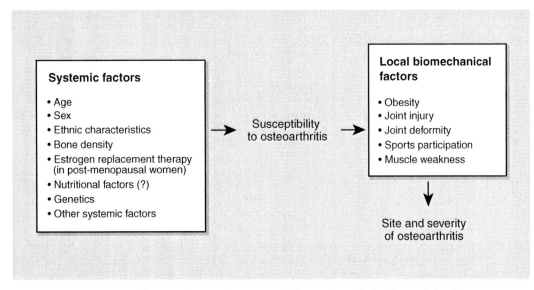

FIGURE 10-2 Pathogenesis of osteoarthritis with putative risk factors. (Modified with permission from Dieppe P. The classification and diagnosis of osteoarthritis. In: Kuettner K, Goldberg V, eds. Osteoarthritic Disorders. Rosemont, IL: American Academy of Orthopaedic Surgeons; 1995:7.)

proprioception. These factors are particularly relevant for the knee joint. Laxity of the knee, especially in the frontal plane, increases the risk of OA. Proprioception, the conscious and unconscious perception of joint position and movement, is critical to the maintenance of joint stability under dynamic conditions. Proprioceptive accuracy at the knee declines with age (30) (particularly in sedentary individuals [31]), and it has been found to be worse in patients with OA of the knee (32). These findings suggest that proprioceptive deficit may increase the risk of knee OA (1).

Injuries that result in articular surface fractures, joint dislocations, and meniscal and ligament ruptures increase the risk of developing OA (1,15,33–35). This risk is further increased by residual joint instability and malalignment, persistent articular surface incongruity, overweight, and strenuous physical activity (1). Joint dysplasias may cause cumulative articular surface stress above a critical threshold that leads to joint degeneration (1). Muscle weakness, notably of the quadriceps muscle, increases the risk of knee OA (1,6,36,37). Modeling of knee OA suggests that each 10 ft-lb increase in knee extensor strength is associated with a 20% reduction in the odds of radiographic disease and a 29% reduction in the odds of symptomatic knee OA. An increase of approximately 20% in knee extensor strength for men and 25% increase for women lowered the odds of having knee OA by 20 to 30% (38).

The risk of OA is increased in several occupations where workers are exposed to repetitious tasks overworking the joints and fatiguing the muscles that protect the joints. Jobs requiring kneeling or squatting along with heavy lifting are associated with particularly high rates of both knee and hip OA. Turning or twisting while doing the activities clearly increases the risk further (1,39,40). The risk of OA related to sports is discussed below.

Physical Activity, Sports, and OA

Physical activity and sports can be related to risk of OA through loading or through injuries. The articular cartilage is highly resistant to stress caused by physical loading. If the load is applied slowly, the cartilage has time to deform and tolerates the stress well. Furthermore, the adjacent muscles contract and absorb much of the energy and stabilize the joint (6,41). However, sudden single or repetitive impacts or torsional loadings can cause damage to articular cartilage and the subchondral bone (42). Normal articular cartilage may rupture if the stresses between the adjacent surfaces are 25 MPa (megapascals, newtons per square meter) or more. For example, the peak articular contact stresses during running and jumping are 4 to 9 MPa. Moderate amounts of these kinds of activities are unlikely to cause damage in healthy joints. This notion is supported also by extensive animal experiments. However, chronic or repetitive stresses <25 MPa may cause articular damage or degeneration (43,44). A number of studies report greatly increased risk of OA with chronic or repetitive loading (e.g., in occupational work [40,45,46]).

Physical loading can be beneficial for cartilage by compressing it, thereby facilitating its nutrition (47,48). This seems to be the case, because unloading and complete physical inactivity are detrimental to cartilage and the adjacent structures of the joint (5,49). The necessary physical activity to maintain normal joint structures may be so small that this need is met by ordinary daily activities. Animal studies show that moderate physical activity causes beneficial structural and functional changes in joints (5). However, only limited evidence suggests that physical activity could directly prevent OA in ambulatory subjects. However, it has been hypothesized that physical activity in childhood may be important for the development of joint cartilage and prevention of future OA (50). Indirectly, physical activity could be of benefit by decreasing the risk of overweight and obesity.

A number of population-based studies indicate that moderate levels of physical activity do not increase the risk for OA (1,33,43,44,48,51). However, the risk was increased in the most active subjects in several of those studies (44). Some estimates of the risk associated with increasing amounts of physical activity are available, namely, at least 4 hours per day of heavy physical activity for radiologic, at least 3 hours per day for symptomatic OA of the knee in one study (52), and running at least 20 miles per week for hip or knee OA in another study (53).

Running is an activity that includes repetitive moderate impact forces but does not cause frequent injuries affecting joints. Several studies on runners suggest no increased risk of OA, except possibly in competitive athletes running high mileages (1,5,33,43,44) However, self-selection to begin, continue, and discontinue running at various levels causes problems in the interpretation of these findings.

The risk of OA is several times higher in sports that include a high rate of injury, especially if combined with high impacts and torsional movements (e.g., soccer and American football) (1,43,51,54). The highest risk is seen in players at the elite level and in women (35). Soft-tissue injuries without direct involvement of the joint also seem to increase the risk for OA (35,55,56). Injuries that lead to instability and sensory denervation of the joint structures show a high rate of development of OA (43). Unfortunately, surgical reconstruction of ruptured ligaments or of the meniscus of the knee joint does not seem to protect against development of OA in this joint (35).

Management of OA

If the title of this section is taken literally, it is grossly misleading. It is important to treat the local osteoarthritic process itself, but it is also necessary to manage the consequences of the primary condition. OA and its immediate effects (pain and limitations of movement) tend to initiate a vicious circle, in which increasing age and decreasing physical and social activities facilitate the effects of the primary condition and tend to cause progressive problems. These include deteriorating aerobic and muscular fitness, weight gain, depressive mood, lack of self-confidence and initiative, decreasing capacity for activities of daily living, increasing dependency, and development of comorbidities. The goal of OA management is to slow down, stop, or even partially reverse the vicious circle. This goal can be achieved by good palliative treatment of OA itself and by comprehensive secondary and tertiary preventive measures.

The measures for managing OA can be divided into three groups: nonpharmacologic measures, pharmacologic (systemic, topical, and intraarticular) measures, and surgical procedures. Because OA is a progressive condition that cannot be cured and because the patients and their problems vary greatly,

OA management should be based on three principles. First, although pharmacologic treatment is necessary at least periodically for most patients, the nonpharmacologic measures should be the primary part of the regimen. Second, the management program and its various measures should be tailored individually to meet the needs and expectations of each patient. Third, because the program should be continuous, patients and their families should be taught to carry out as much of it as possible.

The nonpharmacologic options include education (patient and spouse or family), social support (e.g., telephone contact), physiotherapy (e.g., diathermy, ultrasound, aerobic exercise, muscle strengthening, patellar strapping), weight loss, acupuncture, thermal modalities, aids and appliances, and transcutaneous electrical nerve stimulation (TENS) (10,57–59). Recent evaluation of the evidence indicates that patient education can have a significant beneficial effect on pain but not on disability. Education was about 20% as effective as nonsteroidal antiinflammatory drugs (60). Telephone contact from health care workers also was effective in reducing pain and improving functional capacity (61). Social support given by family members educated to provide it also benefited the patient (62). Two modes of physiotherapy (aerobic conditioning and muscle-strengthening exercises) have proven effective in improving pain and disability in OA of the knee (63). Other modes of physiotherapy (e.g., diathermy, ultrasound, and other forms of heat and cold) have limited or no beneficial effects (57, 59). The effects of occupational therapy have not been thoroughly evaluated, but vast practical experience is favorable. True acupuncture did not produce beneficial effects compared with random needling. TENS may give modest relief of pain (57,59). Even modest weight loss (5 kg) was effective in reducing the risk of developing symptomatic knee OA by 50% and in reducing the severity of joint pain (29).

Exercise in the Management of Patients with OA

The value of exercise for patients with OA is determined by the extent to which exercise meets the needs and expectations of patients and to what extent patients are willing and able to accomplish the necessary exercise regimens.

Patients with OA have several problems that are caused by OA or are related to it. The most common problems caused by OA are pain, localized tenderness, stiffness and limited range of motion, joint instability, periarticular muscle weakness, disability, and fatigue. The problems related to OA (or those frequently found among these patients as indirect consequences of OA) include lower aerobic capacity, muscle strength, flexibility, proprioception, and balance compared with that of healthy subjects (7,33,51,57,64). OA patients are often also less physically active, and their cardiovascular risk factors are higher than those in healthy persons (33,40,51,57,64). Most patients are older, and many are overweight or obese and may have depressive mood and decreased self-confidence. These characteristics of OA patients offer a number of potential goals for exercise programs and at the same time suggest considerable difficulties in their realization.

EFFECTS OF EXERCISE PROGRAMS IN PATIENTS WITH OA

Published studies, meta-analyses, and systematic reviews based on them show evidence of several favorable, clinically significant effects of exercise programs on patients with OA. Systematic reviews of controlled trials show that exercise has (a) small-to-moderate short-term beneficial effects on pain, (b) small beneficial effects on self-reported and observed disability and walking, and (c) moderate-to-large beneficial effects on the patients' global assessment of the effects in patients with knee OA and in fewer studies in patients with hip OA (44,51,58,65–67). The benefits regarding self-reported pain and physical function have been smaller in studies that used blinded outcome assessment than in studies using uncertain or unblinded outcome assessment (67). Evidence of long-term benefits of time-limited exercise programs is scarce and conflicting (68,69). However, no effects of exercise can be expected to last long after cessation of the activity, and exercise should be a continuous part of life in general, particularly when it is indicated for a specified purpose. Aerobic programs increase aerobic capacity, walking time, and self-reported functioning and

decrease pain and the use of medications (33,51). Resistance- training programs have resulted in decrease of pain (70,71), in substantial increases in strength, improved function, and aerobic walking (33,72). Weight training also has resulted in less disability and in less time needed to perform daily activities (72) as well as improved postural sway and thereby balance and ambulation in older patients with OA (73). Some evidence suggests that exercise regimens that strengthen the quadriceps muscle may slow the progression of joint damage in patients with knee OA (37,38). No studies in humans have indicated that exercise exacerbates the symptoms or signs of OA or accelerates cartilage degeneration. In general, exercise programs are safe and well tolerated by individuals with OA, although complications can occur (48).

Scientific evidence clearly indicates that systematic, individualized exercise training can bring significant and multiple benefits for patients with OA and that effective exercise regimens are safe, especially when adequately supervised. The evidence for these benefits is stronger for knee than for hip OA. On the basis of the evidence, exercise is currently recommended as an essential part of comprehensive treatment and secondary prevention of OA (74). However, several issues regarding the planning and implementation of optimally effective, safe and feasible exercise regimens remain. These issues include lack of knowledge of the optimal types of exercise, the dose-response relationships for various benefits, and the administration of the programs (individual, group, or home-based regimens) (44,67,75), as well as problems related to the beginning and continuation of exercise programs (48,51,64). These issues have to be solved by applying the knowledge of exercise physiology and the experience and findings from previous studies. When all specific evidence, more general knowledge, and considerable experience are taken together, there is a solid basis to plan and implement effective, safe, and feasible exercise regimens for patients with OA.

GOALS OF EXERCISE PROGRAMS

The needs of patients with OA and the evidence of attainable benefits of feasible exercise programs permit setting several goals for systematically conducted exercise regimens.

- The primary and most specific goal is to restore and maintain the best possible function of the arthritic joint and to prevent its further degeneration due to inactivity, disuse, or aggravation by excessive loading. This goal includes reducing pain, increasing range of motion, and strengthening the periarticular muscles for stabilization of the joint.
- The second goal, very similar to the first, is to protect the joint from damage by reducing stress on the joint, attenuating joint forces, and improving biomechanics.
- The third goal is to restore, maintain, or improve the patient's capacity to walk and to do other activities of daily living. This goal includes exercises that improve flexibility, balance, proprioception, gait, and muscular and aerobic fitness.
- The fourth goal is to reduce the risks of comorbid conditions that are causally related to inactivity and that can be influenced favorably by moderate and feasible physical activity. Examples of these conditions are overweight and obesity, elevated blood pressure, type 2 diabetes, coronary heart disease and stroke, osteoporosis, a propensity for falls, depressive mood, and poor sleep.

The importance, attainability, timing, and priority order of the goals will vary widely among patients, and all goals may not be relevant to, or attainable by, all patients, at least in the beginning of the exercise program. The exercise regimens related to the fourth goal are covered extensively in specific chapters of this book.

ASSESSMENT OF THE PATIENT'S NEEDS, ABILITIES, RISKS, AND OPPORTUNITIES FOR EXERCISE

Rational and responsible prescription and management of exercise for patients with OA calls for a thorough assessment of their needs, abilities, risks, and opportunities for exercise as related to OA and to their health status and life situation as a whole. Reliable assessment serves planning, implementation, follow-up, evaluation, and adjustment of the exercise program and eventually other components of patient management. The assessment is done for practical purposes to serve each specific individual. However, when assessments are done systematically using standardized tests and are documented appropriately, they build up an evidence-based experience and may be useful for research purposes.

The assessment related to exercise of OA patients shares many of the same principles and elements as that for persons with other diseases discussed in this book. This is true particularly concerning the assessment of cardiorespiratory and metabolic conditions and risks. Therefore, the reader is referred to the corresponding chapters for details on those aspects of assessment. The musculoskeletal aspects of health, fitness, and risk assessment and exercise programing are more specific to OA and are dealt with in greater detail in this chapter.

The assessment of health, abilities, fitness, safety, and opportunities for exercise can be done in many different ways. It can be done in medical settings, fitness facilities, or on the field conducted by the corresponding personnel. It can use highly technologic and numerous tests or mostly simple tests restricted to the most essential ones. It can apply computer-based systems for calculation, interpretation, and feedback of the results or use manual methods. As well, it can charge patients considerable sums of money or just a few dollars. Although these different ways have their merits, drawbacks, and justifications in various circumstances for different patients, the following principles and conditions should always be met (76):

- The assessment provides the essential information for planning, implementation, and follow-up of a potentially effective, feasible, and safe exercise program for the patient but does not include irrelevant and potentially costly or unsafe elements.
- The tests and methods are valid, feasible, and safe for their purposes.
- The testers have mastered all aspects related to the proper conduct of the tests.
- The patient has been informed of all relevant aspects of the tests. Usually, written consent is required. It is advisable to obtain consent in any case.
- The patient has self-prepared for the tests as advised regarding such factors as health condition, medication, meals and drinks, tobacco, alcohol, previous physical and other activities, clothing, warming up, practice, and familiarization with all parts of the procedures.

- The patient has been given relevant results and their interpretation without undue delay. The information should give the patient a realistic and balanced view of the possibilities, limitations, benefits, and risks he or she can expect when participating in the prescribed exercise.

The preparticipation or baseline assessment should include a clinical examination, laboratory tests as indicated for disease risk factors, and performance or health-related fitness tests.

CLINICAL EXAMINATION

Clinical examination has always been and has to remain the key part in assessing an individual's health status and related factors. It cannot be compensated (only complemented) by other examinations and tests. Personal and emergency information, past and present medical history, and pertinent health behaviors can be obtained by one of the many available forms (e.g., 76).

Symptoms and signs of OA are naturally the central focus of the examination, even when the diagnosis has been made previously, because they are the basis for exercise prescription and follow-up. Symptoms of OA of the hip are usually felt in and around the hip at the front and inner part of the thigh down to the knee, in the groin, and in the buttock, and sometimes in the sacroiliac joint. In the early phases of OA, pain is felt occasionally and especially under loading (e.g., while walking or carrying objects). Later on, pain is felt as a "start pain" when one begins to move, and finally, also at rest. The symptoms usually worsen during the course of the day. The pain is accompanied by some degree of limp. The pain in different locations and in different circumstances can be graded in different ways (e.g., by using the visual analog scale, a 10-cm line divided by mm from 0 to 100). The main problem is sometimes stiffness, weakness of the leg, or a feeling of giving away. The limitations caused by the condition in the activities of daily living have to be questioned and recorded carefully (e.g., by using one of the forms developed for these purposes).

In OA of the knee, the first symptom is usually pain that may appear when sitting for a long period, when walking stairs, or when kneeling or squatting. Later symptoms are pain during movement, movement limitations, and muscle weakness.

The symptoms (limp, need for support while walking stairs and in squatting, feeling of giving away, pain, swelling) can be graded using the Lysholm scale (77).

Physical examination of the patient with hip OA includes observation from the front, side, and back when the patient is standing and walking. Observing patients when they rise from a chair is informative about the need for support. Walking on stairs or on a treadmill adds to the information regarding limp, length of the stride, speed and rhythm of movement, malalignment, instability, muscle strength, and need for support. The hip region on both sides is inspected for color, contours and evenness of the anterior spina iliaca when the patient is lying supine. The range of all movements of the hip and the endfeel (the type of resistance at the end of the passive range of motion) may be measured in both active and passive movements by use of a goniometer. With OA, all movements of the hip are restricted. The muscle strength in various movements can be tested against the resistance of the examiner's arm or more accurately using various dynamometers. With hip OA, strength of the thigh muscles is decreased. Standard values for various tests and equipment can be obtained from various guidebooks and manuals. The length difference of the legs is examined clinically, by pelvimeter, or most precisely by radiographic techniques.

The physical examination of the knee is begun by inspecting patients when they are standing (deformities, malalignments, differences between legs) and then while walking (symmetry, length, speed and rhythm of the stride). Squatting gives information on the functional limitations of the knee. Palpation and various tests when patients are lying give information on symptoms, movements and stability of the knee, and strength of the adjacent muscles.

FUNCTIONAL OR HEALTH-RELATED FITNESS TESTS

Vast experience shows that OA at one joint influences the functions of many other joints and organs. In addition, most patients with OA are older, and many are overweight and have other diseases. Therefore, it is often appropriate to complement the clinical examination by more accurate tests of the affected joints and adjacent muscles as well as by tests of more distant functions. A relevant concept that unifies these tests is health-related fitness (HRF), i.e., those components of fitness that are influenced by habitual physical activity and relate to present and future health (78). The emphasis in HRF testing is more on enhancing physical capacity for everyday life than on avoiding specific diseases. This aim corresponds well with that of prescribing exercise for patients with OA. Furthermore, HRF tests are designed to be safe, economic, and easy to administer under conditions available in ordinary communities and to be used specifically in testing unfit and physically inactive persons (79). Therefore, exercising at maximal levels of flexibility, strength, and aerobic power are to be avoided.

HRF includes morphologic (body composition, muscle strength), musculoskeletal (muscular strength and endurance, flexibility), motor (postural control), cardiorespiratory (maximal aerobic power or $\dot{V}O_{2max}$, submaximal cardiorespiratory capacity), and metabolic (carbohydrate and lipid metabolism) fitness (78). All these components are valid targets to test in patients with OA to assess their need for exercise, eventual health risks in general and in connection with exercise, and to follow up the effects of the exercise program. None of the developed HRF tests is specific for OA of the hip or knee in terms of assessing current or future functions or health status of these joints. On the other hand, it is not known which types of exercises are most beneficial for those purposes. Thus, both the "treatment" and the tests of its effectiveness are unspecific to the actual disease but valuable regarding the patient's health and functional capacity as a whole.

Several HRF test batteries have been developed, and some are described in various chapters of this book. Most tests assessing cardiorespiratory and metabolic functions and risks have been thoroughly validated to meet the criteria of HRF tests. However, most of the tests assessing morphologic, musculoskeletal, and motor fitness have been insufficiently validated as HRF tests (80,81). Some of them recently have been shown to be feasible, safe, and valid in terms of demonstrating prudent associations with current or future self-rated perceived health, mobility in stair climbing, back functioning, and back pain (82). The development of HRF tests is an ongoing process, and valid and specific tests for assessing patients with hip and knee OA are needed.

Meanwhile, clinical and machine-based tests that measure relevant symptoms, range of motion, and the extent and type of patients' limitations, muscle strength, stability, balance, and walking ability by repeatable, feasible, and safe ways can be used (76,83).

In patients with hip OA, measuring strength of the extensors (gluteus maximus, hamstring muscles) and flexors (iliopsoas, pectineus, and adductor longus as adductors and lateral rotators, and medial rotators) are key targets. In patients with knee OA, the strength of the knee extensor (quadriceps) and flexor (hamstring) muscles are the key targets. It may be advisable to perform the first round of measurements using methods and ways that are not too strenuous, complicated, or perhaps frightening for the patient. The exercise program should begin with a run-in phase, after which measurements can be repeated and complemented once the patient has become familiar with the exercises and equipment.

In principle, cardiorespiratory capacity and cardiovascular risk of patients with hip and knee OA can be assessed using any of the standard tests. However, pain and muscle weakness often limit the patient's walking or cycling before a true $\dot{V}O_{2max}$ has been reached. The preferred exercise modes (walking on treadmill or cycling on ergometer) depend on the patients' symptoms and available equipment. For cardiorespiratory risk evaluation, submaximal levels usually suffice for OA patients because the intensity of the exercise program has to be set to correspond to their symptom-limited level. Furthermore, most serious symptoms and signs indicating cardiovascular risk related to exercise appear already at submaximal intensities. However, one drawback of submaximal testing is that complete information for using heart rate to adjust exercise intensity may not be obtained. On the other hand, the intensity, duration, and modes of exercise for patients with hip and knee OA have to be adjusted mainly on the basis of their symptoms and perceived degree of effort, especially in the beginning of the program, and not by objective physiologic criteria. Furthermore, many patients with OA use medication that influences, e.g., heart rate. Many walking tests are useful and are recommended to assess aerobic endurance capacity (84,85). These tests give relevant objective and perceived information for both the tester and the patient that relates specifically to walking, since walking is usually one of the key components of their exercise program.

Assessing risk factors for cardiorespiratory and metabolic diseases is done using the same criteria, laboratory tests, and methods described in other parts of this book. Likewise, referring patients for further medical examinations and supervised exercise programs based on the results of the risk assessment follows accepted guidelines (86).

EXERCISE PROGRAMS

Two main elements of successful exercise programs are facts and feelings. Facts refer to the scientific evidence of the physiologic principles of the various exercise regimens and their effects on structures and functions and on symptoms, signs, and risk of diseases. Feelings refer to expectations and experiences of the exercise program and its effects on the patients. These expectations and experiences relate to the effects and acceptability (personal and social), accessibility, affordability, safety, and enjoyability of the program. A patient's feelings determine his or her willingness to begin and to continue to participate in the program. Decreased symptoms (pain, stiffness) and decreased limitations in daily life weigh heavily in a patient's expectations, but many other expectations such as less fatigue, improved mood, company, and losing weight may be important. The task of the planner and supervisor of the exercise program is to create a proper balance between facts and feelings.

Two guiding principles related to facts when planning exercise programs are overload and specificity (please see Chapter 2 for more details). These principles are applied to each main component of the program, namely, range of motion and stretching, muscle strengthening, and aerobic exercises. When structures and functions undergo adaptive changes to tolerate an overload, the load has to be increased gradually. Because these adaptations take time, usually weeks or several months, the meager results in many exercise training programs are partly due to the short duration of training. Specificity means that the load has to be applied to those structures and functions that are the primary targets of training. Thus, although studies have shown improved balance of patients with OA as a result of generic stretching, range-of-motion, resistance,

and aerobic exercises (73), better results can be obtained by using exercise modes that specifically stimulate functions related to maintaining balance (e.g., yoga, tai chi, dance, ball games, and walking or skiing on variable surfaces).

All benefits of exercise are reversible, some within days, some within weeks, and many within months. This phenomenon has two important implications. First, it is unrealistic to expect effects of an exercise program to remain 1 year after its cessation (e.g., if the supervised program is not followed by self-conducted exercises). Second, exercise programs for patients with OA should be planned and implemented so that patients are taught and motivated to continue appropriate exercises and physical activity in general as a permanent life habit.

The amount of adaptive change of many structural and functional effects of exercise shows predictable relationships to dose, i.e., its intensity, duration, frequency, or total volume (87,88). These relationships are the most accurate bases for exercise recommendations to obtain various benefits. The dose-response relationships also hold regarding many biologic effects of exercise on patients with OA. However, because these patients frequently show symptoms, functional limitations, low fitness level, lack of experience of previous exercise training, and comorbidities, general exercise guidelines (89) may not always be applicable to them. Persons supervising their exercise training must know these guidelines and criteria and especially their underlying principles, but the exercise has to be prescribed and adjusted according to the highly variable and often rapidly changing individual needs, abilities, and preferences of the patients. This task is a measure of the professional skills of the responsible health and physical activity personnel.

A comprehensive exercise training program for patients with OA is not only a technical regimen, because education and patient support are also key parts. The first part of an exercise program educates patients about the benefits of, and the need for, regular exercise; about attainable personal goals and the exercise needed to attain them; and about the initial responses to, and symptoms caused by, the exercise that the patient is likely to experience (64). This information has to be individually tailored, and parts of it should be repeated during the program, using appropriate formats, especially including education as part of the training sessions.

An important part of the education is to prepare the patient to adopt regular exercises and other physical activities as a lifestyle.

Patients usually need professional and social support, advice, practical measures, and encouragement to understand and overcome the barriers to exercise and to feel that it is worthwhile to continue. Frequent barriers related directly to exercise are fear of damage to the joints, falls, injuries, pain (during or after the exercise), fatigue, and boredom. All these problems can be lessened effectively by caring verbal support and appropriate practical measures such as teaching relaxation skills, using well-cushioned and well-supporting shoes and orthotics (e.g., wedged insoles) when needed, using pain medication prior to exercise sessions, hip protectors during sessions, and local heat and cold at appropriate times. The body, mind, and soul must be treated together.

Stretching and Range-of-Motion (ROM) Exercises

These exercises are the core of the training program for patients with OA and should be done daily. Although the main emphasis is on the affected joints and their contralateral counterparts, stretching and ROM exercises should also include most other joints and muscle groups. The mobility of the hips and low back reciprocally influence the patients' symptoms and functions. Exercises should be done in a relaxed way in safe, comfortable positions and in sufficiently warm conditions, possibly after local heat application and following active warm-up. The ROM exercises should put the joints through the full ROM until it is limited by pain and/or tissue, especially bony resistance. The movements are repeated several (~10) times and are gradually extended further. It is advisable to repeat these exercises, especially those related to the affected joints, more than once a day. These exercises should be taught to patients by a trained professional, but later they should be done mainly by the patients themselves.

With stretching exercises, relaxed and safe positions are important to allow stretching of muscles so that they do not contract during the stretch. Another key feature is to extend the stretching slowly and gradually to the comfortable limit and to hold the position for at least 10 to 30, even 90 sec. The exercises are repeated three to five times during the session, and key exercises should be done more than once each day.

Muscle-Strengthening Exercises

The goals of the muscle-strengthening exercises are to improve the shock attenuation and stability of the affected joints, to decrease pain, and to improve the functional capacity of the patient. The training should influence not only strength but also endurance and motor skills, to attain its goals. The most important muscles to be trained, especially in patients with knee OA, are the quadriceps muscles. While static or dynamic exercises can be used, isometric exercises may be preferable initially and when joint pain is a key problem. It is safe to avoid using maximal contractions near the limit of the ROM to avoid joint damage. The same holds true with dynamic strengthening exercises. On the other hand, it is important to increase muscle strength over the whole ROM. Concentric movements are preferable to eccentric ones, and impacts should be avoided in resistance and other types of exercises. Movements should be made in good form at slow or moderate speed while maintaining good stability and control through the whole movement to avoid injuries. The intensity of the activity can be adjusted by varying the load, number of repetitions, number of sets of repetitions, and length of the rest between the sets and exercises. The general advice for isotonic strength training is to perform 6 to 10 successive repetitions (a set) at 85% of one repetition maximum (1-RM = the maximal load that a muscle group can lift one time through the whole ROM using correct form). Each decrease of 2.5% in the 1-RM allows one more repetition. These sets are repeated three times for each muscle group, and the exercise is done three to five times for a minimum of twice a week. The load is increased when the subject easily performs the given number of repetitions and sets. If the number of repetitions is increased, and resistance decreased (e.g., 15-RM or 60% of 1-RM for 15 repetitions), muscle endurance would increase more than maximal strength (76). Lighter loads and more repetitions are recommended for older persons in general and for patients with OA. Remember, the exercise dose has to be individually set for patients with OA.

All modes of dynamic or varying resistance training methods are useful, except for plyometric training where the muscle is stretched immediately prior to the contraction (e.g., by jumping from a bench to the ground and then springing back). Although isokinetic training offers some advantages over the other methods relative to ease of performance, risk of muscle soreness and injury, and improvement of skills, availability and equipment costs limit its use (76).

Aerobic Training

Aerobic exercises are used for general conditioning and many modes offer good opportunities for weight control, recreation, socializing, and training of coordination, balance, and stability. Increasing evidence shows that even light aerobic training at 30 to 40% $\dot{V}O_{2max}$ can benefit unfit, sedentary, and older subjects (90,91). Furthermore, low-intensity training increases endurance capacity more than $\dot{V}O_{2max}$, and this is particularly important for performing daily tasks. Patients' perceptions must be given much weight in adjusting the exercise intensity, and a mechanistic application of heart rate criteria may be grossly misleading. Sufficient evidence indicates also that 30 min of daily aerobic activity can be performed in several bouts without compromising its effectiveness (92,93). This is important for many patients with OA to avoid fatigue and excessive loading of the joints.

Perhaps the most important criterion of aerobic training for patients with OA is that it should be done daily, not only during the formal program but also continuously thereafter. An ideal form of aerobic activities is exercise in water. Other suitable modes include walking (not walking on stairs for many patients), cycling (preferably at low pedal load), calisthenics, slow aerobics, cross-country skiing, rowing, nonimpact dancing, and some ball games at a moderate tempo (e.g., badminton, table tennis, and golf). Nordic or stick (pole) walking, using special-purpose poles that are much like downhill ski poles in both hands in roughly the same way as in cross-country skiing, has gained wide popularity, especially in Finland among adults, but particularly among older and disabled persons. Poles, when used effectively, may increase energy expenditure, the number of involved muscles and thus effectiveness of this mode of walking, compared with ordinary walking. As well, the poles increase the safety of Nordic walking under variable conditions. For patients with OA, the poles can be used to reduce loading of the hip and knee joints. These

features may indirectly increase the effectiveness of pole walking as an exercise mode in OA patients.

Safety Precautions

The general safety precautions concerning physical exercise also apply to patients with OA (86,89). Special attention should be given not to load joints that are acutely inflamed or are otherwise unusually painful. The amount, intensity, and mode of exercise naturally have to be adjusted if training increases the symptoms. The substantial day-to-day variation in symptoms of many patients must be given due consideration.

Rheumatoid Arthritis

Rheumatoid arthritis (RA) is the most common inflammatory arthritic disease. It is a chronic, progressive, autoimmune disease with unknown etiology. RA is a systemic disease, but its key feature is inflammation of joint lining or synovium that becomes thick and interferes with joint mobility. The joints are swollen and painful with motion and when palpated, and they are stiff for several hours in the morning because of extra fluid in the joint space. The most commonly affected joints are the ball of the foot, fingers, and wrist, but any joint can be affected. The number of inflamed joints increases with the progression of the disease. The joint cartilage is gradually eroded, and the cartilage, the bone underneath, and the adjacent ligaments are destroyed, leading to deformities and impaired function. The systemic nature of the disease is seen in various inflammatory manifestations in many organs, e.g., the heart, lungs, vasculature, eyes, and peripheral nerves. The diagnosis of RA is based on the criteria established by the American Rheumatism Association (94) (Table 10-1). At least four of the seven criteria in Table 7-1 must be met for diagnosis, and criteria 1 through 4 must have been present for at least 6 weeks. RA is a catabolic state leading to loss of muscle (95) and bone (8,96–98) and consequently to muscular weakness, low endurance, and increased risk of hip fracture (99). Patients with RA also have an increased risk of coronary heart disease, probably related to inflammation.

The prevalence of RA is about the same as that for OA, i.e., 0.5 to 1% in most adult populations

TABLE 10-1   THE 1987 REVISED CRITERIA FOR THE CLASSIFICATION OF RHEUMATOID ARTHRITIS (RA)

Criterion	Definition
1. Morning stiffness	Morning stiffness in and around the joints, lasting at least 1 hour before maximal improvement
2. Arthritis of 3 or more joint areas	At least three joint areas simultaneously have had soft tissue swelling or fluid (not bony overgrowth alone) observed by a physician; the 14 possible areas are right or left PIP, MCP, wrist, elbow, knee, ankle, and MTP joints
3. Arthritis of hand joints	At least one area swollen (as defined above) in a wrist, MCP, or PIP joint
4. Symmetric arthritis	Simultaneous involvement of the same joint areas (as defined in 2) on both sides of the body (bilateral involvement of PIP, MCP, or MTP is acceptable without absolute symmetry)
5. Rheumatoid nodules	Subcutaneous nodules over bony prominences or extensor surfaces or in juxtaarticular regions, observed by a physician.
6. Serum rheumatoid factor	Demonstration of abnormal amounts of serum rheumatoid factor by any method for which the result has been positive in < 5% of normal control subjects
7. Radiographic changes	Radiographic changes typical of rheumatoid arthritis on posteroanterior hand an wrist radiograph, which must include erosions or unequivocal bony decalcification localized in or most marked adjacent to the involved joints (osteoarthritis changes alone do not qualify)

DIP, distal interphalangeal joints; PIP, proximal interphalangeal joints; MCP, metacarpophalangeal joints; MTP, metatarsophalangeal joints.

from which reliable estimates are available (100). About two thirds of patients are women. The disease can begin at any age, but the highest incidence is seen at age 55 to 60 years. The highest prevalence is found at about age 70 years.

The progression of the disease is often classified in four stages. In stage I, first bone changes are seen in radiographs. In stage II, some muscle wasting and limitation of movement are also observed. In stage III, there are joint defects, a large amount of muscle wasting, and bone and cartilage destruction. Stage IV is the end stage, showing the changes of previous phases and fiberlike or bony joining (ankylosis) of the inflamed joints (101). Although the prevalence of RA is relatively low, its burden is high because of its severely debilitating nature. The main symptom, chronic pain, leads often to depressive mood, anxiety, feelings of helplessness, physical inactivity, and decreased social contacts. Especially during the active phases, the patients have reduced appetite and increased catabolism, and consequently they lose weight, es-

pecially muscle tissue. About 10% of patients with RA are estimated to depend on another person for daily activities (100). RA patients represent only 8% of all patients with musculoskeletal disorders, but they consume 40% of all hospital days used by this patient group (102). More than 50% of the patients become work-disabled within 10 years of the disease (103–105), and the fastest decline is seen during the first 3 years (106). In a community-based study, the probability for disability was 7.7 times higher in RA patients than in community controls after adjustment for several potential confounding factors (107), and the impact of RA was greater in younger and middle-aged than in elderly persons. Currently, RA cannot be cured or prevented. All these features emphasize the importance of secondary prevention of RA.

MANAGEMENT OF RA

The systemic nature of RA causes multiple problems for patients. Therefore, the management of RA requires a comprehensive approach including drug and surgical treatment as well as various forms of physical, psychologic, social, and vocational rehabilitation. Secondary preventive measures to preserve the joints and their function should begin immediately after the diagnosis has been made. An important part of the management is to educate the patients and their families to take an active part in the treatment and rehabilitation of the disease.

Exercise in the Management of RA

Because loading of the arthritic joints has been feared to facilitate their destruction, passive methods of treatment were used to manage RA until the 1970s (108), and nonloading exercises were used in the 1970s (109). Several studies showed evidence, however, that dynamic exercise was safe and effective in patients with RA and did not aggravate the clinical condition or increase joint destruction (110–115). Several harmful effects caused by or related to RA are potentially amenable to the beneficial influences of appropriate exercise. These effects include stiffness, pain and limited mobility of the affected joints, loss of muscle mass and strength (95,116–118), decreased bone mass (96–98,119) and aerobic capacity, and increased risk of coronary heart disease. Keep in mind, however, that studies of poorer quality may show better results than trials of better quality (120).

In the preparticipation screening and testing, special emphasis is placed on evaluating the status and function of the affected joint and other joints. Radiographs are important because the findings can be used as objective signs of the development of the disease. Several validated methods can be used to score the radiographs (121,122). One must check neck pain and related symptoms carefully, because a typical lesion in RA is anterior subluxation of the os atlantis due to erosion of the ligament between the arches of the vertebrae. This condition requires special exercises and support by hard collar, but traction of the neck is contraindicated. Functional capacity and quality of life of the patient can be assessed by validated self-administered questionnaires (123–125). Because of the increased risk of CHD in these patients, the CHD risk factors must be assessed. The necessity of an exercise stress test to assess the risk related to exercise is decided on the basis of the symptoms, level of risk factors, and

planned exercise. Nevertheless, at least a submaximal test (e.g., walking) (84,85) is recommended to get a baseline of the patient's aerobic performance capacity.

The goals of exercise and other modes of physical therapy are to decrease pain, to maintain and increase joint function, to prevent and correct deformities, to maintain and increase muscle strength and general performance capacity, to train daily activities, and to educate the patient in the management of the disease. In the beginning, the exercises should be supervised by trained personnel. This is necessary to teach the patients and also to encourage them to continue exercising, because an exercise bout causes some discomfort in most RA patients. In a quarter of them the symptoms last for several days (126). However, patients should begin to do some activities, e.g., mobility exercises, on their own as early as possible. A preferred time for the supervised exercises is around noon, when morning stiffness has disappeared and fatigue has not yet set in.

Mobility exercises that include stretching and warm-up are central parts of the exercise regimen of RA patients to prevent development of contractures as well as to avoid excessive stress on the tendons weakened by inflammation. The movements should be done smoothly and supported by the supervisor or the patient, being careful not to force the movement to the furthest degree. Mobility exercises should be repeated several times each day.

Because of the catabolic nature of RA, strengthening of the muscles both around the affected joints and in general is important. During the acute phase, isometric exercises have been recommended for the periarticular muscles to avoid excessive joint loading. The results have been controversial, showing positive effects (127) or no changes (128–129). On the contrary, a number of studies using dynamic exercises found increases in muscle strength (114,120) and aerobic capacity of patients with chronic or early (115,130,131) RA without detrimental effects on disease activity, pain, or radiologic findings. It seems that patients with active RA benefit from and tolerate well even intensive strength training using isokinetic techniques that seem to be more effective than isometric training (132). Explosive strength also can be increased by using high movement velocities in the training regimen (130).

This finding is important because it suggests that exercise training of RA patients can be used to prevent disease-induced atrophy of type II muscle fibers (133), which seem to be specifically affected by RA (134). Some studies also have shown a decreased number of tender and swollen joints (135,136) and positive changes in self-assessed functional capacity (115,130,131). However, the effects of exercise training on general performance capacity are unclear (120,132,137).

Little research has been done on the effect of exercise on bone mineral density in patients with RA. Recent studies addressing this aspect showed no significant changes as a result of strengthening exercises (130,131), probably because the training did not meet the characteristics of an effective bone-loading stimulus (138).

The intensity of the muscle training has to be adjusted on a strictly individual basis. In weak patients, resistance against gravity, water, or another part of the body often suffices as a training stimulus. Later and in stronger patients, the criteria for training emphasizing strength (60–80% 1-RM) or endurance (30–60% 1-RM) can be applied. The exercises must be performed with proper technique, in good positions, and using appropriate supports when needed.

Aerobic exercise is indicated for RA patients to maintain or improve fitness and to prevent cardiovascular diseases. Aquatic exercises are particularly suitable. Other effective and safe modes include walking, Nordic or pole walking, cycling, and cross-country skiing. The intensity is adjusted individually, and the lower end of the heart rate and other physiologic criteria are usually applied. Several short bouts of exercise during the day are preferable to one longer, continuous exercise bout, to avoid excessive joint loading and fatigue.

As expected, the effects of exercise training disappear gradually when the program is stopped (139). This observation emphasizes the need for continuing regular exercise and less formal physical activity for patients with RA.

Exercise has reached approved status as part of the management of RA. When exercise is used as a medical modality, the requirements for its safety are comparable to those associated with using drugs but higher than those associated with self-initiated recreational exercise. Even minor injuries, unexpected pain and soreness, or other unpleasant perceptions can lead to harmful consequences, e.g., to cessation of the program. This emphasizes the need for careful prescription and monitoring of exercise and avoidance of all risks related to the exercise itself, to the patient, to the supervisor, to the equipment and clothing, and to the environment. RA is a disease with fluctuating course, and patients have episodes when the condition is worse, i.e., flare-ups. Loading the acutely inflamed joint must be avoided, but unloaded movements are necessary during a flare-up. Generally the exercise capacity of the patients decreases during the active phases of the disease because of pain, stiffness, and catabolic state. Patients may be fatigued and unwilling to exercise. These features call for appropriate adjustments of the exercise program.

Summary

- Arthritis in even one joint causes multiple problems for the patient and requires comprehensive management.
- Because arthritis cannot be cured, the patient has to learn to live with it. However, good treatment and secondary prevention, in which the patient plays a central role, can lessen the damage, improve the quality of life remarkably, and prevent worsening of the condition.
- Exercise and physical activity in general, initially supervised and then independent, is one of the key components for preventing functional deterioration of the diseased joints and worsening of other direct and indirect consequences of the disease.
- The mode and dose of the exercise has to be determined individually on the basis of the patient's health status and functional abilities to set a proper balance between effectiveness and safety.
- Exercise and physical activity in general should be continuous habits of the patient. Therefore, one of the primary goals of exercise programs should be to find feasible and satisfying ways for exercise by full consideration of the expectations, abilities, opportunities, limitations, and preferences of the patient.
- Exercise for patients with arthritis is part of a medical regimen and should continue as a lifelong

habit. Therefore, the same criteria for safety with drugs apply with exercise.

REFERENCES

1. Felson DT, Lawrence RC, Dieppe PA, et al. Osteoarthritis: new insights. NIH conference, Part 1: The disease and its risk factors. Ann Intern Med 2000;133:635–646.
2. Mitchell NS, Cruess RL. Classification of degenerative arthritis. Can Med Assoc J 1977;117:763–765.
3. Buckwalter, JA, Mankin HJ. Articular cartilage II. Degeneration and osteoarthritis, repair, regeneration and transplantation. J Bone Joint Surg Am 1997;79A:612–632.
4. Cardone DA, Tallia AF. Osteoarthritis. In: Singleton JK, Sandowski SA, Green-Hernandez C, et al., eds. Primary care. Philadelphia: Lippincott, 1999:543–548.
5. Arokoski JPA, Jurvelin J, Vaatainen U, et al. Normal and pathological adaptation of articular cartilage to joint loading. Scand J Med Sci Sports 2000;10:186–198.
6. Kee CK. Osteoarthritis: manageable scourge of aging. Rheumatology 2000;35:199–208.
7. Birchfield PC. Osteoarthritis overview. Geriatr Nurs 2001;22:124–131.
8. Messier SP, Loeser RF, Hoover JL, et al. Osteoarthritis of the knee: effects on gait, strength, and flexibility. Arch Phys Med Rehabil 1992;73:29–36.
9. Wegener L, Kisner C, Nichols D. Static and dynamic balance responses in persons with bilateral knee osteoarthritis. J Orthop Sports Phys Ther 1997;25:13–18.
10. Manek NJ. Medical management of osteoarthritis. Mayo Clin Proc 2001;76:533–539.
11. Tinetti ME, Doucette J, Claus E, et al. Risk factors for serious injury during falls by older persons in the community. J Am Geriatr Soc 1995;43:1214–1221.
12. Dieppe P. What is the relationship between pain and osteoarthritis. Rheumatol Eur 1998;27:55–56.
13. Townes AS. Osteoarthritis. In: Barker LR, Burton JR, Zieve PD, eds. Principles of Ambulatory Medicine. 5th ed. Baltimore: Williams & Wilkins, 1999:960–973.
14. Oliveria SA, Felson DT, Reed JI, et al. Incidence of symptomatic hand, hip, and knee osteoarthritis among patients in a health maintenance organization. Arthritis Rheum 1995;38:1134–1141.
15. Felson DT, Zhang Y. An update on the epidemiology of knee and hip osteoarthritis with a view to prevention. Arthritis Rheum 1998;41:1345–1355.
16. Petersson IF. Occcurence of osteoarthritis of the peripheral joints in European populations. Ann Rheum Dis 1996;55:659–661.
17. Felson DT. Epidemiology of hip and knee osteoarthritis. Epidemiol Rev 1988;10:1–28.
18. Murray JL, Lopez AD, eds. The Global Burden of Disease: A Comprehensive Assessment of Mortality and Disability from Diseases, Injuries and Risk Factors in 1990 and Projected to 2020. Cambridge, MA: Harvard University Press, 1996.
19. Guccione AA, Felson DT, Anderson JJ, et al. The effects of specific medical conditions on functional limitations of elders in the Framingham Study. Am J Public Health 1994;84:351–358.
20. National Institute of Arthritis and Musculoskeletal and Skin Disease, National Institutes of Health. Arthritis prevalence rising as baby boomers grow older. Available at *www.nih.gov/niams.* 1998.
21. Arthritis: a leading cause of disability in the United States. Natl Acad Aging Soc 2000;5:1–6.
22. Yelin E. The economics of osteoarthritis. In: Brandt KD, Doherty M, Lohmander LS, eds. Osteoarthritis. New York: Oxford University Press, 1998:23–30.
23. Dougados M, Gueguen A, Nguyen M, et al. Longitudinal radiologic evaluation of osteoarthritis of the knee. J Rheumatol 1992;19:378–383.
24. Schouten JS, van den Ouweland F, Valkenburg HA. A 12 year follow up study in the general population on prognostic factors of cartilage loss in osteoarthritis of the knee. Ann Rheum Dis 1992;51:932–937.
25. Manninen P, Riihimaki H, Heliovaara M, Makela P. Overweight, gender, and knee osteoarthritis. Int J Obes Relat Metab Disord 1996;20:595–597.
26. Felson DT, Zhang Y, Hannan MT, et al. Risk factors for incident radiographic knee osteoarthritis in the elderly: the Framingham Study. Arthritis Rheum1997;40:728–733.
27. Karlson EW, Mand LA, Grodstein F, et al. Risk factors for severe hip osteoarthritis in a large female cohort study (abstract). Arthritis Rheum 2000;43(suppl):S152.
28. Felson DT, Zhang Y, Anthony JM, et al. Weight loss reduces the risk for symptomatic knee osteoarthritis in women. The Framingham Study. Ann Intern Med 1992;116:535–539.
29. McGoey BV, Deitel M, Saplys RJ, Kliman ME. Effect of weight loss on musculoskeletal pain in the morbidly obese. J Bone Joint Surg Br 1990;72:322–323.
30. Sharma L. Proprioceptive impairment in osteoarthritis. Rheum Dis Clin North Am 1999;25:299–314.
31. Petrella RJ, Lattanzio PJ, Nelson MG. Effect of age and activity on knee joint proprioception. Am J Phys Med Rehabil 1997;76:235–241.
32. Sharma L, Pai YC, Holtkamp K, Rymer WZ. Is knee joint proprioception worse in the arthritic knee

versus the unaffected knee in unilateral knee os-teoarthritis? Arthritis Rheum 1997;40:1518–1525.

33. Casper J, Berg K. Effects of exercise on osteoarthritis: a review. J Strength Cond Res 1998;12:120–125.

34. Gelber AC, Hochberg MC, Mead IA, et al. Joint injury in young adults and risk for subsequent knee and hip osteoarthritis. Ann Intern Med 2000;133:321–328.

35. Lohmander LS, Roos HP. Osteoarthritis. In: Kjaer M, Krogsgaard M, Magnusson P, et al., eds. Textbook of Sports Medicine. Malden, MA: Blackwell Science, 2003.

36. Slemenda C, Hellman D, Brandt KD, et al. Weight, adiposity and quadriceps weakness as predictors of progression of knee osteoarthritis (OA). Arthritis Rheum 1997;40:S1246.

37. Slemenda C, Heilman DK, Brandt KD, et al. Reduced quadriceps strength relative to body weight: a risk factor for knee osteoarthritis in women? Arthritis Rheum 1998;41:1951–1959.

38. Slemenda C, Brandt KD, Hellman DK, et al. Quadriceps weakness and osteoarthritis of the knee. Ann Intern Med 1997;127:97–104.

39. Felson DT, Hannan MT, Naimark A et al. Occupational physical demands, knee bending, and knee osteoarthritis: results form the Framingham Study. J Rheumatol. 1991;18:1587–1592.

40. Kirkeskov-Jensen L, Eenberg W. Occupation as a risk factor for knee disorders. Scand J Work Environ Health 1996;22:165–175.

41. O'Reilly S, Jones A, Doherty M. Muscle weakness in osteoarthritis. Curr Opin Rheumatol 1997;9:259–262.

42. Thompson R, Oegema TR, Lewis JL, Wallace L. Osteoarthritic changes after acute transarticular load: an animal model. J Bone Joint Surg 1991;73A:990–1001.

43. Buckwalter JA, Lane NE. Athletics and osteoarthritis. Am J Sports Med 1997;25:873–881.

44. Vuori IM. Dose-response of physical activity and low back pain, osteoarthritis, and osteoporosis. Med Sci Sports Exerc 2001;33(suppl):S551–586.

45. Vingard EL, Alfredsson L, Goldie I, Hogstedt C. Occupation and osteoarthrosis of the hip and knee: a register-based cohort study. Int J Epidemiol 1991;20:1025–1031.

46. Panush RS, Inzinna JD. Recreational activities and degenerative joint disease. Sports Med 1994;17:1–5.

47. Ratcliffe A, Beauvais P, Saed-Nejad F. Differential levels of aggregan aggregate components in synovial fluids from canine knee joints with experimental osteoarthritis and disuse. J Orthop Res. 1994;12:464–473.

48. Sharkey NA, Williams NI, Guerin JB. The role of exercise in the prevention and treatment of osteoporosis and osteoarthritis. Nursing Clin North America 2000;35:209–221.

49. Setton L, Zimmeman J, Mow V, et al. Effect of disuse on the tensile properties and composition of canine knee joint cartilage. Transactions of the Orthopaedic Research Society 1990;15:155–159.

50. Helminen HJ, Hyttinen MM, Lammi MJ, et al. Regular joint loading in youth assists in the establishment and strengthening of the collagen network of articular cartilage and contributes to the prevention of osteoarthrosis later in life: a hypothesis. J Bone Miner Metab. 2000;18:245–257.

51. Ettinger WH Jr. Physical activity, arthritis, and disability in older people. Clin Geriatric Med 1998;14:633–640.

52. McAlindon TE, Wilson PWF, Aliabadi P, et al. Level of physical activity and the risk of radiographic and symptomatic knee osteoarthritis in the elderly: the Framingham study. Am J Med 1999;106:151–157.

53. Cheng Y, Macera CA, Davis DR, et al. Physical activity and self-reported, physician-diagnosed osteoarthritis: is physical activity a risk factor? J Clin Epidemiol 2000;3:315–322.

54. Lequesne MG, Dang N, Lane NE. Sport practice and osteoarthritis of the limbs. Osteoarthritis Cartilage 1997;5:75–86.

55. Roos H, Lindberg H, Gardsell P, et al. The prevalence of gonarthrosis and its relation to meniscectomy in former soccer players. Am J Sports Med 1994;22:219–222.

56. Spector TD, Harris PA, Hart DJ, et al. Risk of osteoarthritis associated with long-term weight–bearing sports-a radiologic survey of the hips and knees in female ex-athletes and population controls. Arthritis Rheum 1996;39:988–995.

57. Brandt KD. The importance of nonpharmacologic approaches in management of osteoarthritis. Am J Med 1998;105:39S–44S.

58. Felson DT, Lawrence RC, Hochberg MC, et al. Osteoarthritis: New insights. NIH Conference, Part 2: Treatment approaches. Ann Intern Med 2000;133:726–737.

59. Walker-Bone K, Javaid K, Arden N, Cooper C. Medical management of osteoarthritis. BMJ 2000;321:936–940.

60. Superio-Cabyslay E, Ward MM, Lorig KR. Patient education interventions in osteoarthritis and rheumatoid arthritis: a meta-analytic comparison with nonsteroidal anti-inflammatory drug treatment. Arthritis Care Res 1996;9:292–301.

61. Rene J, Weinberger M, Mazzuca SA, et al. Reduction of joint pain in patients with knee osteoarthritis who have received monthly telephone calls

from lay personnel and whose medical treatment regimens have remained stable. Arthritis Rheum 1992;35:511–515.

62. Keefe FJ, Caldwell DS, Baucom D, et al. Spouse-assisted coping skills training in the management of osteoarthritic knee pain. Arthritis Care Res 1996;9:279–291.

63. Puett DW, Griffin MR. Published trials of non-medicinal and non-invasive therapies for hip and knee osteoarthritis. Ann Intern Med 1994;121:133–140.

64. Resnick B. Managing arthritis with exercise. Geriatr Nurs 2001;22:143–150.

65. Van Baar ME, Assendelft WJJ, Dekker J, et al. Effectiveness of exercise therapy in patients with osteoarthritis of the hip or knee. Arthritis Rheum 1999;42:1361–1369.

66. Van den Ende CHM, Vliet Vlieland TPM, Munneke M, Hazes JMW. Dynamic exercise therapy for rheumatoid arthritis. The Cochrane Library, Issue 2, 2003.

67. Fransen M, McConnell S, Bell M. Exercise for osteoarthritis of the hip or knee. The Cochrane Library, Issue 1, 2004.

68. Deyle GD, Henderson NE, Matekel RI, et al. Effectiveness of manual physical therapy and exercise in osteoarthritis of the knee. A randomised controlled trial. Ann Intern Med 2000;132:173–181.

69. Sullivan T, Allegrante JP, Peterson MG, et al. One-year follow-up of patients with osteoarthritis of the knee who participated in a program of supervised fitness walking and supportive patient education. Arthritis Care Res 1998;11:228–233.

70. Chamberlain MA, Care G, Harfield B. Physiotherapy in osteoarthrosis of the knees. A controlled trial of hospital versus home exercises. Int Rehabil Med 1982;4:101–106.

71. Fisher NM, Pendergast DR, Gresham GE, Calkins E. Muscle rehabilitation: its effect on muscular and functional performance of patients with knee osteoarthritis. Arch Phys Med Rehabil 1991;72:367–374.

72. Ettinger WH Jr, Burns R, Messier SP, et al. A randomized trial comparing aerobic exercise and resistance exercise with a health education program in older adults with knee osteoarthritis. JAMA 1997;277:25–31.

73. Messier SP, Royer TD, Craven TE, et al. Long-term exercise and its effect on balance in older, osteoarthritic adults: results from the Fitness, Arthritis, and Senior Trial (FASR). J Am Geriatr Soc 2000;48:131–138.

74. American College of Rheumatology Subcommittee on Osteoarthritis Guidelines. Recommendations for the medical management of osteoarthritis

of the hip and knee: 2000 update. Arthritis Rheum 2000;43:1905–1915.

75. Brosseau L, MacLeay L, Robinson V, et al. Intensity of exercise for the treatment of osteoarthritis. The Cochrane Library, Issue 2, 2003.

76. Howley TE, Franks BD. Health Fitness Instructor's Handbook. 3rd ed. Champaign, IL: Human Kinetics, 1997.

77. Lysholm J, Gillqvist J. Evaluation of the knee ligament surgery results with emphasis on use of a scoring scale. Am J Sports Med 1982;10:150–154.

78. Bouchard C, Shephard RJ. Physical activity, fitness and health: the model and key concepts. In: Bouchard C, Shephard RJ, Stephens T, eds. Physical Activity, Fitness, and Health. Champaign, IL: Human Kinetics, 1994:77–88.

79. Skinner JS, Oja P. Laboratory and field tests for assessing health-related fitness. In: Bouchard C, Shephard RJ, Stephens T, eds. Physical Activity, Fitness, and Health. Champaign, IL: Human Kinetics, 1994:160–179.

80. Suni J, Oja P, Laukkanen R, et al. Health-related fitness test battery for adults: aspects of reliability. Arch Phys Med Rehab 1996;77:399–405.

81. Suni J, Miilunpalo S, Asikainen T-M, et al. Safety and feasibility of a health-related fitness test battery for adults. Phys Ther 1998;78:134–148.

82. Suni J, Oja P, Miilunpalo S, et al. Health-related fitness test battery for adults: associations with perceived health, mobility, and back function and symptoms. Arch Phys Med Rehab 1998;79:559–569.

83. Maud PJ, Foster C, eds. Physiological Assessment of Human Fitness. Champaign, IL: Human Kinetics, 1995.

84. Fleg JL, Piña IL, Balady GJ, et al. Assessment of functional capacity in clinical and research applications. An advisory from the Committee on Exercise, Rehabilitation, and Prevention, Council of Clinical Cardiology, American Heart Association. Circulation 2000;102:1591–1597.

85. Noonan V, Dean E. Submaximal exercise testing: clinical application and interpretation. Phys Ther 2000;80:782–807.

86. ACSM's Guidelines for Exercise Testing and Prescription. 6th ed. Philadelphia: Lippincott Williams & Wilkins, 2000.

87. Haskell W. Dose-response issues from a biological perspective. In: Bouchard C, Shephard RJ, Stephens T, eds. Physical Activity, Fitness, and Health. Champaign, Il: Human Kinetics, 1994:1030–1039.

88. Dose-response issues concerning physical activity and health: an evidence-based symposium. Med Sci Sports Exerc 2001;33(suppl):S345–S641.

89. American College of Sports Medicine Position Stand. The recommended quantity and quality of exercise for developing and maintaining cardiorespiratory and muscular fitness, and flexibility in healthy adults. Med Sci Sports Exerc 1998;30:975–991.

90. Morris JN, Hardman AE. Walking to health. Sports Med 1997;23:306–332.

91. Asikainen T-M, Miilunpalo S, Oja P, et al. Randomised, controlled walking trials in postmenopausal women: the minimum dose to improve aerobic fitness? Br J Sports Med 2002;36:189–194.

92. Hardman AE. Issues of fractionization of exercise (short vs long bouts). Med Sci Sports Exerc 2001;33(suppl):S421–S7

93. Asikainen T-M, Miilunpalo S, Oja P, et al. Walking trials in postmenopausal women: effect of one vs two daily bouts on aerobic fitness. Scand J Med Sci Sports 2002;12:99–105.

94. Arnett F, Edworthy S, Bloch D, et al. The American Rheumatism Association 1987 revised criteria for the classification of rheumatoid arthritis. Arthritis Rheum 1988;31:315–324.

95. Roubenoff R, Roubenoff RA, Cannon J, et al. Rheumatoid cachexia: cytokine-driven hypermetabolism accompanying reduced body cell mass in chronic inflammation. J Clin Invest 1994;93:2379–2386.

96. Sambrook P, Eisman J, Champion G, et al. Determinants of axial bone loss in rheumatoid arthritis. Arthritis Rheum 19987;30:721–728.

97. Kroger H, Honkanen R, Saarikoski S, Alhava E. Decreased axial bone mineral density in perimenopausal women with rheumatoid arthritis. A population based study. Ann Rheum Dis 1994;53:18–23.

98. Hansen M, Florescu A, Stoltenberg M, et al. Bone loss in rheumatoid arthritis. Influence of disease activity, duration of the disease, functional capacity, and corticosteroid treatment. Scand J Rheumatol 1996;25:367–376.

99. Hooyman J, Melton L, Nelson A, et al. Fractures after rheumatoid arthritis. Arthritis Rheum 1984;27:1353–1361.

100. Gran J. The epidemiology of rheumatoid arthritis. In: Schlumberger HD, ed. Epidemiology of Allergic Diseases. Monographs in Allergy, vol 21. Basel: Karger, 1987:162–196.

101. Ekblom B, Nordemar R. Rheumatoid arthritis. In: Skinner JS, ed. Exercise Testing and Exercise Prescription for Special Cases. 2nd ed. Philadelphia: Lea & Febiger, 1993:113–126.

102. Yelin E, Felts W. A summary of the impact of musculoskeletal conditions in the United States. Arthritis Rheum 1990;33:750–755.

103. Makisara G, Makisara P. Prognosis of functional capacity and work in rheumatoid arthritis. Clin Rheumatol 1982;1:117–125.

104. Borg G, Allander E, Berg E, et al. Auranofin treatment in early rheumatoid arthritis may postpone early retirement. Results from a 2-year double blind trial. J Rheumatol 1991;18:1015–1020.

105. Wolfe F, Andersson J, Hawley D. Rates and predictors of work disability in rheumatoid arthritis: importance of disease, psycho-social and workplace factors. Arthritis Rheum 1994;37:S231 (abstr).

106. Mau W, Bornmann M, Weber H, et al. Prediction of permanent work disability in a follow-up study of early rheumatoid arthritis: results of a tree structured analysis using recpam. Br J Rheumatol 1996;35:652–659.

107. Sokka T, Krishnan E, Hakkinen A, Hannonen P. Functional disability in rheumatoid arthritis patients compared with a community population in Finland. Arthritis Rheum 2003;48:59–63.

108. Alexander G, Hortas C, Bacon P. Bed rest, activity and the inflammation of rheumatoid arthritis. Br J Rheumatol 1983;22:134–140.

109. Jivoff L. Rehabilitation and rheumatoid arthritis. Bull Rheum Dis 1975;26:838–841.

110. Ekblom B, Lovgren O, Alderin M, et al. Effect of short-term physical training on patients with rheumatoid arthritis. Scand J Rheumatol 1975;4:87–91.

111. Minor MA, Hewett JE, Webel RR, et al. Efficacy of physical conditioning exercise in patients with rheumatoid arthritis and osteoarthritis. Arthritis Rheum 1989;32:1396–1405.

112. Ekdahl C, Andersson S, Moritz U, Svensson B. Dynamic versus static training in patients with rheumatoid arthritis. Scand J Rheumatol 1990;19:17–26.

113. Stenstrom C, Lindell B, Swabberg E, et al. Intensive dynamic training in water for rheumatoid arthritis functional class II—a long-term study of effects. Scand J Rheumatol 1991;20:358–365.

114. Hansen T, Hansen G, Langgaard A, Rasmussen J. Longterm physical training in rheumatoid arthritis. A randomised trial with different training programs and blinded observers. Scand J Rheumatol 1993;22:107–112.

115. de Jong Z, Munneke M, Zwinderman AH, et al. Is a long-term high-intensity exercise program effective and safe in patients with rheumatoid arthritis? Results of a randomised controlled trial. Athritis Rheum 2003;48:2393–2395.

116. Ekblom B, Lovgren O, Alderin M, et al. Physical performance in patients with rheumatoid arthritis. Scand J Rheumatol 1974;3:121–125.

117. Ekdahl C, Broman G. Muscle strength, endurance, and aerobic capacity in rheumatoid arthritis: a

comparative study with healthy subjects. Ann Rheum Dis 1992;51:35–40.

118. Hakkinen A, Hannonen P, Hakkinen K. Muscle strength in healthy people and in patients suffering from recent-onset inflammatory arthritis. Br J Rheumatol 1995;34:355–360.

119. Star V, Hochberg M. Osteoporosis in patients with rheumatic diseases. Rheum Dis Clin North Am 1994;3:561–576.

120. Van den Ende CHM, Vliet Vlieland TPM, Munneke M, Hazes JMW. Dynamic exercise therapy for treating rheumatoid arthritis. In: The Cochrane Library, Issue 1, 2004.

121. Larsen A, Dale K, Eek M. Radiographic evaluation of rheumatoid arthritis and related conditions by standard reference films. Acta Radiol 1977;18;481–491.

122. Sharp J. Scoring radiographic abnormalities in rheumatoid arthritis. J Rheumatol 1989;16:568–569.

123. Fries J, Spitz P, Kraines R, Holman H. Measurement of patient outcome in arthritis. Arthritis Rheum 1980;23:137–145.

124. Meenan R, Gertman P, Mason J. Measuring health status in arthritis: the Arthritis Impact Measurement Scales. Arthritis Rheum 1980;23:146–152.

125. Kirvan J, Reeback J. Stanford Health Assessment Questionnaire modified to assess disability in British patients with rheumatoid arthritis. Br J Rheumatol 1986;25:206–209.

126. Nordemar R, Ekblom B, Zachrisson L, Lundqvist K. Physical training in rheumatoid arthritis: a controlled long-term study. Scand J Rheumatol 1981;10:17–23.

127. Machover S, Sapecky A. Effect of isometric exercise on the quadriceps muscle in patients with rheumatoid arthritis. Arch Phys Med Rehabil 1966;47:737–741.

128. Cuddigan J. Quadriceps femoris strength. Rheumatol Rehabil 1973;12:77–83.

129. Luckhurst B, Peppiat J, Reynolds W. The response of the quadriceps muscle to an isometric strengthening program in rheumatoid arthritis. Proceedings World Confederation for Physical Therapy Seventh International Congress 1974:244–249.

130. Hakkinen A, Sokka T, Kotaniemi A, et al. Dynamic strength training in patients with early rheumatoid arthritis increases muscle strength but not bone mineral density. J Rheumatol 1999;26:1257–1263.

131. Hakkinen A, Sokka T, Kotaniemi A, Hannonen P. A randomized two-year study of the effect of dynamic strength training on muscle strength, disease activity, functional capacity and bone mineral density in early rheumatoid arthritis. Arthritis Rheum 2001;44:515–422.

132. Van den Ende CHM, Breedveld FC, le Cessie S, et al. Effect of intensive exercise on patients with active rheumatoid arthritis: a randomised clinical trial. Ann Rheum Dis 2000;59:615–621.

133. Hsieh L, Detenko B, Schumacher H. Isokinetic and isometric testing of knee musculature in patients with rheumatoid arthritis with mild knee involvement. Arch Phys Med Rehabil 1987;68:294–297.

134. Danneskiold-Samsoe B, Grimby G. Isokinetic and isometric muscle strength in patients with rheumatoid arthritis. The relationship to clinical parameters and the influence of corticosteroid. Clin Rheumatol 1986;5:459–467.

135. van den Ende HJ, le Cessie S, Mulder W, et al. Comparison of high and low intensity training in well controlled rheumatoid arthritis. Results of a randomised trial. Ann Rheum Dis 1996;55:798–805.

136. Stenstrom C, Arge B, Sundbom A. Dynamic training versus relaxation training as home exercise for patients with inflammatory rheumatic diseases. A randomised controlled study. Scand J Rheumatol. 1996;25:28–33.

137. Hakkinen A, Sokka T, Lietsalmi AM, et al. Effects of dynamic strength training on physical function, Valpar work sample test, and working capacity in patients with early rheumatoid arthritis. Arthritis Rheum 2003;49:71–77.

138. Vuori I, Kannus P. Exercise for prevention of osteoporotic fracturres. In: An Y, ed.Orthopaedic Issues in Osteoporosis. Boca Raton, FL: CRC Press, 2003:543–555.

139. Hakkinen A, Malkia E, Hakkinen K, et al. Effects of detraining on neuromuscular function in patients with inflammatory arthritis. Br J Rheumatol 1997;36:1075–1081.

11

Osteoporosis

Kerri M. Winters-Stone and Christine M. Snow

The clinical condition of osteoporosis is characterized by bone loss that increases skeletal fragility and fracture risk. Of the 44 million Americans threatened by osteoporosis, approximately 10 million already have the disease, and another 34 million are at risk (1). Women are at particular risk for osteoporosis because of accelerated bone loss of 2.0 to 6.5% per year within the first 5 to 8 years after menopause. Thus, a postmenopausal woman may lose 20% of her skeletal mass in that time span (2–5). As medical awareness and early detection of osteoporosis progresses, more men are being diagnosed (6). While genetics accounts for most skeletal mass, lifestyle factors that include reproductive hormones, nutrition (namely calcium [Ca] and vitamin D), and activity, may account for 20 to 40% of a person's bone mass and thus influence the risk for osteoporosis (7).

There are approximately 1.5 million osteoporosis-related fractures each year in the United States that carry health costs over $13 billion (8). Most (>70%) fractures occur in persons over the age of 70 years. Most commonly, fractures occur at the forearm, spine, or hip. Hip fractures carry the most severe consequences with respect to morbidity and mortality. Currently, annual U.S. health care costs for hip fracture exceed $9 billion (9). Vertebral fractures are also costly and often result in chronic pain and deformity that can be debilitating. Low bone mass of the hip, spine, or forearm increases the risk

of fracture at these sites. It is estimated that each one standard deviation decrease in bone mass increases fracture risk by 10 to 15% (10). However, there is considerable overlap in bone mass among those who fracture and those who do not, suggesting that additional factors contribute (11,12). The classic osteoporotic fracture is one in which a frail skeleton cannot withstand the weight of the body or the application of normal forces during routine movements such as bending, twisting, or coughing. However, most hip fractures (>90%), over half of all spine fractures, and all forearm fractures are not caused by skeletal frailty alone but rather result from trauma associated with a fall. Among community-dwelling elderly, 30 to 50% over age 65 fall, and 25% of all falls result in serious injury, such as fracture (13,14). Thus, the combination of skeletal frailty and a propensity to fall greatly increases an individual's fracture risk profile. Physical risk factors for falls include reduced muscle mass, poor lower extremity strength and power, and instability (15).

Skeletal Physiology

To understand the mechanisms underlying osteoporosis, one must have a basic understanding of skeletal physiology at both the organizational and cellular levels. The skeleton serves several functions, but preservation of serum Ca and mechanical integrity primarily determine skeletal mass. Anatomically, the skeleton is organized into axial (skull, spine, ribs, and sternum) and appendicular (pelvis, clavicles, scapulae, and upper and lower limbs) divisions. The skeleton is further organized according to its composition and related architecture. The two types of skeletal tissue are cortical ("compact") and trabecular ("spongy") bone. The proportion of each tissue varies depending upon the skeletal region's mechanical and metabolic requirements. Cortical bone, predominant in the skull and shafts of long bones, consists of a central canal surrounded by concentric layers of mineralized collagen that create a dense, compact tissue suitably designed to withstand mechanical stresses. Trabecular bone, predominant in flat or cuboid bones and the ends of long bones, consists of an irregular latticelike network of mineralized plates called trabeculae and a plentiful blood supply. Compared with cortical bone, trabecular bone has a greater turnover rate, susceptibility to hormone-induced demineralization, and structural fragility. Sites with a higher proportion of trabecular bone (hip, spine, and wrist) are most susceptible to osteoporotic fracture.

At the cellular level, bone is a dynamic tissue, and its balance is coordinated by the relative activity of its three cell types: osteoclasts, osteoblasts, and osteocytes. *Osteoclasts* are bone-resorbing cells that secrete an acidic medium that solubilizes pockets of bone tissue, mobilizing Ca from the skeleton. *Osteoblasts* are bone-forming cells that deposit a collagenous matrix that is subsequently mineralized to form hard tissue. *Osteocytes* are former osteoblasts whose precise function is unknown but may play some role in cell-to-cell communication.

Bone is in constant turnover where osteoclastic resorption of old, weakened bone tissue is followed by osteoblastic formation of new, stronger material. In the mature skeleton, these processes are referred to as *remodeling* and, when uncoupled, cause net bone gain or loss. With age, resorption slightly exceeds formation, resulting in a 0.5 to 1.0% loss per year after age 30 (16), while certain conditions may accelerate (e.g., estrogen withdrawal) or inhibit (e.g., antiresorptive drugs) resorption (17) or stimulate bone formation (e.g., exercise; [18,19]). In the growing skeleton, *modeling* describes the

process whereby large gains in skeletal mass and development of bony macroarchitecture are made because of increased formation. As such, some have suggested that this is the optimal time to maximize skeletal health via lifestyle factors (20,21). However, since bone is a dynamic tissue throughout life, interventions aimed at fracture reduction may be useful at any life stage.

Effect of Osteoporosis on the Body and Exercise Capacity

Osteoporosis is referred to as the "silent disease" for its inconspicuous presentation in affected individuals. Bone loss is not painful and produces no noticeable symptoms. Often the first sign of disease is a fracture, though advances in detection now permit disease identification before a fracture occurs. Some vertebral fractures escape detection when mistaken for low-back pain. Osteoporotic fractures incur considerable morbidity (22). Bone pain is common in the weeks following fracture, and soft tissue trauma often causes additional discomfort for extended periods of time. Depending on the location and severity of the fracture, mobility can be significantly impaired, and function greatly reduced (23). Reduced mobility and function lead to loss of independence and possible depression (24). Fear of falls and fractures is common in older individuals, and the response to this fear is often reduced activity. In a survey of older women at risk for hip fracture, 80% stated that they would rather be dead than experience the loss of independence and quality of life that results from a serious hip fracture and subsequent nursing home admission (25). While osteoporosis develops quietly, awareness of disease risk and attention to modifiable risk factors can avoid the physical and emotional pain that results from fractures.

In the event of a fracture, pharmaceutical intervention to improve skeletal status is implicated, while lifestyle strategies directed toward reducing fall risk are important. If the fracture requires surgical repair, deconditioning will likely occur during hospitalization and recovery. Following surgery, physical therapy is necessary to restore basic mobility and should continue until relatively pain-free movement is achieved. Once mobile, a limited program of regular exercise can begin, which progresses according to the individual's tolerance and capabilities. This program should aim to restore cardiorespiratory capacity for general health and restore and improve musculoskeletal fitness for fall risk reduction.

Determinants of Fracture: Osteoporosis

The etiology of osteoporosis is complex and no single factor can be implicated as the sole determinant of disease development (Table 11-1). Uncontrollable factors that influence bone mass include genetics, gender, race, age, and secondary disease. A family history of osteoporosis, particularly with related fractures, is a significant risk factor (26). Women are at higher risk because of their smaller skeletal size and susceptibility to estrogen-related bone loss after menopause (27). Approximately 20% of osteoporosis cases are men; this percentage may increase as men live longer and awareness of disease risk in men increases. Osteoporosis is more prevalent among Caucasian and Asian women than African-American and Latino

women, while disease prevalence in other races has not been well described (28). Aging accounts for bone loss of 0.5 to 1.0% per year, beginning near the end of the third decade (29,30). Cumulatively, age-related declines may lead to losses of 15 to 30% of skeletal mass by age 60 and possibly 50% by age 80. Although osteoporosis is most often diagnosed after the age of 50, environmental influences on bone health and disease development begin in childhood and continue throughout adulthood.

Controllable factors that influence bone mass include reproductive hormone levels, dietary adequacy (namely, Ca and vitamin D), and physical activity. Near or at the onset of menopause and resultant estrogen decline, bone loss accelerates from the typical 0.5 to 1.0% up to 2.0 to 6.5% per year (3,4). Estrogen and/or hormone-replacement therapy (combination of estrogen and progesterone; HRT) halts this bone loss and may lead to 2 to 3% gains in bone mass in the first 3 to 5 years of treatment (18). However, some women opt against HRT because of breast cancer risk or concern over harmful side effects (31). For these women, alternative drug therapies may be implicated (i.e., bisphosphonates [Fosamax, Actonel], calcitonin [Miacalcin],

TABLE 11-1 SELECTED RISK FACTORS FOR OSTEOPOROSIS AND FALLS

Osteoporosis	Falls
Being female	Advanced age
Thin and/or small frame	Poor leg strength and/or power
Advanced age	Impaired balance and gait
Family history of osteoporosis	Reduced reaction time
Postmenopause, including early or surgically induced menopause	Poor or impaired vision
Abnormal absence of menstrual periods (amenorrhea)	Poor or impaired hearing
Anorexia nervosa	Postural hypotension
Diet low in calcium	Multiple medication use, medications that affect water balance
Use of certain medications, such as corticosteroids and anticonvulsants	Risky environment: inadequate lighting, uneven flooring, unsecured carpets/rugs, obstacles, tight turns in walking path
Low testosterone levels in men	Personal habits: improper/inappropriate footwear, outdated visual prescriptions, refusal to use assistive devices
Inactive lifestyle	
Cigarette smoking	
Excessive use of alcohol	
Being Caucasian or Asian; African Americans and Hispanic Americans are also at significant risk	

selective estrogen-receptor modulators [Evista]), particularly in those with diagnosed osteoporosis. An analogous role of testosterone in male osteoporosis is unclear. While some osteoporotic men also have low testosterone levels, low testosterone does not inevitably lead to osteoporosis. Evidence suggests that low circulating levels of estrogen in men are potent regulators of bone mass, and declining levels of estrogen in the male may lead to bone loss (32).

Ninety-nine percent of total body Ca is stored in the skeleton, with the remainder distributed among the blood and other peripheral tissues. Stable blood Ca levels are critical to normal physiologic functions, and daily losses of Ca via urine, feces, and sweat must be replaced through the diet. When Ca intake is chronically inadequate, bone mineral is lost, and skeletal integrity is compromised. Intestinal absorption of Ca in humans is poor and worsens with age and estrogen deprivation. To offset daily losses in older individuals (>60 years), intake should increase from the recommended adult intake of 800 to 1000 mg/day to 1200 mg/day and again to 1500 mg/day in women not taking HRT or those over 80 years (33). As maximal absorption is saturated at 500-mg doses, Ca intake achieved through supplementation should be spaced in 500-mg doses throughout the day (34).

Adequate vitamin D is necessary for efficient Ca absorption. While vitamin D is obtained from 10 to 15 min of daily UV exposure and from fortified cow's milk, individuals with lactose intolerance and housebound elderly are at risk for vitamin D deficiency and would benefit from a supplement. Additional nutrients that may influence skeletal health include protein, sodium, and vitamins C and K, but precise evidence on the role of each in osteoporosis development is still debatable. Adherence to a sensible diet and ingestion of a multivitamin supplement, if implicated, may minimize nutritionally related bone loss.

Bone is a dynamic tissue that adjusts its mass according to the stresses placed upon it. In general, inactive women have lower bone mass than their physically active counterparts (35,36). Space flight, immobilization, and bed rest studies report significant bone loss as a result of disuse and loss of weight-bearing mechanical forces on the bone (37). The optimal type and quantity of activity necessary to prevent or reverse declines is yet to be defined (19).

Determinants of Fracture: Falls

Increases in fall risk parallel age-related declines in bone mass. Falls may be attributable to unsafe environments, secondary effects of medical conditions, and/or physiologic decrements (Table 11-1). Hazardous environments are created by the presence of obstacles, narrow pathways with tight turns, uneven flooring, and/or inadequate lighting. Additionally, personal habits such as improper footwear, outdated visual prescriptions, and/or refusal to use assistive devices can lead to instability. Medical conditions or related treatment may impair stability. Dehydration, prescription medication, and neural impairment should be evaluated and corrected to reduce fall risk. Physiologic declines in the neuromuscular system lead to poor postural control and impaired ability to recover from a slip, trip, or stumble. Reduced muscle mass, poor lower-extremity strength and power, and postural instability are independently associated with increased fall risk and lower functional capacity for tasks such as lifting objects or performing household chores (38,39).

Declines in muscle mass are evident by the third decade and become more pronounced after age 60 (40). While these losses have been attributed in part to age-related declines in growth hormone secretion, reduced activity is also a likely contributor (41,42). Directly related to muscle loss are reductions in both strength and power (43). Declines in the force capacity of muscle are not only due to absolute loss of muscle mass, but particularly to the selective loss of fast-twitch (high-force and power-producing) fibers. As participation in activities requiring strength wanes with age, selective atrophy of fast-twitch fibers results in loss of strength and power (44). Loss of muscle strength contributes to instability, while loss of power impairs the ability to counteract a potential fall (45–47). Stability also worsens with age, and while strength declines may partially explain this change, instability is more likely determined by a complex set of inputs from visual, vestibular, and somatosensory systems (48,49). Inactivity accelerates age-related declines in muscle mass, strength, power, and stability, and these declines contribute to increased fall risk (39,50). Thus, along with creation of a safe living environment and minimization of stability-related side effects of medical conditions, physical activity aimed at improving neuromuscular function should lead to fall risk reduction.

Testing and Evaluation

Comprehensive fracture risk assessment should include evaluation of skeletal status and fall risk (Table 11-2). With technologic advances, several new patient-friendly methods of evaluating skeletal status have emerged. Fall risk assessment can range from sophisticated laboratory tests of neurologic capacity to relatively simple, inexpensive field tests that effectively discriminate "fallers" from "nonfallers." For purposes of this text, only the latter methods are discussed in detail.

Prior to performing any performance-based assessments, physician clearance should be obtained if implicated (51). In addition, a complete medical history, physical activity history (e.g., PAR-Q), and resting heart rate (HR) and blood pressure (BP) should be obtained. In those individuals with contraindications (i.e., HR and/or BP), testing should be postponed until proper clearance and/or appropriate medical supervision can be obtained. Proper warm-up including 5 to 10 min of light aerobic activity (e.g., stationary cycling, marching in place) is needed. Stretching should precede and follow maximal testing. If repeat measurements are performed after the initial evaluation, efforts should be made to maintain similar testing conditions. Selection of the appropriate testing method will depend on several factors, including patient acceptability, practicality, validity, reliability, and sensitivity to change.

SKELETAL STATUS

Dual Energy X-Ray Absorptiometry

The current gold standard to evaluate osteoporosis is measurement of bone mineral density (BMD; $g \cdot cm^{-1}$) via dual-energy x-ray absorptiometry (DXA). BMD is inversely related to bone

TABLE 11-2   EVALUATION OF SKELETAL STATUS AND FALL RISK

Skeletal Status	Fall Risk
Bone Mineral Density ($g \cdot cm^{-1}$)	Leg strength
Dual Energy X-Ray Absorptiometry (DXA), gold	One-repetition max (1-RM)
standard	Six-repetition max (6-RM)
BMD at fracture sites	Dynamometry (isokinetic or isometric)
WHO diagnostic criteria	Chair sit-to-stand
Peripheral DXA (pDXA): screening tool	Leg power
BMD at peripheral sites: calcaneus, wrist, finger	Wingate anaerobic power test
Peripheral BMD poor predictor of axial fractures	Leg extensor power
Bone quality	Vertical jump
Quantitative Ultrasound (QUS), screening tool	Timed stair ascent
Broadband attenuation (BUA) and velocity (SOS)	Balance
at peripheral site: calcaneus	Laboratory assessment
Comparable fracture prediction to central DXA	Static: single leg stance: eyes open/closed;
via T-scores, but poor reliability	tandem stance
Bone turnover	Dynamic: tandem walk: forward, backward
Serum or urine markers of formation or	Gait
resorption	Laboratory measures
Additional prediction of fracture risk along	Up-and-Go test
w/DXA	Medical evaluation: vision, hearing, blood pressure,
Formation: osteocalcin, bone specific alkaline	medication interaction
phosphatase	Environment evaluation: lighting, flooring, obstacles,
Resorption: pyrodinoline or deoxypyrodinoline	personal habits
cross-links, N-terminal telopeptide	

fragility and fracture risk (52). As site-specific BMD yields the best indication of fracture risk of a particular skeletal region, BMD should be measured at the hip and spine (10,53). While prediction of axial fractures from peripheral BMD is also strong, fracture risk is best assessed from BMD values at the site of interest (54,55). DXA precision error is quite low (Coefficient of variation <1.0–1.5%), making it an ideal tool to evaluate treatment efficacy and/or strategies designed to alter bone mass. Because of its high rate of turnover, the spine is a particularly sensitive region for monitoring responses (56).

Based on BMD measures, skeletal health is evaluated by comparing individual BMD values to those of both age-matched and young normal reference groups. Age-matched comparisons (Z-scores) describe the individual's BMD value in standard deviations (SD) from others of similar gender, age, and race/ethnicity. While a useful indicator of age-related skeletal status, low BMD typical of older age may indicate "average" for a woman's age, but high risk of disease. For example, an 80-year-old woman with a Z-score of "0," or 100% of age-matched levels, is osteoporotic based on diagnostic criteria. Therefore, Z-scores should not be used to diagnose disease, but only to assess age-expected BMD. In 1994, diagnostic criteria for osteoporosis were established by the World Health Organization and are based on young-normal comparisons (T-scores; 9). T-scores compare an individual's BMD reading in SDs from the average 30-year old of similar age, gender, and race/ethnicity. A T-score equal to or more than 2.5 SD below young-normal indicates osteoporosis; between 1 and 2.5 SD below young-normal indicates osteopenia (low bone mass); and less than 1 SD below young-normal indicates absence of disease. Established osteoporosis is defined as a diagnostic T-score and the presence and/or history of one or more osteoporotic fractures.

DXA-based assessment of osteoporosis is recommended for the following:

1. Postmenopausal women under age 65 with one or more additional risk factors
2. All women ≥65 years of age
3. Postmenopausal women with fractures (to confirm diagnosis and determine disease severity)
4. Women considering therapy for osteoporosis
5. Women on HRT for prolonged periods
6. Men with one or more of the following:

a. Prolonged exposure to certain medications (e.g., steroids for asthma or arthritis, anticonvulsants, certain cancer treatments, and aluminum-containing antacids)
b. Chronic disease of the kidneys, lungs, stomach, or intestines
c. Low levels of testosterone

In addition, pre- or perimenopausal women, particularly those with a family history of osteoporosis and/or >1 risk factor, may wish to have a DXA evaluation. However, insurance often does not cover the cost of DXA for premenopausal women even though early evaluation of BMD could offer the best strategy to prevent age-related decline in bone mass and to delay or offset the onset of osteoporosis.

A less sensitive and specific, yet convenient and increasingly popular DXA measurement in screening situations is peripheral DXA (pDXA), which is performed on the heel, wrist, or finger using a small portable device with conventional DXA technology that emits far less radiation than central DXA (57). While obviously popular for its ability to reach large segments of the population, epidemiologic data does not support the ability of pDXA-derived BMD measurements to effectively predict spine and hip fractures (10,53). Furthermore, changes in peripheral BMD in response to therapeutic treatment are relatively small. Thus, pDXA may not be sensitive enough to monitor or diagnose, but may be a useful screening tool (55).

Quantitative Ultrasound (QUS)

Another technique to evaluate the peripheral skeleton, QUS is gaining popularity due to its low cost, portability, lack of radiation exposure, and potential to assess bone quantity and quality (58). QUS is based on the principles of ultrasound, in which a sonographic pulse is transmitted across the heel. As the number and quality of trabeculae within the calcaneus increase, pulse attenuation increases proportionally. Bone integrity is measured by both broadband ultrasound attenuation and speed of sound; both measures are reduced in osteoporotic patients (59). Recent data suggests that the predictive value of QUS for hip fracture is comparable to that of central DXA. However, these studies are limited to predicting fracture in persons over 70 years, only evaluated hip fracture, and used earlier water-based systems (60,61). Other limitations of QUS include its inability to apply the same WHO diagnostic criteria using a peripheral measure and the poor reliability of day-to-day measures, prohibiting its use as a tool to monitor therapeutic or time-related bone changes (62). As with pDXA, QUS should be used only as a screening tool with recommendations for central DXA evaluation when appropriate.

Biomarkers of Bone Turnover

New evidence suggests that bone turnover, as evidenced by biomarkers of both bone formation and resorption, predicts fracture independent of BMD and may assess microarchitectural integrity of bone (8,63–67). It has been advanced that increased osteoclastic activity associated with high levels of bone turnover in postmenopausal women leads to perforations in trabeculae that may cause their ultimate destruction and/or distortion (68). Biomarkers of bone turnover are elevated in postmenopausal women not receiving HRT and decline in response to antiresorptive therapy (69,70). Biomarkers can be determined from serum or urinary specimens using commercial kits and are becoming more routinely available. The most common markers of bone formation found in serum are osteocalcin and bone-specific alkaline phosphatase, while markers of bone resorption include pyrodinoline or deoxypyrodinoline cross-links and N-telopeptide (urinary markers should be indexed by creatinine to adjust for variations in urine volume). Premenopausal norms are available for most biomarkers. Individuals with both low BMD and high levels of biomarkers of turnover (above premenopausal norms) should be considered at higher risk of fracture than those with either low BMD or high turnover alone (65). As early reductions in biomarkers successfully predict BMD increases in response to therapeutic agents and exercise (71,72), serial measurement of biomarkers may be a low-cost, convenient way to identify responders and nonresponders to intervention strategies.

EVALUATION OF FALL RISK

Falls often have a complex etiology. Thus, proper risk assessment should include the following: medical evaluation of vision, hearing, blood pressure and medication interaction; evaluation of potential hazards in the living environment; and laboratory or clinical evaluation of physical predictors of falls.

Lower-Extremity Strength

Several methods of evaluating muscle strength are available. In healthy individuals, maximal testing using free or machine weights is useful to assess strength and to prescribe exercise intensity for strength-training programs. The one-repetition maximum (1-RM) is the highest weight a muscle group can lift one time and can be safely performed in most adult populations, including the elderly (73). Individuals who are frail or osteoporotic, have cardiovascular risk factors, or are unaccustomed to exercise should avoid maximal testing. Strength evaluation to assess fall risk should focus on the lower extremity. Proper supervision, spotting, and use of machine-based equipment are important to minimize risk of injury. With those individuals for whom 1-RM testing is contraindicated, maximal strength can be estimated by measuring a six-repetition maximum (6-RM). 1-RM can then be estimated by extrapolation using gender-specific equations. Standardized protocols, conversion equations, and age-based norms for both 1-RM and 6-RM are available (74).

Maximal strength can also be measured via dynamometry. Isokinetic dynamometry is usually performed with an isokinetic testing device in a laboratory or clinic; they are not usually available in field settings and private medical offices. Isokinetic testing should be done at slower velocities ($30–60°\cdot\sec^{-1}$) to elicit peak strength; manufacture-based norms are usually available. Isometric strength can be evaluated by hand-held portable dynamometers that test strength in several movements (e.g., hip abduction, knee flexion/extension, ankle plantar/ dorsiflexion). Disadvantages of hand-held dynamometers include high muscle strength for testing staff (to resist patient motion) and modest reproducibility. Nevertheless, they can be useful in field settings, for general evaluation, and in frail populations.

Functional strength can be evaluated by two tests that are easily conducted in a variety of settings and are safe to administer to frail individuals (75). However, these tests may not be sensitive enough to evaluate strength in fitter adults. The timed chair stand measures the time required to rise from and return to a seated position five times. The chair stand measures the number of times an individual can rise from a seated position in 30 seconds; this test has been validated against isokinetic dynamometry. A standardized protocol and age-based norms for individuals 60 to 94 years old have been published (75).

Leg Power

Muscle power declines with age, and reductions indicate impaired function and recovery from slips, trips, or stumbles (46,47). The choice of how to measure leg power depends upon equipment, individual capacity, and testing goals. The Wingate Anaerobic Test (WAnT) measures maximal pedaling or arm-cranking speeds over 30 seconds against a constant force. Standardized or modified protocols and age- and gender-specific norms are available (76) . This test is a valid and reliable measure of power but may not be suitable for unfit, frail, or otherwise high-risk populations. A leg extensor dynamometer (Medical Research Faculty, Nottingham, UK) has been specifically designed to measure maximal leg power and is a valid and reliable measure that is suitable in fit or frail populations.

Simple field measures of power include the vertical jump and stair-ascent tests. Vertical jump is a commonly used test of leg power. Age-based norms are available, but because safety must be ensured, this may not be suitable for frail or unstable persons. The standardized stair-ascent test measures leg power by the time required to ascend six stairs taking three steps at a time. This test can be modified for older and/or frail populations by limiting the number of stairs to three, taken one step at a time. Handrails should be provided and appropriate supervision and safety precautions ensured to avoid injury.

Balance: Static and Dynamic

Balance is the ability to maintain the body's position over its base of support during quiet standing (static) or when in motion (dynamic). Reductions in static and dynamic balance are related to increased risk of falling (77,78), but static balance may indicate only fall risk for elderly who fall without warning rather than during activities of daily living. Laboratory measures of balance include postural sway, center of pressure excursion, Wolfson's postural stress test and Nashner's platform perturbation test (79–81).

Simple clinical measures of static balance include the one-legged stance (OLST) and Romberg tests. The OLST measures the time an individual can stand on one foot without putting the other foot (positioned half-way up the calf of the standing leg) on the floor. It is typically performed with eyes open and with eyes closed and is usually terminated after 30 seconds. The eyes-closed condition is more difficult, but the eyes-open condition is more age sensitive and reliable (82). The Romberg test, also known as tandem stance, measures static balance by having the subject stand in a heel-to-toe position with the dominant foot behind the nondominant foot with eyes open and eyes closed (83). Position maintenance time is recorded until the subject moves his/her feet, opens eyes on eyes-closed trials, or reaches the maximum of 60 seconds.

Tests of dynamic balance evaluate the ability to maintain one's center of gravity while moving over its base of support (e.g., reaching or ambulating). The Tinetti performance-oriented mobility assessment is a battery of simple tests that evaluate several aspects of dynamic balance and gait as a singular Mobility Index that is predictive of falls in the elderly (78). The tandem walk requires subjects to traverse a proscribed distance in a heel-to-toe fashion and discriminates between fallers and nonfallers (84). The Up-and-Go test may be useful to predict the ability to maneuver quickly and attend to tasks in a safe and timely manner. There are several versions of the test, and a length-modified version has age-based norms for persons 60 to 94 years old (75). The Functional Reach test measures the ability of older persons to maintain equilibrium while reaching for an object (85). Functional reach is defined as the maximal distance subjects can reach forward beyond their own arm's length while maintaining a fixed base of support in a standing position. All of these clinical measures are suitable for balance assessment in unfit or frail populations, but may not be sensitive enough to discriminate among younger and/or fitter individuals.

Gait

Normal gait is altered with age, resulting in wider and shorter strides, longer periods of double support, and slower speeds (86). Sophisticated laboratory gait measures use sensitive pressure transducers and video and digitizing equipment.

The gait-testing portion of the Tinetti Mobility Index, the Up-and-Go test, and walking velocity are all useful indicators of gait and mobility.

Exercise to Reduce Fracture Risk

Exercise presents a particularly attractive strategy to reduce fractures. In addition to its cost-effectiveness, only exercise has the potential to simultaneously reduce the risk of multiple chronic diseases (e.g., osteoporosis, cardiovascular disease, type 2 diabetes) and improve mental health (87). With respect to fractures, targeted exercise has the potential to improve or preserve skeletal health and to reduce fall risk. All training programs should follow the principle of progression and include proper warm-up and cool-down periods. A particular program should be tailored to the individual's personal interests, exercise capacity, physical weaknesses, and skeletal competence as judged by DXA. For example, a healthy nonosteoporotic, postmenopausal woman may engage in osteogenic and fall-reduction exercise at moderate-to-high intensity, whereas a frail osteoporotic woman should aim to maintain a level of physical function and reduce her risk of falls. Those unaccustomed to exercise should be supervised during the initial stages. Programs using high-intensity exercise or machine-based equipment require adequate supervision.

EXERCISE TO IMPROVE SKELETAL STATUS

Observations of bone loss in response to space flight, bed rest or immobilization highlight the importance of weight-bearing forces to maintain skeletal mass (37). It logically followed that increased weight bearing should stimulate osteogenesis. Over the past decade, several exercise interventions have studied the optimal mode, intensity, duration, and frequency of exercise necessary to positively affect bone. Unfortunately, the data are sparse compared with what is known for other physiologic systems. As well, the interventions are often too varied to adequately compare. However, general and conservative recommendations can be made (Table 11-3).

Traditional modes include weight-bearing (e.g., walking, jogging, stair stepping, aerobic dance), resistance, and impact (e.g., jumping) exercise. Skeletal responsiveness to exercise is age dependent and seems to be most effective at optimizing skeletal health and perhaps preventing osteoporosis when adopted during the growing years (20,21). After maturity, exercise-induced gains in bone mass are still positive but are attenuated (88–91). In later adulthood, preservation of mass is the most achievable response (73,92). The studies in this chapter are limited to those in adults over 50 years, the approximate age of menopause. Of those studies reviewed here, most were conducted in nonosteoporotic postmenopausal women; not all studies controlled for HRT status. Few studies included men, and in those that did, men responded as well as or slightly better than women (93,94). A recent meta-analysis reported a modest effect ($\sim +1.0\%$) of either strength or endurance exercise (aerobic and impact/stepping, but not walking) on hip and spine BMD in postmenopausal, nonosteoporotic women (19). HRT use slightly augmented exercise gains. Though seemingly small, a 1% increase maintained over time may translate into a significant reduction in fracture risk. This estimate is particularly true when a regular exercise program is initiated early and sustained for the lifetime.

Contrary to common medical recommendations, walking interventions exert only a modest preservative effect on spine BMD, even when weight is added in the form of a weighted belt (95,96). It is thought that the skeleton has already adjusted its mass to withstand forces produced by habitual walking. While walking may suffice for cardiorespiratory improvement, its failure to affect the musculoskeletal system prevents its recommendation to specifically reduce fracture risk. To stimulate osteogenesis, additional loads must exceed the daily strains experienced during usual activities. Hence, higher-intensity aerobic exercise, such as jogging or dancing (particularly when some form of stepping routine is included) preserves or slightly improves both hip and spine BMD (94,97,98). Thus, an appropriate exercise prescription is weight-bearing activity performed at 70 to 85% of maximal HR sustained for 30 to 45 min. Impact exercise alone (e.g., jumping) has yielded equivocal results in postmenopausal women (92,99,100) but may offer a quick and simple means to specifically preserve bone

TABLE 11-3 EXERCISE PRESCRIPTION FOR REDUCING FRACTURE RISK IN POPULATIONS OF VARYING SKELETAL STATUS[a]

Population	Goal	Mode	Intensity	Duration	Suggested exercises
Nonosteoporotic men and women	• ↑ or maintain spine and hip BMD	• Aerobic	• Initial: 60–70% HRmax • Target: 70–85% HRmax	• 15–60 min/session	• Weight-bearing aerobic + stepping (brisk walking/jogging, hiking, stair climbing)
		• Resistance	• Initial: 50–60% 1-RM • Target: 70–85% 1-RM	• 10–15 reps, 1–3 sets • 6–10 reps, 2–3 sets	• Free: squat, forward & side lunge, heel-toe raise, upright row, bicep curl, tricep ext., shoulder raise • Machine: leg press, hip/knee ext/flex, hip abd/add, trunk ext, bench press, military press, biceps curl, lat pull-down
	• ↓ Fall risk	• Impact	• Jumps performed from floor, height ~1–2"	• 10–15 reps, 3–5 sets	• Two-footed in place on firm surface
		• Resistance	• Same as above	• Same as above	• Same as above, except emphasize lower-body strength (including hip abductors); focus on exercises that emphasize functional movement (chair sit-to-stand, side lunge, heel/toe raise)
		• Balance	• N/A	• N/A	• Stand on one leg: eyes open/closed, tandem walk: forward/backward
Osteopenic men and women	• ↑ or maintain spine and hip BMD	• Aerobic	• Same as above	• Same as above	• Weight-bearing aerobic + stepping (brisk walking/jogging, hiking, stair climbing)
		• Resistance	• Same as above with slower progression	• Same as above	• Same as above but lifts that put undue pressure on the spine, such as lateral raises, are contraindicated. Avoid hyperflexion/extension and twisting movements
	• ↓ Fall risk	• Impact	• Jumps performed from floor, height ~1–2"	• 10–15 reps, 3–5 sets	• Two-footed in place on firm surface
		• Resistance + balance	• Same as above for fall risk	• Same as above for fall risk reduction	• Same as above for fall risk reduction. Avoid risky movements. Ensure safe exercise environment
Osteoporotic men and women	• ↓ Fall risk	• Resistance + balance	• Same as above; depending on functional capacity	• Same as above for fall risk reduction	• Same as above for fall risk reduction. Avoid risky movements. Ensure safe exercise environment.

Abbreviations: HR, heart rate; ext, extension; flex, flexion; lat, latissimus dorsi; abd, abduction; add, adduction.
[a]Recommended frequency of exercise is 2–3 days per week, although recently it was reported that resistance training 1–2 day per week produces similar neuromuscular gains to 3 days/week (107).

mass at the hip, particularly if added to an exercise program designed to reduce fall risk (92,100). Women who regularly engaged in resistance exercise plus 50 two-footed jumps from the ground maintained hip bone mass after five continuous years of exercise; this included women not on HRT and those with low BMD (92).

Resistance training has received considerable study drawing on the hypothesis that strong muscular contractions transmit high force to the bone, resulting in osteogenic adaptation. Unfortunately, resistance-training programs vary tremendously with respect to mode (machine vs. free-weight vs. resistive tubing), intensity, and duration; this variability precludes recommending any single program. However, programs of sufficient intensity have successfully preserved or slightly improved hip and spine BMD in nonosteoporotic, postmenopausal women (73,92,101,102). Free-weight and machine-based programs appear to be equally effective, but the most favorable results occur with sufficiently high loads. Intensities above 70% 1-RM (weight could also be set as $\leq$10 RM) most effectively preserve bone; under supervised conditions, this intensity is well tolerated and safe, even in older adults (73,103).

Exercise studies in women with low BMD are few. Two studies specifically targeting osteopenic women reported either preservation of spine BMD from walking plus stepping exercises (104) or increases in both hip (6%) and spine (2%) BMD from a similar regimen of higher intensity (105). While it could be concluded that the principle of initial values explains the large increase in BMD in the latter study, when HRT users and nonusers were separated, HRT users showed much greater gains. Thus, they may have artificially inflated the average increase of the small sample ($N = 16$). More importantly, both programs showed successful bone adaptation and skeletal tolerance in women with low BMD. Currently, there is no quantitative estimate of the upper-tolerance limit of exercise-induced loads to avoid fracture in osteoporotic women. However, practical and conservative recommendations suggest avoiding the following: high-impact exercise (e.g., jumping), spinal flexion against resistance (e.g., maintain straight back), high compressive forces on the spine (e.g., avoid overhead loads or high loads distal from the body's central axis), or exercises that produce quick trunk rotation (e.g., twisting movements such as golf).

EXERCISE TO REDUCE FALL RISK

Strategies to reduce fall risk are important because falls are a leading contributor to fractures and other injuries. Nonosteoporotic individuals can engage in osteogenic exercise but should also aim to reduce fall risk to reduce the risk of fracture. Osteoporotic or frail individuals, however, may not tolerate osteogenic exercise, but would benefit from programs aimed to reduce fall risk. While causes of falls are multifactorial and complex, modifying certain physical risk factors through exercise (including strength and power, stability/balance and gait) may feasibly reduce fall risk and fall incidence. Again, exercise intervention trials have varied greatly in mode, intensity, duration, and frequency of training, but general recommendations can be given (Table 11-3).

Because of the relationship between reduced muscle mass, strength, power, and impaired gait and balance, most exercise intervention programs include strengthening exercise with or without additional balance training. Strength-training programs are largely successful at increasing muscle mass and dramatically improving muscle strength in older populations (73,100,101,103,106,107). These studies also confirm that community-dwelling, otherwise healthy older adults can participate in a moderate-to- high-intensity resistance-training program with little risk of injury. As most hip fractures result from falls to the side (108), it is prudent to include lower-extremity strengthening exercises that target muscles involved in lateral movement. Using weighted vests as resistance, Shaw et al. (100) demonstrated 33% gains in hip abductor strength from a lower-body strength training program that included side stepping and side lunges.

Assuming proper progression during the initial stage of the exercise program, older adults should aim to perform two to three sets of 8 to 12 repetitions at an intensity of 70 to 85% of 1-RM (or weight that can be lifted 8–12 times to modest fatigue), similar to what is recommended to maintain bone mass (103). Machines or free weights can be used to target major muscle groups (hips, knees, ankles, shoulders, back, arms, trunk), although machines may be safer for weak persons or first-time exercisers. Though dramatic increases in strength (+174%) have been reported in nonagenarians engaged in high-intensity, supervised strength training (106), frail populations can also benefit from modest-intensity strengthening exercise of two to three sets of 10 to 12 repetitions using body weight, resistive tubing, or light (5–10 lb) ankle or wrist weights (109,110) that may be more amenable and feasible in this population. Modest strength training with balance training has reduced falls (109). Programs using weighted vests, resistive tubing, or small weights may improve adherence, as these exercises can be performed at home and are inexpensive. Furthermore, adherence may be encouraged by the recent report that resistance training 1 day/week produced comparable gains to the same program performed 3 days/week (107). Thus, older individuals should not be discouraged by the recommendation to strength train, as the training may be done at home, need not involve expensive or intimidating equipment, and requires only a modest time commitment.

Leg power may also be an important determinant of falls that can be modified via exercise. Power is the ability to develop force quickly and may partially determine the ability to recover from a slip, trip, or stumble (46,47). Power declines with age more rapidly than strength. While strength-training programs will usually increase power somewhat, optimal gains are achieved through specific emphasis on explosive movements. Plyometric exercise (jumping and bounding type movements) are traditionally used by athletes to improve power but are not recommended for older adults. However, simple vertical jumping has also improved power (88,91), even in older adults (100). Thus, in nonosteoporotic individuals, a simple jumping program may be added to a strength-training regimen to target both hip BMD and leg power. Jumping should be added only after 4 to 6 months of consistent training for lower-extremity strength and power.

Balance improvement should also be an aim of fall risk reduction strategies. While sophisticated laboratory-based balance-training programs show improvements in static and dynamic balance and reductions in sway (111,112), these programs are often not accessible to the broader population. Because lower-limb strength has been correlated with static and dynamic balance, strength-training programs should produce some improvements in balance (100,107). In conjunction with general strengthening exercise, specific balance exercises (e.g., single-leg stance with eyes open or closed, tandem walking forward or backward, and negotiating nonlinear pathways with turns) have been shown to reduce falls (109,110). These strength and balance programs also improved gait and reaction time.

In summary, exercise can reduce fracture risk by preserving or slightly improving BMD and reducing risk factors associated with falls. Few exercise programs described above used a singular mode of exercise, but rather used multimode exercise designed to target several risk factors for fracture in a comprehensive program. Several programs were also home based or could be adapted for home use. Based on these successful programs, exercise prescription and programing are offered (Table 11-3). Comprehensive, practical training programs offer a sensible strategy for reaching a large segment of the population by effectively lowering their risk of fracture.

EFFECT OF TRAINING ON OSTEOPOROSIS AND FRACTURES

Unfortunately, no exercise intervention to date has answered the question of whether exercise effectively reduces fractures. However, because exercise can preserve skeletal mass and reduce falls, one may assume that exercise effectively reduces fracture risk. It is clear, though, that habitual participation in exercise is central to retaining musculoskeletal benefits of exercise and to reduce the risk of fracture. Improvements in BMD and fall risk factors reverse when training is withdrawn and often in half the time spent training (91,97). This reversibility underscores the importance of creating effective, efficient, and enjoyable programs that meet the physiologic, financial, and practical needs of the individual.

Summary

- Fractures in later life are commonly attributed to osteoporosis and falls.
- While certain contributors to both osteoporosis and falls cannot be changed, several can be

addressed such as reproductive hormones, poor nutrition, and inactivity.

- Exercise can favorably alter both bone mass and fall risk in older adults.
- Evaluation of fracture risk should include assessment of *both* skeletal status (preferably DXA) and fall risk (leg strength, balance, and gait).
- Comprehensive exercise programs aimed at reducing fracture risk should include a strength and balance training component. Older and frail individuals can safely participate in light- to moderate-intensity strength training.
- Specifics of the program (mode, intensity, duration) will depend upon several factors including the individual's age, fitness, bone health, physical limitations, and health-related goals.
- Regular exercise participation must continue to maintain benefits that reduce fracture risk.

REFERENCES

1. National Osteoporosis Foundation Report. America's Bone Health: The State of Osteoporosis and Low Bone Mass. Washington, DC: 2002.
2. Dalen N, Olsson KE. Bone mineral content and physical activity. Acta Orthop Scand 1974;45:170–174.
3. Gallagher JC, Goldgar D, Moy D. Total bone calcium in normal women: effect of age and menopause status. J Bone Miner Res 1987;2:491–496.
4. Krolner B, Nielsen S. Bone mineral content of the lumbar spine in normal and osteoporotic women: cross-sectional and longitudinal studies. Clin Sci 1982;62:329–336.
5. Nilas L, Gotfredsen A, Hadberg A, et al. Age-related bone loss in women evaluated by the single and dual photon technique. Bone Miner 1988;4:95–103.
6. Orwoll ES. Osteoporosis in men. Endocrinol Metab Clin North Am 1998;27:349–367.
7. Pocock NA, Eisman JA, Hopper JL, et al. Genetic determinants of bone mass in adults. A twin study. J Clin Invest 1987;80:706–710.
8. Melton LJ, Thamer M, Ray NF, et al. Fractures attributable to osteoporosis: report from the National Osteoporosis Foundation. J Bone Miner Res 1997;12:16–23.
9. World Health Organization. Assessment of fracture risk and its application to screening for osteoporosis. WHO technical report series 843. Geneva: WHO, 1994.
10. Cummings SR, Black DM, Nevitt MC. Bone density at various sites for prediction of hip fractures. Lancet 1993;341:72–75.
11. Cummings SR, Nevitt MC. A hypothesis: the causes of hip fractures. J Gerontol 1989;44:M107–111.
12. Kanis JA. Diagnosis of osteoporosis and assessment of fracture risk. Lancet 2002;359:1929–1936.
13. Blake AJ, Morgan K, Bendall MJ, et al. Falls by elderly people at home: prevalence and associated factors. Age Ageing 1988;17:365–372.
14. O'Loughlin JL, Robitaille Y, Boivin JF, et al. Incidence of and risk factors for falls and injurious falls among the community-dwelling elderly. Am J Epidemiol 1993;137:342–354.
15. Greenspan SL, Meyers ER, Maitland LA, et al. Fall severity and bone mineral density as risk factors for hip fracture in ambulatory elderly. JAMA 1994;271:128–133.
16. Hui SL, Zhou L, Evans R, et al. Rates of growth and loss of bone mineral in the spine and femoral neck in white females. Osteoporos Int 1999;9:200–205.
17. Riggs BL. Endocrine causes of age-related bone loss and osteoporosis. Novartis Found Symp 2002;242:247–259.
18. Cummings SR, Karpf DB, Harris F, et al. Improvement in spine bone density and reduction in risk of vertebral fractures during treatment with antiresorptive drugs. Am J Med 2002;112:281–289.
19. Wolff I, van Croonenborg JJ, Kemper HC, et al. The effect of exercise training programs on bone mass: a meta-analysis of published controlled trials in pre- and postmenopausal women. Osteoporosis Int 1999;9:1–12.
20. Fuchs RK, Bauer JJ, Snow CM. Jumping improves hip and lumbar spine bone mass in prepubescent children: a randomized controlled trial. J Bone Miner Res 2001;16:148–156.
21. McKay HA, Petit MA, Schutz RW, et al. Augmented trochanteric bone mineral density after modified physical education classes: a randomized school-based exercise intervention study in prepubescent and early pubescent children. J Pediatr 2000;136:156–162.
22. Chrischelles E, Butler CD, Davis CS, Wallace RB. A model of lifetime osteoporosis impact. Arch Intern Med 1991;151:2026–2032.
23. Miller W. Survival and ambulation following hip fracture. J Bone Joint Surg 1978;60A:930–934.
24. Gignac MA, Cott C, Badley EM. Adaptation to chronic illness and disability and its relationship to perceptions of independence and dependence. J Gerontol B Psychol Sci Soc Sci 2000;55:P362–372.
25. Salkeld G, Cameron ID, Cumming RG, et al. Quality of life related to fear of falling and hip

fracture in older women: a time trade off study. BMJ 2000;320:341–346.

26. Keen RW, Hart DJ, Arden NK, et al. Family history of appendicular fracture and risk of osteoporosis: a population-based study. Osteoporosis 1999;10:161–166.

27. Arendt EA. Gender differences in musculoskeletal health. J Gend Specif Med 2000;3:58–64.

28. Pollitzer WS, Anderson JJ. Ethnic and genetic differences in bone mass: a review with a hereditary vs environmental perspective. Am J Clin Nutr 1989;50:1244–1259.

29. Geusens P, Dequeker A, Verstraeten A, et al. Age-, sex-, and menopause-related changes of vertebral and peripheral bone population study using dual and single photon absorptiometry and radiogrammetry. J Nucl Med 1986;27:1540–1549.

30. Riggs BL, Wahner HW, Melton LJ, et al. Rates of bone loss in appendicular and axial skeletons of women: evidence of substantial vertebral bone loss before menopause. J Clin Invest 1986;77:1487–1491.

31. Writing Group for the Women's Health Initiative Investigators. Risks and benefits of estrogen plus progestin in healthy postmenopausal women: principal results from the Women's Health Initiative randomized controlled trial. JAMA 2002;288:321–333.

32. Khosla S, Melton LJ 3rd, Riggs BL. Clinical review 144: estrogen and the male skeleton. J Clin Endocrinol Metab 2002;87:1443–1450.

33. National Institutes of Health Consensus Conference, Optimal calcium intake. JAMA 1994;272:1942–1948.

34. Heaney RP. Calcium in the prevention and treatment of osteoporosis. J Intern Med 1992;231:169–180.

35. Fehling PC, Alekel L, Clasey J, et al. A comparison of bone mineral densities among female athletes in impact loading and active loading sports. Bone 1995;17:205–210.

36. Robinson TL, Snow-Harter C, Taaffe DR, et al. Gymnasts exhibit higher bone mass than runners despite similar prevalence of amenorrhea and oligomenorrhea. J Bone Miner Res 1995;10:26–35.

37. Baldwin KM, White TP, Arnaud SB, et al. Musculoskeletal adaptations to weightlessness and development of effective countermeasures. Med Sci Sports Exerc 1996;28:1247–1253.

38. Drinkwater BL, Grimston SK, Raab-Cullen DM, et al. ACSM position stand on osteoporosis and exercise. Med Sci Sports Exerc 1995;27:i–vii.

39. Myers AH, Young Y, Langlois JA. Prevention of falls in the elderly. Bone 1996;18:87–102S.

40. Poehlman ET, Toth MJ, Gardner AW. Changes in energy balance and body composition at menopause: a controlled longitudinal study. Ann Intern Med 1995;123:673–675.

41. Carter WJ. Effect of anabolic hormones and insulin-like growth factor-I on muscle mass and strength in elderly persons. Clin Geriatr Med 1995;11:735–748.

42. Horber FF, Kohler SA, Lippuner K, et al. Effect of regular physical training on age-associated alteration of body composition in men. Eur J Clin Invest 1996;26:279–285.

43. Larsson L. Histochemical characteristics of human skeletal muscle during aging. Acta Physiol Scand 1983;117:469–471.

44. Larsson L, Grimby G, Karlsson J. Muscle strength and speed of movement in relation to age and muscle morphology. J Appl Physiol 1979;46:451–456.

45. Lord SR, Clark RD, Webster IW. Postural stability and associated physiological factors in a population of aged persons. J Gerontol 1991;46:M69–76.

46. Maki BE. Gait changes in older adults: predictors of falls or indicators of fear. J Am Geriatr Soc 1997;45:313–320.

47. Skelton DA, Kennedy J, Rutherford OM. Explosive power and asymmetry in leg muscle function in frequent fallers and non-fallers aged over 65. Age Ageing 2002;31:119–125.

48. Balogun JA, Akindele KA, Nihinlola JO, et al. Age-related changes in balance performance. Disabil Rehabil 1994;16:58–62.

49. Tinetti ME, Doucette J, Claus E, et al. Risk factors for serious injury during falls by older persons in the community. J Am Geriatr Soc 1995;43:1214–1221.

50. Fiatarone MA, Evans WJ. The etiology and reversibility of muscle dysfunction in the aged. J Gerontol 1993;48(spec no.):77–83.

51. American College of Sports Medicine. Guidelines for Exercise Testing and Prescription. 6th ed. Philadelphia: Lippincott Williams & Wilkins, 2000.

52. Bouxsein ML, Courtney AC, Hayes WC. Ultrasound and densitometry of the calcaneus correlate with the failure loads of cadaveric femurs. Calcif Tissue Int 1995;56:99–103.

53. Marshall D, Johnell O, Wedel H. Meta-analysis of how well measures of bone mineral density predict occurrence of osteoporotic fractures. BMJ 1996;312:1254–1259.

54. Eckstein F, Lochmuller EM, Lill CA, et al. Bone strength at clinically relevant sites displays substantial heterogeneity and is best predicted from site-specific bone densitometry. J Bone Miner Res 2002;17:162–171.

55. Faulkner KG. Bone densitometry: choosing the proper skeletal site to measure. J Clin Densitom 1998;1:279–285.

56. Eastell R. Treatment of postmenopausal osteoporosis. N Engl J Med 1998;338:736–746.

57. Patell R, Blake GM, Fogelman I. Radiation dose to the patient and operator from a peripheral dual x-ray absorptiometry system. J Clin Densitom 1999;2:397–401.

58. Njeh CF, Boivin CM, Langton CM. The role of ultrasound in the assessment of osteoporosis: a review. Osteoporos Int 1997;7:7–22.

59. Nairus J, Ahmadi S, Baker S, et al. Quantitative ultrasound: an indicator of osteoporosis in perimenopausal women. J Clin Densitom 2000;3:141–147.

60. Hans D, Dargent-Molina P, Schott AM, et al. Ultrasound measurements for the prediction of osteoporotic fractures in elderly women: the EPIDOS prospective study. Lancet 1996;348:511–514.

61. Pluijm SMF, Graafmans WC, Bouter LM, et al. Ultrasound measurements for the prediction of osteoporotic fractures in elderly people. Osteoporosis Int 1999;9:550–556.

62. Gluer C-C. Quantitative ultrasound techniques for the assessment of osteoporosis—expert agreement on current status. J Bone Miner Res 1997;12:1280–1288.

63. Garnero P, Hausherr E, Chapuy MC, et al. Markers of bone resorption predict hip fracture in elderly women: The EPIDOS prospective study. J Bone Miner Metab 1996;11:1531–1538.

64. Garnero P, Dargent-Molina P, Hans D, et al. Do markers of bone resorption add to bone mineral density and ultrasonographic heel measurement for the prediction of hip fracture in elderly women? The EPIDOS prospective study. Osteoporosis Int 1998;8:563–569.

65. Riggs BL, Melton LJ, O'Fallon WM. Drug therapy for vertebral fractures in osteoporosis: evidence that decreases in bone turnover and increases in bone mass both determine antifracture efficacy. Bone 1996;18:197S–201S.

66. Riggs BL, Melton LJ 3rd. Bone turnover matters: the raloxifene treatment paradox of dramatic decreases in vertebral fractures without commensurate increases in bone density. J Bone Miner Res 2002;17:11–14.

67. Saakar S, Mitlak BH, Wong M, et al. Relationships between bone mineral density and incident vertebral fracture risk with raloxifene therapy. J Bone Miner Res 2002;17:1–10.

68. Parfitt AM, Mathews CH, Villanueva AR, et al. Relationships between surface, volume, and thickness of iliac trabecular bone in aging and in osteoporosis. Implications for the microanatomic and cellular mechanisms of bone loss. J Clin Invest 1983;72:1396–1409.

69. Chesnut CH 3rd, McClung MR, Ensrud KE, et al. Alendronate treatment of the postmenopausal osteoporotic woman: effect of multiple dosages on bone mass and bone remodeling. Am J Med 1995;99:144–152.

70. Hamwi A, Ganem AH, Grebe C, et al. Markers of bone turnover in postmenopausal women receiving hormone replacement therapy. Clin Chem Lab Med 2001;39:414–417.

71. Ravn P, Hosking D, Thompson D, et al. Monitoring of alendronate treatment and prediction of effect on bone mass by biochemical markers in the early postmenopausal intervention cohort study. J Clin Endocrinol Metab 1999;84:2363–2368.

72. Winters KM, Lougheed CY, Snow CM. Reductions in bone turnover predict exercise-induced increases in bone mineral density in mature premenopausal women. J Bone Miner Res 2001;16(suppl 1):S411.

73. Nelson ME, Fiatarone MA, Morganti CM, et al. Effects of high-intensity strength training on multiple risk factors for osteoporotic fractures. A randomized controlled trial. JAMA 1994;272:1909–1914.

74. Heyward, V. Advanced Fitness Assessment and Exercise Prescription. 4th ed. Champaign, IL: Human Kinetics, 2002.

75. Rikli RE, Jones CJ. Senior Fitness Test Manual. Champaign, IL: Human Kinetics, 2000.

76. Inbar O, Bar-Or O, Skinner JS. The Wingate Anaerobic Test. Champaign, IL: Human Kinetics, 1996.

77. Overstall PW, Exton-Smith AN, Imms FJ, et al. Falls in the elderly related to postural imbalance. BMJ 1977;1:261–264.

78. Tinetti ME. Performance-oriented assessment of mobility problems, I. Elderly patients. J Am Geriatrics Soc 1986;34:119–126.

79. Wolfson L, Whipple R, Amerman P, et al. Stressing the postural response: a quantitative method for teaching balance. J Am Geriatr Soc 1986;34:845–850.

80. Murray MP, Seireg AA, Sepic SB. Normal postural stability and steadiness: quantitative assessment. J Bone Joint Surg 1975;57A:510–516.

81. Nashner LM. Adapting reflexes controlling the human posture. Exp Brain Res 1976;26:59–72.

82. Stones MJ, Kozma A. Balance and age in the sighted and blind. Arch Phys Med Rehabil 1987;66:85–89.

83. Graybiel A, Frgly AR. A new quantitative ataxia test battery. Acta Otolaryngol 1966;61:292–312.

84. Dargent-Molina P, Favier F, Grandjean H, et al. Fall-related factors and risk of hip fracture: the EPIDOS prospective study. Lancet 1996;348:145–149.

85. Duncan PW, Weiner DK, Chandler J, et al. Functional reach: a new clinical measure of balance. J Gerontol Med Sci 1990;45:M192–M197.

86. Wolfson L, Whipple R, Amerman P, et al. Gait assessment in the elderly: a gait abnormality rating scale and its relation to falls. J Gerontol 1990;45: M12–19.

87. American College of Sports Medicine. Position stand: exercise and physical activity for older adults. Med Sci Sports Exerc 1998;30:992–1008.

88. Heinonen A, Kannus P, Sievanen H, et al. Randomised controlled trial of effect of high-impact exercise on selected risk factors for osteoporotic fractures. Lancet 1996;348:1343–1347.

89. Lohman T, Going S, Pamenter R, et al. Effects of resistance training on regional and total bone mineral density in premenopausal women: a randomized prospective study. J Bone Miner Res 1995;10:1015–1024.

90. Snow-Harter C, Bouxsein ML, Lewis BT, et al. Effects of resistance and endurance exercise on bone mineral status of young women: a randomized exercise intervention trial. J Bone Miner Res 1992;7:761–769.

91. Winters KM, Snow CM. Detraining reverses positive effects of exercise on the musculoskeletal system in premenopausal women. J Bone Miner Res 2000;15:2495–2503.

92. Snow CM, Shaw JM, Winters KM, et al. Long-term exercise using weighted vests prevents hip bone loss in postmenopausal women. J Gerontol A Biol Sci Med Sci 2000;55:M489–491.

93. Maddalozzo GF, Snow CM. High intensity resistance training: effects on bone in older men and women. Calcif Tissue Int 2000;66:399–404.

94. Welsh L, Rutherford OM. Hip bone mineral density is improved by high-impact aerobic exercise in postmenopausal women and men over 50 years. Eur J Appl Physiol Occup Physiol 1996;74:511–517.

95. Brooke-Wavell K, Jones PR, Hardman AE, et al. Commencing, continuing and stopping brisk walking: effects on bone mineral density, quantitative ultrasound of bone and markers of bone metabolism in postmenopausal women. Osteoporosis Int 2001;12:581–587.

96. Nelson ME, Fisher EC, Dilmanian FA, et al. A 1-y walking program and increased dietary calcium in postmenopausal women: effects on bone. Am J Clin Nutr 1991;53:1304–1311.

97. Dalsky G, Stocke KS, Ehsani AA. Weight-bearing exercise training and lumbar bone mineral content in postmenopausal women. Ann Intern Med 1988;108:824–828.

98. Kohrt WM, Ehsani AA, Birge SJ. Effects of exercise involving predominantly either joint-reaction or ground-reaction forces on bone mineral density in older women. J Bone Miner Res 1997;12:1253–1261.

99. Bassey EJ, Rothwell MC, Littlewood JJ, et al. Pre- and postmenopausal women have different bone mineral density responses to the same high-impact exercise. J Bone Miner Res 1998;13:1805–1813.

100. Shaw JM, Snow CM. Weighted vest exercise improves indices of fall risk in older women. J Gerontol A Biol Sci Med Sci 1998;53:M53–58.

101. Kerr D, Morton A, Dick I, et al. Exercise effects on bone mass in postmenopausal women are site-specific and load-dependent. J Bone Miner Res 1996;11:218–225.

102. Pruitt LA, Taaffe DR, Marcus R. Effects of a one-year high-intensity versus low-intensity resistance training program on bone mineral density in older women. J Bone Miner Res 1995;10:1788–1795.

103. Evans WJ. Exercise training guidelines for the elderly. Med Sci Sports Exerc 1999;31:12–17.

104. Kronhed AC, Moller M. Effects of physical exercise on bone mass, balance skill and aerobic capacity in women and men with low bone mineral density, after one year of training—a prospective study. Scand J Med Sci Sports 1998;8(5 Pt 1):290–298.

105. Chien MY, Wu YT, Hsu AT, et al. Efficacy of a 24-week aerobic exercise program for osteopenic postmenopausal women. Calcif Tissue Int 2000;67:443–448.

106. Fiatarone MA, Marks EC, Ryan ND, et al. High-intensity strength training in nonagenarians. Effects on skeletal muscle. JAMA 1990;263:3029–3034.

107. Taaffe DR, Duret C, Wheeler S, et al. Once-weekly resistance exercise improves muscle strength and neuromuscular performance in older adults. J Am Geriatr Soc 1999;47:1208–1214.

108. Greenspan SL, Myers ER, Kiel DP, et al. Fall direction, bone mineral density, and function: risk factors for hip fracture in frail nursing home elderly. Am J Med 1998;104:539–545.

109. Campbell AJ, Robertson MC, Gardner MM, et al. Randomised controlled trial of a general practice programme of home based exercise to prevent falls in elderly women. BMJ 1997;315:1065–1069.

110. Lord SR, Ward JA, Williams P, et al. The effect of a 12-month exercise trial on balance, strength, and falls in older women: a randomized controlled trial. J Am Geriatr Soc 1995;43:1198–1206.

111. Kollmitzer J, Ebenbichler GR, Sabo A, et al. Effects of back extensor strength training versus balance

training on postural control. Med Sci Sports Exerc 2000;32:1770–1776.

112. Wolf SL, Barnhart HX, Ellison GL, et al. The effect of tai chi Quan and computerized balance training on postural stability in older subjects. Atlanta FICSIT Group. Frailty and injuries: cooperative studies on intervention techniques. Phys Ther 1997;77:371–381 (discussion 382–384).

RELATED WEB SITES

American Society for Bone and Mineral Research
www.asbmr.org
Professional society of academic and clinical experts promoting both research and practice guidelines in the field of osteoporosis and other bone diseases.

Better Bones and Balance
www.bonesandbalance.com
A commercial Web site with patient information about exercise to reduce fracture risk, and home video and exercise equipment for purchase.

Bone Key Osteovision
www.bonekey-ibms.org
This site serves as a central repository of knowledge in the field of bone, cartilage, and mineral metabolism for clinicians and researchers.

International Osteoporosis Foundation
www.osteofound.org
An international organization for research and health professionals with interest in osteoporosis.

National Osteoporosis Foundation
www.nof.org
Both public and professional organization providing information, materials and public advocacy.

National Institutes of Health Osteoporosis and Related Diseases Resource Center
www.osteo.org
Comprehensive resource center for both the public and medical professionals interested in osteoporosis and related bone diseases.

National Institute of Aging
www.nia.nih.gov
Branch of the NIH specifically devoted to aging research; also provides health information and materials including the free "Exercise: A Guide from the NIA" that gives step-by-step instructions for strength training in older adults.

12

Chronic Pain States

Angela K. Lyden, Kirsten Ambrose, and Daniel J. Clauw

Chronic pain and fatigue are common somatic symptoms. Approximately 30% of the U.S. population suffers from chronic pain (1), and about 15% report chronic fatigue (2). In most cases, there is no "organic" cause that can be identified to account for these symptoms (3).

Chronic Multisymptom Illnesses

Population-based studies show that although pain, fatigue, or memory or mood disturbances can occur in isolation in individuals, they commonly cluster, such that individuals who have chronic pain are more likely to have comorbid fatigue or other somatic symptoms. This clustering of symptoms gives rise to syndromes such as fibromyalgia (FM), chronic fatigue syndrome (CFS), and irritable bowel syndrome (IBS) (4,5). The term *chronic multisymptom illnesses* (CMI) has been used to describe this overlapping constellation of symptoms and syndromes (Fig. 12-1) (6,7).

Although the terms used to describe CMI are relatively new, the conditions are not. For centuries, medical literature has included symptom complexes nearly identical to those now labeled FM and CFS (8). Many terms previously used to

describe these conditions (e.g., myofibrositis or fibrositis, or chronic Epstein-Barr virus) were attempts to link the symptom complex to an underlying pathophysiologic process. The more generic terms used today recognize that we know what does *not* cause these illnesses. For example, it is fairly certain that there is no "-*itis*" (i.e., inflammation) of the muscles in FM, and that CFS is not caused by an infection (9,10).

While criteria exist for FM (11) and CFS (12), they are not necessarily intended for clinical use to diagnose individual patients. Many persons who are diagnosed with FM or CFS may not fulfill the classification criteria. For example, while the FM criteria reflect only those individuals who report constant and widespread pain, the symptoms that define these illnesses fall along a continuum: some individuals rarely experience pain, others experience pain intermittently, and yet others experience pain continuously enough to meet established criteria. The same holds true for CFS, in that many more individuals meet criteria for chronic idiopathic fatigue than for CFS. Research suggests these subsyndromal patients share the same seminal features as those with FM/CFS without meeting the classification criteria. Although this chapter focuses on the data collected in individuals at one end of this continuum (i.e., those who have symptoms at a frequency or severity to meet criteria for FM or CFS),

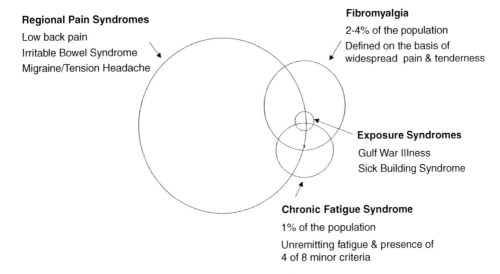

Regional Pain Syndromes

Low back pain
Irritable Bowel Syndrome
Migraine/Tension Headache

Fibromyalgia

2-4% of the population
Defined on the basis of
widespread pain & tenderness

Exposure Syndromes

Gulf War Illness
Sick Building Syndrome

Chronic Fatigue Syndrome

1% of the population

Unremitting fatigue & presence of
4 of 8 minor criteria

FIGURE 12-1 Relationships between chronic multisymptom illnesses.

many persons experience less severe symptomatology and may respond to similar treatments. Of note, FM is often used as an example because of the larger knowledge base. However, statements in this chapter apply to all patients with CMI, regardless of their cardinal symptom (i.e., pain or fatigue).

SYMPTOM DEVELOPMENT

Much has been learned about the neurobiologic mechanisms that may underlie symptom expression in CMI (Fig. 12-2). As with many illnesses, CMI may occur when a person who is genetically predisposed comes in contact with certain environmental exposures that could trigger the development of symptoms. Many environmental exposures that are generally accepted triggers of CMI fall under the category of "stressors," including physical trauma (especially to the axial skeleton), infections, and emotional distress (13,14). For each of these, studies show that in a small subset of individuals exposed to that particular stressor, symptoms can continue well after cessation of the original exposure, leading to chronic illness. Although studies of *groups* suggest that many stressors are capable of triggering the development of these illnesses, there are no concrete data establishing a linear relationship between the "triggering event" and the sustained presence of symptoms in an individual.

Symptom Maintenance: Peripheral Mechanisms

The precise mechanisms responsible for continued symptom expression beyond the initial stressor are unknown but are complex and multifactored (5,14). Considering that most CMI patients report "muscle pain," much of the early research focused on the most obvious: neuromuscular deficiencies and adaptations. Bennett et al. (15) described reduced aerobic exercise tolerance and lower muscle blood flow in FM patients than in sedentary and exercising controls, but did not find any correlation with either exercise performance or reported symptoms. Mengshoel et al. (16) found that FM patients had reduced muscle strength and a relative inability to perform dynamic and static muscle endurance activities. This was secondary to pain and fatigue, induced or exacerbated by exercise. In healthy individuals, the increased metabolic demands of working muscles suffer because of impaired microcirculation and depletion of energy compounds in the muscle. Mengshoel et al. (16) argued that these changes were similarly seen in FM subjects but that they occurred at an earlier stage, thus inhibiting

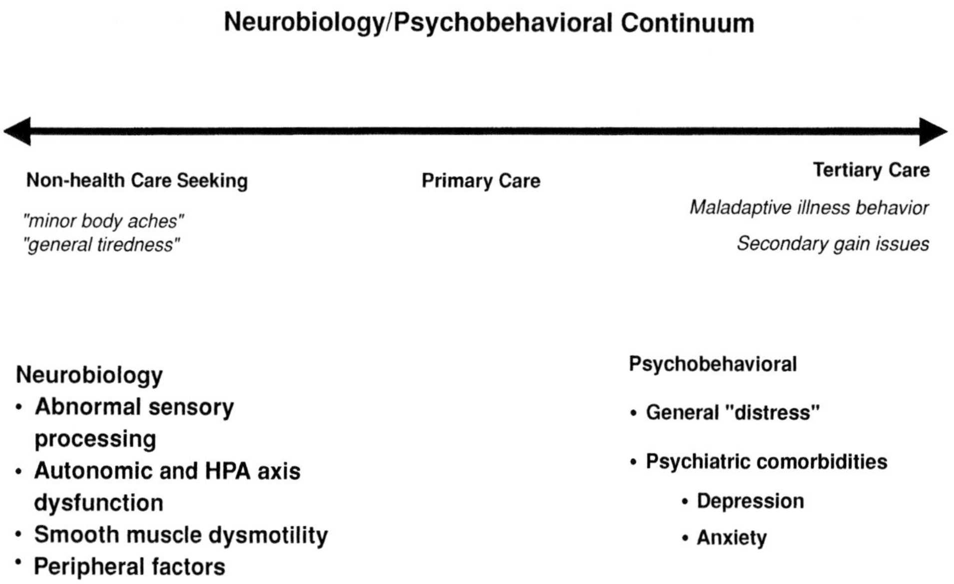

Neurobiology/Psychobehavioral Continuum

Non-health Care Seeking

"minor body aches"
"general tiredness"

Primary Care

Tertiary Care

Maladaptive illness behavior
Secondary gain issues

Neurobiology
- **Abnormal sensory processing**
- **Autonomic and HPA axis dysfunction**
- **Smooth muscle dysmotility**
- **Peripheral factors**

Psychobehavioral
- **General "distress"**
- **Psychiatric comorbidities**
  - **Depression**
  - **Anxiety**

FIGURE 12-2 Neurobiology/psychobehavioral continuum.

their ability to exercise. Borman et al. (17) also found reduced muscle strength and endurance in FM patients and attributed this reduced work capacity to generalized deconditioning and fatigue rather than pain. Poor effort by patients was yet another explanation for reduced work capacity (18).

Later studies, however, determined that muscle energy metabolism was no different in FM patients than in healthy controls (20). Hakkinen et al. (19) compared three groups, sedentary healthy controls (HC), FM controls (FMC), and FM patients trained (FMT) over the course of a 21-week, 2×/week strength-training program. In addition to significant and comparable strength gains in the FMT and HC groups, they found normal training-induced hypertrophy in a cross-sectional area of the quadriceps femoris muscle group and significant increases in strength and neural activation of the trained muscles. These adaptations would be expected following a normally prescribed strength-training program and lend support to normal muscle metabolism in FM patients. Simms et al. (20) showed that any deficiencies in strength were more likely affected by muscle deconditioning than by flaws in muscle metabolism. Geel et al. (21) demonstrated normal resting muscle high-energy metabolism, with a significantly lower metabolic re-

sponse to fatiguing exercise. Global deconditioning was the proposed explanation for less depletion of phosphate stores following dynamic muscle work, with arguments for a peripheral pathophysiology remaining unconvincing. Studies emerged that targeted dysregulation in the central nervous system (CNS), particularly pain processing, as a precursor to symptoms in CMI. Current opinion suggests that aberrant CNS processing maintains symptom expression in CMI (10,22–24), specifically sensory processing, autonomic and neuroendocrine functioning, and psychobehavioral factors.

Symptom Maintenance: Central Mechanisms

Sensory Processing. Patients with FM do not have a low sensory detection threshold, i.e., they cannot detect electrical, thermal, or pressure stimuli at lower levels than healthy controls. However, the point at which these stimuli reliably evoke the report of pain is lowered (25,26). Using functional magnetic resonance imaging, Gracely et al. (27) showed that similar subjective levels of experimental pressure pain intensity led to similar activation patterns in the brains of both FM patients and controls, i.e., similar absolute pressure stimuli resulted in greater activation in patients and no comparable regions of activation in controls. Evidence also suggests that dysregulation in central analgesic systems may propagate CMI symptom expression. One potential explanation for increased pain sensitivity in CMI is decreased activity of the descending antinociceptive pathways. Under normal conditions, these pathways inhibit the upward transmission of pain. Kosek et al. (28) demonstrated that isometric muscle contractions exerted an analgesic effect on pressure pain threshold in healthy controls, whereas FM patients responded with a paradoxically lowered pain threshold. Although the endogenous opioid system functions normally in FM patients (29), diffuse noxious inhibitory control (DNIC) or widespread analgesia in response to intense noxious stimuli may not. Early studies found that DNIC manipulation in response to ischemic pain decreased sensitivity to painful pressure in controls, but not in FM patients (30).

Hypothalamic–Pituitary–Adrenal Axis (HPA Axis).

Another area of interest involves the major components of the "stress response," an array of biochemical cascades and effector systems that allow the body to respond and adapt to stimuli. Data indicate that the HPA axis functions differently in subsets of patients with FM and related disorders (31), such that each disorder differs slightly with respect to the precise perturbation. In all instances, hypothalamic function is only "abnormal" in a small subset of patients. In FM, most studies reveal low 24-hour urinary free cortisol, exaggerated ACTH release in response to a corticotropin-releasing hormone challenge, and abnormal diurnal secretion of cortisol. Van Denderen et al. (32) reported similar basal cortisol levels in FM patients and controls, with the expected postexercise rise in controls and a paradoxical decrease in patients; this suggested an adrenal insufficiency in response to maximal exercise in FM patients. While current data suggest attenuated "stress response activity," differences between patients and controls are typically seen in group means, with considerable overlap in individual values.

Autonomic Functioning.

Perhaps the most consistent finding regarding autonomic function in FM is an impaired sympathetic ability to respond to a stressor (e.g., exercise, muscle contraction, noise) (32–34). More recent studies support dysautonomia and a blunted sympathetic response to tilt-table testing (35,36).

Psychologic Factors.

The influence of psychiatric, psychologic, and behavioral factors in CMI has long been debated. Approximately 20 to 40% of FM patients seen in tertiary care have a current identifiable mood disorder (37). As with nearly every chronic illness, a myriad of psychosocial factors play a role in illness expression among CMI patients: behavioral pathways (sick role behavior and maladaptive coping mechanisms); cognitive pathways (victimization and loss of control); and social pathways (interference with role functioning and deterioration of social/support networks). These influences play a prominent role in symptom chronicity and disability (38,39).

Treatment

Given the diverse expression of CMI, it is unrealistic to expect a single treatment paradigm or algorithm to be effective. Rather, management of CMI and affiliated symptoms should be thought of as a fluid approach including the patient and a multidisciplinary team. The best multimodal approaches often include education about the illness, pharmacotherapy, cognitive–behavioral therapy (or attention to mental health needs), and exercise.

Education.

Individuals with mild symptoms often respond to illness-specific information, notably, that CMI is a nonprogressive condition that does not cause damage or inflammation. These patients may fall near the "pure neurobiology" end of the continuum (Fig. 12-2), and they usually possess adequate strategies for improving symptoms and maintaining function. Patients must learn to distinguish information from misinformation. Support of evidenced-based treatment strategies is preferred over products and devices backed only with testimonials. For example, widespread availability of the internet has generated numerous Web sites touting miracle cures for FM and CFS, including coffee enemas, intravenous vitamin drips, and "special" elimination diets among the potential treatments purported to cure CMI. Health care providers should educate their patients to identify valid and reputable information.

Pharmacologic Therapies.

Patients often present with a long list of current and past medications, and in some cases have difficulty determining which ones have helped. The best-studied class of drugs for CMI is tricyclic antidepressants, particularly low doses of amitriptyline and cyclobenzaprine for sleep and pain symptoms (40). While this class of drugs does not directly affect exercise performance, early pharmaceutical management of cardinal symptoms is often beneficial prior to introducing exercise as a potential therapeutic tool. Other classes of compounds (e.g., tramadol, gabapentin, and other classes of antidepressants) may also be effective analgesics.

Cognitive–Behavioral Therapy (CBT). The theoretical basis of CBT is grounded in the idea that pain and suffering result from a complex integration of pathophysiology, cognition, affect, and behavior (41). Through a series of learned skills and behaviors (e.g., relaxation, pacing, pleasant activity scheduling, cognitive reappraisal, goal setting), patients establish a sense of control over their illness, thereby increasing function and reducing pain.

Exercise. Exercise has been widely regarded as beneficial for CMI patients and is recommended as an integral component of long-term symptom management. Although several studies demonstrate improved fitness and improved symptom report following aerobic exercise interventions, methodological differences make interstudy comparison difficult.

Clinical Effects of Exercise

CARDIOVASCULAR TRAINING ADAPTATIONS AND EFFECTS ON SYMPTOMS

In one of the first exercise interventions for FM, McCain et al. (42) used a 20-week cycling program to improve cardiovascular fitness and symptom report in 42 patients. Subjects were randomized to either a cardiovascular-training group (3×/week at a heart rate [HR] >150 bpm) or a flexibility-training group (3×/week, HR <115 bpm). Individuals in the cardiovascular-training group improved their cardiovascular fitness significantly more than individuals in the flexibility-training group, and 12 of 18 subjects in the cardiovascular-training group reported reduced tenderness. When queried on global FM status, 50% of the cardiovascular- and 60% of the flexibility-training groups reported overall improvement. Neither program affected sleep quality or overall pain distribution. This was the first evidence that FM patients could participate safely in an aerobic exercise-training program, that they could train enough to improve cardiovascular fitness, and that their symptoms improved with exercise.

While the most commonly used exercise modalities include walking (43,44) and cycling (42), aerobic dance (45) and game activities (46) have also been studied. Subjects seem to respond equally to a variety of different activities, although riding the stationary bike has been associated with greater initial local-muscle fatigue (47) and localized gluteal tenderness. Recent studies have included aquatic workouts (48,49) similar to those used in rheumatoid arthritis and osteoarthritis. These programs are well tolerated, especially in warm-water pools (85–88°F). Jentoft et al. (48) designed land- and pool-based programs that were 60 min, with about 25 min of aerobic training (40–50% of the time was spent at a HR that was 60–80% of age-predicted maximal HR). They demonstrated that both programs significantly improved cardiovascular capacity. Both programs elicited improvements in pain, fatigue, and/or anxiety/depression, with patients in both groups maintaining their poststudy status through the follow-up period. While pool exercise may have exerted additional positive effects on self-reported mood states and pain, there was little difference in clinical outcomes between these programs.

Mengshoel et al. (45) demonstrated that submaximal capacity improved after 20 weeks of twice-weekly, low-impact aerobic dance sessions. At baseline, the median steady-state HR was 165 bpm, which dropped significantly to 142 bpm for the same power output after training. Subjects did not report improvements in overall general pain (visual analog scale [VAS] score), but did report a significant decrease in exercise-induced pain during dynamic and static upper-extremity work.

A common finding with aerobic exercise is that FM patients resemble sedentary healthy controls for absolute fitness, but that they may perceive aerobic exercise to be more difficult at the same power output. Some investigators have shown that patient groups report higher commensurate ratings of perceived exertion, fatigue, and pain than do controls at comparable power outputs (50,51). Nielens et al. (50) showed that cardiovascular performance was similar between a group of FM patients and an age-matched group of controls, but that a novel perceived exertion index (calculated from the 10-point Borg scale and HR) was greater in patients at a similar work index. Martin et al. (52) showed increased tenderness in FM subjects following a 6-week exercise program that included 20 min of walking at a pace that elevated HR to 60 to 80% of age-predicted max HR and 20 min each of flexibility and strength training. Perhaps due to the brevity of the intervention, this group did not see a change in overall health. Nevertheless, the modest improvements in tenderness and aerobic fitness were promising. Strength improvements were not detected, but the subjects' ability to tolerate a comprehensive program without symptom exacerbation is noteworthy.

STRENGTH TRAINING ADAPTATION AND EFFECTS ON SYMPTOMS

Historically, FM patients and practitioners have avoided strength training because of the primary complaint of musculoskeletal pain. In light of recent CNS findings and the overall deconditioned state of many FM patients, this line of thinking has been challenged. Like healthy sedentary individuals, FM patients can not only tolerate strength training, but also can benefit from a carefully prescribed strength-training program. Rooks et al. (53) had FM patients exercise for 60 min per session, 3×/week, beginning with pool-based training for the first 4 weeks and graduating to land-based training for the remaining 16 weeks. Including static and dynamic movements of major muscle groups using machines, hand weights, and body weight, they showed that women with FM could safely improve strength without exacerbating FM-related symptoms or developing musculoskeletal injuries.

Another group had similar findings with a progressive 21-week strength-training program that compared FM subjects with healthy sedentary controls (19,54). Progressing through weights from low intensities and high repetitions to higher intensities and lower repetitions over the 21 weeks,

both groups showed comparable improvements in overall muscle strength. While pain and tenderness did not change, subjective perceptions of mood, fatigue, and neck pain improved in the patient group (54).

VARIATIONS IN EXERCISE INTENSITY AND PROGRAM DESIGN

In aggregate, the data suggest that both aerobic and anaerobic exercises are beneficial for CMI patients. Questions regarding intensity and structure are less well established. While McCain et al. (42) demonstrated that FM patients could exercise at a vigorous intensity without increasing symptoms or illness severity, several studies later suggested that lower-intensity aerobic exercise promotes similar improvements in symptoms and well-being without the potential exacerbation of pain and fatigue. Meyer et al. (55) compared high (85% HR reserve by week 10) to low (60% HR reserve by week 10) intensity aerobic exercise in FM patients. As with many exercise studies in this population, there was a problem with compliance. Twenty-one subjects were divided among the two intensity groups and a control group. After 24 weeks, only 8 subjects (38%) remained. They were then reassigned to groups based on weekly activity logs, such that there were 5 in a low-intensity group (50% HR reserve) and 3 in a high-intensity group (75% HR reserve). While the small number of subjects precludes definite conclusions, the authors report that the 5 subjects in the low-intensity group had significantly lower Fibromyalgia Impact Questionnaire (FIQ) scores (35% decrease) than the 3 high-intensity subjects (8% increase). Pain report also tended to be lower in the low-intensity group and higher in the high-intensity group. One caveat of this study is the discrepancy between the original exercise prescription and the actual program "performed" (56). When left to their own devices, FM patients tend to self-select an exercise intensity that is low to moderate.

Home-based exercise programing has also been studied in FM patients. Using similar exercise prescriptions, Ramsay et al. (64) presented one group with a single didactic experience, i.e., written instructions to take home. Another group met once per week for 12 weeks with a physiotherapist and was encouraged to continue exercises at home. While there were significant gains in psychologic well-being, the authors reported that they were "modest and ill-sustained," and neither group improved their pain report over baseline. Meiworm et al. (65) and Busch et al. (66) showed favorable results with their home-based programs, improving performance and pain, and function and illness severity, respectively.

Whether improvement in physical fitness translates into an improved symptom profile is debatable. The literature suggests that greater levels of physical activity are related to a greater perceived control of symptoms and health-related quality of life (42,45–47,58–60), although effects on specific symptoms (pain and fatigue) tend to be less robust than effects on more global measures of well-being. Some indices of pain, particularly clinical pain, are typically not as amenable to change following exercise training (45,46). The Cochrane report (56) states that protocols meeting ACSM guidelines for aerobic training "produce short-term improvements in pain pressure threshold of FM tenderpoints." However, considering that tender points are highly influenced by levels of distress and are not necessarily measures of pain or tenderness per se (1,62–63), these results may reflect a change in affective status rather than an alteration in sensory processing. A review by Koltyn (61) addressed the issue of exercise-induced hypoalgesia (reduced sensitivity to painful stimuli). In pain-free individuals, hypoalgesia was consistently induced following high-intensity exercise. Further research is necessary, however, to establish the appropriate balance, or "dose," of intensity and duration of exercise in individuals with chronic pain.

There are no data on the use of lifestyle physical activity in FM patients. In obese and healthy populations, lifestyle activity programs have been used to increase daily energy expenditure and to lower disease risk profiles. Given the lack of correlation between physical fitness and symptom severity, it seems likely that CMI patients would respond favorably to increased lifestyle physical activity. The advantages of such a program are that they allow freedom of choice in activity, time, and intensity and, importantly, they shift responsibility to the patient. Whether performing lifestyle physical activity or a strict exercise prescription, patients should

learn what to expect with regard to potential feelings of fatigue and discomfort during and after exercise. Self-monitoring during exercise (e.g., using HR or perceived exertion) to prevent overexertion while ensuring that some level of effort is achieved is particularly important.

Almost every exercise study of CMI reports that subjects improve for the duration of the study, but very few studies demonstrate significant adherence to continued exercise afterward. This should be addressed in future studies, as long-term adherence seems to be the most salient aspect of exercise or activity for FM patients. Another interesting note is that serious adverse events do not occur with greater frequency in FM patients than in the general population, although FM-related events (e.g., symptom flares) are not well documented in studies. The 1996 Surgeon General's report (67) promoting more lifestyle physical activity substantially broadens the opportunities for FM patients to incorporate exercise and/or physical activity into their lives.

Recommendations for Exercise and Activity

The particular combination of symptoms that constitute the CMI spectrum can pose significant challenges to both the patient and the exercise professional. Consider the activity and exercise one does as a drug, and titrate the dose up to the individual's maximal tolerated levels (Fig. 12-3). While not always quantified in studies, many FM patients report a transient increase in their cardinal symptom when starting a novel activity, exercise or otherwise. Their natural response to any increase in pain and fatigue may be to stop, or severely curtail, their activity. This behavior pattern perpetuates a futile cycle: promoting maladaptive illness behaviors, diminishing productivity, and reducing quality of life. Programs with the greatest chance for success will consider potential barriers and implement sound reinforcement and relapse-prevention strategies early in the education-exercise process.

Patient characteristics that affect adoption and maintenance of routine exercise participation include (*a*) readiness to adopt a new behavior

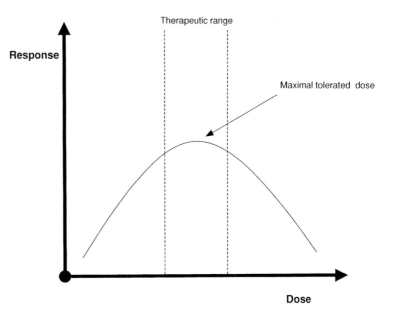

Response

Therapeutic range

Maximal tolerated dose

Dose

FIGURE 12-3 Therapeutic dosing of exercise for chronic multisymptom illnesses (CMIs) following a pharmacotherapy model.

that may, at first, increase discomfort; *(b)* readiness to accept a self-management approach to their illness (68); *(c)* unrealistic or discordant expectations; *(d)* fear of increased pain and fatigue; *(e)* past experience with exercise and activity; and *(f)* available social support (e.g., family, friends).

Program characteristics likely to influence adoption and maintenance of exercise participation include *(a)* intensity of exercise, *(b)* any factor viewed as "stressful" (e.g., time consuming, parking difficulties, inconvenient), *(c)* available social support (e.g., exercise professional, doctor, nurse and family, friends), and *(d)* progression rate (either too fast or too slow).

While these lists are not exhaustive, they provide a general idea of what to consider when developing exercise programs for individuals with CMI. Readiness to adopt a self-management approach to pain is an important consideration for overall symptom management and a precursor to behavior change (69). A program that focuses largely on education may most benefit these patients. Education about their illness itself, as well as education on how and why a combination of therapies should be used may be most beneficial. Given that any newfound knowledge about illness is likely to be lost by 12 weeks

(70), a paced approach with verbal and written information will maximize knowledge retention or at least availability. One hopes that this tactic will also lessen unrealistic expectations of a monotherapy "magic bullet."

When considering which characteristics of an exercise program influence results, the literature and clinical experience suggest that a lower intensity (<75% of age-predicted maximal HR) is more likely to be tolerated by CMI patients, at least initially. Equally important is the rate of progression. Whereas a healthy individual may progress from 15 to 30 min in 4 weeks, a patient with CMI might take twice that time or longer. An important corollary is lack of progression. The actual rate may be less relevant than reducing maladaptive behaviors or beliefs by continual, forward progress. Pain and fatigue may worsen initially, but will likely abate within a few days to a few weeks. To avoid entrance into a futile cycle, one must encourage continuing with the program, albeit at a reduced level. While there are no good data on how to properly manage a flare of symptoms within the context of an exercise program, clinical experience suggests a reduction by half (usually of quantity, with a commensurate lowering of intensity), with a gradual return to preflare levels within 3 days to 1 week (Fig. 12-4).

Flare Management

• Reduce volume by half

• Gradual return to preflare levels over
  3 days to 1 week

Example—Current exercise program
is 40 minutes per week, spread over
4 days of one 10-minute session per day.

Day 1–5 minutes, with relaxation activity for
5 minutes

Day 2–7 minutes, with relaxation activity for 4–5
minutes

Day 3–9 minutes

Day 4–10 minutes; inclusion of relaxation
activites serves as a "placeholder" for the remaining
exercise minutes.

FIGURE 12-4 Flare management.

ADHERENCE

Compliance and long-term adherence to exercise behaviors are difficult for CMI patients. This problem is seen for many illnesses and their associated behaviors, regardless of the degree of health risk. For example, to maintain virologic suppression, AIDS patients must follow a pill-taking regimen with ≥95% accuracy. Nevertheless, 40 to 60% of these patients are less than 90% compliant (71). Similarly, Kushner (73) reported 30% compliance to a lipid-lowering diet with potential for improving disease risk factors. General reasons given for failure to adhere to health behaviors vary: boredom, forgetfulness, interference of life events, fear of pain or injury, discordant expectations and goals, etc. (71,72,74). Patients with CMI face similar challenges and attrition rates with regard to adopting exercise behaviors.

The high recidivism rate is perhaps the biggest shortcoming among exercise interventions in CMI patients. Although some trials report fairly high compliance rates (66), others report high numbers of dropouts (56,65). Unfortunately, any benefits conferred by regular exercise participation are lost once the patient stops (47,56,65). Possible contributing factors to high dropout rates include those common to other populations: lack of time, family commitments, and lack of convenience. More specific to patients with CMI are baseline pain and fatigue and fear of postexertional pain and fatigue. Patients report feeling "broken down" for more than 24 hours after a training session and have referred to exercise as "time consuming," "painful," and "stressful" (58).

A recent finding suggested that 55% of dropouts from a comprehensive pain rehabilitation center left treatment early because of "discrepant expectations" (69). One study showed only 25% of subjects continuing regular physical activity a year or more after the study (47). The 16 studies described in the Cochrane report (57) as "high quality training studies," reported an average attrition rate of 25%. A number of trials have incorporated educational or behavioral elements to traditional training programs (59,60,70) in an attempt to improve long-term adherence and to bolster the effects of regular exercise. A meta-analysis by Rossy et al. of 49 FM treatment outcome studies (75) concluded that nonpharmacologic treatments (i.e., exercise and CBT) were optimal intervention strategies, along with appropriate pharmacologic treatment for pain and sleep symptoms.

With a recalcitrant population (62% disability), Burkhardt et al. (60) demonstrated that while pain and physical fitness parameters remained unaffected by a combined program of education and exercise or by an education-alone program, both groups significantly improved quality-of-life measures and self-efficacy for function relative to a delayed-treatment control group (60). At 4- to 8-month follow-up, the combination group fared more favorably than the education-alone group. Overall, 71% of subjects replied favorably to the question of the impact of the intervention on their symptoms. Buckelew et al. (59) also showed that a combination group (exercise plus biofeedback) maintained improvements in tenderness and self-efficacy for function at 2-year follow-up.

RELAPSE PREVENTION

Relapse prevention strategies are used in a wide variety of illness and behavior scenarios to promote progression through a given program or practice. In general, relapses are frequently unexpected and can result from symptom flares, unforeseeable life events or simply forgetfulness. Other influences on the adoption or resumption of an exercise program are the history of pain or injury or the expectation of future pain or injury (74). The danger of a relapse lies in the patient's inability to cope and subsequent failure to return to activity. With this in mind, prevention strategies such as adopting an exercise program with flexible goals, identifying potential high-risk situations before they occur, developing coping skills to deal with those situations, and educating individuals on specific techniques that facilitate readoption of the program (74) are designed to tackle these issues.

While not formally studied, many CBT lessons could be applied to the adoption and maintenance of exercise behaviors. Two such lessons include pacing and cognitive reappraisal. The construct of pacing instructs patients to break tasks into manageable, time-based segments. For example, a household task that usually requires 1 hour to complete is broken into six 10-min segments to avoid excess pain and fatigue. The same concept can be applied to exercise. Multiple short sessions, as opposed to one long one, provide a means of interspersing exercise throughout the day in intervals convenient to the individual, without the added apprehension or potential for perceived failure that might accompany longer, single bouts of activity. The idea behind cognitive reappraisal is that thinking drives emotion, and thinking is alterable. In the context of a symptom flare, patients can be taught to change how they react. Rather than feeling guilt or helplessness, they learn to restructure their thoughts and, consequently, their actions to prevent a lapse in their daily activity or exercise program. Similarly, restructuring a failure in terms of success can mitigate potential pitfalls before they arise.

Social support is provided from a variety of individuals and groups in the patient's life. Family and friends are crucial in promoting positive health behaviors. However, it is the professional (doctor, nurse, and exercise professional) who imparts a tremendous influence on the patient. This does not have to imply extra or longer office visits. After an orientation session, brief ongoing phone calls can help individuals maintain their exercise behaviors (76,77). With the wide availability of the internet, e-mail is another potential avenue for social support. More recently, the palm pilot has appeared as

a tool to promote patient education, goal setting, progress tracking, symptom reporting, and adherence (78). This technology could be further used to assess reasons for and degree of relapse and subsequently adjust the patient's activity level to ease reentry into the program.

Assessing Outcomes

Outcome measures can describe achieved objectives and provide evidence of therapeutic efficacy. Primary outcomes are those measures directly influenced by treatment and are quantified by changes in a particular variable. They can reflect illness-specific domains (pain) or general physiologic adaptations ($\dot{V}O_{2max}$) to training. Process measures are those variables that affect primary outcomes (e.g., adherence to the intervention). According to the Cochrane report (57), outcome measures commonly reported in exercise treatment trials for FM can be divided into seven domains: clinical pain (visual analog scale, body map); tenderness (tender point count, total myalgic score, dolorimetry); physical function by objective (cardiorespiratory fitness) and subjective (self-reported physical function, FIQ physical impairment subscale) measures; musculoskeletal performance (strength, endurance); global well-being and perceived improvement (physician-rated change, FIQ total score); self-efficacy; fatigue and sleep (FIQ fatigue subscale, visual analog scale); and psychologic function (depression and anxiety scales, FIQ). Choosing appropriate outcome measures is tantamount to the program design and depends highly on the goals of the individual and of the intervention. Inclusion of primary outcomes and process measures ensures a more accurate representation of a program's impact on the patient and the illness.

EXERCISE TESTING

Standard practice in exercise rehabilitative settings is to perform an exercise tolerance test. This is a way to evaluate the individual and the program and can be an educational and motivational tool. In CMI patients, the information gained from testing, in conjunction with a medical and exercise history, can be used to assist the individual to achieve health and lifestyle goals.

Aerobic Fitness

The decision to perform a maximal or submaximal test depends on the reason for the test and the availability of equipment and personnel. Among FM patients, performance on maximal exercise tests varies. Most investigators report that some of their subjects fail to achieve a physiologic maximum (52,79,80). Sietsema et al. (79) reported peak $\dot{V}O_2$ values for patients and controls of 21 ± 9 and 27 ± 8 mL·kg^{-1}·min^{-1}, respectively, with fewer patients reaching criteria for near-maximal effort. Only 7 of 18 FM patients (vs. 8 of 8 controls) attained either a plateau in $\dot{V}O_2$ or 80% of age-predicted maximal HR. Limiting the analysis to the 7 FM patients, peak $\dot{V}O_2$ values were similar to those of controls (26.8 ± 9 mL·kg^{-1}·min^{-1}). Gursel et al. (81) reported similar peak $\dot{V}O_2$ values for patients and controls. In contrast to varied maximal tests, submaximal exercise performance may be fairly close to normal in FM patients. Data from Sietsema et al. (79) reflect comparable anaerobic thresholds in patients and controls (13 ± 4 and 15 ± 3 mL·kg^{-1}·min^{-1}).

Testing mode depends on available equipment. Patients with FM have performed adequately on Balke and Naughton treadmill protocols (45,58) as well as numerous cycle ergometer protocols. Regardless of mode, common sense suggests that "start low, go slow" is important when testing CMI patients. The primary concern is an adequate warmup and a tolerable rate of increase to minimize premature local muscle fatigue and pain, frequent endpoints of many tests.

An often-performed test is the 6-min walk (6MW) test. This test is better used as a functional test, rather than as a measure of cardiorespiratory fitness. Pankoff et al. (80) had FM patients perform a series of 6MW tests. Subjects performed three 6MW tests on consecutive days. There were significant differences between walk 1 (478 ± 61 m) and walk 2 (492 ± 57 m) and between walk 1 and walk 3 (495 ± 60 m). Following a 4-week multidisciplinary intervention, three more 6MW tests were performed, with no significant differences in distance traveled (507 ± 67, 505 ± 63, and 509 ± 62 m). With a different group of FM patients, Pankoff et al. (80) had subjects complete a 6MW test, the FIQ, and a peak $\dot{V}O_2$ test before and after a 12-week exercise program. Correlations between the 6MW test and peak $\dot{V}O_2$ were insignificant *(a)* before the intervention, *(b)* after significant improvements in both the 6MW and peak $\dot{V}O_2$ tests, and *(c)* for change scores of both measures.

Although the 6MW test responds to change in patients with FM, it is not a good measure of cardiorespiratory fitness and may represent a more composite measure of global improvement. Considering that the 6MW test can be influenced by motivation and encouragement and that performance is stabilized after two walks, this test may be useful for self-monitoring among patients or as a more clinical outcome measure.

Muscular Fitness

Over the years, researchers in FM have used a variety of methods and machines to evaluate muscular fitness (e.g., handgrip manometers, dynamometers). Hagberg et al. (82) developed a test to measure static endurance in patients with myofascial shoulder pain. Patients were required to hold an arm in a predetermined, fixed position while balancing a sheet of paper on a pen. Endurance time was calculated when the subject could no longer hold the pen steady, causing the paper to fall. This was a simple way to correlate endurance time with pain and fatigue. Recent studies have used more sophisticated methods, such as weight machines and dynamometers, to obtain a single measure of strength or to extrapolate results for a training study (17–20,54).

An important consideration for both muscle strength and aerobic training is that activities involving largely eccentric contractions result in delayed-onset muscle soreness (DOMS) more frequently than do those involving concentric contractions. Typically, the individual with DOMS reports pain, stiffness, and strength loss, with accompanying loss of function. In FM patients, this common side effect of exercise can derail even the most intact exercise program.

Summary

FM and other CMIs are complex conditions with neurobiologic factors playing some role in symptom expression. These symptoms (e.g., pain, unremitting fatigue, and memory and/or cognitive difficulties) can also be tied to a host of psychiatric comorbidities and psychosocial factors. Current understanding of these factors does not allow the identification of mechanisms operative in individual patients, so health care practitioners must focus on treating symptoms. A multimodal treatment scheme, including pharmacotherapy, cognitive–behavioral therapy, and exercise therapy may represent the best approach for managing patients with these conditions.

Either independently or as part of a more comprehensive program, exercise has been repeatedly shown to be an effective therapy with little ill effect and numerous benefits for patients with CMI. Unfortunately, exercise is often underused because of poor physician understanding of how it should be prescribed, lack of confidence on the part of the patient, poor insurance coverage, etc. Using a program catered to the individual's situation, regular exercise or physical activity teaches patients with CMI that they can exercise safely and effectively. More importantly, an individualized approach will calm the patient's fears about inducing a flare-up (83). A beginning exercise program should include attainable goals and ample support. Consistency and participation in an increasingly active lifestyle are the key factors to facilitating sustained benefits and continued commitment to health.

REFERENCES

1. Wolfe F, Ross K, Anderson J, et al. Aspects of fibromyalgia in the general population: sex, pain threshold, and fibromyalgia symptoms. J Rheumatol 1995;22:151–156.
2. Buchwald D, Umali P, Umali J, et al. Chronic fatigue and the chronic fatigue syndrome: prevalence in a Pacific northwest health care system. Ann Intern Med 1995;123:81–88.
3. Renfro L, Feder HM Jr, Lane TJ. Yeast connection among 100 patients with chronic fatigue. Am J Med 1989;86:165–168.
4. Doebbeling BN, Clarke WR, Watson D, et al. Is there a Persian Gulf War syndrome? Evidence from a large population-based survey of veterans and non-deployed controls. Am J Med 2000;108:695–704.
5. Clauw DJ, Chrousos GP. Chronic pain and fatigue syndromes: overlapping clinical and neuroendocrine features and potential pathogenic mechanisms. Neuroimmunomodulation 1997;4:134–153.
6. Fukuda K, Nisenbaum R, Stewart G, et al. Chronic multisymptom illness affecting air force veterans of the gulf war. JAMA 1999;280:981–988.
7. Nisenbaum R, Barrett DH, Reyes M, et al. Deployment stressors and a chronic multisymptom illness among Gulf War veterans. J Nerv Ment Dis 2000;188:259–266.
8. McKenzie R, Straus SE. Chronic fatigue syndrome. Adv Intern Med 1995;40:119–153.
9. Straus SE. Studies of herpes virus infection in chronic fatigue syndrome. Ciba Found Symp 1993;173:132–139.
10. Yunus MB. Towards a model of pathophysiology of fibromyalgia: aberrant central pain mechanisms with peripheral modulation. J Rheumatol 1992:19:846–850 (editorial).
11. Wolfe F, Smythe HA, Yunus MB, et al. The American College of Rheumatology 1990 criteria for the classification of fibromyalgia. Report of the Multicenter Criteria Committee. Arthritis Rheum 1990;33:160–172.
12. Holmes GP, Kaplan JE, Gantz NM, et al. Chronic fatigue syndrome: a working case definition. Ann Intern Med 1988;108:387–389.
13. Buskila D, Neumann L, Vaisberg G, et al. Increased rates of fibromyalgia following cervical spine injury: a controlled study of 161 cases of traumatic injury. Arthritis Rheum 1997;40:446–452.
14. Hudson JI, Goldenberg DL, Pope HG Jr, et al. Comorbidity of fibromyalgia with medical and psychiatric disorders. Am J Med 1992;92:363–367.
15. Bennett RM, Clark SR, Goldberg L, et al. Aerobic fitness in patients with fibrositis: a controlled study of respiratory gas exchange and 133xenon clearance from exercising muscle. Arthritis Rheum 1989;32:454–460.
16. Mengshoel AM, Forre O, Komnaes HB. Muscle strength and aerobic capacity in primary fibromyalgia. Clin Exp Rheumatol 1990;8:475–479.
17. Borman P, Celiker R, Hascelik Z. Muscle performance in fibromyalgia syndrome. Rheumatol Int 1999;19:27–30.
18. Norregaard J, Bulow PM, Lykkegaard JJ, et al. Muscle strength, working capacity and effort in patients with fibromyalgia. Scand J Rehabil Med 1997;29:97–102.
19. Hakkinen A, Hakkinen K, Hannonen P, et al. Force production capacity and acute neuromuscular responses to fatiguing loading in women with fibromyalgia are not different from those of healthy women. J Rheumatol 2000;27:1277–1282.
20. Simms RW, Roy S, Skrinar G, et al. Lack of association between fibromyalgia syndrome and abnormalities in muscle energy metabolism. Arthritis Rheum 1994;37:794–800.
21. Geel SE, Robergs RA. The effect of graded resistance exercise on fibromyalgia symptoms and

muscle bioenergetics: a pilot study. Arthritis Rheum 2002;47:82–86.

22. Russell IJ, Orr MD, Littman B, et al. Elevated cerebrospinal fluid levels of substance p in patients with the fibromyalgia syndrome. Arthritis Rheum 1994;37:1593–1601.

23. Harvey CK. Fibromyalgia. Part II: Prevalence in the podiatric patient population. J Am Podiatr Med Assoc 1993;83:416–417.

24. Crofford LJ, Engleberg NC, Demitrack MA. Neurohormonal perturbations in fibromyalgia. Baillieres Clin Rheumatol 1996;10:365–378.

25. Donald F, Esdaile JM, Kimoff JR, et al. Musculoskeletal complaints and fibromyalgia in patients attending a respiratory sleep disorders clinic. J Rheumatol 1996;23:1612–1616 [see Comments].

26. Arroyo JF, Cohen ML. Abnormal responses to electrocutaneous stimulation in fibromyalgia. J Rheumatol 1993;20:1925–1931.

27. Gracely RH, Petzke F, Wolf JM, et al. Functional magnetic resonance imaging evidence of augmented pain processing in fibromyalgia. Arthritis Rheum 2002;46:1333–1343.

28. Kosek E, Ekholm J, Hansson P. Modulation of pressure pain thresholds during and following isometric contraction in patients with fibromyalgia and in healthy controls. Pain 1996;64:415–423.

29. Price D, Staud R, Robinson M, et al. Enhanced temporal summation of second pain and its central modulation in fibromyalgia patients. Pain 2002;99:49–59.

30. Kosek E, Hansson P. Modulatory influence on somatosensory perception from vibration and heterotopic noxious conditioning stimulation (HNCS) in fibromyalgia patients and healthy subjects. Pain 1997;70:41–51.

31. Crofford LJ. Neuroendocrine abnormalities in fibromyalgia and related disorders. Am J Med Sci 1998;315:359–366.

32. van Denderen JC, Boersma JW, Zeinstra P, et al. Physiological effects of exhaustive physical exercise in primary fibromyalgia syndrome (PFS): is PFS a disorder of neuroendocrine reactivity? Scand J Rheumatol 1992;21:35–37.

33. Elam M, Johansson G, Wallin BG. Do patients with primary fibromyalgia have an altered muscle sympathetic nerve activity? Pain 1992;48:371–375.

34. Qiao ZG, Vaery H, Mrkrid L. Electrodermal and microcirculatory activity in patients with fibromyalgia during baseline, acoustic stimulation and cold pressor tests. J Rheumatol 1991;18:1383–1389.

35. Clauw DJ, Radulovic D, Heshmat Y, et al. Heart rate variability as a measure of autonomic dysfunction in fibromyalgia and chronic fatigue syndrome. Arthritis Rheum 1995;38:R25.

36. Clauw DJ, Radulovic D, Antonetti D, et al. Tilt table testing in fibromyalgia. Arthritis Rheum 1996;39:R20.

37. Boissevain MD, McCain GA. Toward an integrated understanding of fibromyalgia syndrome. II. Psychological and phenomenological aspects. Pain 1991;45:239–248.

38. Pulliam CB, Gatchel RJ, Gardea MA. Psychosocial differences in high risk versus low risk acute low-back pain patients. J Occup Rehabil 2001;11:43–52.

39. Epker J, Gatchel RJ, Ellis E III. A model for predicting chronic TMD: practical application in clinical settings. J Am Dent Assoc 1999;130:1470–1475.

40. Godfrey RG. A guide to the understanding and use of tricyclic antidepressants in the overall management of fibromyalgia and other chronic pain syndromes. Arch Intern Med 1996;156:1047–1052.

41. Turk DC. A cognitive-behavioral perspective of the therapy process. In: Turk DC, Meichenbaum D, Genest M, eds. Pain and behavioral medicine: a cognitive-behavioral perspective. New York: Guilford Press, 1983:3–17.

42. McCain GA, Bell DA, Mai FM, et al. A controlled study of the effect of a tonic pain stimulus on pain threshold in patients with FM, and effects of a supervised cardiovascular fitness training program on the manifestations of primary fibromyalgia. Arthritis Rheum 1988;31:1135–1141.

43. Nichols DS, Glenn TM. Effects of aerobic exercise on pain perception, affect, and level of disability in individuals with fibromyalgia. Phys Ther 1994;74:327–332.

44. Martin L, Nutting A, MacIntosh BR, et al. An exercise program in the treatment of fibromyalgia. J Rheumatol 1996;23:1050–1053.

45. Mengshoel AM, Komnaes HB, Forre O. The effects of 20 weeks of physical fitness training in female patients with fibromyalgia. Clin Exp Rheumatol 1992;10:345–349.

46. Wigers SH, Stiles TC, Vogel PA. Effects of aerobic exercise versus stress management treatment in fibromyalgia: a 4.5 year prospective study. Scand J Rheumatol 1996;25:77–86.

47. Klug GA, McAuley E, Clark S. Factors influencing the development and maintenance of aerobic fitness: lessons applicable to the fibrositis syndrome. J Rheumatol 1989;19(suppl):30–39.

48. Jentoft ES, Kvalvik AG, Mengshoel AM. Effects of pool-based and land-based aerobic exercise on women with fibromyalgia/chronic widespread muscle pain. Arthritis Rheum 2001;45:42–47.

49. Mannerkorpi K, Nyberg B, Ahlmen M, et al. Pool exercise combined with an education program for patients with fibromyalgia syndrome: a prospective, randomized study. J Rheumatol 2000;27:2473–2481.

50. Nielens H, Boisset V, Masquelier E. Fitness and perceived exertion in patients with fibromyalgia syndrome. Clin J Pain 2000;16:209–213.

51. Burckhardt CS, Clark SR, Padrick KP. Use of the modified Balke treadmill protocol for determining the aerobic capacity of women with fibromyalgia. Arthritis Care Res 1989;2:165–167.

52. Martin L, Nutting A, MacIntosh BR, et al. An exercise program in the treatment of fibromyalgia. J Rheumatol 1996;23:1050–1053.

53. Rooks DS, Silverman CB, Kantrowitz FG. The effects of progressive strength training and aerobic exercise on muscle strength and cardiovascular fitness in women with fibromyalgia: a pilot study. Arthritis Rheum 2002;47:22–28.

54. Hakkinen A, Hakkinen K, Hannonen P, et al. Strength training induced adaptations in neuromuscular function of premenopausal women with fibromyalgia: comparison with healthy women. Ann Rheum Dis 2001;60:21–26.

55. Meyer BB, Lemley KJ. Utilizing exercise to affect the symptomatology of fibromyalgia: a pilot study Med Sci Sports Exerc 2000;32:1691–1697.

56. Busch A, Schacter CL, Peloso PM, et al. Exercise for treating fibromyalgia. (Cochrane Review). In: *The Cochrane Library* [3], Oxford: Update Software, 2002.

57. van Santen M, Bolwijn P, Verstappen F, et al. A randomized clinical trial comparing fitness and biofeedback training versus basic treatment in patients with fibromyalgia. J Rheumatol 2002;29:575–581.

58. Buckelew SP, Conway R, Parker J, et al. Biofeedback/relaxation training and exercise interventions for fibromyalgia: a prospective trial. Arthritis Care Res 1998;11:196–209.

59. Burckhardt CS, Mannerkorpi K, Hedenberg L, et al. A randomized, controlled clinical trial of education and physical training for women with fibromyalgia. J Rheumatol 1994;21:714–720.

60. Karper WB, Hopewell R, Hodge M. Exercise program effects on women with fibromyalgia syndrome. Clin Nurs Spec 2001;15:67–73.

61. Koltyn KF. Exercise-induced hypoalgesia and intensity of exercise. Sports Med 2002;32:477–487.

62. Croft P, Schollum J, Silman A. Population study of tender point counts and pain as evidence of fibromyalgia. BMJ 1994;309:696–699 [see Comments].

63. Wolfe F, Ross K, Anderson J, et al. The prevalence and characteristics of fibromyalgia in the general population. Arthritis Rheum 1995;38:19–28.

64. Ramsay C, Moreland J, Ho M, et al. An observer-blinded comparison of supervised and unsupervised aerobic exercise regimens in fibromyalgia. Rheumatology 2000;39:501–505.

65. Meiworm L, Jakob E, Walker UA, et al. Patients with fibromyalgia benefit from aerobic endurance exercise. Clin Rheumatol 2000;19:253–257.

66. Busch AJ, Schacter CL, Sheppard MS. Home-based videotaped program of aerobics for fibromyalgia. Arthritis Rheum 1999;46:S220.

67. United States Department of Health and Human Services. Physical activity and health: a report of the Surgeon General. Atlanta, GA: US Department of Health and Human Services, Centers for Disease Control and Prevention, National Center for Chronic Disease Prevention and Health Promotion, 1996.

68. Kerns RD, Haythornthwaite J, Williams DA, et al. Can matching chronic pain patients to psychological treatments improve outcomes? Oral presentation. 16th annual meeting of the American Pain Society, New Orleans, LA, 1997.

69. Nelson PJ, Bee SM, Evans MM, et al. Characteristics of dropouts from a pain rehabilitation program: support for "pain stages of change" model. IASP abstracts: 10th world congress on pain, San Diego, CA 2002;10:448.

70. Gowans SE, deHueck A, Voss S, et al. A randomized, controlled trial of exercise and education for individuals with fibromyalgia. Arthritis Care Res 1999;12:120–128.

71. Bartlett JA. Addressing the challenges of adherence. J Acquired Immune Defic Syndr 2002;29(suppl 1):S2–10.

72. Smith CF, Burke LE, Wing RR. Vegetarian and weight-loss diets among young adults. Obes Res 2000;8123–8129.

73. Kushner RF. Long-term compliance with a lipid-lowering diet. Nutr Rev 1993;51:16–18.

74. Dishman R. Consensus, problems, and prospects. In: Dishman R, ed. Advances in Exercise Adherence. Champaign, IL: Human Kinetics, 1994;1–28.

75. Rossy LA, Buckelew SP, Dorr N, et al. A meta-analysis of fibromyalgia treatment interventions. Ann Behav Med 1999;21:180–191.

76. King AC, Taylor CB, Haskell WL, et al. Strategies for increasing early adherence to and long-term maintenance of home-based exercise training in healthy middle-aged men and women. Am J Cardiol 1988;61:628–632.

77. Juneau M, Rogers F, De Santos V, et al. Effectiveness of self-monitored, home-based, moderate-intensity exercise training in middle-aged men and women. Am J Cardiol 1987;60:66–70.

78. Davidson MH. Strategies to improve adult treatment panel III: guideline adherence and patient compliance. Am J Cardiol 2002;89:8C–20C.

79. Sietsema KE, Cooper DM, Caro X, et al. Oxygen uptake during exercise in patients with primary fibromyalgia syndrome. J Rheumatol 1993;20:860–865.

80. Pankoff B, Overend T, Lucy D, et al. Validity and responsiveness of the 6 minute walk test for people with fibromyalgia. J Rheumatol 2000;27:2666–2670.

81. Gursel Y, Ergin S, Ulus Y, et al. Hormonal responses to exercise stress test in patients with fibromyalgia syndrome. Clin Rheumatol 2001;20:401–405.

82. Hagberg M, Kvarnstrom S. Muscular endurance and electromyographic fatigue in myofascial shoulder pain. Arch Phys Med Rehabil 1984;65:522–525.

83. Ax S, Gregg VH, Jones D. Coping and illness cognitions: chronic fatigue syndrome. Clin Psychol Rev 2001;21:161–182.

13

Spinal Cord Injury

Thomas W. J. Janssen and Maria T. E. Hopman

A spinal cord lesion is a partial or total disruption of the structural and functional integrity of the spinal cord, often caused by some sort of trauma, resulting in impairments such as paralysis, loss of sensation, and autonomic nervous system dysfunction. Spinal cord lesions above the first thoracic spinal segment result in tetraplegia, i.e., (partial) loss of neurologic innervation of upper limbs, trunk, abdomen, pelvis, and lower limbs. Spinal cord injury (SCI) at or below the first thoracic segment defines the condition of paraplegia, with the degree of dysfunction approximately proportional to the level of the lesion.

SCI results in sudden and drastic changes in health status and lifestyle of the individual, which may lead to a loss of health and fitness. Whereas some decades ago, individuals with SCI died at an early age because of respiratory and other complications, they now have a longer life expectancy, and attention has to be focused on improving their quality of life.

Confinement to a wheelchair following SCI is associated with inactivity and degenerative symptoms such as muscle atrophy, loss of bone integrity below the lesion level, and changes in the cardiovascular and respiratory systems. To improve general health, physical fitness, and functional ability and to reduce the risk for secondary complications, regular participation in exercise is recommended. Arm exercise, electrically stimulated (ES) leg exercise, or a combination of both are the proper exercise modes.

This chapter presents an overview of the effects of SCI on cardiorespiratory and musculoskeletal function, as well as the exercise responses of those with SCI to different modes of exercise. Recommendations for exercise testing in SCI are made, and special considerations are discussed. Finally, suggestions for training protocols for individuals with SCI are presented, and the adaptations to training are discussed.

Effect of SCI on the Body

MUSCLE

As a result of the lesion, dramatic muscle atrophy of the paralyzed muscles develops soon after the injury (1). This muscular atrophy is reflected by a reduction in cross-sectional area and a loss of muscle fibers (2) and can be accompanied by an increased amount of perimysial tissue. Paralyzed muscles below the lesion show a transformation in fiber distribution toward a predominance of type II muscle fibers (3). These alterations in fiber type expression are accompanied by pronounced metabolic changes such as reduced oxidative enzyme activity and/or mitochondrial content (4). These "typical" changes in muscle fiber composition and metabolic profile are most likely adaptations to reduced neuromuscular activity as well as to the lack of mechanical loading, reduced stretch, reduced oxygen demand, and possibly hormonal changes.

BONE

Osteoporosis and concomitant increased risk for fractures is a common problem in SCI (5,6) The greatest bone loss occurs in the 2-year post-SCI period, followed by a markedly reduced rate of bone loss (7).

CIRCULATION

Not only muscle fibers, but also the vascular system in the legs appears to atrophy as a result of the inactivity of the paralyzed legs after SCI. Using echo Doppler ultrasonography, several investigators report smaller diameters of the common femoral artery in those with SCI (~5–6 mm) than in age-, sex-, and body size-matched controls (~8–10 mm) (8–10). Blood flow in the femoral artery in individuals with SCI is 30 to 50% of that in able-bodied (AB) controls (8,10,11). These circulatory adaptations are most likely physiologic adjustments to the low oxygen demand in the paralyzed leg muscles; i.e., oxygen delivery is geared to oxygen demand by functional and structural adaptations of the vessels.

The opposite, increased vessel diameter and blood flow, has been shown for the arm vasculature in individuals with SCI as an adaptation to long-term arm work. Shenberger et al. (12) reported larger diameters of the brachial artery in individuals with paraplegia than in AB controls. The mechanism behind this may be hypoxia and related chronic enhancement of shear forces inducing endothelial cell-mediated alterations in the release of growth factors, nitric oxide, and other vasodilating factors leading ultimately to structural adaptations of the vascular wall (13).

In SCI, venous capacity is decreased by about 40%, and venous outflow resistance increases to about 130% of AB values (14,15). These results indicate that venous distensibility has decreased as a result of increased stiffness of the venous wall and/or the tissue that surrounds the venous system in the lower limbs. In addition, the total cross-sectional area of the leg venous system is smaller. This supports the hypothesis of venous atrophy as an adaptation to the paralysis and inactivity and dismisses the concept of venous blood pooling in the legs of those with SCI. These vascular adaptations seem to occur very rapidly after the SCI.

HEART

The morphology of the heart is changed in individuals with SCI, particularly those with tetraplegia. A smaller left ventricular heart mass (~25% reduction) and left ventricular dimensions have been found consistently in those with tetraplegia (16), whereas smaller left ventricular dimensions have been reported only in sedentary individuals with paraplegia (9,17). The effect of SCI on cardiac function is unknown.

CORONARY HEART DISEASE (CHD) RISK FACTORS

The risk of CHD appears to be higher in those with SCI than in the AB population (18); this may be due in part to adoption of a sedentary lifestyle with consequent degenerative changes in the cardiovascular system (19,20). The high risk of CHD among sedentary individuals with SCI is indicated by poor blood lipid profiles, such as lower high-density lipoprotein cholesterol, higher total and low-density lipoprotein cholesterol, and higher triglyceride concentrations than in more active persons with SCI and sedentary and active AB individuals (19,21–23). Since activity level and cardiopulmonary fitness of those with SCI appear to be related to CHD risk factors as in the AB population, upper-body exercise training may improve the health status and reduce CHD risk of persons with SCI just as leg exercise training benefits AB individuals.

PULMONARY SYSTEM

In persons with cervical lesions below C4, motor innervation of the diaphragm and sternocleidomastoid muscle is intact, and they can breathe independently. The loss of innervation of respiratory muscles depends on the level and completeness of the lesion and induces another, probably less efficient, breathing pattern in individuals with complete and incomplete lesions. With tetraplegia, the lung volume is changed. In particular, the vital capacity is decreased (24,25), most likely because of decreased expiratory reserve capacity and increased residual volume (24,26). The maximal expiratory flow is also decreased (24). Paralysis of the intercostal muscles results in changes in the mechanics of the lungs and thorax, such as reduced lung compliance and a strong restrictive ventilatory impairment (25). With tetraplegia, inspiratory force is about 60% of that in age-matched AB subjects (27). The efficiency of the unaffected muscles may be decreased because of instability of the chest wall and an inactive lifestyle (27). The respiratory muscle dysfunction in individuals with tetraplegia can be described as "muscle weakness" (low maximal strength) and as "muscle fatigue" (low endurance capacity) of the respiratory muscles. Both appear to be significantly lower in individuals with tetraplegia than in AB individuals (28).

Training of inspiratory muscles may be an important addition to the treatment of persons with tetraplegia to improve performance in exercise and daily activities as well as to improve quality of life by preventing pulmonary/respiratory infections.

SCI and Exercise

To enhance physical fitness and health status and to prevent secondary complications of SCI, participation in exercise on a regular basis is recommended; this will be either arm exercise, ES-assisted leg cycling exercise (ES-LCE) or a combination of both.

ARM EXERCISE

The three major modes of arm exercise are arm cranking, wheelchair propulsion, and hand biking. There are differences in efficiency and muscle function among the three modes of arm exercise. In general, dynamic arm exercise has a lower efficiency than dynamic leg exercise (e.g., biking; 7–13 vs. 18–23%). Maximal oxygen intake ($\dot{V}O_{2max}$) during arm exercise is about 70% of that during cycling exercise with the legs in the AB population (29).

RESPONSES TO SUBMAXIMAL ARM EXERCISE

The appropriate circulatory adjustment during exercise in AB subjects is regulated by the central nervous system (autonomic nervous system and reflex mechanisms) and by local mechanisms and humoral influences. The redistribution of blood during arm exercise in individuals with SCI is impaired because of a lack of sympathetic vasoconstriction below the lesion and a loss of motor innervation of the leg muscles, resulting in muscle pump inactivity (30,31). This causes an inability to redistribute blood below the lesion and, consequently, a lower increase in mean systemic and ventricular filling pressure during arm exercise in SCI than in AB subjects (Fig. 13-1). According to the Frank-Starling mechanism, the lower ventricular filling pressure will cause the myocardium to contract on a less efficient part of the ventricular function curve. As a result, stroke volume (SV) is lower in individuals with SCI than in AB controls, who have an effective redistribution of blood.

The lower SV in persons with paraplegia is compensated by an increase in heart rate (HR). Responsibility for this compensatory mechanism may stem from the sympathetic innervation of the heart and humoral influences (32). Consequently, cardiac output, or $\dot{Q}$, (the product of HR and SV) is similar to that in AB subjects at a given submaximal $\dot{V}O_2$. Individuals with high thoracic SCI (>T6) or cervical spinal cord lesions have a disturbed sympathetic innervation of the heart and the increase in HR is limited to a maximum of about 120 to 130 beats·min^{-1} (based on vagal withdrawal).

RESPONSES TO MAXIMAL ARM EXERCISE

In spite of the observed compensatory tachycardia, the lower SV in individuals with paraplegia limits the augmentation of $\dot{Q}$ during maximal exercise. Consequently, the insufficient muscle blood flow leads to an early onset of peripheral fatigue as a result of limited oxygen supply, and maximal performance is reduced. As a consequence of the loss of motor innervation below the SCI lesion, the smaller active muscle mass during arm exercise may also reduce $\dot{V}O_{2max}$ in comparison with that seen in AB subjects, who use trunk and leg muscles for stabilization during arm exercise and as a fulcrum from which to push. In addition, the limited active muscle mass associated with SCI may restrict the cardiovascular load, the intrinsic cardiac adaptations

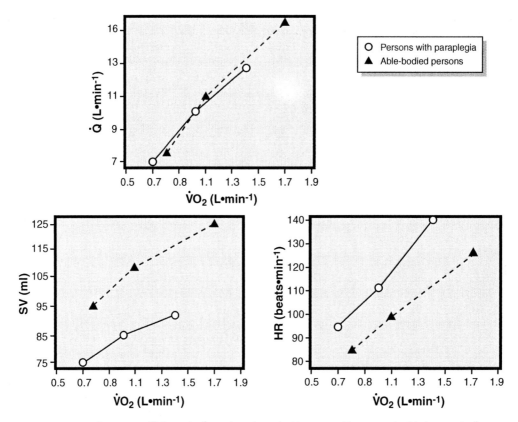

FIGURE 13-1 Cardiac output ($\dot{Q}$) in L·min^{-1}, stroke volume (SV) in mL, and heart rate (HR) in beats·min^{-1} versus oxygen uptake ($\dot{V}O_2$) in L·min^{-1} during submaximal arm exercise in persons with paraplegia and able-bodied persons. (Redrawn from Coutts KD, Rhodes EC, McKenzie DC. Maximal exercise responses of tetraplegics and paraplegics. J Appl Physiol 1983;55:479–482.)

to exercise, and the absolute fitness level that may be achieved through exercise training; these factors produce a lower maximal performance than that found in similarly trained AB subjects (33–35).

As a result of the gained insight in the circulatory problems caused by paraplegia, researchers have tried to find a way to support the redistribution of blood and to improve circulatory adjustment to physical performance. A study by Hopman et al. (36) found no increase in $\dot{V}O_{2peak}$, or peak performance, using several conditions to improve the blood redistribution during arm exercise (simulation of the leg muscle pump by ES of the leg muscles, applying counterpressure to the legs and abdomen by an anti-G suit, and exercising in the supine position to promote venous return). This suggests that the limitation in $\dot{V}O_{2peak}$ in this pop-

ulation is located peripherally (i.e., the small muscle mass and the metabolic machinery within the muscle) rather than centrally (oxygen supply). It cannot be ruled out that training with one of these supportive devices may benefit the fitness status of SCI individuals.

SPECIFIC CONSIDERATIONS

The higher the level and more complete the SCI, the more widespread is the loss of somatic and autonomic nervous system function. The more skeletal muscles that are paralyzed, the lower will be the functional independence and the ability to perform voluntary exercise at metabolic rates high enough to stimulate the cardiopulmonary system and, subsequently, the lower will be the cardiopulmonary fitness level that may be achieved through exercise training. In individuals with higher-level SCI, paralysis of the intercostal muscles can severely limit pulmonary ventilation, which further reduces exercise capability and leads to secondary pulmonary problems.

The active arm muscles are fatigued quickly because of their relatively small mass, a potentially inadequate blood flow, a limited aerobic energy supply, and a greater component of anaerobic energy supply with the accumulation of metabolites in the muscles (37). The early fatigue of the arm muscles during both wheelchair locomotion and exercise training can discourage many wheelchair users from leading active lives. Unfortunately, a sedentary lifestyle leads to a further decrement in physical fitness and even greater reduction of functional capability. Aging further decreases cardiovascular, pulmonary, and muscular function, which can eventually lead to a loss of independence and an increase in medical complications. An active lifestyle that incorporates specific exercise training and/or sports programs is needed to break this debilitating cycle of sedentary lifestyle and loss of fitness and to enhance functional independence and quality of life.

RESPONSES TO ELECTRICAL STIMULATION-INDUCED EXERCISE

Using paralyzed lower-limb muscles to exercise could alleviate some of the problems discussed above (i.e., small active muscle mass) and may improve rehabilitation. During the past two decades, ES has been used increasingly to induce exercise in paralyzed lower-limb muscles. Typically, electrical pulses from a stimulator are used in conjunction with skin surface electrodes placed over motor points to induce tetanic contractions of controlled intensity. Therefore, ES-LCE can potentially use a large muscle mass that otherwise would be dormant. In addition, this exercise augments the circulation by activating the skeletal muscle pump and increasing metabolic demand. Thus ES-exercise modes can often improve the health and fitness of persons with SCI to levels often higher than can be attained with arm exercise alone. Persons with tetraplegia will most likely find this induced exercise mode particularly advantageous because

of the small muscle mass that is under voluntary control.

Another important advantage of ES-LCE is that central hemodynamic responses are superior to those for voluntary arm exercise. For example, Figoni et al. (38) found significantly higher SV (92 vs. 58 mL·beat^{-1}) at the same $\dot{V}O_2$ of 1 L·min^{-1} for 6 men with tetraplegia performing ES-LCE and arm-cranking exercise. A probable mechanism for these responses is that ES-LCE activated the skeletal muscle pump and enhanced venous return, increasing cardiac preload and subsequently SV. Figoni et al. (38) found a 25% lower HR and a 19% lower rate–pressure product (HR × systolic blood pressure [SBP]) during ES-LCE, suggesting that the higher cardiac volume load was achieved with lower myocardial $\dot{V}O_2$. Therefore, ES-LCE is potentially more effective than arm cranking for cardiopulmonary training of individuals with tetraplegia and has a lower cardiovascular risk.

RESPONSES TO COMBINED ARM AND LEG EXERCISE

Various upper-extremity activities provide those with SCI the opportunity to engage in purposeful exercise programming that improves overall fitness. However, exercise movements using the arms allow significantly less work effort than those involving the legs. ES-LCE is used in rehabilitation centers to improve physical fitness of SCI individuals and produces beneficial peripheral adaptations such as increased lower-extremity muscle mass and circulation. As a combined exercise (arm cranking and ES-LCE are performed concurrently), there is a larger active muscle mass, which in turn elicits greater cardiorespiratory demands. In addition, the simulation of the muscle pump by ES-LCE improves venous return, which may improve circulation to both upper- and lower-body muscles. Hooker et al. (39) found greater increases in $\dot{V}O_2$, HR, SV, and $\dot{Q}$ during the combination of arm and ES-LCE than with arm exercise alone in persons with tetraplegia. Raymond et al. (40) demonstrated that during submaximal and maximal exercise, a greater metabolic stress was elicited during combined arm and leg exercise than during arm exercise alone. They showed that SV was higher during combined arm and leg exercise than with arm exercise alone and that HR did not differ between the two modes of exercise. From this, they concluded that blood redistribution had improved and that venous return had increased. They speculated that arm and leg exercise combined may improve aerobic fitness in persons with SCI more effectively than either of the two alone.

SCI and Exercise Testing

Exercise testing enables assessment of cardiopulmonary fitness by evaluating exercise capacity and metabolic and cardiopulmonary responses. In AB individuals, leg exercise (treadmill walking/running or leg cycle ergometry) is typically used for stress testing, and the large muscle mass contracting rhythmically stimulates maximal metabolic and cardiopulmonary responses for valid functional evaluation of these systems. The primary factors that restrict maximal power output (PO) and $\dot{V}O_{2max}$ during leg exercise are associated with the central circulation, which limits the delivery of sufficient oxygen to the large exercising muscle mass (41). In contrast, upper-body exercise (arm-crank and wheelchair exercise) activates a relatively small muscle mass. The primary limiting factors may be peripheral, and local fatigue of the heavily stressed arm musculature can occur rapidly despite the delivery of sufficient blood and oxygen (42). Because of the lower PO capability and the early onset of fatigue, arm exercise may not provide sufficient stimulus to drive the metabolic and cardiopulmonary systems to full output, making valid functional evaluation of these systems difficult. Since the highest level of $\dot{V}O_2$ that can be obtained for maximal effort arm exercise is somewhat lower than the true physiologic maximum expected for leg exercise in AB individuals, the term $\dot{V}O_{2peak}$, rather than $\dot{V}O_{2max}$, is typically used.

ARM EXERCISE TESTING

Clinical exercise testing of wheelchair users with SCI typically involves arm-crank ergometers (ACEs) since they are commercially available and the exercise intensity can be accurately set to desired levels. Wheelchair ergometers (WERGs), which are stationary devices that enable close simulation of wheelchair locomotion, are also used (43,44). So-

phisticated WERGs that have been custom designed and constructed for exercise physiology and biomechanical research studies permit precise measurement of various operational torques, forces, and velocity for determining PO and propulsion characteristics (45). Although excellent for their intended purposes, these WERGs have drawbacks: they are relatively unavailable, are expensive to construct, and do not allow the use of one's own wheelchair. However, another type of WERG that may be advantageous consists of a person's own wheelchair mounted on a commercially available roller system. Setting exercise intensity accurately requires a roller system that enables measurement of propulsive force and velocity. Another mode that can be useful for exercise testing and training is operating a wheelchair on a motor-driven treadmill (46,47). Exercise intensity can be regulated by adjusting velocity and grade or by applying additional resistive force via a pulley system (46). This system enables better simulation of actual wheelchair locomotion, but is not practical for most wheelchair users.

Sawka et al. (48) compared WERG to ACE exercise at the same *submaximal* PO levels and found that WERG exercise generally elicited a higher $\dot{V}O_2$, respiratory minute volume, $\dot{Q}$, SV, SBP, and HR. Other studies found that *maximal* effort WERG and ACE exercise elicited a similar $\dot{V}O_{2peak}$, but a significantly lower maximal PO for WERG exercise (49,50). Because of similar maximal aerobic metabolic rates, it appears that both WERG and ACE will yield similar results for exercise testing of wheelchair users. However, the concept of "exercise specificity" suggests that WERG exercise may be more appropriate for individuals who propel their wheelchairs for sporting events or when wheelchair locomotion capability needs to be assessed, since it more closely resembles actual wheelchair locomotion. The lower metabolic rate and cardiopulmonary responses found for submaximal ACE exercise, as well as the greater maximal PO achieved, suggest that arm cranking may be superior to hand-rim stroking as a means of wheelchair locomotion. Indeed, Smith et al. (51) found a significantly lower $\dot{V}O_2$ (−32%) and HR (−19%) when operating an arm crank-propelled wheelchair than with hand-rim propulsion under the same locomotive conditions; this has been confirmed by additional studies (50,52). Recently, hand biking has become popular among wheelchair users, mainly for sports. Arm-cranking exercise tests may be most appropriate to assess their exercise capacity (53).

TESTING PROTOCOLS: ARM EXERCISE

The fundamental principles followed for lower-body exercise testing of AB individuals may be used for upper-body exercise testing of individuals with SCI. Tests are usually progressive in exercise intensity and have well-defined *submaximal* or *maximal* effort endpoint criteria. Either a *continuous* or *discontinuous* protocol may be used. Discontinuous submaximal protocols are preferable for stress testing individuals with SCI, since they are relatively safe and comfortable. A suitable protocol would be to have exercise bouts that are 4 to 6 min in duration, separated by 5 to 10 min of rest. For WERG and ACE tests, velocity is typically held constant (e.g., a wheel velocity of 3 $km \cdot h^{-1}$ and a crank rate of 50 rpm, respectively) while the resistance increases during the test. With WERG, 5 W appears to be an appropriate initial PO, as it is frequently encountered during daily wheelchair locomotion. Increments of 5 to 10 W are appropriate for SCI individuals, and PO can be limited to 25 to 35 W for submaximal tests (43,54). For ACE, submaximal PO levels vary from 20 to 80 W, depending on fitness status and lesion level. Steady-state (submaximal) physiologic responses can be determined during the last minute of each 4- to 6-min exercise bout. Criteria for maximal exercise test termination include *(a)* voluntary cessation, *(b)* symptoms of cardiovascular or pulmonary abnormalities (e.g., chest discomfort, inappropriate ECG changes, marked hypertension or hypotension, dyspnea), *(c)* achievement of the maximal PO level required for the test, and *(d)* attainment of a predetermined HR. However, for individuals with high-level SCI, the HR criterion may be less useful because of the interruption of sympathetic pathways to the heart and limited ability for cardioacceleration.

Peak PO and $\dot{V}O_{2peak}$ may be predicted from the submaximal data by extrapolating them to the estimated maximal HR levels. In AB individuals, maximal HR during leg exercise is often estimated by use of the formula 220 minus age. However, this method would be less valid for those who have high-level SCI, since their cardioacceleratory mechanism can be markedly impaired. In addition, the maximal HR achieved for arm exercise may be 10 to 20 $beats \cdot min^{-1}$ lower than that for leg exercise (as found in AB individuals), because of the smaller active muscle mass. Thus, values obtained by use of the formula 220 $beats \cdot min^{-1}$ minus age to estimate maximal HR may need to be reduced by 10 to 20 $beats \cdot min^{-1}$ for WERG and ACE exercise (48,55).

For accurate determination of peak metabolic and cardiopulmonary data, maximal exercise testing should be conducted. For this, the discontinuous submaximal test can be extended to maximal effort by increasing the number of exercise bouts. Drawbacks to this protocol are that much time is required to complete the test and the multiple bouts of exercise could lead to fatigue and underestimation of peak PO and $\dot{V}O_{2peak}$. Therefore, if maximal testing is desired and submaximal data are not needed, a continuous, maximal exercise protocol can be used. This shorter protocol begins at a low-to-moderate PO as a warm-up, and PO increases every 1 to 2 min until maximal effort is reached (56,57). With ACE, PO increments can vary from 3 to 5 W for individuals with tetraplegia up to 10 W for individuals with paraplegia, with typical maximal PO levels varying from 30 to 50 W for persons with tetraplegia up to 150 W for well-trained individuals with paraplegia.

Exercise testing fitness criteria are based upon the magnitudes of metabolic and cardiopulmonary responses elicited at given PO levels, as well as the maximal PO achieved. At given submaximal POs, well-trained and fit individuals typically exhibit lower HR and ventilation responses, indicating greater cardiopulmonary fitness, lower relative stress, and more functional reserve. In individuals with high-level SCI, however, care must be taken not to interpret the low exercise HR responses as an indication of superior cardiovascular fitness. As indicated above, cardioacceleration in these individuals is limited by insufficient sympathetic stimulation, and most observed increases in HR are due to vagal withdrawal. Nevertheless, HR can still be used to indicate fitness in this population when expressed as a percentage of HR reserve (i.e., the functional range between resting and maximal HR) (58). At maximal exercise, peak values for PO, $\dot{V}O_2$, pulmonary ventilation, $\dot{Q}$, and SV would be expected to be higher for fit individuals. Therefore, more fit

TABLE 13-1 SUGGESTED PROTOCOLS FOR ARM-EXERCISE TESTING, SUBMAXIMAL TESTS, AND MAXIMAL TESTS, USING ARM-CRANKING EXERCISE (ACE AT 50–60 rpm) AND WHEELCHAIR ERGOMETRY (WERG AT 3 km/h)

	Paraplegia	Tetraplegia
ACE Submaximal	Exercise for 4–6 min at levels between 20 and 80 W	Exercise for 4–6 min at levels between 5 and 40 W
ACE Maximal	Starting between 0–10 W, increment 10 W every min	Starting between 0 and 5 W, increment 3–5 W every min depending on level and completeness of the lesion and fitness status of the subject
WERG Submaximal	Exercise for 4–6 min at 25–35 W	Exercise for 4–6 min at levels between 5 and 25 W
WERG Maximal	Starting at 5 W, with increments of 10 W per min	Starting at 0–5 W, with increments of 5 W per min

individuals would have greater metabolic and cardiopulmonary reserve, and given submaximal tasks would be less stressful since they are performed at a lower percentage of peak $\dot{V}O_2$. See Table 13-1 for an overview of testing protocols.

To provide normative values, Janssen et al. (59) reanalyzed data from five studies in which SCI individuals performed maximal exercise on a wheelchair ergometer or with the wheelchair on a treadmill. Ranges in physical capacity parameters were extensive, and normative values for individuals with tetraplegia and paraplegia were established and are shown in Table 13.2.

SPECIAL CONSIDERATIONS

A problem in studying physiologic and circulatory responses during arm exercise in persons with SCI is the great variety in spinal cord lesions with respect to level and completeness. This results in heterogeneity in physiologic and functional behavior. Generally, the higher the level and extent of the SCI, the greater the concomitant autonomic and sensomotor dysfunction. An important level is the sixth thoracic vertebra. Persons with spinal cord lesions between the first and the sixth thoracic vertebrae may have disturbed cardiac sympathetic innervation. Parasympathetic innervation will not be disturbed (vagal nerve) and may even overrule. This will have consequences for HR during rest and exercise (i.e., cardioacceleration depends largely on withdrawal of vagal tone), resulting in low HRs.

Persons with lesions below the sixth thoracic vertebra will have intact sympathetic innervation to the heart, but the sympathetic innervation to the splanchnic and renal areas may still be missing, depending on the level of the lesion. The splanchnic vascular bed plays an important role in redistributing blood during exercise. Renal innervation may be important for hormonal control of the circulation during exercise.

An important technical limitation during arm exercise is the ability to assess blood pressure by the standard cuff method in an exercising arm. Generally, measurements are obtained during short breaks or immediately after cessation of exercise. The validity of these measurements, however, is doubtful. There is a need for alternative methods to measure blood pressure during arm exercise by persons with SCI, since this provides important additional information on their hemodynamics.

ES-INDUCED LEG-EXERCISE TESTING

The two most commonly used ES-induced leg-exercise modes in individuals with SCI are resistance exercise and endurance exercise. Most research on ES resistance exercise has been directed toward the paralyzed quadriceps muscles because of their responsiveness to ES, proportional increase in force output with increasing ES current, and relative ease of exercise implementation. However, this ES technique can be adapted to provide resistance exercise for other paralyzed/weakened

TABLE 13-2   PHYSICAL CAPACITY NORMS FOR MEN WITH TETRAPLEGIA (TP) AND PARAPLEGIA (PP) DURING ARM EXERCISE IN A WHEELCHAIR (INCLUDING THOSE WITH INCOMPLETE LESIONS)

Variable		Classification[a]				
		Poor	Fair	Average	Good	Excellent
$\dot{V}O_{2peak}$ (L·min^{-1})	TP	<0.51	0.52–0.79	0.80–0.96	0.97–1.19	>1.19
	PP	<1.33	1.34–1.72	1.73–2.00	2.01–2.31	>2.31
$\dot{V}O_{2peak}$ (mL·kg^{-1}·min^{-1})	TP	<7.60	7.61–10.00	10.01–13.39	13.40–16.94	>16.94
	PP	<16.50	16.51–22.70	22.71–29.20	29.21–34.35	>34.35
PO_{max} (W)	TP	<11.6	11.6–20.0	20.1–26.8	26.8–37.5	>37.5
	PP	<52.7	52.8–70.4	70.5–82.1	82.2–97.8	>97.8
PO_{max} (W·kg^{-1})	TP	<0.14	0.15–0.26	0.27–0.34	0.35–0.44	>0.44
	PP	<0.69	0.70–0.92	0.93–1.13	1.14–1.42	>1.42
P_{30} (W)	TP	<18.7	18.8–25.4	25.5–39.1	39.2–68.4	>68.4
	PP	<75.0	75.0–92.9	93.0–114.1	114.2–133.4	>133.4
P_{30} (W·kg^{-1})	TP	<0.25	0.25–0.33	0.34–0.54	0.55–0.93	>0.93
	PP	<1.05	1.05–1.22	1.23–1.58	1.59–1.85	>1.85
F_{iso} (N)	TP	<60.3	60.3–105.6	105.7–119.4	119.5–185.0	>185.0
	PP	<158.5	158.5–206.9	207.0–258.5	258.6–290.1	>290.1
F_{iso} (N·kg^{-1})	TP	<0.87	0.87–1.27	1.28–1.65	1.66–2.48	>2.48
	PP	<2.14	2.14–2.61	2.62–3.41	3.42–3.84	>3.84

From Janssen TWJ, Dallmeijer AJ, Veeger DJ, et al. Normative values and determinants of physical capacity in individuals with spinal cord injury. J Rehabil Res Dev 2002;39:29–39.

P_{30}, mean power output during 30 sec all-out sprinting; F_{iso}, isometric arm extension strength; N, Newton.

[a]Classification based on percentiles: Poor (<20%), Fair (20–40%), Average (40–60%), Good (60–80%), Excellent (>80%).

muscles. For endurance exercise, a leg cycle ergometer (LCE) was developed in 1982 (60). Computer-controlled ES is used to induce contractions of the paralyzed quadriceps, hamstring, and gluteal muscle groups during proper angle ranges of the pedals to maintain smooth cycling. To control the cyclic ES pattern and current intensity, a microprocessor receives pedal position and velocity feedback information from sensors. As muscle fatigue progresses during exercise, ES current intensity automatically increases to a maximum of about 140 mA to recruit nonfatigued muscle fibers to try to maintain 50 rpm. When maximal current is reached and additional muscle fiber recruitment is no longer possible, the pedaling rate declines and ultimately falls below 35 rpm, at which time exercise is automatically terminated. Peak cardiopulmonary variables can be measured during the last stage of stimulation.

The primary requirement for using ES is that the muscles to be exercised are paralyzed because of upper motor neuron damage and that the motor units are intact and functional. The existence of stretch reflex activity and spasticity indicates which individuals are potential candidates for ES exercise. However, if they retain some sensate skin, ES may cause discomfort or pain, and the high stimulation current that is required to induce forceful contractions may not be tolerated. Prior to an ES-exercise testing or program, a thorough medical examination is essential, including x-rays of the paralyzed limbs, range-of-motion testing, neurologic examination, and an ECG.

Since the muscles, bones, and joints of the paralyzed lower limbs tend to deteriorate, ES-induced contractions should be kept as smooth as possible, and the contraction force generated should be limited to a safe level to prevent injury. In individuals with lesions at or above T6, ES exercise may provoke autonomic dysreflexia, with episodic dangerously high blood pressure. Therefore, blood pressure must be monitored periodically, especially during the initial ES-exercise testing sessions. Such exercise should be discontinued immediately if any response is observed that places the individual at risk.

SCI and Exercise Training

Normal daily wheelchair activity may not provide sufficient exercise to train the muscular and cardiopulmonary systems and make supplemental exercise training necessary to improve physical fitness (61,62). Such training programs can increase cardiopulmonary fitness and reserve capability and make activities of daily living (e.g., wheelchair locomotion and making transfers) less stressful, since they would be performed at lower percentages of maximal PO, $\dot{V}O_{2peak}$, and HR reserve (63,64). This could possibly contribute to improved functional independence and rehabilitation outcome. In a 3-year study, Janssen et al. (64) demonstrated that a decline of only 5 to 10 W in PO capability of sedentary wheelchair users with tetraplegia could result in a loss of independence. In contrast, cohorts who regularly participated in sports activities and increased their physical fitness generally maintained their independence and performed daily activities with less stress. Thus, regular exercise training may reduce the stresses of wheelchair locomotion and those of other daily life activities, retard the decline in physical capability that typically accompanies aging, and lower some of the risks associated with secondary cardiovascular disabilities.

ARM-EXERCISE TRAINING

To promote muscular and cardiopulmonary fitness and to enhance performance, arm exercise training for wheelchair users with SCI should follow the principles of overload and specificity that AB persons do. The reader should see Chapters 2 and 3 for general information.

Arm-exercise training protocols may be continuous or discontinuous. If enhanced cardiopulmonary fitness is the primary goal, PO should be adjusted to allow moderate levels of exercise for relatively long durations (15–60 min for continuous bouts and 3–10 min for each of several discontinuous bouts) without excessive fatigue or respiratory distress. Exercise should be done two to five times per week. Traditionally, ACE exercise has been used for

endurance training of wheelchair users with SCI. This exercise mode is readily available and improves cardiopulmonary fitness (65,66). Although WERG exercise elicits similar peak metabolic and cardiopulmonary responses, it has the advantage of more closely resembling actual wheelchair activity and may better enhance wheelchair locomotive performance. If enhancing muscular power is the primary goal, higher POs should be used, and exercise bouts should be shorter (e.g., a few seconds to a few minutes). The large anaerobic energy component causes a marked accumulation of blood lactate. This form of exercise is useful for wheelchair athletes who want to improve sprinting performance and for most other wheelchair users, since many daily life activities (e.g., transfers, overcoming architectural barriers) require intense, short-duration efforts.

When developing an aerobic arm-exercise training protocol for individuals with SCI, an effective training intensity may be more difficult to set and one must know the HR during peak exercise. The HR response expressed either as a percentage of HR reserve or maximal HR can be a useful indicator of exercise stress in the SCI population, but the actual value used would depend on the exercise response characteristics of the individual (67,68). Therefore, to set arm-exercise intensity for various individuals with SCI, direct determination of peak values for HR, PO, $\dot{V}O_2$, ventilation, and blood lactate concentration (during exercise testing) is desirable. In individuals who do not exhibit a clear relationship among these variables (which is more common in those with tetraplegia), training at a percentage of maximal PO may be preferable (69). When laboratory testing is not available, intensity criteria may be established according to the subjective rating of perceived exertion (e.g., the Borg scale) and the actual exercise endurance capability. In most cases, several trials will be needed for each individual to set training intensity effectively. See Table 13.3 for suggested training protocols.

ES-INDUCED LEG CYCLE TRAINING

ES-exercise training can be applied in a functional way (walking or cycling) or as a form of resistance training. Individuals should be informed of the potential benefits and risks of ES-exercise training and clearly understand that ES *will not* regenerate damaged neurons or cure paralysis. As with voluntary

TABLE 13-3   SUGGESTED AEROBIC TRAINING PROTOCOLS FOR CONTINUOUS ARM-EXERCISE TRAINING (15–60 MIN) OR DISCONTINUOUS ARM-EXERCISE TRAINING (3–10 MIN EACH BOUT) PERFORMED TWO TO FIVE TIMES A WEEK

	Paraplegia	Tetraplegia
ACE/Hand biking	• Between 60 and 90% of the HR reserve • Subjectively, Borg scale (1–10), between 6 and 9	• Between 60 and 90% of the HR reserve • Between 50 and 90% of the maximal PO achieved • Subjectively, Borg scale (1–10), between 6 and 9.
WERG	• Between 60 and 90% of the HR reserve • Subjectively, Borg scale (1–10), between 6 and 9.	• Between 60 and 90% of the HR reserve • Between 50 and 90% of the maximal PO achieved • Subjectively, Borg scale (1–10), between 6 and 9

exercise training, it should also be understood that any health and fitness benefits derived from ES-exercise training will be lost several weeks after this activity is discontinued. Results discussed below are mainly based on studies using ES-LCE. Studies indicate that ES-LCE elicits relatively high aerobic metabolic and cardiopulmonary responses as well as favorable central and peripheral hemodynamic responses from individuals with SCI (70–72). ES-LCE offers individuals with SCI a potential tool for training at an aerobic metabolic rate similar to that with jogging, but they would have to be highly trained in ES-LCE to achieve such high metabolic responses for long durations. Most individuals with SCI perform ES-LCE at metabolic levels equivalent to walking ($\dot{V}O_2 \sim 1$ L·min^{-1}). This can be quite beneficial for those with tetraplegia, as this rate is higher than most can achieve with arm exercise (59).

Adaptations to Training in SCI

PHYSIOLOGIC ADAPTATIONS TO ARM-EXERCISE TRAINING

Studies on individuals with SCI indicate that endurance-type arm-exercise training markedly increases PO capability, $\dot{V}O_{2peak}$, and cardiopulmonary performance by 10 to 20% within 7 to 20 weeks (73–75). Using WERG exercise, Miles et al. (76) reported that eight wheelchair athletes increased their maximal PO by 31%, $\dot{V}O_{2peak}$ by 26%, and peak respiratory minute volume by 32%

after 6 weeks of interval training, three times per week. These gains were even more remarkable considering that the athletic subjects had relatively high levels of fitness before training.

Although arm-exercise training limits the absolute level of aerobic fitness that can be achieved, some cardiopulmonary benefits can be expected for most persons, depending on the initial fitness level and the size of the muscle mass available for exercise. Many of the observed gains in arm-exercise performance are due to peripheral adaptations such as improved capillary density and/or metabolic capability within muscles, but central circulatory adaptations cannot be ruled out. Nevertheless, regular arm-exercise training appears to increase maximal PO and $\dot{V}O_{2peak}$ and may also decrease levels of physiologic responses for given submaximal exercise tasks and daily life, including wheelchair locomotion (64,77).

Habitual arm exercise training and sports participation may also reduce the risk for acquiring CHD. Cross-sectional studies on sedentary and physically active wheelchair users showed that the more active individuals had better blood lipid profiles, as indicated by a lower total cholesterol level, a lower low-density lipoprotein-cholesterol level, and a higher high-density lipoprotein-cholesterol level (21,22,78).

ADAPTATIONS TO ES-LCE TRAINING

Studies on ES-LCE exercise training have demonstrated several physiologic adaptations that probably reflect both peripheral (skeletal muscle) and cardiopulmonary benefits. Generally, significant improvements in exercise performance and in peak $\dot{V}O_2$ and SV are seen after 1.5 to 6 months of ES-LCE training (71,72,79). Improved cardiopulmonary fitness resulting from ES-LCE training was also indicated by better responses during submaximal exercise and at rest. Under resting conditions, an increase in SBP, HR, and cardiac index was found in individuals with tetraplegia after ES-LCE training; this helped them to alleviate their chronic hypotension and improve cardiovascular stability (80,81). In contrast, beneficial *reductions* in resting blood pressure and HR are commonly found in those with paraplegia (80). For a given submaximal $\dot{V}O_2$ or PO, improved responses such as lower HR, blood lactate concentration, and arterial blood pressure, as well as faster $\dot{V}O_2$ kinetics, were found (80,82). Like those typically obtained for AB individuals, these responses suggest that oxygen delivery to the muscle improved and/or the aerobic capacity of the muscles was enhanced as result of ES-LCE training. Gains in cardiopulmonary fitness may ultimately translate into reduced risk for cardiopulmonary complications, as well as less stressful performance of daily life tasks.

ES-LCE training elicits hypertrophy of the skeletal muscles used, as indicated by increased thigh circumference and quadriceps muscle area (83,84). In addition, Baldi et al. (85) found that ES-LCE exercise training prevented the occurrence of gluteal muscle atrophy seen in a nonexercising control group during the first 6 months postinjury. Moreover, possibly due to advantageous central hemodynamic responses, ES-LCE can also result in a (partial) reversal of the commonly found cardiac atrophy in individuals with tetraplegia (81,86). Thus, ES-LCE exercise training appears to have a marked effect on reversing the disuse atrophy of paralyzed skeletal muscles (or retarding its rate of progression) and on reversing cardiac atrophy.

Not only muscle atrophy, but also the atrophy of the vascular system commonly seen in individuals with SCI below the level of the lesion can be counteracted by ES-LCE (10,87,88). Several investigators report an increase in the diameter of the femoral artery, increased lower-limb blood flow, or increased capillarization after ES-LCE training. Recently, Gerrits et al. (88) demonstrated that even after 6 weeks of ES-LCE training, the diameter significantly increased by 10 to 15%; this coincided with an approximately 40% increase in resting arterial inflow. Clearly, vascular properties of the paralyzed lower limbs of persons with SCI can change very soon after the start of ES leg training. These adaptations most likely result from increased oxygen demand in the previously inactive muscles.

PRESSURE SORES

Skin-related secondary disabilities, especially pressure sores, are a common problem for individuals with SCI, resulting in great discomfort and significant medical care costs. Individuals with SCI are at increased risk for pressure sores because of such factors as reduced mobility, reduced microcirculation, impaired sympathetic function, and atrophy of the paralyzed muscles. In addition, due to impaired sensation, individuals are often not aware of the necessity to relieve pressure. Theoretically, ES-induced exercise can assist in pressure-sore risk reduction, since it has been shown to increase muscle mass, capillary density, and skin and muscle blood flow (see above). Since ES-LCE exercise involves induced contractions of the gluteal muscles, this activity may be especially effective for reducing pressure sore risk. Although not confirmed by controlled experimental studies, Petrofsky (89) reported that the incidence of pressure sores was reduced by 90% in a group of individuals with SCI participating in a 2-year ES-exercise program.

Special Considerations for SCI and Exercise

EXERCISE AND THERMAL STRESS

During prolonged exercise and heat stress, an extra load is added to the circulatory system. The temperature and cardiovascular regulating systems have to adjust to extra endogenous and exogenous heating to maintain a constant internal body temperature. This results in increased blood flow to the active muscles for oxygen supply and increased skin blood flow for heat transport and heat loss. The enhanced skin blood flow may result in blood volume displacement into cutaneous veins, which may lower cardiac filling pressure and SV. For SCI individuals with an impaired redistribution of blood during exercise, heat stress imposes an extra stress on the already affected circulatory system.

To prevent hyperthermia or hypothermia, careful consideration should be given to ambient temperature, relative humidity, and clothing worn, as well as to exercise intensity and duration. Many individuals with SCI have a limited thermoregulatory capacity due to inadequate sweat secretion and impaired vasoregulation, so that overheating occurs more easily than in the AB population (90,91). This is especially true in a hot, humid environment in which prolonged strenuous exercise can cause severe dehydration, dangerously elevated body temperature, and possibly heat stroke and circulatory collapse. Under these conditions, frequent and adequate fluid replacement is essential. Exercise in cold environments may result in excessive heat loss, also exacerbated by impaired cardiovascular system control. If there are symptoms of hyperthermia or hypothermia, exercise should be discontinued, and clothing and environmental conditions should be appropriately adjusted.

AUTONOMIC DYSREFLEXIA

Occasionally, some individuals with high-level SCI exhibit a sudden and inappropriate episode of extreme hypertension due to autonomic dysreflexia, caused by loss of central control (i.e., inhibition) of sympathetic spinal reflexes and a subsequent exaggerated sympathetic response to noxious stimuli such as skin trauma, bowel impaction, and bladder overdistension. This situation is quite hazardous and can be fatal if not corrected in a timely manner (92). To help avoid this condition, those with SCI should follow proper health practices to eliminate noxious stimuli and to seek medical treatment when appropriate. The bladder should be emptied just prior to exercise and during prolonged exercise bouts, and blood pressure should be monitored at regular intervals (at least during initial exercise sessions). Exercise should be discontinued immediately if there are adverse reactions, and appropriate action taken to alleviate the problem (tilting up for hypertension and reclining for hypotension and syncope).

Summary

In summary, individuals with SCI experience a wheelchair-bound lifestyle, and their daily life is often composed of dramatically low levels of activity, leading to varying degrees of physical deconditioning. For these individuals, performing exercise on a regular basis is of the highest importance. Several aspects should be considered for testing and training of individuals with SCI:

- SCI individuals experience disturbed blood redistribution during exercise because of lack of sympathetically induced vasoconstriction and leg muscle pump activity. The most important practical implications are a low SV and a compensatory high HR during exercise.
- Individuals with lesion levels above T6 depend almost entirely on vagal withdrawal for their increase in HR during exercise, which limits peak HR to about 130 beats·min^{-1}. Therefore, training intensities should be expressed as HR reserve.
- Arm exercise, the most commonly used mode of exercise for testing and training SCI individuals, activates only a small muscle mass, which limits the cardiopulmonary load. A good alternative (or addition) is ES-induced leg exercise. The latter has the advantage of activating a larger muscle mass and inducing both central and peripheral training effects.
- As with voluntary exercise training in AB individuals, duration, frequency, and intensity are the most important determinants for training outcome in SCI. Moreover, any health and fitness benefits derived from ES or arm-exercise training in SCI will be lost several weeks after this activity is discontinued.
- SCI individuals have a limited thermoregulatory capacity because of inadequate sweat secretion and impaired vasoregulation. Therefore, overheating occurs more rapidly.

REFERENCES

1. Burnham R, Martin T, Stein R, et al. Skeletal muscle fibre type transformation following spinal cord injury. Spinal Cord 1997;35:86–91.
2. Gordon T, Mao J. Muscle atrophy and procedures for training after spinal cord injury. Phys Ther 1994;74:50–60.

3. Grimby G, Broberg C, Krotkiewska I, et al. Muscle fiber composition in patients with traumatic cord lesion. Scand J Rehabil Med 1976;8:37–42.

4. Martin TP, Stein RB, Hoeppner PH, et al. Influence of electrical stimulation on the morphological and metabolic properties of paralyzed muscle. J Appl Physiol 1992;72:1401–1406.

5. Garland DE, Maric Z, Adkins RH, et al. Bone mineral density about the knee in spinal cord injured patients with pathologic fractures. Contemp Orthop 1993;26:375–379.

6. Ragnarsson KT, Sell GH. Lower extremity fractures after spinal cord injury: a retrospective study. Arch Phys Med Rehabil 1981;62:418–423.

7. Garland DE, Stewart CA, Adkins RH, et al. Osteoporosis after spinal cord injury. J Orthop Res 1992;10:371–378.

8. Hopman MTE, van Asten WN, Oeseburg B. Changes in blood flow in the common femoral artery related to inactivity and muscle atrophy in individuals with long-standing paraplegia. Adv Exp Med Biol 1996;388:379–383.

9. Huonker M, Schmid A, Sorichter S, et al. Cardiovascular differences between sedentary and wheelchair-trained subjects with paraplegia. Med Sci Sports Exerc 1998;30:609–613.

10. Nash MS, Montalvo BM, Applegate B. Lower extremity blood flow and responses to occlusion ischemia differ in exercise-trained and sedentary tetraplegic persons. Arch Phys Med Rehabil 1996;77:1260–1265.

11. Taylor PN, Ewins DJ, Fox B, et al. Limb blood flow, cardiac output and quadriceps muscle bulk following spinal cord injury and the effect of training for the Odstock functional electrical stimulation standing system. Paraplegia 1993;31:303–310.

12. Shenberger JS, Leaman GJ, Neumyer MM, et al. Physiologic and structural indices of vascular function in paraplegics. Med Sci Sports Exerc 1990;22:96–101.

13. Hudlicka O, Price S. The role of blood flow and/or muscle hypoxia in capillary growth in chronically stimulated fast muscles. Pflügers Arch 1990;417:67–72.

14. Hopman MTE, Nommensen E, van Asten WN, et al. Properties of the venous vascular system in the lower extremities of individuals with paraplegia. Paraplegia 1994;32:810–816.

15. Frieden RA, Ahn JH, Pineda HD, et al. Venous plethysmography values in patients with spinal cord injury. Arch Phys Med Rehabil 1987;68:427–429.

16. Kessler KM, Pina I, Green B, et al. Cardiovascular findings in quadriplegic and paraplegic patients and in normal subjects. Am J Cardiol 1986;58:525–530.

17. Washburn RA, Savage DD, Dearwater SR, et al. Echocardiographic left ventricular mass and physical activity: quantification of the relation in spinal cord injured and apparently healthy active men. Am J Cardiol 1986;58:1248–1253.

18. Le CT, Price M. Survival from spinal cord injury. J Chronic Dis 1982;35:487–492.

19. Dearwater SR, LaPorte RE, Robertson RJ, et al. Activity in the spinal cord-injured patient: an epidemiologic analysis of metabolic parameters. Med Sci Sports Exerc 1986;18:541–544.

20. Heldenberg D, Rubinstein A, Levtov O, et al. Serum lipids and lipoprotein concentrations in young quadriplegic patients. Atherosclerosis 1981;39:163–167.

21. Dallmeijer AJ, Hopman MTE, van der Woude LH. Lipid, lipoprotein, and apolipoprotein profiles in active and sedentary men with tetraplegia. Arch Phys Med Rehabil 1997;78:1173–1176.

22. Janssen TWJ, van Oers CAJM, van Kamp GJ, et al. Coronary heart disease risk indicators, aerobic power, and physical activity in men with spinal cord injuries. Arch Phys Med Rehabil 1997;78:697–705.

23. LaPorte RE, Adams LL, Savage DD, et al. The spectrum of physical activity, cardiovascular disease and health: an epidemiologic perspective. Am J Epidemiol 1984;120:507–517.

24. Forner JV. Lung volumes and mechanics of breathing in tetraplegics. Paraplegia 1980;18:258–266.

25. De Troyer A, Heilporn A. Respiratory mechanics in quadriplegia. The respiratory function of the intercostal muscles. Am Rev Respir Dis 1980;122:591–600.

26. Hjeltnes N. Cardiorespiratory capacity in tetra- and paraplegia shortly after injury. Scand J Rehabil Med 1986;18:65–70.

27. Grassino A. A rationale for training respiratory muscles. Int Rehabil Med 1984;6:175–178.

28. Hopman MTE, van der Woude LHV, Dallmeijer AJ, et al. Respiratory muscle strength and endurance in individuals with tetraplegia. Spinal Cord 1997;35:104–108.

29. Sawka MN. Physiology of upper body exercise. Exerc Sport Sci Rev 1986;14:175–211.

30. Davis GM. Exercise capacity of individuals with paraplegia. Med Sci Sports Exerc 1993;25:423–432.

31. Hopman MTE, Oeseburg B, Binkhorst RA. Cardiovascular responses in paraplegic subjects during arm exercise. Eur J Appl Physiol Occup Physiol 1992;65:73–78.

32. Rowell LB, O'Leary DS. Reflex control of the

circulation during exercise: chemoreflexes and mechanoreflexes. J Appl Physiol 1990;69:407–418.

33. Davis GM, Shephard RJ. Cardiorespiratory fitness in highly active versus inactive paraplegics. Med Sci Sports Exerc 1988;20:463–468.

34. Figoni SF. Exercise responses and quadriplegia. Med Sci Sports Exerc 1993;25:433–441.

35. Hopman MTE, Kamerbeek IC, Pistorius M, et al. The effect of an anti-G suit on the maximal performance of individuals with paraplegia. Int J Sports Med 1993;14:357–361.

36. Hopman MTE, Dueck C, Monroe M, et al. Limits to maximal performance in individuals with spinal cord injury. Int J Sports Med 1998;19:98–103.

37. Glaser RM. Exercise and locomotion for the spinal cord injured. Exerc Sport Sci Rev 1985;13:263–303.

38. Figoni SF, Glaser RM, Hendershot DM, et al. Hemodynamic responses of quadriplegics to maximal arm-cranking and FES leg cycling exercise. 10th annual IEEE conference of the Engineering in Medicine and Biology Society, New Orleans, 1988;1636–1637.

39. Hooker SP, Figoni SF, Rodgers MM, et al. Metabolic and hemodynamic responses to concurrent voluntary arm crank and electrical stimulation leg cycle exercise in quadriplegics. J Rehabil Res Dev 1992;29:1–11.

40. Raymond J, Davis GM, Climstein M, et al. Cardiorespiratory responses to arm cranking and electrical stimulation leg cycling in people with paraplegia. Med Sci Sports Exerc 1999;31:822–828.

41. Reybrouck T, Heigenhauser GF, Faulkner JA. Limitations to maximum oxygen uptake in arms, leg, and combined arm-leg ergometry. J Appl Physiol 1975;38:774–779.

42. Shephard RJ, Bouhlel E, Vandewalle H, et al. Muscle mass as a factor limiting physical work. J Appl Physiol 1988;64:1472–1479.

43. Glaser RM, Foley DM, Laubach LL, et al. An exercise test to evaluate fitness for wheelchair activity. Paraplegia 1979;16:341–349.

44. Brattgard SO, Grimby G, Hook O. Energy expenditure and heart rate in driving a wheel-chair ergometer. Scand J Rehabil Med 1970;2:143–148.

45. Niesing R, Eijskoot F, Kranse R, et al. Computer-controlled wheelchair ergometer. Med Biol Eng Comp 1990;28:329–338.

46. Janssen TWJ, van Oers CAJM, Hollander AP, et al. Isometric strength, sprint power, and aerobic power in individuals with a spinal cord injury. Med Sci Sports Exerc 1993;25:863–870.

47. van der Woude LH, Veeger HE, Rozendal RH, et al. Wheelchair racing: effects of rim diameter and speed on physiology and technique. Med Sci Sports Exerc 1988;20:492–500.

48. Sawka MN, Glaser RM, Wilde SW, et al. Metabolic and circulatory responses to wheelchair and arm crank exercise. J Appl Physiol 1980;49:784–788.

49. Glaser RM, Sawka MN, Brune MF, et al. Physiological responses to maximal effort wheelchair and arm crank ergometry. J Appl Physiol 1980;48:1060–1064.

50. Martel G, Noreau L, Jobin J. Physiological responses to maximal exercise on arm cranking and wheelchair ergometer with paraplegics. Paraplegia 1991;29:447–456.

51. Smith PA, Glaser RM, Petrofsky JS, et al. Arm crank vs handrim wheelchair propulsion: metabolic and cardiopulmonary responses. Arch Phys Med Rehabil 1983;64:249–254.

52. van der Woude LH, de Groot G, Hollander AP, et al. Wheelchair ergonomics and physiological testing of prototypes. Ergonomics 1986;29:1561–1573.

53. Janssen TWJ, Dallmeijer AJ, Van der Woude LHV. Physical capacity and race performance of handcycle users. J Rehabil Res Dev 2001;38:33–40.

54. Lasko-McCarthey P, Davis JA. Protocol dependency of VO2max during arm cycle ergometry in males with quadriplegia. Med Sci Sports Exerc 1991;23:1097–1101.

55. Stenberg J, Åstrand PO, Ekblom B, et al. Hemodynamic response to work with different muscle groups, sitting and supine. J Appl Physiol 1967;22:61–70.

56. Bar-Or O, Zwiren LD. Maximal oxygen consumption test during arm exercise—reliability and validity. J Appl Physiol 1975;38:424–426.

57. Coutts KD, Rhodes EC, McKenzie DC. Maximal exercise responses of tetraplegics and paraplegics. J Appl Physiol 1983;55:479–482.

58. Janssen TWJ, van Oers CAJM, Veeger HEJ, et al. Relationship between physical strain during standardised ADL tasks and physical capacity in men with spinal cord injuries. Paraplegia 1994;32:844–859.

59. Janssen TWJ, Dallmeijer AJ, Veeger DJ, et al. Normative values and determinants of physical capacity in individuals with spinal cord injury. J Rehabil Res Dev 2002;39:29–39.

60. Petrofsky JS, Phillips CA, Heaton HHI, et al. Bicycle ergometer for paralyzed muscles. J Clin Eng 1984;9:13–19.

61. Hjeltnes N, Vokac Z. Circulatory strain in everyday life of paraplegics. Scand J Rehabil Med 1979;11:67–73.

62. Janssen TWJ, van Oers CAJM, van der Woude LHV, et al. Physical strain in daily life of wheelchair users with spinal cord injuries. Med Sci Sports Exerc 1994;26:661–670.

63. Dallmeijer AJ, van der Woude LHV, Hollander AP, et al. Changes in physical capacity and performance

of activities of daily living during rehabilitation in persons with spinal cord injuries. Med Sci Sports Exerc 1999;31:1330–1335.

64. Janssen TWJ, van Oers CAJM, Rozendaal EP, et al. Changes in physical strain and physical capacity in men with spinal cord injuries. Med Sci Sports Exerc 1996;28:551–559.

65. Davis G, Plyley MJ, Shephard RJ. Gains of cardiorespiratory fitness with arm-crank training in spinally disabled men. Can J Sport Sci 1991;16:64–72.

66. Hjeltnes N. Capacity for physical work and training after spinal injuries and strokes. Scand J Soc Med Suppl 1982;29:245–251.

67. Hooker SP, Greenwood JD, Hatae DT, et al. Oxygen uptake and heart rate relationship in persons with spinal cord injury. Med Sci Sports Exerc 1993;25:1115–1119.

68. Janssen TWJ, van Oers CA, Veeger HE, et al. Relationship between physical strain during standardised ADL tasks and physical capacity in men with spinal cord injuries. Paraplegia 1994;32:844–859.

69. McLean KP, Jones PP, Skinner JS. Exercise prescription for sitting and supine exercise in subjects with quadriplegia. Med Sci Sports Exerc 1995;27:15–21.

70. Figoni SF, Glaser RM, Hooker SP, et al. Peak hemodynamic responses of SCI subjects during FNS leg cycle ergometry. 12th annual RESNA conference on rehabilitation technology, Washington, DC, 1989;97–98.

71. Mohr T, Andersen JL, Biering-Sorensen F, et al. Long-term adaptation to electrically induced cycle training in severe spinal cord injured individuals. Spinal Cord 1997;35:1–16 [erratum appears in Spinal Cord 1997;35:262].

72. Pollack SF, Axen K, Spielholz N, et al. Aerobic training effects of electrically induced lower extremity exercises in spinal cord injured people. Arch Phys Med Rehabil 1989;70:214–219.

73. Knutsson E, Lewenhaupt-Olsson E, Thorsen M. Physical work capacity and physical conditioning in paraplegic patients. Paraplegia 1973;11:205–216.

74. DiCarlo SE, Supp MD, Taylor HC. Effect of arm ergometry training on physical work capacity of individuals with spinal cord injuries. Phys Ther 1983;63:1104–1107.

75. Nilsson S, Staff PH, Pruett ED. Physical work capacity and the effect of training on subjects with long-standing paraplegia. Scand J Rehabil Med 1975;7:51–56.

76. Miles DS, Sawka MN, Wilde SW, et al. Pulmonary function changes in wheelchair athletes subsequent to exercise training. Ergonomics 1982;25:239–246.

77. Dallmeijer AJ, Hopman MTE, van As HH, et al. Physical capacity and physical strain in persons with tetraplegia; the role of sport activity. Spinal Cord 1996;34:729–735.

78. Brenes G, Dearwater S, Shapera R, et al. High density lipoprotein cholesterol concentrations in physically active and sedentary spinal cord injured patients. Arch Phys Med Rehabil 1986;67:445–450.

79. Krauss JC, Robergs RA, Depaepe JL, et al. Effects of electrical stimulation and upper body training after spinal cord injury. Med Sci Sports Exerc 1993;25:1054–1061.

80. Faghri PD, Glaser RM, Figoni SF. Functional electrical stimulation leg cycle ergometer exercise: training effects on cardiorespiratory responses of spinal cord injured subjects at rest and during submaximal exercise. Arch Phys Med Rehabil 1992;73:1085–1093.

81. Danopulos D, Kezdi P, Stanley EL, et al. Changes in cardiovascular circulatory dynamics after a twelve week active bicycle rehabilitation in young tetraplegics. J Neurol Orthop Med Surg 1986;7:179–184.

82. Barstow TJ, Scremin AM, Mutton DL, et al. Changes in gas exchange kinetics with training in patients with spinal cord injury. Med Sci Sports Exerc 1996;28:1221–1228.

83. Pacy PJ, Hesp R, Halliday DA, et al. Muscle and bone in paraplegic patients, and the effect of functional electrical stimulation. Clin Sci 1988;75:481–487.

84. Sloan KE, Bremner LA, Byrne J, et al. Musculoskeletal effects of an electrical stimulation induced cycling programme in the spinal injured. Paraplegia 1994;32:407–415.

85. Baldi JC, Jackson RD, Moraille R, et al. Muscle atrophy is prevented in patients with acute spinal cord injury using functional electrical stimulation. Spinal Cord 1998;36:463–469.

86. Nash MS, Bilsker S, Marcillo AE, et al. Reversal of adaptive left ventricular atrophy following electrically-stimulated exercise training in human tetraplegics. Paraplegia 1991;29:590–599.

87. Chilibeck PD, Jeon J, Weiss C, et al. Histochemical changes in muscle of individuals with spinal cord injury following functional electrical stimulated exercise training. Spinal Cord 1999;37:264–268.

88. Gerrits HL, de Haan A, Sargeant AJ, et al. Peripheral vascular changes after electrically stimulated cycle training in people with spinal cord injury. Arch Phys Med Rehabil 2001;82:832–839.

89. Petrofsky JS. Functional electrical stimulation: a two-year study. J Rehabil 1992;58:29–34.

90. Hopman MTE, Oeseburg B, Binkhorst RA. Cardiovascular responses in persons with paraplegia to prolonged arm exercise and thermal stress. Med Sci Sports Exerc 1993;25:577–583.

91. Sawka MN, Latzka WA, Pandolf KB. Temperature regulation during upper body exercise: able-bodied and spinal cord injured. Med Sci Sports Exerc 1989;21:S132–140.

92. Wheeler G, Cumming D, Burnham R, et al. Testosterone, cortisol and catecholamine responses to exercise stress and autonomic dysreflexia in elite quadriplegic athletes. Paraplegia 1994;32:292–299.

RELATED WEB SITES
Spinal Cord Injuries

Spinal Cord Injury Information Network
www.spinalcord.uab.edu

Spinal Injuries
www.spinalinjury.org

National Spinal Cord Injury Association
www.spinalcord.org

National Institute of Neurological Disorders and Stroke Spinal Cord Information Page
www.ninds.nih.gov/health_and_medical/disorders/sci.htm

Christopher and Dana Reeve Paralysis Resource Center
www.paralysis.org

Paralyzed Veterans of America
www.pva.org

University of Michigan Health Systems Health Topics A–Z: Spinal Cord Injury
www.med.umich.edu/1libr/aha/umscord.htm

University of Michigan Health Systems Model Spinal Cord Injury Care System
www.med.umich.edu/pmr/model_sci

Wheelchair Mobility

Wheelchair Mobility
www.wheelchairmobility.com

Metabolic Conditions

14

Diabetes Mellitus

Arthur S. Leon and Otto A. Sánchez

About 15 million (5%) Americans are estimated to have diabetes mellitus (DM), half of whom are unaware that they have the condition (1). The prevalence of impaired fasting glucose, a precursor of DM, is about 7%. These two conditions combined affect about 29 million persons (1). DM is the sixth leading cause of mortality in the United States, directly responsible for 40,000 deaths annually. However, this figure grossly underestimates its contribution to mortality, because most victims of DM die of associated cardiovascular complications (2).

Description

DM is actually a heterogeneous group of metabolic disorders having in common an absolute or relative insufficiency of insulin secretion. This peptide hormone is synthesized by the beta (β) pancreatic islet cells and promotes the transport of glucose across cell membranes in insulin-responsive tissues (e.g., adipose tissue and skeletal muscle) and its subsequent oxidation for energy production. Thus, insulin insufficiency reduces the body's ability to use glucose as fuel. The ability of muscle to synthesize glycogen from glucose is also defective, and hepatic glucose release is increased, resulting in elevated blood glucose (hyperglycemia), the clinical hallmark of DM. When plasma glu-cose exceeds 160 to 180 mg/dL, it usually spills over into the urine, resulting in *glycosuria*. This is accompanied by increased frequency of urination and volume of urine excreted *(polyuria)*. The associated loss of large amounts of body water increases thirst and water intake *(polydipsia)*. However, dehydration may still result because of excess fluid loss due to hyperosmolarity of the glucose-containing urine. These four metabolic abnormalities (hyperglycemia, glycosuria, polyuria, and polydipsia) are the principal clinical symptoms and signs of DM.

Types of Diabetes Mellitus

There are two major clinical types of DM. Type 1 DM, formerly known as insulin-dependent DM, is generally caused by immune system-mediated destruction of pancreatic β cells. Type 2 DM, previously referred to as non-insulin-dependent DM, is characterized by cellular insulin resistance with a relative insulin insufficiency, even in the presence of hyperinsulinemia. Other less common types of DM are secondary to various medical conditions or syndromes adversely affecting pancreatic function. The onset of DM during pregnancy is referred to as *gestational DM;* it is subsequently reclassified if it persists after pregnancy. Table 14-1 compares major characteristics of type 1 and type 2 DM.

TABLE 14-1   COMPARISON OF TYPE 1 AND TYPE 2 DIABETES MELLITUS

Characteristics	Type 1	Type 2
Former designation	IDDM	NIDDM
Age of onset	Usually <35 years	Usually >40 years
Clinical onset	Abrupt	Gradual
Family history	Not always	Yes
HLA association[a]	Yes	No
Body composition	Normal or thin	Usually obese (central type)
Blood insulin levels	Reduced or absent	Normal or increase
Cell insulin resistance	Absent or minor	Present
Tendency for ketosis (without replacement insulin)	Yes	No
Treatment for control of hyperglycemia	Insulin, diet, ± exercise	Weight loss, diet, oral hypoglycemic drugs or insulin

[a] Association with specific genetically determined histocompatibility leukocyte antigen (HLA) types.

IDDM, insulin-dependent diabetes mellitus; NIDDM, non-insulin-dependent diabetes mellitus; HLA, histocompatibility leukocyte antigen.

Etiology

There is evidence that mumps and Coxsackie B viruses may cause type 1 DM by invading and destroying pancreatic β islet cells. A strong possibility also exists that viral-damaged islet cells act as antigens, which results in antibody production in susceptible individuals that can destroy remaining β cells through an autoimmune process (3). An inherited predisposition for both types of DM is also well established. For example, if both parents have type 2 DM, their children have a 4 to 6 times greater chance of developing type 2 DM than offspring of nondiabetic parents (4). Individuals with a genetic predisposition to type 2 DM generally progress gradually from normal glucose tolerance to overt DM over several years. Initially, impaired

cellular glucose uptake and phosphorylation and impaired glycogen synthesis often precede type 2 DM, especially in offspring of patients with type 2 DM (5). In addition to the inherited metabolic impairments, most pre-type 2 DM individuals accumulate fat in the abdominal region (6). This contributes to insulin resistance in liver and skeletal muscle, perhaps by the accelerated release of fatty acids from abdominal adipose tissue (7). Increased secretion of cytokines by adipose cells also may interfere with insulin receptor functions and induce insulin resistance (8). The resistance to insulin action stimulates increased insulin secretion to maintain normal blood glucose levels. The resulting compensatory hyperinsulinemia can induce a constellation of metabolic and cardiovascular disorders referred to as the metabolic syndrome (9), which is characterized by insulin resistance, hypertriglyceridemia, reduced high-density lipoprotein (HDL) cholesterol and elevated blood pressure. This constellation of risk factors contributes to a high prevalence of cardiovascular disease (10). Epidemiologic studies consistently show that obesity is a major risk factor for type 2 DM, as about 80% of people with this disease are obese (6). In addition, central or abdominal body fat (e.g., waist circumference >40 inches in men and >34 inches in women) has been shown in prospective studies to predict future DM, independent of relative body weight (11). The incidence of glucose intolerance and type 2 DM increases with age, with most patients over 40 years of age (1). The usual age-associated reductions in physical activity and lean body mass and increase in adiposity most likely contribute significantly.

Clinical Aspects of Diabetes

DIAGNOSTIC CRITERIA

Current diagnostic criteria for DM are based on blood glucose levels, i.e., a fasting level of 125 mg·dL^{-1} or above or one above 200 mg·dL^{-1} following an oral glucose challenge (Table 14-2). Fasting levels between 110 and 125 mg·dL^{-1} are defined as *impaired fasting glucose*. Blood glucose levels between 140 and 200 mg·dL^{-1} 2 hours after an oral glucose challenge are referred to as *impaired glucose tolerance* (IGT) (12).

TABLE 14-2   DIAGNOSTIC CRITERIA FOR DIABETES MELLITUS

1. Normal values: fasting[a] plasma glucose $\leq$ 110 mg·dL^{-1} (6.1 mmol·L^{-1}) or 2-h plasma glucose during an OGTT $\leq$ 140 mg·dL^{-1} (7.8 mmol·L^{-1})
2. Symptoms of diabetes plus casual plasma glucose concentration $\geq$ 200 mg·dL^{-1} (11.1 mmol·L^{-1}). (Casual is defined as any time of day without regard to time since the last meal. The classic symptoms of diabetes include polyuria, polydipsia, and unexplained weight loss).
   or
3. FPG $\geq$ 125 mg·dL^{-1} (7.0 mmol·L^{-1}).
   or
4. 2-h plasma glucose $\geq$ 200 mg·dL^{-1} (11.1 mmol·L^{-1}) during an OGTT. The test should be performed as described by the WHO, using a glucose load containing the equivalent of 75 g of anhydrous glucose dissolved in water.

OGTT, oral glucose tolerance test.
[a]Fasting is defined as no energy intake for the last 8 hours.

BLOOD GLUCOSE MONITORING

Once DM is diagnosed, monitoring blood glucose (glycemic) status is essential to evaluate the efficacy of therapy. The recommended approach is self-monitoring of blood glucose (SMBG) by automated procedures. SMBG should be performed three to four times per day by all those on insulin and by type 2 DM patients on oral hypoglycemic agents, especially those not achieving optimal glycemic goals during therapy (13,14). Glycosylated hemoglobin is a laboratory test to evaluate long-term blood sugar control. It measures the percentage of total hemoglobin glycosylated into its HbA$_{1c}$ fraction, which in healthy persons should be below 6%, and reflects the individual's usual serum glucose level over the previous 2 to 3 months (15).

ACUTE DIABETIC COMPLICATIONS

The natural history of DM is extremely variable, making it difficult to predict specific outcomes in any given person (16). Many diabetic individuals from all socioeconomic strata remain free of significant complications and carry on active, productive lives for many decades, despite even severe type 1 DM, including professional athletes. However, despite good DM control, some patients have acute and chronic complications. Acute situations may occur any time with DM and are usually temporary and remediable.

Hypoglycemia

Hypoglycemia or low blood sugar is the most common complication for diabetic patients receiving insulin or an oral hypoglycemic agent (OHA). It results from an overdose of a glucose-lowering agent relative to the patient's dietary and physical activity status. Usual precipitating factors are insufficient food intake to cover the blood glucose-lowering effect of the drug or more physical activity than is customary for the individual. Although symptoms of hypoglycemia usually develop when plasma glucose is <50 mg·dL^{-1}, they also may occur at higher levels in response to a rapid drop during treatment. Resulting symptoms are of sympathetic and central nervous system origin and include hunger, weakness, trembling, sweating, confusion, bizarre behavior, and headaches. A DM patient with such symptoms should immediately consume 10 to 15 g of carbohydrates. Table 14-3 lists foods and beverages containing 10 to 15 g per serving. If the diabetic individual does not do this, loss of consciousness may result. Occasionally, a patient with subclinical DM develops hypoglycemia as an initial

TABLE 14-3   FOOD AND BEVERAGES CONTAINING 10 TO 15 GRAMS OF CARBOHYDRATES PER SERVING FOR MANAGEMENT OF HYPOGLYCEMIA

Food or Beverage	Quantity
Glucose tablets	2–3
Sugar cubes, large	2
Honey	2 teaspoons
Lifesavers	7
Dried fruit	$1/4$ cup
Fresh fruit	1 exchange
Bread	1 exchange
Orange juice	$1/2$ cup
Milk	1 cup
Sports drink 5–10% carbohydrate	1 cup
Soft drink (not diet)	$1/2$ cup

presenting symptom because of inappropriate timing or quantity of insulin released by the β cells following meals. Because of this potential danger, DM individuals should wear appropriate alert tags for identification.

Diabetic Ketoacidosis

Diabetic ketoacidosis was a common life-threatening complication prior to the discovery of insulin. Currently, only about 1% of type 1 DM patients die of this complication. An insufficiency of insulin results in increased lipolysis of adipose tissue triglycerides (TG), raising free fatty acids (FFAs) in the blood, which results in their accelerated use for fuel. However, since the liver has a limited capacity to use the excess acetyl-coenzyme A generated from β-oxidation of FFA, ketone bodies are formed. Accumulation of ketone bodies in the blood and their excretion in the urine causes metabolic acidosis (ketoacidosis), which leads to further loss of water and electrolytes and can result in coma and circulatory collapse.

Skin Problems

Many skin and mucosal problems may occur in those with DM. These include localized infections such as furuncles and carbuncles (abscesses), which may be the initial presenting symptoms of type 2 DM. Abscesses also may occur at insulin injection sites because of careless techniques. Pruritus vulvae due to a yeast infection (moniliasis) is another frequent skin problem in diabetic women.

LATE (CHRONIC) COMPLICATIONS

The incidence of chronic complications increases with duration of DM, especially in the absence of optimal glycemic control (16). Late complications are main contributors to premature mortality with DM. These may be classified as *microvascular* (small vessel) complications, *macrovascular* (moderate or large vessel) atherosclerotic complications, and *neuropathies.*

Microvascular Complications

One of the most prevalent microvascular complications is diabetic retinopathy (DR), occurring in about 25 to 50% of all DM patients (17). DR is characterized by the presence of microaneurysms of the retinal capillaries that can result in retinal hemorrhage, followed by scarring and new vessel formation (proliferative retinopathy), leading to retinal detachment, progressive visual impairment, and blindness.

Nephropathy is observed in about 40 to 50% of type 1 DM patients (20). This condition is the leading cause of end-stage renal disease requiring long-term renal dialysis and/or a kidney transplant and is a common cause of death in persons under age 40 years with type 1 DM. The initial manifestation of diabetic nephropathy is the presence of albumin in the urine (proteinuria), which should be closely monitored by the attending physician to assess kidney damage.

Macrovascular (Atherosclerotic) Complications

An accelerated form of atherosclerosis is common in both major types of DM, as well as with IGT (18). Atherosclerosis is the underlying cause of myocardial infarctions, strokes, and peripheral arterial disease in diabetic patients. Typically, atherosclerotic cardiovascular complications appear only after many years of type 1 DM and are usually preceded by microvascular disease. However, older individuals with type 2 DM or IGT may present with severe atherosclerosis of the coronary and peripheral vessels relatively soon after the initial diagnosis of DM. In the Framingham Heart Study, the incidence of cardiovascular disease (CVD) among diabetic men and women was about two to three times that of matched nondiabetic individuals (19). Over 60% of all deaths in diabetic patients in Western societies are attributed to CVD (19). An interaction of multiple factors appears to be involved, e.g., dysfunction of artery wall endothelial linings (20–22), lipid disturbances, hyperinsulinemia in type 2 DM patients, blood pressure elevation, and procoagulant hemostatic disturbances. Endothelial dysfunction results in an imbalance between vasodilatory and vasoconstrictive factors favoring vasoconstriction, as well as platelet aggregation. Elevated blood pressure and abnormalities in the blood lipid–lipoprotein profile (elevated TG and reduced HDL cholesterol) commonly associated with DM accelerate the atherosclerotic process as they do in nondiabetic individuals (20). Diabetic nephropathy and renal failure can cause further elevations in blood pressure and dyslipidemias, which further accelerates atherosclerosis.

Neuropathies

Almost any nerve pathway (peripheral motor or sensory, central, or autonomic) can be affected by DM (23). Neurologic symptoms, ranging in severity from mild to incapacitating, include numbness, tingling or pain in the lower extremities, muscle wasting and weakness, foot drop, absent ankle jerk reflex, postural hypotension, gastrointestinal symptoms, difficulty emptying the bladder (neurogenic bladder), and impotence (14). Blunting of sympathetic nervous system activity may make it difficult for those with DM to recognize symptoms of hypoglycemia. Silent myocardial ischemia and silent myocardial infarction also may be related to autonomic system neuropathy.

Reduced muscle strength is more common in patients with long-term DM than in matched control subjects (24). Muscle atrophy, alterations in contractile proteins, motor neuropathy, and impaired blood flow to skeletal muscles are important contributing factors to skeletal muscle weakness (25,26). Furthermore, the combination of DM, physical inactivity, and the effects of aging might contribute to the loss of muscle strength in older diabetic individuals. Muscle weakness can contribute to a loss of independent living at an earlier age than for nondiabetic individuals.

Management of DM

Treatment of DM is a lifetime affair to regulate its metabolic effects. The ultimate goal of treatment is glycemic control to eliminate symptoms related to hyperglycemia and the prevention or reduction in severity of chronic complications, allowing the patient to achieve a more normal lifestyle (13,14).

The three essential therapeutic approaches for glycemic control are medications, diet, and regular exercise. Optimal diabetic management also includes control of other atherogenic risk factors, particularly cigarette smoking, abnormal blood lipid levels, hypertension, obesity, and physical inactivity, to prevent CVD complications.

MEDICATIONS TO CONTROL HYPERGLYCEMIA

Insulin and oral hypoglycemic agents are pharmacologic approaches to control blood glucose, if a program of weight reduction, diet, and exercise do not. Detailed descriptions on using these drugs are available elsewhere (13,14) and are briefly reviewed here.

Insulin Therapy

Few developments in medicine have changed the course of a disease as drastically as the discovery of insulin. The principal indications for insulin therapy are *(a)* to treat or prevent episodes of ketoacidosis with type 1 DM and *(b)* to control symptoms associated with the metabolic derangements accompanying marked hyperglycemia in patients with either type of DM (14). Insulin requirements are established by progressively increasing subcutaneous doses as guided by repeated blood glucose determinations. Optimal control requires sufficient insulin administration to allow proper use of nutrients for energy or storage, relief of diabetic symptoms, and maintenance of near-normal blood sugar levels without frequent hypoglycemic reactions.

The type of insulin is classified by the time required after injection to achieve peak activity and by the duration of action, i.e., fast-, intermediate-, or prolonged-acting. Intermediate- or prolonged-acting insulin is often combined with a fast-acting insulin for optimal glucose control. Because "tight glucose control" can significantly reduce the incidence of retinopathy, neuropathy, and nephropathy (27), the American Diabetes Association (ADA) recommends maintaining blood glucose and Hb_{A1c} near normal levels (Table 14-4) by frequent SMBG, while administering multiple daily insulin injections (13). In type 1 DM patients, an intermediate-acting insulin (e.g., lente or NPH insulin) or a long-acting insulin (e.g., ultralente or glargine), representing about half of the daily insulin requirement, is generally administered in two doses, 10 to 12 hours apart. The remainder is generally given 20 to 45 min before every meal as a short-acting insulin; the dose depends on the preprandial blood glucose and the anticipated carbohydrate intake (14,28). Frequent (4–8 times a day) SMBG is essential for such a regimen to be safe and successful. Different insulin

TABLE 14-4   IDEAL GOALS FOR DESIRED GLYCEMIC CONTROL

	Normal Range	Goal	Additional Action Suggested
Average preprandial glucose, mmol·L^{-1} (mg·dL^{-1})	<5.0 (100)	4.4–6.7 (80–120)	<4.4 (80) or >7.8 (140)
Average bedtime glucose, mmol·L^{-1} (mg·dL^{-1})	<6.1 (110)	5.5–7.8 (100–140)	<5.5 (100) or >8.8 (160)
Hb$_{A1c}$, %	<6	<7	>8

regimes exist, and treatment should be individualized.

Type 2 DM patients presenting with marked hyperglycemia often require insulin for initial therapy, particularly those with marked weight loss. Insulin may be administered along with hypoglycemic agents if glucose control cannot be achieved with these agents alone. In type 2 DM patients, insulin generally needs to be administered only once a day to control hyperglycemia.

Various insulin pump models can significantly improve control of DM and make life easier and more normal for persons with type 1 DM (29). These instruments consist of a pager-size pump worn outside the body on a pouch or a belt clip. They are preprogramed to infuse insulin subcutaneously throughout the day and to administer insulin in boluses when blood glucose levels are expected to rise (e.g., after meals or snacks). Individualized algorithms based on preprandial plasma glucose values and anticipated carbohydrate intake determine the amount required. Adjustments also can be made before engaging in physical activities. These devices require the patient to be trained by a knowledgeable health care team to properly use the pumps and avoid complications (29).

Oral Hypoglycemic Agents (OHAs)

OHAs can effectively control blood sugar levels in many patients with type 2 DM who fail to respond or adhere to a dietary and exercise program (14,28). OHAs differ in their mechanisms of action (Table 14-5). Sulfonylurea drugs, the most common type, stimulate the pancreatic β islet cells to release more insulin. They also improve peripheral insulin sensitivity and inhibit secretion of

TABLE 14-5   CURRENT AVAILABLE TYPES OF ORAL HYPOGLYCEMIC AGENTS

Type (Examples)	Mechanism of Action	Usual Daily Dose	No. of Doses a Day	Contraindications
1. Sulfonylureas (e.g., tolbutamide)	Increase insulin release from pancreatic β cells	500–2000 mg	2–3	Renal or hepatic disease
2. Biguanides (e.g., metformin)	Decrease hepatic glucose production	500–1000 mg	2–3	Renal or hepatic disease, past history of lactic acidosis from any cause
3. α-Glucosidase inhibitors (e.g., acarbose)	Decrease intestinal absorption of glucose	500–1000 mg	1	Renal or hepatic disease
4. Thiazolidinediones (e.g., rosiglitazone pioglitazone)	Reduce insulin resistance by binding to nuclear peroxisome proliferator-activator receptor γ	4–8 mg	1	Hepatic disease and congestive heart failure

the insulin antagonist, glucagon, from the α islet cells of the pancreas (28). Biguanides lower blood glucose by decreasing hepatic glucose production. Thiazolidinediones, also known as PPARγ (peroxisome proliferators-activator receptor γ) agents lower blood glucose by increasing insulin sensitivity and decreasing hepatic glucose production. α-Glucosidase inhibitors lower blood glucose by decreasing intestinal absorption of carbohydrates.

DIETARY APPROACHES

General Principles

Diet has traditionally been the cornerstone for managing both types of DM. Detailed dietary guidelines have been published (30) and include reducing excess weight to improve glycemic control and reducing other coronary heart disease (CHD) risk factors; substitution of complex carbohydrates for dietary saturated fat, while minimizing the use of simple sugars, salt, and alcohol; eating nutritionally sound meals; and spreading food intake over 24 hours to cover insulin administration (Table 14-6).

Weight Management

Because many individuals with type 2 DM are obese, metabolic improvement or satisfactory glycemic control and enhanced peripheral insulin sensitivity generally result from losing excess

---

TABLE 14-6 RECOMMENDED DIETARY GOALS FOR PATIENTS WITH DIABETES

1. If obese, reduce calories and increase physical activity to gradually attain and maintain ideal weight.
2. Liberalize intake of complex carbohydrates.
3. Reduce intake of total fat, saturated fat, and cholesterol.
4. Minimize intake of simple carbohydrates, except those that occur naturally in fruits and vegetables.
5. Consume nutritionally sound meals using the food exchange list.
6. Individuals on insulin should spread their food intake throughout the waking part of the day.
7. Limit use of salt and alcohol.
8. There is insufficient evidence that any specific supplement of vitamins or minerals will improve metabolic alterations or prevent chronic complications.
9. There is no evidence that a diet providing 15–20% of energy from protein would contribute to diabetic nephropathy.

---

weight. Thus, reduced total energy intake and increased physical activity to achieve and maintain proper body weight are important goals in the management of DM.

Diet Composition

The current recommendations of the ADA are for carbohydrates to provide 60 to 70% of daily energy requirements, with an associated dietary fiber intake of 25 to 30 g·day^{-1} (30). This should be provided primarily by increased consumption of whole-grain cereals and bread, starchy roots, legumes and other vegetables, and fruits. The ADA has liberalized the consumption of table sugar or sucrose and of fruit containing simple carbohydrates by diabetic individuals. However, high sucrose intake may impair insulin sensitivity and adversely affect lipid metabolism for at least 6 weeks (31). Thus, the current consensus is that sucrose and other simple sugars should account for ≤10% of total dietary energy and come primarily from fruit and vegetable sources (30). Currently, sucrose supplies about 16% of the energy in the usual American diet.

An important health concern of the previously traditional low-carbohydrate diabetic diet is that it was high in total fat, saturated fat, and cholesterol. This eating pattern contributes to elevated total and LDL cholesterol levels in blood, thereby accelerating the atherosclerotic process and risk of CVD complications. Current ADA recommendations are to reduce total fat content to ≤30% of daily energy intake, with an equal proportion of energy from saturated, polyunsaturated, and monounsaturated fatty acids (30). Dietary cholesterol should be <300 mg·day^{-1}. These recommendations are in line with the American Heart Association step I diet and the National Research Council's dietary recommendations (32). For type 2 DM patients with hyperlipidemias, the ADA advocates further restriction of dietary fats to ≤20% of daily energy intake and of dietary cholesterol to 100 to 150 mg·day^{-1} (30). Protein intake should be similar to that recommended for nondiabetic individuals (0.8 g·kg^{-1} or about 15% of energy intake) in the absence of significant renal disease. However, a significant amount should come from plant instead of animal sources to reduce intake of associated saturated fat and cholesterol. For those with poor glycemic control, protein requirements may be increased to 1 g·kg^{-1} of body weight to avoid a negative amino acid balance due

found statistically significant differences in weight loss in only a minority of the studies (86). The review panel noted that the short duration of the interventions and small sample sizes probably contributed to the lack of statistically significant differences in some studies. In a similar vein, a meta-analysis covering 25 years of weight-loss research reported that average weight losses were similar in studies comparing diet plus exercise (11.0 kg) with diet alone (10.7 kg) (90). Wing (91) has suggested that the failure of diet plus exercise regimens to result in more substantial weight loss than dietary modification alone is due to the fact that individuals in the diet plus exercise programs compensated for the energy deficit due to exercise by reducing physical activity at other times in the day or by eating somewhat more.

EXERCISE AND DIETARY MODIFICATION IN THE MAINTENANCE OF WEIGHT LOSS

The 1999 ACSM roundtable examined six randomized controlled trials that addressed the issue of whether exercise plus dietary modification maintained weight loss better than dietary modification alone (86). Two of the six studies showed significant long-term effects favoring exercise plus dietary modification, and the other four were inconclusive. Based on the relatively strong trends of the two positive studies, the panel concluded that exercise plus dietary modification provided benefits over dietary modification alone in maintaining weight loss. The panel went on to note that correlational studies and studies of successful weight losers consistently show that physical activity is strongly associated with better long-term maintenance of weight loss (86).

RESPONDERS AND NONRESPONDERS

When examining the effectiveness of exercise on weight loss across individuals, remember that there likely will be "responders" and "nonresponders" to the same exercise program (22,82). At least part of the variability of response to exercise training appears to be due to genetic predisposition. In a study of exercise and weight loss in identical twins, Bouchard et al. (92) reported that the variance for

changes in body weight was 6.8 times greater between twin pairs than within twin pairs.

Exercise Prescription

A broad-based intervention combining increased exercise with reduced dietary intake and behavior therapy appears most likely to be successful (62). This section considers the exercise component of this strategy, with recommendations regarding the amount, intensity, and type to be used. Suggestions for exercise adherence are also presented.

AMOUNT OF EXERCISE

For the general adult population, the current public health recommendation from the ACSM/CDC is that every U.S. adult should accumulate 30 min or more of moderate-intensity physical activity on most, preferably all, days of the week (93). This is often interpreted as a minimum of 150 min per week and equates to a physical activity-related EE of approximately 1000 kcal/week (18). Although this may be a reasonable initial goal for many obese individuals, it appears that more exercise may be needed for long-term weight loss and maintenance. Thus, ACSM recommends that for long-term weight loss, obese adults should eventually progress to between 200 and 300 min of physical activity per week, or the equivalent of at least 2000 kcal/week (18). Table 15-3 provides information on EE for various modes of physical activity at various body weights.

Progressing to 200 to 300 min of weekly physical activity may present a significant challenge for a large proportion of obese individuals, many of whom are sedentary and unfit. Many obese simply cannot perform large amounts of exercise, at least initially. Many cannot walk 1 mile continuously (43). Thus, it is important to progress gradually and stay attuned to the level of activity that individuals are willing to adopt and maintain. By way of reference, a minimum of 17 to 20 weeks of progression has been suggested for the endurance component of an exercise prescription for an apparently healthy individual prior to achieving 200 min of endurance exercise per week (i.e., 5 days per week × 40 min per session) (82).

Fortunately, research suggests that daily exercise goals designed to promote weight loss need not be achieved in single bouts of continuous exercise, but can be accumulated in a series of shorter bouts. Jakicic et al. (94) found that intermittent short bouts of exercise were just as effective as continuous bouts in reducing body mass of obese women over an 18-month period. The use of intermittent rather than continuous exercise bouts may appeal to certain segments of the obese population.

EXERCISE INTENSITY

There is little definitive research on the effects of exercise intensity on weight loss and prevention of weight regain. Observational data from the National Weight Control Registry suggest that individuals who have lost weight and maintained their weight loss performed approximately 25% of their total weekly exercise at a vigorous intensity (95). On the other hand, in a 24-week walking study with overweight women in which exercise intensity was manipulated (86, 67, or 56% of maximal heart rate) and total exercise volume was equated, no differential effect of exercise intensity on body weight or body composition was observed (96). Noting the paucity of data from randomized controlled trials in this area, the 2001 ACSM position stand on weight loss strategies concludes that sufficient amounts of moderate-intensity (55–69% of maximal heart rate) exercise appear to be beneficial in obesity management and that limited evidence supports the need for including more vigorous ($\geq 70\%$ of maximal heart rate) forms of exercise for long-term management of body weight (18).

TYPES OF EXERCISE

Exercises that use large muscle groups, are rhythmic and aerobic, can be done over prolonged periods of time, and are associated with a relatively low risk of injury should form the cornerstone of the exercise component of an obesity-management program. Walking, various forms of cycling, swimming, rowing, various types of dancing, and machine-based stair climbing would qualify as cornerstone activities. These exercise modalities also provide for individual variability relative to skill level and enjoyment. It may be desirable to have obese individuals engage in more than one activity to reduce repetitive orthopedic stresses and involve more muscle groups (82).

Walking should probably be considered first when prescribing exercise (9). Walking has the advantage of being a familiar activity that can be done most anywhere at any time, requires no specialized equipment or skill, and has been used successfully in obesity management (95,97). At the same time, remember that exercise tolerance during walking is often reduced in the obese (98). Mattson et al. (99) have cautioned that although brisk walking may be experienced as a light-to-moderate–intensity activity by normal-weight individuals, it appears to be a moderate-to-high–intensity activity for many obese. Thus, particular attention should be paid to intensity considerations when prescribing walking. Initial emphasis should be on increasing duration rather than intensity, with the goal of optimizing EE (82).

It has been suggested that low-intensity, non-weight-bearing activities like cycling and swimming result in greater ease of performance, causing greater long-term EE and weight loss (79). Hence, aquatic activities may be an attractive alternative to walking for many obese persons. Due to buoyancy, exercise performed in water reduces loading on joints, permitting obese individuals to increase exercise volume with less risk of injury. Also, water exercise can reduce thermoregulatory problems and chafing often experienced by the obese.

Current thinking regarding exercise prescription recommends that resistance training supplement the endurance-exercise program (18,100). The 2001 ACSM position stand (18) notes that there is no scientific evidence showing resistance exercise to be superior to endurance exercise for weight loss. Nevertheless, resistance exercise improves muscular strength and endurance, which may be especially beneficial in maintaining functional tasks by the obese (e.g., getting out of a chair, lifting one's own body weight). This may facilitate adoption of a more active lifestyle in sedentary obese individuals. In terms of the resistance training prescription, ACSM recommends that individuals *(a)* perform a minimum of 8 to 10 separate exercises that train the major muscle groups (arms, shoulders, chest, abdomen, back, hips, and legs); *(b)* perform a minimum of one set of 8 to 12 repetitions of each exercise to the point of volitional fatigue; and *(c)* perform the exercises 2 to 3 days per week (82). Resistance training can be accomplished using a variety of training devices such as free weights, weight machines, and elastic bands. For obese subjects, a person's own body weight can often function as the resistance for calisthenic-type exercises.

Another perspective that merits consideration when prescribing exercise for obesity relates to so-called lifestyle activities. Adherence to formal exercise programs is typically poor among the obese (101). Lifestyle activity, which can be accumulated through daily activities at home and at work, may be an effective option for increasing EE and modifying body weight in the obese. Andersen et al. (102) compared structured aerobic activity and moderate-intensity lifestyle activity and reported that lifestyle activity resulted in weight loss that was comparable to that resulting from aerobic exercise after both 16 and 68 weeks of intervention. Lifestyle-activity recommendations should be focused on such routine

activities as walking, stair climbing, and performing tasks while standing and moving around the job or house. However, further research is necessary to determine the effectiveness of specific forms of lifestyle activity in terms of body composition changes (18).

There are insufficient data to determine whether traditional, structured, group-exercise programs or less formal home-based exercise programs are more effective models for obesity management. Group-exercise programs can enhance safety and surveillance, provide opportunities for social reinforcement, and increase contact time with professional staff. On the other hand, group programs are often associated with inconvenient hours, increased cost, and extended travel time (82). Home-based exercise programs have the advantages of lower cost, increased practicality, convenience, and

TABLE 15-7 PRACTICAL RECOMMENDATIONS FOR ENHANCING ADHERENCE TO EXERCISE

Recommendation	Comment
Recruit physician support[a]	A strong recommendation from their primary care physician has been shown to be the most important factor in determining patients' participation in exercise
Reduce risk of injury[a]	Excess intensity ($\geq$85% $\dot{V}O_{2max}$), frequency ($\geq$5 days per week), or duration ($\geq$45 min per session) increase the risk of orthopedic injury
Advocate exercising with others[a]	Poorer long-term adherence has been reported in programs in which an individual exercises alone
Emphasize variety and enjoyment in the exercise program[a]	The most successful exercise programs are those that are pleasurable and offer variety
Provide positive reinforcement through periodic testing[a]	Favorable changes in aerobic fitness, body composition, blood pressure, and blood lipids measured across time can serve as powerful motivators that produce renewed interest and dedication
Recruit support among family and friends[a]	Lack of social support is frequently found to be a precursor to exercise noncompliance; spousal support appears to play a key role
Include recreational games in the exercise program[a]	Recreational games that minimize skill and competition and maximize participation can be a useful augmentation to structured exercise
Establish regularity of workouts[a]	Exercising at the same time of day helps make exercise habitual
Use progress charts to record exercise achievements[a]	Daily and cumulative exercise achievements provide positive feedback for reinforcing health-related behaviors
Provide access to qualified, enthusiastic exercise professionals[a]	Having well-trained, compassionate, sensitive, innovative, and enthusiastic exercise professionals is an important variable affecting exercise adherence
Don't make weight loss the only endpoint; encourage obese subjects to become more physically active and fit, even if they never become thin[b]	There are important health-related benefits to physical activity even in the absence of large reductions in body weight

[a]Based on American College of Sports Medicine. ACSM's Guidelines for Exercise Testing and Prescription. 6th ed. Baltimore: Lippincott Williams & Wilkins, 2000:245–249.
[b]Based on Leermakers EA, Dunn AL, Blair SN. Exercise management of obesity. Med Clin North Am 2000;84:419–440.

the potential to promote independence and self-responsibility for health and fitness needs (103).

Whether a group or home-based program is recommended, injury prevention is an especially important consideration when prescribing exercise for the obese, because physical injury is one reason for discontinuing exercise (104). Recommendations to reduce the risk of injury include gradual progression of exercise intensity and duration, use of low-impact or non-weight-bearing exercises, consideration of a person's injury history, selection of appropriate exercise environments and apparel to avoid heat-related complications, and incorporation of resistance and flexibility training into the exercise prescription.

ADHERENCE

As noted, adherence to formal exercise programs is typically poor among the obese (101,105). Long-term follow-up results show a return to baseline weight for most in the absence of continued behavior intervention (106,107). Given that exercise appears to be an important behavior for long-term weight control in obese persons, exercise prescriptions should pay special attention to issues affecting adherence. Some practical recommendations for enhancing adherence to exercise are shown in Table 15-7. Selective incorporation of several of these techniques is recommended, but it is not necessary to use all of them (82).

Summary

- Given the increasing prevalence of obesity in all segments of the U.S. population, contact with this special population by exercise professionals will likely increase.
- Obesity results from an imbalance over time between EI and EE. This imbalance involves interactions between genetic, metabolic, behavioral, environmental, and cultural factors.
- Guidelines published by nationally recognized organizations such as the ACSM and the AHA recommend standard exercise testing methods and protocols with the obese, using low-impact (treadmill walking) or non-weight-bearing (cycle ergometer) protocols.

- Physical activity should be a cornerstone in obesity management (along with a sensible diet and behavioral techniques).
- For long-term weight loss, obese adults should eventually progress to between 200 and 300 min of physical activity per week, or the equivalent of at least 2000 kcal·wk^{-1}. These benchmarks can be achieved through structured exercise or increased activities of daily living, using continuous exercise or intermittent physical activity, and performed at a variety of intensities.
- Weight loss should not be the only endpoint. Obese individuals should be encouraged to become more physically active and fit, even if they never become thin.

REFERENCES

1. Mokdad AH, Bowman BA, Ford ES, et al. The continuing epidemics of obesity and diabetes in the United States. JAMA 2001;286:1195–200.
2. World Health Organization. Obesity: preventing and managing the global epidemic. Report of a WHO consultation on obesity. Geneva: WHO, 1998.
3. US Department of Health and Human Services, NCHS. Third National Health and Nutrition Examination Survey (NHANES), Table 2: prevalence of overweight and obesity among adults: United States, 1999. Washington, DC: Centers for Disease Control and Prevention, 1999.
4. World Health Organization. Obesity epidemic puts millions at risk from related diseases. Geneva: WHO, 1997.
5. Crespo CJ, Smit E, Troiano RP, et al. Television watching, energy intake, and obesity in US children: results from the third National Health and Nutrition Examination Survey, 1988–1994. Arch Pediatr Adolesc Med 2001;155:360–365.
6. Bray G. Historical framework for the development of ideas about obesity. In: Bray G, Bouchard C, James W, eds. Handbook of Obesity. 2nd ed. New York: Marcel Dekker, 1998:1–30.
7. Metropolitan Life Insurance Company . Metropolitan height and weight tables. New York: Metropolitan Life Insurance Company, 1983:2–9.
8. Rao S, Donahue M, Pi-Sunyer FX, et al. Obesity as a risk factor in coronary artery disease. Am Heart J 2001;142:1102–1107.
9. Buskirk ER. Obesity. In: Skinner JS, ed. Exercise Testing and Exercise Prescription for Special Populations. 2nd ed. Baltimore: Lippincott, Williams & Wilkins, 1993:185–210.

10. National Institutes of Health, National Heart, Lung, and Blood Institute. Clinical guidelines on the identification, evaluation, and treatment of overweight and obesity in adults: the evidence report. Bethesda, MD, 1998.

11. Allison DB, Saunders SE. Obesity in North America. An overview. Med Clin North Am 2000;84:305–332.

12. Roche AF, Sievogel RM, Chumlea WC, et al. Grading body fatness from limited anthropometric data. Am J Clin Nutr 1981;34:2831–2838.

13. Khaodhiar L, Blackburn GL. Results of expert meetings: obesity and cardiovascular disease. Obesity assessment. Am Heart J 2001;142:1095–1101.

14. Lew EA, Garfinkel L. Variations in mortality by weight among 750,000 men and women. J Chronic Dis 1979;32:563–576.

15. Barrett-Connor EL. Obesity, atherosclerosis, and coronary artery disease. Ann Intern Med 1985;103:1010–1019.

16. Hoffmans MD, Kromhout D, de Lezenne Coulander C. The impact of body mass index of 78,612 18-year old Dutch men on 32-year mortality from all causes. J Clin Epidemiol 1988;41:749–756.

17. Power C, Lake JK, Cole TJ. Measurement and long-term health risks of child and adolescent fatness. Int J Obes Relat Metab Disord 1997;21:507–526.

18. American College of Sports Medicine. Appropriate intervention strategies for weight loss and prevention of weight regain for adults. Med Sci Sports Exerc 2001;33:2145–2156.

19. Després JP, Moorjani S, Ferland M, et al. Adipose tissue distribution and plasma lipoprotein levels in obese women. Importance of intra-abdominal fat. Arteriosclerosis 1989;9:203–210.

20. Pouliot MC, Després JP, Nadeau A, et al. Visceral obesity in men. Associations with glucose tolerance, plasma insulin, and lipoprotein levels. Diabetes 1992;41:826–834.

21. Rissanen J, Hudson R, Ross R. Visceral adiposity, androgens, and plasma lipids in obese men. Metabolism 1994;43:1318–1323.

22. Rippe JM, Crossley S, Ringer R. Obesity as a chronic disease: modern medical and lifestyle management. J Am Diet Assoc 1998;98:S9–15.

23. Pouliot MC, Després JP, Lemieux S, et al. Waist circumference and abdominal sagittal diameter: best simple anthropometric indexes of abdominal visceral adipose tissue accumulation and related cardiovascular risk in men and women. Am J Cardiol 1994;73:460–468.

24. Visscher TL, Seidell JC. The public health impact of obesity. Annu Rev Public Health 2001;22:355–75.

25. Ohrvall M, Berglund L, Vessby B. Sagittal abdominal diameter compared with other anthropometric measurements in relation to cardiovascular risk. Int J Obes Relat Metab Disord 2000;24:497–501.

26. Richelsen B, Pedersen SB. Associations between different anthropometric measurements of fatness and metabolic risk parameters in non-obese, healthy, middle-aged men. Int J Obes Relat Metab Disord 1995;19:169–174.

27. Flegal KM, Carroll MD, Kuczmarski RJ, et al. Overweight and obesity in the United States: prevalence and trends, 1960–1994. Int J Obes Relat Metab Disord 1998;22:39–47.

28. Downey M. Results of expert meetings: obesity and cardiovascular disease. Obesity as a disease entity. Am Heart J 2001;142:1091–1094.

29. Harnack LJ, Jeffery RW, Boutelle KN. Temporal trends in energy intake in the United States: an ecologic perspective. Am J Clin Nutr 2000;71:1478–1484.

30. Norris J, Harnack L, Carmichael S, et al. US trends in nutrient intake: the 1987 and 1992 National Health Interview Surveys. Am J Public Health 1997;87:740–746.

31. Briefel RR, McDowell MA, Alaimo K, et al. Total energy intake of the US population: the third National Health and Nutrition Examination Survey, 1988–1991. Am J Clin Nutr 1995;62:1072S–1080S.

32. Bray GA. The energetics of obesity. Med Sci Sports Exerc 1983;15:32–40.

33. Hill JO, Wyatt HR, Melanson EL. Genetic and environmental contributions to obesity. Med Clin North Am 2000;84:333–346.

34. Bouchard C, Blair SN. Introductory comments for the consensus on physical activity and obesity. Med Sci Sports Exerc 1999;31:S498–501.

35. Powers S, Howley E. Exercise Physiology: Theory and Application to Fitness and Performance. 4th ed. New York: McGraw-Hill, 2001.

36. Rissanen AM, Heliovaara M, Knekt P, et al. Determinants of weight gain and overweight in adult Finns. Eur J Clin Nutr 1991;45:419–430.

37. French SA, Jeffery RW, Forster JL, et al. Predictors of weight change over two years among a population of working adults: the Healthy Worker Project. Int J Obes Relat Metab Disord 1994;18:145–154.

38. Slattery ML, McDonald A, Bild DE, et al. Associations of body fat and its distribution with dietary intake, physical activity, alcohol, and smoking in blacks and whites. Am J Clin Nutr 1992;55:943–949.

39. Rippe JM, Hess S. The role of physical activity in the prevention and management of obesity. J Am Diet Assoc 1998;98:S31–38.

40. Physical activity trends—United States, 1990–1998. MMWR Morb Mortal Wkly Rep 2001;50:166–169.

41. Surgeon General's report on physical activity and health. From the Centers for Disease Control and Prevention. JAMA 1996;276:522.

42. Caspersen CJ, Merritt RK. Physical activity trends among 26 states, 1986–1990. Med Sci Sports Exerc 1995;27:713–720.

43. Leermakers EA, Dunn AL, Blair SN. Exercise management of obesity. Med Clin North Am 2000;84:419–440.

44. Vogler GP, Sorensen TI, Stunkard AJ, et al. Influences of genes and shared family environment on adult body mass index assessed in an adoption study by a comprehensive path model. Int J Obes Relat Metab Disord 1995;19:40–45.

45. Bouchard C. The Genetics of Obesity. Boca Raton, FL: CRC Press, 1994.

46. Troiano RP, Frongillo EA, Jr, Sobal J, et al. The relationship between body weight and mortality: a quantitative analysis of combined information from existing studies. Int J Obes Relat Metab Disord 1996;20:63–75.

47. Manson JE, Willett WC, Stampfer MJ, et al. Body weight and mortality among women. N Engl J Med 1995;333:677–685.

48. Lindsted K, Tonstad S, Kuzma JW. Body mass index and patterns of mortality among Seventh-day Adventist men. Int J Obes 1991;15:397–406.

49. Lee IM, Manson JE, Hennekens CH, et al. Body weight and mortality. A 27-year follow-up of middle-aged men. JAMA 1993;270:2823–2828.

50. Lee CD, Blair SN, Jackson AS. Cardiorespiratory fitness, body composition, and all-cause and cardiovascular disease mortality in men. Am J Clin Nutr 1999;69:373–380.

51. Eckel RH. Obesity and heart disease: a statement for healthcare professionals from the Nutrition Committee, American Heart Association. Circulation 1997;96:3248–3250.

52. Manson JE, Colditz GA, Stampfer MJ, et al. A prospective study of obesity and risk of coronary heart disease in women. N Engl J Med 1990;322:882–889.

53. Rimm EB, Stampfer MJ, Giovannucci E, et al. Body size and fat distribution as predictors of coronary heart disease among middle-aged and older US men. Am J Epidemiol 1995;141:1117–1127.

54. Goodpaster BH, Thaete FL, Simoneau JA, et al. Subcutaneous abdominal fat and thigh muscle composition predict insulin sensitivity independently of visceral fat. Diabetes 1997;46:1579–1585.

55. Ross R, Fortier L, Hudson R. Separate associations between visceral and subcutaneous adipose tissue distribution, insulin and glucose levels in obese women. Diabetes Care 1996;19:1404–1411.

56. Després JP, Lemieux S, Lamarche B, et al. The insulin resistance-dyslipidemic syndrome: contribution of visceral obesity and therapeutic implications. Int J Obes Relat Metab Disord 1995;19(suppl 1):S76–86.

57. Must A, Spadano J, Coakley EH, et al. The disease burden associated with overweight and obesity. JAMA 1999;282:1523–1529.

58. Després JP. Dyslipidaemia and obesity. Baillieres Clin Endocrinol Metab 1994;8:629–660.

59. Denke MA, Sempos CT, Grundy SM. Excess body weight. An under-recognized contributor to dyslipidemia in white American women. Arch Intern Med 1994;154:401–410.

60. Reeder BA, Angel A, Ledoux M, et al. Obesity and its relation to cardiovascular disease risk factors in Canadian adults. Canadian Heart Health Surveys Research Group. Can Med Assoc J 1992;146:2009–2019.

61. Denke MA, Sempos CT, Grundy SM. Excess body weight. An underrecognized contributor to high blood cholesterol levels in white American men. Arch Intern Med 1993;153:1093–1103.

62. Poirier P, Després JP. Exercise in weight management of obesity. Cardiol Clin 2001;19:459–470.

63. Stamler R, Stamler J, Riedlinger WF, et al. Weight and blood pressure. Findings in hypertension screening of 1 million Americans. JAMA 1978;240:1607–1610.

64. Kannel WB, Brand N, Skinner JJ Jr, et al. The relation of adiposity to blood pressure and development of hypertension. The Framingham Study. Ann Intern Med 1967;67:48–59.

65. Albu J, Pi-Sunyer FX. Obesity and diabetes. In: Bray G, Bouchard C, James W, eds. Handbook of Obesity. New York: Marcel Dekker, 1998:697–707.

66. Colditz GA, Willett WC, Rotnitzky A, et al. Weight gain as a risk factor for clinical diabetes mellitus in women. Ann Intern Med 1995;122:481–486.

67. Chan JM, Rimm EB, Colditz GA, et al. Obesity, fat distribution, and weight gain as risk factors for clinical diabetes in men. Diabetes Care 1994;17:961–969.

68. Lee IM, Paffenbarger RS Jr. Quetelet's index and risk of colon cancer in college alumni. J Natl Cancer Inst 1992;84:1326–1331.

69. Giovannucci E, Ascherio A, Rimm EB, et al. Physical activity, obesity, and risk for colon cancer and adenoma in men. Ann Intern Med 1995;122:327–334.

70. Giovannucci E, Colditz GA, Stampfer MJ, et al. Physical activity, obesity, and risk of colorectal adenoma in women (United States). Cancer Causes Control 1996;7:253–263.

71. Ursin G, Longnecker MP, Haile RW, et al. A meta-analysis of body mass index and risk of premenopausal breast cancer. Epidemiology 1995;6:137–141.

72. Pi-Sunyer FX. Medical complications of obesity. In: Brownell KD, Fairburn C, eds. Eating Disorders and Obesity. New York: Guilford Press, 1995:401–405.

73. Hart DJ, Spector TD. The relationship of obesity, fat distribution and osteoarthritis in women in the general population: the Chingford Study. J Rheumatol 1993;20:331–335.

74. Foss ML, Lampman RM, Schteingart D. Physical training program for rehabilitating extremely obese patients. Arch Phys Med Rehabil 1976;57:425–429.

75. Donnelly JE, Jacobsen DJ, Jakicic JM, et al. Estimation of peak oxygen consumption from a submaximal half mile walk in obese females. Int J Obes Relat Metab Disord 1992;16:585–589.

76. Buskirk ER, Taylor HL. Maximal oxygen intake and its relation to body composition, with special reference to chronic physical activity and obesity. J Appl Physiol 1957;11:72–78.

77. Farrell PA, Gustafson AB, Kalkhoff RK. Assessment of methods for assigning treadmill exercise workloads for lean and obese women. Int J Obes 1985;9:49–58.

78. Moody DL, Kollias J, Buskirk ER. Evaluation of aerobic capacity in lean and obese women with four test procedures. J Sports Med Phys Fitness 1969;9:1–9.

79. Goran M, Fields DA, Hunter GR, et al. Total body fat does not influence maximal aerobic capacity. Int J Obes Relat Metab Disord 2000;24:841–848.

80. Wasserman K, Hansen J, Sue D, et al. Principles of Exercise Testing & Interpretation. 3rd ed. Baltimore: Lippincott Williams & Wilkins, 1999.

81. Chung NK, Pin CH. Obesity and the occurrence of heat disorders. Milit Med 1996;161:739–742.

82. American College of Sports Medicine. ACSM's Guidelines for Exercise Testing and Prescription. 6th ed. Baltimore: Lippincott Williams & Wilkins, 2000.

83. DeVore P. Exercise testing of obese subjects. Physician Sports Med 1980;8:47–51.

84. McInnis KJ, Bader DS, Pierce GL, et al. Comparison of cardiopulmonary responses in obese women using ramp versus step treadmill protocols. Am J Cardiol 1999;83:289–291.

85. Fletcher GF, Balady GJ, Amsterdam EA, et al. Exercise standards for testing and training: a statement for healthcare professionals from the American Heart Association. Circulation 2001;104:1694–1740.

86. Grundy SM, Blackburn G, Higgins M, et al. Physical activity in the prevention and treatment of obesity and its comorbidities. Med Sci Sports Exerc 1999;31:S502–508.

87. Ross R, Freeman JA, Janssen I. Exercise alone is an effective strategy for reducing obesity and related comorbidities. Exerc Sport Sci Rev 2000;28:165–170.

88. Sopko G, Leon AS, Jacobs DR Jr, et al. The effects of exercise and weight loss on plasma lipids in young obese men. Metabolism 1985;34:227–236.

89. Ross R, Dagnone D, Jones PJ, et al. Reduction in obesity and related comorbid conditions after diet-induced weight loss or exercise-induced weight loss in men. A randomized, controlled trial. Ann Intern Med 2000;133:92–103.

90. Miller WC, Koceja DM, Hamilton EJ. A meta-analysis of the past 25 years of weight loss research using diet, exercise or diet plus exercise intervention. Int J Obes Relat Metab Disord 1997;21:941–947.

91. Wing RR. Physical activity in the treatment of the adulthood overweight and obesity: current evidence and research issues. Med Sci Sports Exerc 1999;31:S547–552.

92. Bouchard C, Tremblay A, Després JP, et al. The response to exercise with constant energy intake in identical twins. Obes Res 1994;2:400–410.

93. Pate RR, Pratt M, Blair SN, et al. Physical activity and public health. A recommendation from the Centers for Disease Control and Prevention and the American College of Sports Medicine. JAMA 1995;273:402–407.

94. Jakicic JM, Winters C, Lang W, et al. Effects of intermittent exercise and use of home exercise equipment on adherence, weight loss, and fitness in overweight women: a randomized trial. JAMA 1999;282:1554–1560.

95. Klem ML, Wing RR, McGuire MT, et al. A descriptive study of individuals successful at long-term maintenance of substantial weight loss. Am J Clin Nutr 1997;66:239–246.

96. Duncan JJ, Gordon NF, Scott CB. Women walking for health and fitness. How much is enough? JAMA 1991;266:3295–3299.

97. Yamanouchi K, Shinozaki T, Chikada K, et al. Daily walking combined with diet therapy is a useful means for obese NIDDM patients not only to reduce body weight but also to improve insulin sensitivity. Diabetes Care 1995;18:775–778.

98. Pacy PJ, Webster J, Garrow JS. Exercise and obesity. Sports Med 1986;3:89–113.

99. Mattsson E, Larsson UE, Rossner S. Is walking for exercise too exhausting for obese women? Int J Obes Relat Metab Disord 1997;21:380–386.

100. Hills AP, Byrne NM. Exercise prescription for weight management. Proc Nutr Soc 1998;57:93–103.

101. Dishman R, Sallis JF Jr. Determinants and interventions for physical activity and exercise. In: Bouchard C, Shephard RJ, Stephens T, eds. Physical Activity, Fitness, and Health. Champaign, IL: Human Kinetics, 1994:214–238.

102. Andersen RE, Wadden TA, Bartlett SJ, et al. Effects of lifestyle activity vs structured aerobic exercise in obese women: a randomized trial. JAMA 1999;281:335–340.

103. DeBusk RF, Haskell WL, Miller NH, et al. Medically directed at-home rehabilitation soon after clinically uncomplicated acute myocardial infarction: a new model for patient care. Am J Cardiol 1985;55:251–257.

104. Wallace J. Obesity. In: Durstine L, ed. ACSM's Exercise Management for Persons with Chronic Diseases and Disabilities. Champaign, IL: Human Kinetics, 1997:106–111.

105. Perri MG, McAllister DA, Gange JJ, et al. Effects of four maintenance programs on the long-term management of obesity. J Consult Clin Psychol 1988;56:529–534.

106. Wadden TA, Sternberg JA, Letizia KA, et al. Treatment of obesity by very low calorie diet, behavior therapy, and their combination: a five-year perspective. Int J Obes 1989;13:39–46.

107. Perri MG, Nezu AM, Patti ET, et al. Effect of length of treatment on weight loss. J Consult Clin Psychol 1989;57:450–452.

108. Franklin B, Buskirk E, Hodgson J, et al. Effects of physical conditioning on cardiorespiratory function, body composition and serum lipids in relatively normal-weight and obese middle-aged women. Int J Obes 1979;3:97–109.

109. Profant GR, Early RG, Nilson KL, et al. Responses to maximal exercise in healthy middle-aged women. J Appl Physiol 1972;33:595–599.

110. Weber MA, Neutel JM, Smith DH. Contrasting clinical properties and exercise responses in obese and lean hypertensive patients. J Am Coll Cardiol 2001;37:169–174.

RELATED WEB SITES

The Weight-Control Information Network (WIN)
www.win.niddk.nih.gov
This is a national information service of the National Institute of Diabetes and Digestive and Kidney Diseases (NIDDK), National Institutes of Health (NIH), dedicated to providing health professionals and consumers with science-based information on obesity, weight control, and nutrition.

The Combined Health Information Database (CHID)
www.chid.nih.gov
Abstracts, including thousands of references to articles, books, and audiovisual, and educational materials for health care professionals and consumers are available as the weight control subfile.

North American Association for the Study of Obesity (NAASO)
www.naaso.org
An interdisciplinary society whose purpose is to develop, extend, and disseminate knowledge in the field of obesity. Publishes Obesity Research, the official journal of NAASO.

USDA Nutrient Database
www.nal.usda.gov/fnic/cgi-bin/nut_search.pl
Allows public access to information on the nutrient content of thousands of foods.

American College of Sports Medicine
www.acsm.org
Contains healthy activity updates.

Shape Up America!
www.shapeup.org
Designed to provide the public with current information on safe weight management and physical fitness.

Respiratory Conditions

16

Asthma

Alan R. Morton and Kenneth D. Fitch

The relationship of asthma to exercise can be described as paradoxical. Most asthmatics will experience bronchoconstriction during, but mostly after, exertion, a fact known for nearly nineteen centuries (1).Conversely, current opinion considers exercise to be an integral component of the total management of asthma. The first documented exercise prescription was given to the Archbishop of Edinburgh by Professor Cardan of Pavia in 1551. The 40-year-old cleric, severely incapacitated by asthma, was recommended to take a daily horseback ride and in conjunction with other appropriate measures was greatly improved (2). Another notable asthmatic who benefited from exercise was Theodore Roosevelt, later president of the United States. Advised by his physician to undertake a strenuous exercise program during adolescence, Roosevelt did so with enthusiasm and became a fine athlete at Harvard, only mildly inconvenienced by asthma (3).

This chapter reviews the relationship of exercise to asthma, exercise testing, and exercise prescription, including anticipated benefits for asthmatic persons and drugs to reduce, prevent, and relieve exercise-induced asthma (EIA) or bronchoconstriction (EIB).

Definition and Incidence

Asthma is "a chronic inflammatory disorder of the airways in which many cells and cellular elements play a role, in particular mast cells, eosinophils, T lymphocytes, macrophages, neutrophils, and epithelial cells. In susceptible individuals, this inflammation causes recurrent episodes of wheezing, breathlessness, chest tightness, and coughing, particularly at night or in the early morning. These episodes are usually associated with widespread but variable airflow obstruction that is often reversible spontaneously or with treatment. The inflammation also causes an associated increase in the existing bronchial hyperresponsiveness to a variety of stimuli" (4).

Asthma is one of the most common respiratory disorders. Its incidence is highest in the first decade of life, and it occurs among members of all races, with the first episode occurring at any age. It is more common in boys than girls (3:2 ratio) but more common in older women than in older men. At any one time, asthmatic symptoms occur in between 4 and 16% of the population, depending on the country. The prevalence of asthma is escalating, and more than 300 million are suffering from asthma in the world today (5). In the United States, it affects 14 to 15 million people, who collectively have more than 100 million days of restricted activity and 470,000 hospitalizations annually. Asthma results in more than 5000 deaths a year in the United States (4). Airflow limitation is principally caused by mucosal edema, impaired mucociliary function, and contraction of airway smooth muscle. EIA/EIB

may be defined as a clinical syndrome characterized by temporary narrowing of the airways following moderate-to-severe exercise. Occasionally,
exercise is the only stimulus to provoke this narrowing. Anderson and Henriksen (6) suggest that the
term *exercise-induced bronchoconstriction* (EIB) be
reserved for persons who have postexercise narrowing and no clinical diagnosis of asthma. EIA/EIB
has been defined functionally as a 15% or greater
postexercise reduction of the forced expiratory volume in the first second (FEV_1) compared with
preexercise values, after standard submaximal exercise stress (7). Crapo et al. (8) suggest that a 10%
decrease in FEV_1 is sufficient for a positive diagnosis, while Rundell et al. (9) suggest that for elite
athletes who perform in cold environments, a drop
of 7% in the postexercise FEV_1 indicates EIA/EIB.
Currently, the most generally accepted figure is
10%.

It is customary to use an exercise challenge of
6 to 8 min at 65 to 75% of predicted maximal oxygen uptake ($\dot{V}O_{2max}$), which is approximately 75
to 85% of predicted maximal heart rate (HR_{max}).
Following such an exercise challenge, 80 to 90% of
asthmatics can be expected to develop EIA/EIB.
The resultant postexercise bronchoconstriction can
be classified as follows:

- Mild   10–24% fall in FEV_1
- Moderate   25–39% fall in FEV_1
- Severe   40% or greater fall in FEV_1

Causes of EIA/EIB

Despite early recognition of the association between exercise and asthma and extensive research
on EIA during the last 50 years, no mechanism that
satisfactorily explains its occurrence has been proposed and received general acceptance. A number
of initiating stimuli have been postulated, but the
best hypothesis is that EIA is caused by the release
of some bronchoconstrictor substance, probably in
response to the changes in osmolarity of the periciliary fluid. This change is thought to result from the
loss of fluid from the airways during conditioning
of inspired air (10).

Conditioning the air refers to the warming, humidifying, and filtering of inspired air and is important to prevent damage to delicate alveolar tissue

that can occur when it is exposed to cold dry air.
Most conditioning occurs in the nose, pharynx, and
the first seven generations of bronchi. The asthmatic should inhale through the nose during rest
and light exercise to maximize this warming and
humidification process. Even when dry air at 0°C
is inspired through the nose, it is modified so that
it has been humidified and warmed to 37°C by the
time it reaches the alveolar membrane. This saturation of alveolar air occurs by absorbing water from
the airways during its passage from the nose to alveolar regions. This "dries" the airways, thereby con-
centrating the ions in the periciliary fluid. Asthmatics appear to be unusually sensitive to these changes
in osmolarity.

The released bronchoactive mediators may
include histamine, leukotrienes, prostaglandins
and neuropeptides released from the mast cells,
macrophages, eosinophils, epithelial cells, and sensory nerves (11). They may act directly on smooth
muscle, stimulate lung irritant receptors (which
in turn causes bronchoconstriction via vagal influences), and/or produce the inflammation reaction
via such constituents as neutrophil chemotactic factor. Cooling of the airways may enhance the response to water loss (12).

Relationship of Exercise to Asthma

Although breathlessness is normal during high-
intensity exercise, it is abnormal if it occurs during
or after light exercise. Unfortunately, many asthmatics do not realize this fact and are unaware that
they develop EIA. They assume that dyspnea is
just lack of fitness, fail to seek medical advice, and
perform at a disadvantage because they lack appropriate medication. Although this has often been observed, the problem still exists according to Hammerman et al. (13), who found that 12% of 755
athletes studied in 10 Pittsburgh high schools had
undiagnosed asthma.

At least 80 to 90% of asthmatics develop
EIA/EIB after standardized exercise tests (14), and
almost all asthmatics occasionally develop airway
narrowing with physical exertion. Exercise, therefore, may be used as a challenge test to confirm the
diagnosis of asthma. It is also used to categorize

EIA/EIB severity. In addition, exercise is widely used in asthma research to determine (*a*) the efficacy of various medications to prevent and/or reverse asthma and (*b*) the effects of agents that reduce and aggravate EIA/EIB, such as face masks and certain environmental conditions.

Between episodes of asthma, the cardiorespiratory system is normal in many asthmatics and does not interfere with physical performance. The vast number of asthmatics who are classified as elite athletes is testimony to this fact. An asthmatic's exercise performance and the ability to endure will certainly be impaired, however, if he or she participates while airways are constricted. Narrowed airways will limit ventilation and thus oxygen uptake and can result in lower arterial oxygen saturation and a higher level of carbon dioxide in the blood. When hyperinflation occurs, usually as a result of early airway closure, it is an attempt to use the assistance of increased elastic recoil to maintain adequate airflow. However, ventilation at high lung volumes requires the respiratory muscles to operate at a mechanical disadvantage, utilizing the less efficient part of the length-tension range. This can lead to respiratory muscle fatigue.

PROVOCATION OF ASTHMA BY EXERCISE

When exercise provokes a bout of asthma, there is a characteristic response. First, there is bronchodilation, which may last the duration of the activity or may persist for a few minutes. This bronchodilation is followed by narrowing of the airways, an event that accelerates as soon as exercise is finished. The narrowed airway increases the resistance of airflow, reaching a peak 2 to 10 min after exercise cessation.

Airway narrowing is probably due to not only contraction of smooth muscle surrounding the airway but also to airway inflammation, especially during a late or second response to exercise. When the airway wall is thickened because of inflammation, there will be an exaggerated reduction in the size of the airway lumen as a result of a given degree of muscle shortening (15)

Bronchoconstriction usually reverses spontaneously, and the resistance to airflow gradually returns to preexercise levels within 45 to 60 min (16). When there is no spontaneous recovery, medication may be needed to reverse the EIA/EIB.

The pattern of change in airway resistance with exercise is usually evaluated by measuring the change in FEV_1. The relative instability of the airways, that is, the susceptibility for change in airway diameter is indicated by the lability index, which is computed by summing the exercise-induced percentage increase in FEV_1 during bronchodilation and the postexercise maximal percentage decrease in FEV_1 during bronchoconstriction (Fig 16-1). A lability index above 20 is usually considered abnormal (17).

The above indicates that most asthmatics do not exhibit EIA/EIB until after exercise has ceased. The few who develop it during activity will be at a greater disadvantage during sport. The longer the event, the more severe the EIA/EIB in these asthmatics, and the greater the limitation placed on delivery of oxygen to active tissue. Symptoms that may develop during an episode of EIA/EIB include wheezing, shortness of breath, chest tightness, cough, increased production of mucus, and the inability to continue exercise.

Another exercise response that some asthmatics, particularly children, display is termed the *late or second reaction*. This may not develop for 3 to 4 hours after cessation of exercise and may take 3 to 9 hours to reach its peak. This late response is probably due to an inflammatory reaction due to such mediators as neutrophil chemotactic factor (18).

About 50% of asthmatics exhibit a refractory period after exercise. During this period, a second bout of exercise will provoke an airway response that is less than 50% of the initial response (19). This refractory period may last an hour or longer, but refractoriness is usually lost within 2 to 4 hours. Refractoriness is lost if the asthmatic is treated with a nonsteroidal antiinflammatory medication (e.g., naproxen, indomethacin or diclofenac) for several days in an attempt to overcome an injury (20,21). This may indicate that refractoriness is mediated via a prostaglandin.

A disturbing feature of vigorous exercise training in very cold environments has been reported (22–24). Asthma, asthmalike symptoms, and hyperresponsiveness are much more common among cross-country skiers and other similar winter sports athletes than in the general population and nonskiers. This is possibly due to breathing large volumes of very cold air during training and competition.

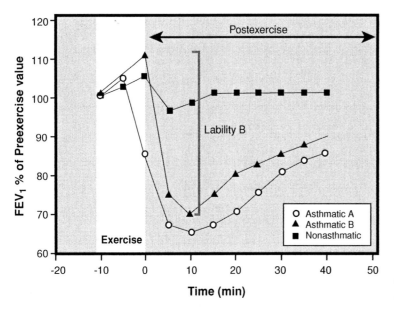

FIGURE 16-1 Typical changes in forced expiratory flow in 1 second in asthmatic and nonasthmatic subjects.

EXERCISE IN THE MANAGEMENT OF ASTHMA

Regular exercise is an important component of disease management because of its beneficial effects on respiratory and circulatory function and on the psychologic development of asthmatics, which is reflected in its effect on their social life. These training benefits are manifested in the improved working capacity due to an increased $\dot{V}O_{2max}$, as well as improved skill and efficiency during motor tasks. This means that the same daily tasks can be performed with less ventilation and thus less drying of the airways. In general, asthmatics should be able to participate in regular exercise and sports with minimal restriction, if correctly medicated.

MODIFICATION OF THE ASTHMATIC RESPONSE TO EXERCISE

Selection of Exercise

The asthmatic's response to exercise is extremely variable from person to person and even in the same person at different times. There is evidence showing that the type (16,25–27), duration (16,28,29), and intensity (29) of exercise, as well as the type of exercise loading (30), the environmental condi-

tions (10,31,32), and pharmacologic intervention, can all modify responses to a bout of exercise.

Briefly, evidence indicates that if modes of exercise are ranked by asthmogenicity, swimming and walking would be the least asthmogenic, progressing through cycling and kayaking to running, which provokes the most severe asthma. There is evidence that exercise of short duration induces less EIA than prolonged activity, but this increasing airway response with a longer duration plateaus at about 6 to 8 min. There is also increased airway resistance at higher exercise intensities up to about 65 to 75% of $\dot{V}O_{2max}$ or about 75 to 85% of predicted HR_{max}.

At least for changes in type, duration, and intensity, these differences in response can be partially explained by differences in ventilatory requirements. For instance, the more intense and the longer the duration of activity, the larger the minute ventilation required and thus the greater the loss of fluid from the airways; this results in more airway drying and a greater increase in osmolarity of the periciliary fluid. Studies that have used various exercise modes but have standardized the effort to ensure equal ventilation and air humidity have found similar asthmogenicity with running, walking, cycling, and arm cranking (17). Swimming allows one to inhale moist air from just above the surface of the water and may explain some of its lower asthmogenicity than other modes of activity.

Although the amount of water loss can account for much of the variability in response, it does not appear to be the only factor involved. Inbar et al. (33) showed that when the water content of inspired air was kept constant (using dry air) and a similar ventilation was induced, swimming still produced a smaller reduction in lung function than running. They also found that if asthmatics breathing dry air and breathing moist air were compared while swimming, there was no significant difference. Bar-Yishay et al. (34) showed a small but significant difference in the asthmogenicity of swimming and running, even under conditions of the same metabolic stress and respiratory heat loss. The fact that the effects of changes in exercise duration plateau at 6 to 8 min and intensity peaks at 75 to 85% HR_{max} is also difficult to explain by the osmolarity theory alone. That is, one would expect that the longer one exercises and the higher the intensity, the greater the total ventilation and total water loss. One explanation might be that there is a maximal amount of airway narrowing possible for a given individual. Once this level has been reached, further stimuli produce no further change.

A comparison of the efficacy of salbutamol, ipratropium bromide, and cromolyn sodium to prevent bronchospasm induced by exercise and hyperosmolar challenges also suggests that hyperosmolarity, though playing a role in EIA, may not be the sole factor involved (35).

Use of Aids to Warm and Humidify Inspired Air

Under resting conditions, breathing through the nose warms and humidifies the air to ensure that when inspired air reaches the delicate alveolar membrane, it is warmed to 37°C and completely saturated with water vapor. As the metabolic rate is raised with increasing exercise intensity, there is a change in ventilation from about 6 $L \cdot min^{-1}$ at rest to levels above 200 $L \cdot min^{-1}$ in some elite athletes performing maximal exercise. The protection from EIA/EIB that could be expected by breathing through the nose is limited to light-to-moderate exercise, as the size of the nostrils allows a max-

imum of about 40 to 100 $L \cdot min^{-1}$ of nasal ventilation (36). Nasal resistance to airflow increases with exercise and eventually reaches critical ventilation (usually about 50 $L \cdot min^{-1}$), at which time respiration is switched from the nose to the mouth. To facilitate the benefits of nasal breathing, Bar-Or (17) recommends a nasal vasoconstrictor for those with allergic rhinitis.

There have been a number of aids suggested to maintain a warmer and moister inspirate during exercise to try to minimize the asthmatic response. For instance, surgical face masks and similar devices have been used with benefit during training sessions, especially during cold weather. There are also a number of commercially produced cold air breathing aids such as BLO.GO and Lungplus Sport, developed in Sweden. Although these aids can be useful during training, they are usually impractical to use during competition. Breathe Right external nasal dilators can be used with some benefit to asthmatic athletes during both training and competition.

When and Where to Exercise

Asthma may be provoked by many factors other than exercise. It is wise to avoid as many of these other provoking agents as possible during exercise, because the effects may be cumulative. For instance, because breathing cold dry air is a potent stimulus for EIA, one should either avoid exercise during the coldest part of the day (early morning or evening) or exercise indoors. Because air pollution can provoke an episode of asthma, exercise should be avoided during those daily periods when pollution is highest. Exercising near busy roadways and factories is also contraindicated. At times when air pollution levels are high, asthmatics should perform their exercise-training programs indoors.

Asthmatics who are allergic to certain grasses and pollens should avoid outdoor exercise when pollen counts are high. Those who are allergic to house dust mites are more liable to EIA if indoor exercise programs are conducted in venues that provide an environment with a high population of mites. Asthmatics must avoid smoke-filled rooms when exercising. Smoking should not be permitted in any indoor sporting arena because of the effects of passive smoking. If an asthmatic exercises by swimming and is susceptible to the effects of cold water, a heated pool should be used.

Warm-Up

A thorough warm-up has a threefold benefit for the asthmatic participant. Firstly, the usual benefits attributed to warm-up prior to vigorous exercise apply. Secondly, a warm-up, which may or may not provoke EIA, can reduce the severity and duration of EIA triggered by a second exercise session. For asthmatics who experience a refractory period following an initial bout of EIA, (19) a warm-up can be scheduled so that they have time to recover from the EIA that it triggers and then be in the refractory state during the competitive event. Reiff et al. (37) found that a prolonged warm-up period of low-intensity exercise can induce refractoriness to EIA without itself inducing marked bronchoconstriction. Anderson (38) suggests that those who demonstrate a refractory period and who are required to perform vigorous exercise at regular intervals throughout the day or those who exercise for long periods may have an advantage. She claims that these asthmatics can prevent a second EIA attack with a reduction or even elimination of further medication. Thirdly, there is some evidence that a thorough warm-up included as part of an exercise session can reduce the EIA that occurs as a result of that session (39).

Medications

An asthmatic's response to exercise can be modified most by the judicious use of medication. This requires that asthmatics and their physicians determine the best medication program to control their chronic asthma and then determine which preexercise medication(s) and dose(s) provide the best protection from EIA/EIB. A discussion of the various medications follows. Asthmatic athletes should ask their physician to provide two written asthma management plans, one to control chronic asthma and the other to prevent and treat EIA. One must gain maximal control over chronic asthma if the incidence and severity of EIA/EIB is to be minimized. Severe bouts of EIA/EIB are an indication of "under-treated asthma" (40). In a recent study, Hammerman et al. (13) found that 85% of high school athletes who knew they had asthma still experienced EIB, suggesting that their asthma was inadequately controlled.

Drugs for EIA

During the last 35 years, several pharmacologically different groups of drugs have been developed to assist the asthmatic by minimizing EIA. They appear to act via several different sites and mechanisms, including smooth muscle relaxation, inhibition of release of bronchoconstrictor mediators, reduction of mucosal edema and permeability, and alteration of vagal tone. The β_2 agonists, khellin derivatives, methyl xanthines, glucocorticosteroids, leukotriene receptor antagonists, and belladonna alkaloids are discussed below.

β_2 AGONISTS

These sympathomimetic amines are the most effective drugs to prevent (if administered preexercise) and to reverse EIA/EIB (41). β_2-Adrenoceptor stimulants have replaced their predecessors, e.g., ephedrine (an α-receptor stimulant) and isoproterenol (isoprenaline) that stimulate both β_1 and β_2 receptors.

Metaproterenol (orciprenaline), albuterol (salbutamol), terbutaline, rimiterol, reproterol, pirbuterol, and bitolterol are about equally effective when administered by the aerosol route (42). About 90% of asthmatics obtain clinical protection from preexercise β_2 agonists. Because of the much lower dosage, greater rapidity of action, and fewer side effects, the aerosol route is always preferred to oral administration, except in very young children who cannot manipulate hand-held aerosols. The correct inhaler technique must be used, because many asthmatics use faulty technique, reducing the effectiveness of the medication. A "spacer" (which is a plastic inhalational chamber used in conjunction with hand-held nebulizers), greatly facilitates the amount of the drug reaching the lungs.

The usual dose is one to two activations shortly before exercise. A similar dose may be administered if EIA/EIB supervenes. Principal side effects (e.g., tremor, nervousness, tachycardia, and palpitations) are more frequent following oral administration. Chronic asthma must be well controlled by an inhaled steroid. β_2 agonists are not used to treat asthma other than as an emergency measure. Recent research has shown that regular use of a β_2 agonist may diminish its bronchodilator effect and thus lead to an inability to provide emergency bronchodilator treatment during an acute asthma attack (43).

Long-acting β_2 agonists (salmeterol and formoterol) are effective for about 12 hours and are particularly useful to prevent EIA/EIB if the physical activity or event lasts for a few hours or if a number of heats or games are to be played in the same day. Salmeterol cannot be used for exacerbations or as a reliever (rescue) medication because of its slow onset of action. However, formoterol can be used because it is both rapidly acting and long acting (39).

KHELLIN DERIVATIVES (MAST CELL STABILIZERS)

Cromolyn sodium (sodium cromoglycate), in clinical use for 35 years, remains the principal example and is totally or partially effective in 70% of asthmatics (45). Intrinsic asthmatics are generally less responsive. A newer khellin derivative, nedocromil sodium, appears to be equipotent with cromolyn but perhaps more effective in intrinsic asthma (46)

Children appear to be more responsive to cromolyn than adults, as are asthmatics who do not experience airway obstruction prior to exercise. In persons with airway obstruction, the administration of cromolyn should be preceded by inhaling a β agonist.

The infrequent late response (i.e., postexercise bronchoconstriction occurring some hours after exercise) is blocked by cromolyn but not by β agonists (38).

METHYL XANTHINES

Theophylline and, to a lesser degree, aminophylline (theophylline ethylene diamine) are usually prescribed for regular oral administration to attain and maintain serum concentrations at 10 to 20 $\mu g \cdot mL^{-1}$ to control asthma and EIA (47). With such therapy, the protection achieved against EIA approximates that of cromolyn. However, because

of more effective aerosol agents with rapid action and fewer side effects, theophylline is no longer considered to have a significant role in the pharmacologic amelioration of EIA (42).

GLUCOCORTICOSTEROIDS

Recent theories that asthma is an inflammatory disease (4) fit comfortably with the excellent therapeutic effect of glucocorticosteroids to treat chronic and life-threatening asthma. In such circumstances, oral and intravenous administrations are used. The nonhalogenated corticosteroids with topical antiinflammatory properties (budesonide and fluticasone) provide excellent protection against EIA (48,49). The principal value of aerosol glucocorticosteroids is to control asthma by regular administration, supplemented by inhaled β agonists before exercise. Inhaled glucocorticosteroids are probably underused. Those with severe EIA/EIB and those with poorly controlled EIA/EIB should increase their intake of steroids. Some athletes obtain an excellent response to regularly inhaled glucocorticoids that obviates the need for preexercise inhaled β agonists.

LEUKOTRIENE RECEPTOR ANTAGONISTS

Leukotrienes are derived from arachidonic acid and are potent mediators of inflammation (especially cysteinyl leukotrienes) and also powerful bronchoconstrictors. Leukotriene receptor antagonists are a group of drugs that provide significant protection against bronchoconstriction induced by leukotrienes. Monolukast sodium and zafirlukast are two leukotriene receptor antagonists administered orally that are used to prevent asthma and EIA in children and adults. These agents provide moderate protection against EIA akin to cromolyn but are customarily administered in combination with inhaled glucocorticoids and β agonists.

BELLADONNA ALKALOIDS

Ipratropium bromide, a quaternary ammonium derivative of atropine with potent anticholinergic properties but minor atropine-like side effects, is beneficial in asthma and EIA with certain patients (50). The principal indication to add ipratropium bromide is the case of an asthmatic with severe and incompletely blocked EIA despite preexercise cromolyn and a β agonist (51).

During the last decade, there was increased use of inhaled glucocorticosteroids to prevent and treat asthma and EIA. These agents are combined with preexercise β agonists with the addition of either cromolyn or a leukotriene receptor antagonist, if necessary. Ipratropium bromide may benefit a few of those still unresponsive. Inhaled β agonists provide effective protection against EIB in those who experience asthma only with exercise.

For those asthmatics who may be subjected to sports drug testing, the World Anti-doping Agency (WADA) and the International Olympic Committee (IOC) permit the use of only four inhaled β_2 agonists: albuterol (salbutamol), formoterol, salmeterol, and terbutaline subject to prior notification to the relevant medical authority (52). All other β agonists are prohibited by inhalation. Oral β_2 agonists (because of anabolic effects) and oral glucocorticosteroids are prohibited. Khellin derivatives, methyl xanthines, inhaled glucocorticosteroids, belladonna alkaloid, and leukotriene receptor antagonists are permitted.

At the 2002 Olympic Winter Games, athletes who needed to inhale a permitted β agonist were required to submit evidence of their asthma and EIA/EIB to an independent panel of experts. This evidence included a clinical history and spirographic evidence of either EIA/EIB ($\geq 10\%$ fall in FEV_1 after exercise challenge), a positive response to an inhaled bronchodilator ($\geq 12\%$ increase in FEV_1), or a positive response (PD20 ≤ 1 mg/mL) after either a methacholine or histamine challenge. If an athlete's data did not satisfy the panel of his/her need to use an inhaled β_2 agonist, the eucapnic voluntary hyperpnea (EVH) challenge (53) was used to confirm that the athlete had EIA/EIB. It is anticipated that the policy of requiring justification to inhale a β agonist by these or similar criteria will be included in WADA's list of prohibited substances valid from January, 2003.

Exercise Testing

The best EIA test for athletes is a "sports-specific" challenge in which respiratory data are collected before and after an actual game or event per-

formed under the usual game or event climatic conditions (54). The usual laboratory test is an exercise challenge. Regardless of the reason for conducting tests on asthmatics, a pretest medical history should be obtained. This history should emphasize the cardiorespiratory system (particularly relating to EIA/EIB), the current list of medications, habitual activity level, and any sporting involvement.

For males older than 40 years and females older than 50 years or those who fall into the high-risk category for coronary artery disease, the testing and exercise precautions set out in the guidelines of the American College of Sports Medicine must be observed (55). Those procedures are in addition to the ones outlined below.

EXERCISE TESTING TO DISPROVE OR CONFIRM EIA

Briefly, the test involves examining airway resistance, as reflected by changes in FEV_1 before and after a bout of exercise. Tests to determine whether one is susceptible to EIA should include the following procedures to optimize the response:

1. The test should be a single-stage, continuous test lasting at least 6 to 8 min.
2. The intensity should be such that one works at 65 to 75% $\dot{V}O_{2max}$, which is approximately 75 to 85% HR_{max}.
3. Ensure that all inhaled air enters via the mouth and is not subject to the warming and humidifying processes of the nose. This is facilitated if the subject wears a nose clip.
4. To determine the severity and duration of EIA, preexercise lung function measurements of FEV_1 and FVC (at least) are obtained. Repeat the same lung function measurements immediately after and at frequent intervals (every 5 min) for 40 min after exercise. Exercise and postexercise values should be expressed as a percentage of the preexercise value.
5. Nonasthmatics will show only a slight change in these measures. A drop in FEV_1 of 10% or more indicates an episode of EIA/EIB (38,56). Other EIA diagnostic tests such as specific conductance (SGaw), the rate of flow at 50% of vital capacity (FEF_{50}), or the average flow

rate between 25 and 75% of vital capacity (FEF$_{25-75}$) are also in common use. These tests require a 35% postexercise reduction to diagnose EIA (17). Reductions in FEF$_{50}$ or FEF$_{25-75}$ indicate small airway involvement, whereas drops in FEV$_1$ indicate large airway involvement.

6. If possible, tests should be conducted under environmental conditions conducive to triggering EIA, i.e., a cold, dry environment.

7. Although EIA can be provoked by all modes of exercise, running is preferred during testing because it is the most asthmogenic.

8. Subjects should abstain from medication prior to testing. Cromolyn sodium, methyl xanthines, and antihistamines should be withheld for a minimum of 24 hours, inhaled glucocorticosteroids for at least 24 hours but preferably 48 to 96 hours, anticholinergics for 8 hours, and β_2 agonists for a minimum of 6 and 24 hours for short- and long-acting preparations, respectively.

9. Vigorous exercise should be avoided for at least 12 hours prior to testing to ensure that the subject is not in a refractory state or likely to have test results influenced by a late or second response to the initial bout of exercise.

10. Food (particularly chocolate and such caffeinated drinks as coffee, tea, and cola) should be avoided for at least 6 hours before testing, because caffeine is a methyl xanthine and has some bronchodilatory effect (57,58). Ingestion of water is not restricted.

Where the fitness level of the subject is unknown, the starting workload should be low. The workload is then increased gradually over the next 2 to 3 min until the target HR is achieved. The last 5 min of the test should be completed at this workload.

The eucapnic voluntary hyperpnea (EVH) challenge is becoming established as an excellent alternative to an exercise challenge because it is easy to generate higher ventilation rates while maintaining normal end-tidal carbon dioxide levels (53,59). This 6-minute test requires the subject to hyperventilate dry gas, at room temperature, containing 5% carbon dioxide so as to maintain arterial carbon dioxide levels within the range found during exercise. The target ventilation rate is 30 times the FEV$_1$, equivalent to about 85% of maximum voluntary ventilation. This test was considered the optimum challenge to confirm that an athlete at the 2002 Winter Olympics had EIA/EIB, a positive test result was a fall in FEV$_1$ of 10% or more from baseline.

Mannitol and hypertonic saline challenges are also used to identify those with EIA/EIB (60,61).

FITNESS ASSESSMENT IN ASTHMATICS

When selecting tests to assess the fitness of asthmatics, one needs to know whether they require a fitness evaluation to participate in some competitive event or sport, or whether it is for general fitness to maintain an optimal normal healthy lifestyle. In each case, the test items selected should be the same as those for the nonasthmatic. In both situations, however, emphasis must be placed on determining the pulmonary function and aerobic power of asthmatic subjects. Asthmatics should also have their EIA severity assessed.

As a minimal requirement, the pulmonary function test should include FEV$_1$, FVC (forced vital capacity), and FEV$_1$% (FEV$_1$/FVC $\times$ 100). Whenever possible, flow volume loops should be obtained together with data usually determined during these tests, including flow rates at different lung volumes (especially FEF$_{25-75}$ and FEF$_{50}$). Other recommended pulmonary function tests include maximal voluntary ventilation (maximal breathing capacity) and determination of the resting lung subdivisions, that is, tidal volume (TV), inspiratory reserve volume (IRV), expiratory reserve volume (ERV), inspiratory capacity (IC), expiratory capacity (EC), vital capacity (VC), residual volume (RV), and functional residual capacity (FRC). There are many portable electronic devices that provide most of these pulmonary function scores on a visual display, as well as in a printed and graphic report. The rating of perceived exertion (RPE) using the Borg scale (62) and rating of breathlessness or dyspnea during exercise (63) should be assessed at given workloads.

Fitness tests for asthmatics should be conducted when they demonstrate unobstructed lung volumes. To ensure this, all tests (except EIA severity) should be performed 5 min after inhalation of two doses of a β_2 agonist.

Testing is of greatest benefit if repeated on a regular basis to determine not merely status, but change in status because of change in activities or medication.

Exercise Prescription

TRAINING FOR COMPETITION

When an asthmatic competes in a sporting event, the training program will be similar to that used by nonasthmatics in the same sport. The asthmatic should inhale adequate preventive medication prior to each training session and competitive event. World championship level performances have been recorded by asthmatics in most sporting events. These athletes train as hard as nonasthmatics, using the same procedures. Occasionally, a training session or even a game or competitive event may be missed if there is a severe episode of asthma.

TRAINING FOR GENERAL FITNESS

Regular fitness training programs appear to be effective for improving work capacity, increasing efficiency, and lessening dyspnea without affecting the disease process. The general fitness program for improved daily living (the wellness program) should emphasize general aerobic fitness and follow the guidelines described by the American College of Sports Medicine concerning exercise prescription for asymptomatic adults (55). Activities to produce neuromuscular relaxation and exercises for breathing control are often valuable. The breathing exercises involve diaphragmatic (abdominal) breathing and activities that require breathing against resistance to increase the strength and endurance of the respiratory muscles. Abdominal breathing can be demonstrated by having the subject place a hand on the abdomen. The abdomen (and the hand) should rise with each inspiration and descend with each exhalation, while keeping the upper thorax relatively still. The abdomen appears to swell because of the downward movement of the diaphragm, which increases intraabdominal pressure. Deep, slow breathing while exhaling against pursed lips helps to keep the small airways open, because these airways tend to collapse (close) when intrapleural pressure exceeds pressure within the airway.

The mode of exercise selected is also important. The success of any training program relies on regular and frequent participation. One of the major stimulants to exercise regularity is an adequate level of enjoyment. Therefore, despite the asthmogenicity of various activities, those of major interest to the individual should be prescribed. The exercise leader should attempt to influence the asthmatic to select aerobic activities. Swimming is less asthmogenic and helps to increase heart and lung volumes (64). The one physical activity that most physicians advise against is scuba diving. Though a great many asthmatics dive without incident, the threat of barotrauma while surfacing following the advent of air trapping due to small airway closure is a real danger. The present medical regulations in some countries prohibit anyone with a history of asthma from this activity, but this rule appears excessively stringent. One method that has gained acceptance is to challenge the prospective scuba diver with an inhaled isotonic saline challenge (60) and to approve only those who have a negative response. In those who sporadically experience EIA, there often appears to be little indication when bronchoconstriction is likely to occur. It is suggested, therefore, that preventive medication be administered before training or competition.

When suffering from an acute respiratory infection, the asthmatic has a greater susceptibility to EIA; this susceptibility may last up to 6 weeks after the acute infection. Whenever possible, therefore, exercising asthmatics should avoid others with such respiratory infections as influenza and the common cold. They should also be sure to have a warm shower and dress in warm clothing as soon as possible after an exercise session, because many asthmatics are susceptible to sudden changes in temperature.

Regular assessment of fitness is a valuable way to motivate the asthmatic and thus maintain training regularity. It also provides an indication of the training program's effectiveness and helps to redirect the program when changes are needed.

When the exercise program is performed in a formal fitness class situation (e.g., a health club or during school physical education), the exercise leader (teacher) should know which participants are asthmatic. The leader should construct a register of asthmatics together with an indication of their best peak expiratory flow rate (PEFR) reading,

80 and 50% of their best PEFR, their usual medication, and their doctors' names and phone numbers. The leader should have an inexpensive peak flow meter available to assess the severity of any bronchoconstriction that occurs. These results allow decisions to be made concerning the advisability of continued participation in a given session and the need for medical assistance.

Many schools require children on medication to keep their medication in a central administrative office or nurse's station. This is considered unwise in the case of asthmatics, who should have free and easy access to their metered-dose inhaler (65).

WHEN TO AVOID OR CEASE EXERTION

If an asthmatic has taken the prescribed preexercise medication and is still exhibiting bronchoconstriction, it is probably unwise to attempt vigorous exercise. While some asthmatics under these conditions find that exercise opens the airways and may alleviate the situation, most get worse. School children reporting to a physical education class or a sports event with airway constriction should be excused for that session. Some can run through mild attacks of EIA, whereas others cannot. As a general rule, asthmatics should cease participating in a game or vigorous exercise session if EIA develops during that activity. If inhalation of a β_2 agonist reverses the bronchoconstriction, asthmatics can resume the exercise or sporting event. If it is not successful, they should refrain from further participation.

Performing vigorous activity with moderate or severe bronchoconstriction can lead to a severe drop in arterial oxygen saturation, carbon dioxide accumulation, and hyperinflation of the lungs with an increased residual volume. This results in severe dyspnea and general discomfort, possible worsening of the resistance to airflow, and respiratory muscle fatigue. If an asthmatic regularly measures PEFR and is aware of his or her normal unobstructed level, a peak flow measure at the time of concern can be a good guide to the advisability of either commencing or continuing activity. It should be at least 80% of his or her "best" value. The availability of inexpensive peak flow meters means that school physical education departments and individual asthmatics

can afford their own instruments and have them available for such use.

Benefits of Regular Exercise

PHYSICAL AND PHYSIOLOGIC BENEFIT

While regular and frequent aerobic exercise at moderate-to-high intensity does not prevent asthma, it does provide the same physiologic benefits for the asthmatic as for the nonasthmatic. For instance, one study (58) showed that asthmatics had significantly improved posture, physical work capacity, and swimming ability, as well as a reduced amount of body fat after 5 months of intensive swimming training. However, their susceptibility to EIA when challenged with a standard treadmill running test was unchanged. This confirms that bronchial hyperresponsiveness is not relieved by enhanced aerobic fitness through training. A similar finding was reported in a study (66) of 9- to 14-year-old boys participating in two 90-min training sessions per week consisting of a short warm-up period, stretching exercises, calisthenics, strengthening exercises, breathing exercises, interval training, and such team games as soccer. Swim training was also included.

Both studies also found a reduction in medication required to control the chronic asthma of the subjects and in the number of asthma episodes. These results suggest that regular aerobic training improves clinical asthma, but like pubertal remissions, the underlying defect remains. These findings are confirmed by some investigators (27,67) but not others (68,69)

Training outcomes of particular importance to the asthmatic are increased physical exercise capacity, as determined by $\dot{V}O_{2max}$ and the $\dot{V}O_2$ at which one can exercise before lactate begins to accumulate in the blood. This event appears to coincide with the respiratory compensation threshold, at which time there is a sudden and disproportionate increase in ventilation.

Residual volume is usually reduced with training because of a decreased amount of air trapped in the lungs (70). Other respiratory system benefits include a more efficient pattern of respiration involving slower and deeper breathing (71), which maximizes alveolar ventilation and minimizes the proportion of total ventilation accounted for by dead space volume (better VD/VT). The proportion of abdominal breathing may also increase.

Training increases the maximal attainable rate of ventilation, while reducing the inspired volume required to perform a given level of submaximal work. This decreased respiration means less air has to be "conditioned" and, as a result, there is a smaller change in osmolarity of the periciliary fluid and less EIA/EIB.

All of the above training-induced changes result in asthmatics being able to perform a given task with a smaller disturbance of their internal environment. This means that the aerobically trained asthmatic can cope better than the untrained asthmatic with the same degree of mild or moderate airway obstruction. Research has also indicated that a rise in aerobic fitness increases the tolerance and threshold levels of asthmatics, so that a higher level of provocation is required to produce symptoms (58,72,73). It has been shown to decrease absenteeism as a result of the disease and to decrease the medication requirement (12,58).

SOCIAL AND PSYCHOLOGIC BENEFITS

Another important benefit of regular exercise is that parents of the asthmatic develop a better insight into their child's disease and his or her capabilities and become less protective. Children cite increased freedom and permission to participate in physical and social activities as evidence of changes in parental thinking (58).

Possibly, psychologic and sociologic benefits of increased aerobic fitness, along with an improvement in self-image and greater recognition and acceptance by both peer groups and parents, help to remove the "cripple" stigma from which many asthmatics suffer. Thus, asthmatics must practice and improve their skills in sports to gain greater status and recognition by others. The young asthmatic must realize that with dedication and application, most asthmatics can compete quite well with nonasthmatic peers, provided that adequate training and preevent medication programs are followed.

Medical records kept on Australian Olympic participants over the past 25 years have demonstrated a threefold increase in athletes with asthma from 7% in 1976 to 21% in 2000. Australian athletes with asthma have won gold medals at all but three Olympic Summer Games since 1956. Asthmatics participate in the complete spectrum of Olympic sporting events (74). Voy reported that 67 (11.2%) of 597 U.S. athletes participating in the 1984 summer Olympics suffered EIA and won 41 medals (15 gold, 20 silver, and 6 bronze) (75). This figure increased to 12.4% in Atlanta 1996 and 19% at the 2000 Olympic Games.

Notifications of β-agonist use at the 1996 and 2000 Olympic Games were 3.6 and 5.5% of all athletes, respectively. However, notifications were very skewed, ranging from 10% or more in athletes from New Zealand, Great Britain, Australia, United States, Ireland, Switzerland, Denmark, and Finland. In contrast, either no or <0.5% of athletes from Russia, Belarus, China, Japan, Kenya, Nigeria, Argentina, and Brazil requested permission from the IOC to inhale a β_2 agonist (74). This wide discrepancy is in accord with the large 1998 ISAAC study that examined asthmalike symptoms in >460,000 children aged 13 to 14 years in 56 countries (76).

Summary

Exercise can induce an episode of asthma, and yet, regular physical activity is an important component in disease management. The severity of EIA can be easily assessed, and the regular measurement of FEV_1 to indicate the state of the airways is recommended. There are a number of effective medications to prevent and to reverse EIA. The use of preexercise medication allows most asthmatics to perform in exercise and sporting events with little disadvantage.

REFERENCES

1. Adams F, ed. and trans. The Extant Works of Aretus, The Cappadocium. London: Sydenham Society, 1856:316.
2. Major RH. A note on the history of asthma. In: Underwood EA, ed. Science, Medicine and History, vol 2. London: Oxford University Press, 1953:522.
3. Szanton VL. Theodore Roosevelt, the asthmatic. Ann Allergy 1969;27:485–489.

4. National Heart, Lung and Blood Institute. Guidelines for the diagnosis and management of asthma, Bethesda: National Institute of Health. Publication no.97.451, 1997.

5. National Asthma Council Australia. Asthma Management Handbook 2002. Melbourne: National Asthma Council Australia Ltd, 2002.

6. Anderson SD, Henriksen JM. Management of exercise-induced asthma. In: Carlsen KH, Ibsen T, eds. Exercise-Induced Asthma and Sports in Asthma. Copenhagen: Munksgaard Press, 1999.

7. Godfrey S. Introduction: symposium on special problems and management of allergic athletes. J Allergy Clin Immunol 1984;73(suppl):630–633.

8. Crapo RO, Casaburi R, Coates AL, et al. Guidelines for methacholine and exercise challenge testing—1999. Am J Respir Crit Care Med 2000;161:309–329.

9. Rundell KW, Wilber RL, Szmedra J, et al. Exercise-induced asthma screening of elite athletes: field versus laboratory exercise challenge. Med Sci Sports Exerc 2000;32:309–316.

10. Hahn A, Anderson SD, Morton AR, et al. A re-interpretation of the effect of temperature and water content of the inspired air in exercise-induced asthma. Am Rev Respir Dis 1984;130:575–579.

11. Anderson SD, Holzer K. Exercise-induced asthma: is it the right diagnosis in elite athletes? J Allergy Clin Immunol 2000;106:419–428.

12. Bundgaard A, Ingemann-Hansen T, Halkjaer-Kristensen J, et al. Short term physical training is bronchial asthma. Br J Dis Chest 1983;77:147–152.

13. Hammerman SI, Becker JM, Rogers J, et al. Asthma screening of high school athletes: identifying the undiagnosed and poorly controlled. Ann Allergy Asthma Immunol 2002;88:380–384.

14. Anderson SD, Silverman M, Konig P, et al. Exercise-induced asthma: a review. Br J Dis Chest 1975;69:1–39.

15. James AR, Pare PD, Hogg JC. The mechanics of airway narrowing in asthma. Am Rev Respir Dis 1989;139:242–246.

16. Jones RS, Buston MH, Wharton MJ. The effect of exercise on ventilatory function in the child with asthma. Br J Dis Chest 1962;56:78–86.

17. Bar-Or, O. Pediatric Sports Medicine. New York: Springer-Verlag, 1983.

18. Lee TH, Nagakura J, Papageorgiou N, et al. Exercise-induced late asthmatic reactions with neutrophil chemotactic activity. N Engl J Med 1983;308:1502–1505.

19. Schoeffel RE, Anderson SD, Gillam I, et al. Multiple exercise and histamine challenge in asthmatic patients. Thorax 1980;35:164–170.

20. O'Byrne PM, Jones GL. The effect of indomethacin on exercise-induced bronchoconstriction and refractoriness after exercise. Am Rev Respir Dis 1986;134:69–72.

21. Wilson BA, Bar-Or O, O'Byrne PM. The effects of indomethacin on refractoriness following exercise both with and without bronchoconstriction. Eur Respir J 1994;12:2174–2178.

22. Larsson K, Ohlsen P, Larsson L, et al. High prevalence of asthma in cross country skiers. Br Med J 1993;307:1326–1329.

23. Wilber RL, Rundell KW, Szmedra L, et al. Incidence of exercise-induced bronchospasm in Olympic winter sport athletes. Med Sci Sports Exerc 2000;32:732–737.

24. Nystad W, Harris J, Sundgot Borgen J. Asthma and wheezing among Norwegian elite athletes. Med Sci Sports Exerc 2000;32:266–270.

25. Fitch KD, Morton AR. Specificity of exercise in exercise-induced asthma. Br Med J 1971;4:577–581.

26. Fitch KD, Godfrey S. Asthma and athletic performance. JAMA 1976;236:152–157.

27. Sly RM. Exercise related changes in airway obstruction: frequency and clinical correlates in asthmatic children. Ann Allergy 1970;28:1–16.

28. Morton AR, Lawrence SR, Fitch KD, et al. Duration of exercise in the provocation of exercise-induced asthma. Ann Allergy 1983;51:530–534.

29. Silverman M, Anderson SD. Standardization of exercise tests in asthmatic children. Arch Dis Child 1972;47:882–889.

30. Morton AR, Hahn AG, Fitch KD. Continuous and intermittent running in the provocation of asthma. Ann Allergy 1982;48:123–129.

31. Strauss RH, McFadden ER Jr, Ingram RH, et al. Enhancement of exercise-induced asthma by cold air. N Engl J Med 1977;297:743–746.

32. Bar-Or O, Neuman I, Dotan R. Effects of dry and humid climates on exercise-induced asthma in children and pre-adolescents. J Allergy Clin Immunol 1977;60:163–168.

33. Inbar O, Dotan R, Dlin RN, et al.: Breathing dry or humid air and exercise-induced asthma during swimming. Eur J Appl Physiol 1980;44:43–50.

34. Bar-Yishay E, Gur I, Inbar O, et al. Difference between swimming and running as stimuli for exercise-induced asthma. Eur J Appl Physiol 1982;48:387–397.

35. Boulet LP, Turotter H, Tennina S. Comparative efficacy of salbutamol, ipratropium and cromoglycate in the prevention of bronchospasm induced by exercise and hyperosmolar challenges. J Allergy Clin Immunol 1989;83:882–887.

36. Morton AR, King K, Papalia SM, et al. Comparison of maximal oxygen consumption with oral and nasal breathing. Aust J Sci Med Sports 1995;27:51–55.

37. Reiff DB, Nozhat B, Choudry Pride NB, et al. The effect of prolonged submaximal warm-up exercise on exercise-induced asthma. Am Rev Respir Dis 1989;139:379–384.

38. Anderson SD. Exercise-induced asthma. In: Middleton E, Reed C, Ellis E, et al., eds. Allergy: Principles and Practice. St. Louis: C V Mosby, 1988, 1156–1175.

39. Schnall RP, Landau LI. Protective effects of repeated short sprints in exercise-induced asthma. Thorax 1980;35:828–832.

40. Morton AR. Asthma. In: Bloomfield J, Fricker PA, Fitch KD, eds. Science and Medicine in Sport. 2nd ed. Carlton, Victoria, Australia: Blackwell Science, 1995:616–627.

41. Anderson SD, Seale JP, Rozea P, et al. An evaluation of pharmacotherapy for exercise-induced asthma. J Allergy Clin Immunol 1979;64:612–624.

42. Fitch KD. The use of anti-asthmatic drugs: do they affect sports performance? Sports Med 1986;3:136–150.

43. Hancock RJ, Bubbarao P, Kamada D, et al. B2-agonist tolerance and exercise-induced bronchospasm. Am J Respir Crit Care Med 2002;165:1068–1070.

44. Seberova E, Hartman P, Ververla J, et al. Formoterol given by Turbuhaler has as rapid an onset of action as salbutamol given by pMDI. [Abstract] Am J Respir Crit Care Med 1999;159:A639.

45. Koenig P. The use of cromolyn in the management of hyperactive airways and exercise. J Allergy Clin Immunol 1984;73(suppl):686–689.

46. Morton AR, Ogle SL, Fitch KD. Effects of nedocromil sodium, cromolyn sodium and a placebo in exercise-induced asthma. Ann Allergy 1992;68:143–148.

47. Ellis EF. Inhibition of exercise-induced asthma by theophylline. J Allergy Clin Immunol 1984;73(suppl):690–692.

48. Henriksen JM, Dahl R. Effects of inhaled budesonide alone and in combination with low dose terbutaline in children with exercise-induced asthma, Am Rev Respir Dis 1983;128:993–997.

49. Thio BJ, Slingerland GL, Nagelkerke AF, et al. Effects of single-dose fluticasone on exercise-induced asthma in asthmatic children: a pilot study. Pediatr Pulmonol 2001;32:115–121.

50. Chan-Yeung H. The effect of Sch 1000 and disodium cromoglycate on exercise-induced asthma. Chest 1977;71:320–323.

51. Thomson NC, Patel KR, Kerr JW. Sodium cromoglycate and ipratropium bromide in exercise induced asthma. Thorax 1978;33:694–699.

52. WADA/IOC. WADA/IOC 2001 list of prohibited substances and prohibited methods. WADA/IOC. Montreal/Lausanne, September, 2001.

53. Anderson SD, Argyros G, Magnussen H, et al. Provocation by eucapnic voluntary hyperpnea to identify exercise-induced bronchoconstriction. Br J Sports Med 2000;35:344–347.

54. Rundell KW, Im J, Mayers LB, et al. Self-reported symptoms and exercise-induced asthma in the elite athlete. Med Sci Sports Exerc 2001;33:208–213.

55. American College of Sports Medicine. Guidelines for Exercise Testing and Exercise Prescription. 6th ed. Philadelphia: Lea & Febiger, 2000.

56. Godfrey S. Exercise-induced asthma. Allergy 1978;33:229–237.

57. Becker AB, Simons KJ, Gillespie RN, et al. The bronchodilator effects and pharmakinetics of caffeine in asthma. N Engl J Med 1984;310:743–746.

58. Fitch KD, Morton AR, Blanksby BA. Effects of swimming training on children with asthma. Arch Dis Child 1976;51:190–194.

59. Anderson SD, Camps J, Perry CP, et al. Prevalence of exercise-induced bronchoconstriction (EIB) in young athletes identified by eucapnic hyperpnea (EVH). [Abstract] Respirology 2001;6(March suppl):A10.

60. Brannan JD, Anderson SD, Koskela H, et al. Responsiveness to mannitol in asthmatic subjects with exercise and hyperventilation-induced asthma. Am J Respir Crit Care Med. 1998;158:1120–1126.

61. Smith CM, Anderson SD. Inhalation provocation tests using non-isotonic aerosols. J Allergy Clin Immunol 1989;84:781–790.

62. Borg GAV. Psychophysical bases of perceived exertion. Med Sci Sports Exerc 1982;14:377–381.

63. Borg G, Ottoson D, eds. The Perception of Exertion in Physical Work. New York: Macmillan, 1986.

64. Eriksson BO, Engstrom I, Karlberg P, et al. A physiological analysis of former girl swimmers. Acta Paediatr Scand 1971;60(suppl 217):68–72.

65. Altenburger KM. More concerning asthma and exercise. Pediatrics 1990;85:385–386.

66. King MJ, Noakes TD, Weinberg EG. Physiological effects of a physical training program in children with exercise-induced asthma. Pediatr Exerc Sci 1989;1:137–143.

67. Bundgaard A, Ingemann-Hansen T, Schmidt A, et al. Exercise-induced asthma after walking, running, cycling. Scand J Clin Lab Invest 1982;42:15–18.

68. Nickerson BG, Daisy B, Bautista BA, et al. Distance running improves fitness in asthmatic children

without pulmonary complications or changes in exercise-induced bronchospasm. Pediatrics 1983;71: 147–152.

69. Orenstein DM, Reed ME, Grogan FT, et al. Exercise conditioning in children with asthma. J Pediatr 1985;106:556–560.

70. Mertens DJ, Shephard RJ, Kavanagh T. Long-term exercise therapy for chronic obstructive lung disease. Respiration 1978;35:96–107.

71. Wolf CR, Suero JT. Alterations in lung mechanics and gas exchange following training in chronic obstructive lung disease. Dis Chest 1969;55: 37–44.

72. Afzelius-Frisk I, Grimby G, Lindholm N. Physical training in patients with asthma. Poumon Coeur 1977;33:33–37.

73. Sly RM, Harper RT, Rosselot I. The effect of physical conditioning upon asthmatic children. Ann Allergy 1972;30:86–94.

74. Fitch K: Personal communication.

75. Voy R. The U. S. Olympic Committee experience with exercise-induced bronchospasm 1984. Med Sci Sports Exerc 1986;18:328–330.

76. Worldwide variation in prevalence of symptoms of asthma, allergic rhinoconjunctivitis and atopic eczema: ISAAC. The International Study of Asthma and Allergies in Childhood (ISAAC) Steering Committee, Lancet 1998;351:1225–1232.

RELATED WEB SITES

Virtual Hospital
www.vh.org

National Asthma Council Australia (NAC), Asthma Management Handbook
www.nationalasthma.org.au/publications/amh/ amhintro.htm

National Heart, Lung, and Blood Institute
www.nhlbi.nih.gov/guidelines/asthma/asthgdln.htm

17

Cystic Fibrosis

Frank J. Cerny and David M. Orenstein

Cystic fibrosis (CF) is the most common profoundly life-shortening inherited disease of whites and is transmitted as an autosomal recessive trait. The gene causing the disease has been described (1) and appears to be responsible for the production of a protein labeled the CF transmembrane conductance-regulator (CFTR) protein. This protein participates in controlling the flux of chloride and sodium into and out of the cells lining the airways and the other epithelial surfaces. The alteration in the CFTR results in abnormal ion flux, abnormally high negative transmembrane electrical charges, and relative dehydration of intraluminal fluids in affected organs. The primary organs affected are the lungs, pancreas, intestines, and sweat glands (2,3). Decreased water in the airways leads to abnormally thick secretions that impede breathing. The defect also prevents the normal secretion of digestive enzymes through the pancreatic ducts into the intestines. In the 1950s, the mean survival age was under 5 years. Even today, the patient may not survive infancy in severe cases. With aggressive therapy, however, most affected individuals survive into adulthood, with the present median age of survival being over 30 years (4).

Symptoms of CF vary among patients (5,6). Pulmonary symptoms include recurrent or persistent cough, wheezing, and dyspnea. Because these symptoms are similar to those of asthma, the correct diagnosis may be overlooked for months or years.

Frequent lower airway infection (particularly with *Staphylococcus aureus, Haemophilus influenzae,* or mucoid *Pseudomonas aeruginosa*) is typical in CF. Gastrointestinal (GI) involvement may present at birth with intestinal obstruction (meconium ileus) or, somewhat later, with failure to thrive. Obstruction of the pancreatic ducts leads to trypsin, amylase, and lipase deficiencies in 90% of patients, resulting in frequent, bulky, and foul-smelling stools with a high lipid content. Treatment of the digestive complications of CF includes supplemental pancreatic enzymes with meals and supplementation with fat-soluble vitamins.

The diagnosis of CF is made definitively by analysis of sweat sodium and chloride (4). The defect results in abnormally high concentrations of these ions in the sweat, with a clear separation between affected (>60 mEq·L^{-1}) and unaffected (<40 mEq·L^{-1}) individuals during childhood; there is a low incidence of false-positive results into adulthood (7). Sweat testing must be performed in a laboratory experienced in the techniques of pilocarpine iontophoresis with quantitative analysis of sodium and/or chloride. These laboratories are most often associated with CF Centers certified by the Cystic Fibrosis Foundation. The rate of false-positive and false-negative test results is very high in inexperienced hands, which can lead to tragic results. DNA testing is now possible and is part of the routine neonatal screening in a handful of states, but it is not yet capable of identifying all affected persons. DNA screening is currently slower and more expensive than sweat testing, but is becoming the definitive test for identifying those with the disease.

The pulmonary complications of the disease are related to the plugging of the airways by the excessive, thick mucous secretions. Repeated airway infections, a hallmark of the disease, also result in inflammation and bronchiectasis, associated with further increases in secretions. Other pulmonary complications may include hemoptysis, atelectasis, allergic aspergillosis, pneumothorax, pulmonary hypertension, cor pulmonale, and respiratory failure (8). The extent of involvement is assessed by radiographs and most sensitively by pulmonary-function testing.

The bronchial plugging eventually results in elevated airway resistance and considerable trapping of air in the lungs such that they become hyperinflated. Over time, there is a mismatching of ventilation and perfusion and deterioration in arterial blood gases. The progressive, chronic hypoxemia can result in cor pulmonale (pulmonary hypertension). The continuing airway obstruction and hyperinflation increase the flow-resistive and the elastic work of breathing, respectively. In most patients, the progressive deterioration in lung function is not reflected in an altered exercise blood gas response until pulmonary reserves fall below a critical threshold. Once this threshold of lung dysfunction is reached, exercise-induced decreases in arterial oxygen and increases in arterial carbon dioxide are noted (9–11). The lung hyperinflation alters lung mechanics such that the respiratory pattern during exercise becomes abnormal (12,13). The increased work of breathing results in long-term increases in resting oxygen consumption (14,15)

The greatest impact on patient morbidity and mortality is from pulmonary complications (8). Treatment of these complications includes control of pulmonary infections with antibiotics and pulmonary hygiene to remove mucus. The underlying pulmonary infection and inflammation worsen periodically. These pulmonary exacerbations may require hospitalization with intravenous antibiotics and chest physical therapy. Patients with mild exacerbations may be treated at home with oral, aerosolized, or even intravenous antibiotics.

The removal of secretions by chest physical therapy has been a standard part of the treatment of CF patients for many years (16). Chest physical therapy consists of postural drainage, chest percussion, forced expirations (17), exercise (18), and high-frequency chest wall oscillation (19). These techniques appear to be effective in inducing sputum expectoration only if cough is induced (20–22) and may be used in combination for greater effect (20,23,24). After decades of use, these chest physical therapy techniques have only recently been shown to be effective in preventing or attenuating deterioration of pulmonary function (25–27).

Airway reactivity is frequently associated with CF and may require treatment with bronchodilators or other drugs that may influence airway function. Corticosteroids (both oral [28] and inhaled [29,30]) and nonsteroidal antiinflammatory agents have been suggested as possible treatment for the airway inflammation of CF (31–33) but studies have shown mixed results in terms of both efficacy and toxicity, and their role is not yet clear.

With the identification of the specific defect in CF, new treatments are being developed and are currently undergoing clinical trials. Finally, there is speculation that therapies eventually will be developed that can replace the defective CFTR protein, alter the defective gene, or even replace it with a normal gene, a procedure that would replace defective airway cells with normally functioning airway cells.

The following section presents (a) the rationale for exercise testing of patients with CF, (b) protocols for the exercise test, (c) the expected pulmonary response to exercise in a healthy and a CF population, (d) a basis for the interpretation of the test and for prescribing exercise, and (e) various strategies for incorporating exercise into the therapeutic regimen of patients.

Why an Exercise Test?

It has been estimated that even at maximal exercise in a healthy population, the lungs are required to use only about 80% of their total capacity for gas exchange; the remaining 20% has been called the pulmonary reserve. As CF compromises lung function, this reserve is decreased and eventually disappears (9,10). By encroaching into these reserves, a progressive, incremental exercise test can be useful to estimate the short- and long-term effects of the lung disease on the appropriateness of the response to exercise. If a program of exercise is being considered or if advice regarding participation in activities is being sought, the exercise test can be useful to identify the level of activity that can be accomplished safely. Tables of energy expenditure for a variety of activities can be used to obtain a qualitative determination of effort for various activities (34). By matching these estimates with the heart rate (HR) response to the exercise test, one can estimate the patient's response to activities of daily living. The exercise threshold above which acute respiratory insufficiency may be observed can be identified through the exercise test. Finally, the effects of disease progression, treatment, or exercise therapy can be evaluated with the exercise test.

The Exercise Test

PATIENTS YOUNGER THAN 7 YEARS

Most patients younger than 7 years cannot cooperate sufficiently for a formal laboratory test with careful monitoring of cardiopulmonary adaptation. The noninvasive monitoring of arterial hemoglobin oxygen saturation (SaO_2) with an oximeter should be a part of any exercise evaluation of patients with CF. Exercise-induced respiratory compromise in infants and children 1 to 3 years old may be detectable by careful observation during feeding, periods of crying, or normal activity. Most children in this age range will not suffer oxyhemoglobin desaturation, but objective documentation of suspected compromise can be accomplished with an oximeter probe attached to the scapha of the ear. Most children will tolerate the ear or finger probe well and do not mind the slight restriction of activity due to the 6- to 8-foot cable connection.

In children from 3 to 6 years of age, a more quantitative estimate of exercise tolerance can be made by using a motor-driven treadmill (35). With support, even children this age can walk on the treadmill while SaO_2% and electrocardiogram (ECG) are monitored. It is difficult to standardize the test in this age group, and the attainment of high work levels is difficult. Young patients rarely exceed an HR of 160 beats per minute for this test. Because most children this age do not carry out sustained activity at HRs higher than 50 to 60% of maximum (36), the information obtained is still useful to describe whether the pulmonary response to exercise is normal and to determine safe levels of activity.

PATIENTS OLDER THAN 7 YEARS

Before the exercise test for these patients, each should undergo a clinical evaluation and pulmonary function tests if these have not been done recently. We have found that FEV_1 correlates best with exercise tolerance and that a scoring system using six resting pulmonary function tests also correlates well (10). There is large individual variation, and although the resting lung function may identify a group of patients at increased risk for exercise-induced desaturation, the exercise test itself is the only tool that can determine with certainty what will happen to oxygen saturation during exercise or what exercise level will be tolerated.

Patients should be dressed appropriately for testing. A loose-fitting T-shirt, shorts, and sneakers are best. Long pants with wide cuffs can become tangled in the cycle pedals or cause the patient to trip on the treadmill. The skin sites for the chest ECG electrodes should be cleaned and lightly abraded to ensure good contact. All procedures should be carefully explained to make the test less frightening and to optimize cooperation.

Several testing protocols can be selected depending on the reason for the exercise evaluation.

Incremental Tests

If the primary purpose of the test is to determine peak exercise capacity, a progressive incremental test using 1-min work periods should be used. If one is interested in the adaptive response to exercise in addition to determining the patient's functional work capacity, 2-min stages are recommended. The 2-min stage allows observation of various parameters during a quasi-steady-state in the last 30 sec of each stage. If 3-min stages are chosen, the test may become unnecessarily long. For those who have a treadmill available or prefer its use, increments in elevation of 2 to 2.5% grade every 2 min are comfortable for most patients and result in an increase in HR of approximately 10 beats per work stage. The speed of the treadmill should be selected so that a moderately fast walk must be assumed and should allow most patients, including those with severe dysfunction, to exercise at two to three levels.

TABLE 17-1 POWER OUTPUT/OXYGEN UPTAKE RELATIONSHIPS ON CYCLE ERGOMETER

Power Output (W·kg^{-1})	Oxygen Uptake (mL·kg^{-1}· min^{-1}) ($\overline{X} \pm$ SE)	Minute Ventilation (mL·kg^{-1}·min^{-1})
0.3	10.2 ± 0.45	0.30 ± 0.01
0.6	13.8 ± 0.28	0.43 ± 0.01
0.9	17.2 ± 0.34	0.54 ± 0.02
1.2	20.0 ± 0.23	0.66 ± 0.02
1.5	22.9 ± 0.037	0.79 ± 0.02
1.8	26.7 ± 0.048	0.94 ± 0.03
2.1	31.2 ± 0.56	1.10 ± 0.03
2.4	35.2 ± 1.02	1.20 ± 0.04
2.7	39.9 ± 1.16	1.31 ± 0.05

Unpublished results, Cerny FJ. Children's Lung Center, Children's Hospital of Buffalo.

For smaller children, this speed ranges from 2 to 3 km·h^{-1}; in adolescents, from 4 to 5 km·h^{-1}; and in adults, 6 to 7 km·h^{-1}.

Most published studies of exercise in CF patients have used the cycle ergometer, which is quieter and less intimidating than the treadmill, safer (patients may fall on the treadmill), and more easily mastered. The patient moves less, making collection of expired gases and measurement of blood pressure and SaO$_2$% by oximetry considerably easier. Power output also depends less on body weight when using the cycle ergometer. In choosing an ergometer for the laboratory, one should consider the need for fitting small children and the need for relatively small increments in power output. Electronically braked ergometers are more expensive than mechanically braked units but have the advantage that power output is relatively independent of pedaling rate. Lower peak oxygen consumption is obtained on the cycle than would be measured using the treadmill because fewer muscles are involved.

On the cycle ergometer, several different protocols can be used. We prefer either of the following:

1. Power output increments of 0.3 watts per kg (W·kg^{-1}) yield results similar to those with the treadmill protocol discussed above. The initial power output should be 0.3 W·kg^{-1} for small or severely compromised patients and 0.6 W·kg^{-1} for others.
2. Godfrey's protocol is based on height, starting with as low a power output as possible on the cycle and 1-min increments of 10, 15, and 20 W for children shorter than 125 cm, between 125 and 150 cm, and those taller than 150 cm, respectively (37). Power output relationships to oxygen consumption and predicted values for maximal exercise are shown in Tables 17–1 and 17–2, respectively.

Other Tests

When it is not necessary to record a peak or maximal exercise value, the above protocols may be modified. When one is interested in the cardiopulmonary adaptation to exercise, measurements should be taken during a steady state. In most circumstances, steady state can be assumed to have been reached between 4 and 5 min after the start of exercise or after a change in exercise level. This time may be somewhat prolonged in patients with severe lung disease (38,39). These tests are generally done to allow special measurements during exercise, such as lung diffusing capacity and cardiac output, or when information is needed at a particular work level (e.g., to simulate job requirements). The one- or two-level test is also useful to evaluate the effects of supplemental oxygen on exercise response.

When periodic check-ups are needed or when the effects of therapy must be determined at frequent intervals, a full incremental test may not be required. In these cases, a shorter test with fewer power outputs can be used. For example, if the exercise prescription asks that the patient exercise below an HR of 150 beats·min^{-1} and arterial oxygen

TABLE 17-2 PREDICTED VALUES AT PEAK POWER OUTPUT USING GODFREY'S PROGRESSIVE CYCLE ERGOMETER PROTOCOL

	Power Output (W)	Oxygen Uptake ($L \cdot min^{-1}$)	Minute Ventilation ($L \cdot min^{-1}$)
Male:	$3.54 \times ht - 377$	$0.045 \times ht - 4.64$	$1.82 \times ht - 192$
Female:	$2.17 \times ht - 197$	$0.031 \times ht - 2.28$	$1.03 \times ht - 88$

Unpublished results, Orenstein DM, Henke KG, Reed ME, Wachnowsky D.
   ht, height in cm.

desaturation is observed at this point during the initial evaluation, follow-up evaluations need take the patient only to a HR of 150. The effects of exercise therapy can be documented by frequent 2- to 3-stage submaximal tests. When sophisticated exercise testing equipment is unavailable or unnecessary, several field tests can be used to assess exercise capacity and the response to exercise. These tests include the 6-min walking test that can be performed in a corridor (40) and a shuttle test that uses increases in pace required to move between two specified points to effect increments in work requirements (41).

Monitoring during the Test

To establish a safe exercise prescription, one must monitor SaO_2 or arterial oxygen pressure (PaO_2) during exercise; this is virtually mandatory in patients with an FEV_1 <50% of the predicted normal value. We recommend the ear oximetric measurement of SaO_2 because it is convenient and noninvasive. Regarding the interpretation of SaO_2 measurements, for patients high on the O_2 dissociation curve (>80 mm Hg PaO_2), relatively large and potentially clinically significant drops in PaO_2 may be reflected in a decrease of only 1 to 2% SaO_2.

In healthy individuals, end-tidal PCO_2 reflects $PaCO_2$ and can be a useful parameter to monitor during exercise. Healthy individuals have a negligible alveolar-to-arterial (A-a) gradient, making alveolar or end-tidal CO_2 a good estimate of arterial CO_2. However, the gradient is increased in patients with lung disease, making it likely that end-tidal CO_2 underestimates arterial CO_2. The measurement of end-tidal CO_2 can still be valuable in reflecting changes in arterial CO_2.

A description of the pulmonary response to exercise requires the measurement of minute ventilation ($\dot{V}_E$), either directly by collecting exhaled air in a gasometer or indirectly by integrating expiratory flow measured with a Pneumotach. The energy expenditure (oxygen consumption, $\dot{V}O_2$) during exercise can be quantified by measuring the mixed expired fractions of O_2 and CO_2.

To assess the cardiovascular responses to exercise, ECG, HR, and blood pressure should be monitored throughout the test. Measurement of HR also allows prescription of activity using HR to monitor the intensity of the exercise.

Termination of the test is based on one or a combination of the criteria discussed by Hebestreit and Bar-Or in Chapter 5. In addition, particular attention should be paid to decreases in SaO_2 below 80% and clinical observations of pallor, extreme dyspnea, or other signs of respiratory decompensation.

Safety Precautions

Equipment in the laboratory should be properly maintained and calibrated. Oxygen and resuscitation supplies (e.g., drugs, intravenous sets) and equipment (e.g., defibrillator and bag respirator) should be readily available. Emergency codes and procedures, including drug availability and dosages, should be posted. Personnel should be trained and, if possible, certified in cardiopulmonary resuscitation (42).

Response to Exercise in Patients with CF

Exercise capacity of CF patients has been shown to be related to severity of lung disease (12,23,25,43, 44) and can be affected by nutritional status (45). There is no evidence that cardiac dysfunction contributes to the disease-related changes in exercise tolerance (46,47). In addition, the slope of the

HR response to exercise in patients is similar to that of healthy subjects (9), changing only in intercept with clinical status (43). The reduced exercise tolerance is due to pulmonary limitations, as evidenced by the strong relationship between pulmonary dysfunction and exercise capacity (9–11,44,48). The strength of this general relationship also is shown by parallel changes in lung function and exercise tolerance in patients hospitalized for acute exacerbation of their lung disease (43). Exercise capacity or response to exercise, however, cannot be predicted simply from lung function because of the variability in the response (11) and because the relationship is not linear, showing nearly normal exercise capacity until lung dysfunction is severe (9,10).

The increase in $\dot{V}_E$ by CF patients during exercise is exaggerated, especially with increasing severity of pulmonary dysfunction (9). The progressive deterioration of blood-gas matching with CF, as measured by the ratio of alveolar ventilation ($\dot{V}_A$) to cardiac output ($\dot{Q}$), requires an increased $\dot{V}_E$ to maintain $\dot{V}_A$. In a few, very severely obstructed patients, dyspnea may force an end to exercise before $\dot{V}_E$ has risen significantly above normal.

In spite of the higher $\dot{V}_E$, some patients with severe dysfunction cannot maintain arterial O_2 and CO_2 levels (9–11). The higher $\dot{V}_E$ in these patients is accomplished by an increased breathing frequency and a small tidal volume. The hyperinflation already seen at rest in CF patients likely minimizes the probability of further increases during exercise. The combination of gas exchange abnormalities and mechanical inefficiency results in exercise limitations that depend on disease severity.

Interpretation of the Exercise Test and Exercise Prescription

When corrected for weight or body surface area, maximal $\dot{V}O_2$ changes little in healthy persons from the age of 7 to adulthood. Values for peak work capacity or $\dot{V}O_{2peak}$ measured in a clinical setting generally are lower than those measured in a school or research setting. Average values for $\dot{V}O_{2peak}$ in a clinical setting range from 38 to 44 mL·kg^{-1}·min^{-1} for boys and 34 to 38 mL·kg^{-1}·min^{-1} for girls on the cycle ergometer. These $\dot{V}O_2$ levels correspond to power outputs of approximately 2.7 to 3.0 W·kg^{-1} and 2.1 to 2.4 W·kg^{-1} for males and females, respectively. Values for $\dot{V}O_{2peak}$ from a treadmill test are approximately 10% higher. The coefficient of variation for these values is about 10%.

The linear relationship between HR and $\dot{V}O_2$ can be used to prescribe and monitor exercise therapy. There is considerable variation between individuals in this relationship, so the exercise test should be used to establish the specific relationship for each patient. By knowing the unique individual relationship between $\dot{V}O_2$ and HR, one can require that the patient exercise at an established HR to accomplish the therapeutic goals based on energy expenditure. The relationship will change as conditioning progresses, so that a higher $\dot{V}O_2$ will be achieved at the same HR, i.e., any given submaximal work rate is done at a lower HR.

THE EXERCISE PROGRAM

Any conditioning program must consider the usual elements of endurance, flexibility, and strength. It is not yet known if any exercise program can prevent or slow the deterioration of lung function in patients with CF, but it is known that aerobic exercise programs can increase cardiopulmonary fitness (49,50), and it is thought that certain types of exercise may facilitate sputum expectoration. The primary concerns for the patient with CF, therefore, are improvement of cardiovascular reserves and promotion of sputum expectoration. Cough and sputum expectoration should be encouraged in all patients, but particularly in those whose cough is productive.

The prescription of endurance (aerobic) exercise must be individualized. In choosing the type of activities for the exercise prescription, the types of activities the patient enjoys must be ascertained and used as a base. Compliance with a program will be poor if the patient finds the exercise boring (51). A second important factor to ensure compliance is to promote the use of exercise partners, whether they be other members of the family or friends. Special outing clubs or sporting groups may help to promote regular activity. Patients should not engage in highly competitive sports in which there may be pressure to exercise beyond what may be safe. Competitive activities should allow some means of self-regulation whereby the patient can slow down without feeling a lot of pressure. Diving, whether underwater or in the sky, should be engaged in only after careful consideration of the potential for negative consequences (e.g., alveolar rupture). This is because the airway obstruction of CF might result in the trapping of air in alveolar areas of the lung. Since these areas do not communicate with the atmosphere, they would expand and contract much like a balloon with the atmospheric pressure changes while diving. Large atmospheric pressure changes might then result in rupture of some of these alveolar areas.

The exercise prescription in young children can be filled simply by encouraging participation in normal activity. The family can be a partner in this by assuming an active lifestyle. This type of partnership also helps ensure that exercise will become part of the patient's lifestyle. As the patient enters the teen years, the exercise prescription can concentrate on more specific activities.

Some strength training can be prescribed for patients with CF. The effects of strenuous body building on patients with CF are unknown, but one study showed that a regular program of weight lifting resulted in improvements in strength and marginal improvements in selected pulmonary function tests (52). As with children in general, we recommend that the more strenuous types of lifting be avoided, particularly by children, through adolescence.

As with other groups, it has been difficult to devise exercise programs to which CF patients will adhere over an extended period (53). Exercise compliance can be improved through strong social support, positive perceptions of competency and self-esteem, and enjoyment of activity. For CF patients, the time required for other treatments makes compliance with exercise even more difficult. Support from the family and health care team can be important in improving exercise adherence through the introduction of behavior change strategies.

In summary, one should choose activities that the patient enjoys, that will specifically improve cardiovascular endurance and strength, and that will allow the use of family or friend support.

EXERCISE INTENSITY

There is a level of exercise intensity below which no training effect will be achieved. There is also a level above which the extra effort required will result in little additional benefit. The exercise prescription should be chosen to ensure that the middle intensities of effort are reached. For cardiovascular benefit, this level is usually between 50 and 70% of the individual's maximal capacity. Guidelines for the calculation of appropriate target HRs are available (54). However, because CF patients may be limited by ventilatory factors before their HR has reached its maximum, one cannot prescribe exercise intensity based on age-predicted maximal HR, but must use each patient's own measured maximum. The target HR should be below the point at which desaturation was observed during the exercise test. In patients who exhibit desaturation as soon as exercise begins or at HRs below 120 beats per min, supplemental oxygen should be considered to keep the SaO_2 above 90% and to allow exercise at HRs of 120 to 130 beats per min.

Strength exercises should be prescribed so that the weight or resistance chosen will allow the patient to do a minimum of 10 repetitions at a time. If this cannot be done, the resistance is too high. Three sets of each exercise should be done at each session. A reasonable session would include 5 to 10 different exercises. Two series of 5 to 10 exercises should be available so that the patient can alternate between these series on different days (e.g., one series would be done on Monday and Friday and a different series on Wednesday and Sunday).

EXERCISE DURATION

Accepted guidelines for cardiovascular exercise prescription suggest doing continuous activity for about 30 min a day; the minimal recommended duration is 10 to 15 min. There should also be additional time to warm up before and to cool down after the main exercise period. Many patients with moderate-to-severe lung dysfunction who are less fit or who have a severely limited work capacity may tolerate light exercise for only 5 min at the start. The exercise time should increase to 10 or 15 min over a period of 1 to 2 weeks. In many cases, the exercise may have to be completed in two sessions.

EXERCISE FREQUENCY

These exercises should be done a minimum of 3 days per week. Ideally, these activities should be done 5 to 6 days per week by patients with little or only mild dysfunction. For patients with more severe dysfunction, rest days must be inserted.

In-Patient Therapy

All patients admitted to the hospital with an acute exacerbation of their disease and those admitted for elective intensive therapy should be considered for exercise therapy. For those few patients restricted to their beds, the exercise can be simple resistive exercises using the body's own weight. These exercises include leg lifts, arm lifts, and modified sit-ups. Ambulatory patients (whether on or off supplemental oxygen) should have a preliminary exercise assessment to determine the degree of monitoring needed during the therapy sessions. Patients who desaturate during their exercise test, regardless of their peak exercise capacity, should be monitored by ear oximetry during exercise. Patients who do not desaturate during the initial evaluation can exercise in the physical therapy department where less-careful monitoring is necessary. All patients who can should be encouraged to move around the ward. Leg, heart, and ventilatory muscle function should not be allowed to deteriorate while lung function is improving.

EXPECTED BENEFITS OF REGULAR EXERCISE IN CF PATIENTS

Except in circumstances in which heavy exercise is done several times a day (55,56), there is no convincing evidence that exercise training will improve lung function, as measured by standard pulmonary function tests. Specific respiratory muscle training will improve respiratory muscle function (57), but how these improvements affect lung dysfunction or exercise capacity is not known. Engaging in regular cardiovascular endurance activities will improve respiratory muscle endurance and exercise capacity (49,50) and may slow the progressive deterioration of lung function and reduce breathlessness (58) in CF patients. Recent evidence indicates that exercise inhibits the luminal sodium conductance, possibly increasing water content of the mucus in CF patients, providing evidence for the possible beneficial effects of exercise in some patients (59). Studies on the potential benefits of long-term regular exer-

cise have not been able to show positive effects on lung function or even always on exercise capacity because of problems of compliance and high individual variability (21,50,51,60–64). However, a close examination of available data indicates that many individual patients can benefit greatly by regular exercise. All patients with CF can safely perform some form of exercise, and exercise should be encouraged as part of the regular routine for these patients.

Summary

Cystic fibrosis is an inherited disease that affects ion transport in the cells of the lungs, pancreas, intestines, and sweat glands. Patients die from lung disease related to thick mucous accumulations in the airway that block the flow of air and promote lung inflammation. These patients can exercise safely, and activity should be encouraged as part of their treatment. Appropriate exercise prescription should be made after an exercise test to determine whether the patient's arterial oxygen levels decrease during exertion. Aerobic exercise can be prescribed at intensities that will not result in a decrease in arterial oxygen or inspired air should be supplemented with oxygen to prevent a decrease in patients in whom this occurs. Exercise promotes the expectoration of the disease-related accumulation of mucus by reducing the viscosity of the mucus and promoting coughing.

REFERENCES

1. Riordan JR, Rommens JM, Kerem B, et al. Identification of the cystic fibrosis gene: cloning and characterization of complementary DNA. Science 1989;245:1066–1073.
2. Quinton P. Cystic fibrosis: a disease in electrolyte transport FASEB J 1990;4:2709–2713.
3. Welsh M. Abnormal regulation of ion channels in cystic fibrosis epithelia. FASEB J 1990;4:2718–2726.
4. Cystic Fibrosis Foundation. Patient registry 2001 annual report. Bethesda, MD: CF Foundation, 2001.
5. Davis P, SantAgnese P. Diagnosis and treatment of cystic fibrosis: an update. Chest 1984;85:802–809.
6. Wood RE, Boat TF, Doershuk CF. Cystic fibrosis. Am Rev Respir Dis 1976;114:753–759.
7. Davis P, Del Rio S, Muntz J, et al. Sweat chloride concentration in adults with pulmonary diseases. Am Rev Respir Dis 1966;93:62–72.

8. Hillman B. Respiratory complications: the chief danger in CF. J Respir Dis 1981;2:75–89.

9. Cerny FJ, Pullano TP, Cropp GJA. Cardiorespiratory adaptations to exercise in cystic fibrosis. Am Rev Respir Dis. 1983;126:217–220.

10. Cropp GJA, Pullano TP, Cerny FJ, et al. Exercise tolerance and cardiorespiratory adjustments at peak work capacity in cystic fibrosis. Am Rev Respir Dis 1982;126:211–216.

11. Henke K, Orenstein D. Oxygen saturation during exercise in cystic fibrosis. Am Rev Respir Dis 1984;129:708–711.

12. Cerny F J. Ventilatory control during exercise in children with cystic fibrosis (CF). [Abstract] Am Rev Respir Dis 1981;123:195.

13. Coates AL, Canny G, Zinman R, et al. The effects of chronic airflow limitation, increased dead space, and the pattern of ventilation on gas exchange during maximal exercise in advanced cystic fibrosis. Am Rev Respir Dis 1988;139:1524–1531.

14. Hirsch J, Zhang S, Rudnick M, et al. Resting oxygen consumption and ventilation in cystic fibrosis. Pediatr Pulmonol 1989;6:19–26.

15. Katsardis CV, Desmond KJ, Coates AL. Measuring the oxygen cost of breathing in normal adults and patients with cystic fibrosis. Respir Physiol 1986;65:257.

16. Mellins RB. Pulmonary physiotherapy in the pediatric age group. Am Rev Respir Dis 1974;110:137–142.

17. Thoma J, Cook T, Brooks D. Chest physical therapy management of patients with cystic fibrosis. Am J Respir Crit Care Med 1995;151:846–850.

18. DeCesare JA, Graybill CA. Physical therapy for the child with respiratory dysfunction. In: Irwin S, Tecklin J, eds. Cardiopulmonary Physical Therapy. 2nd ed. St. Louis: CV Mosby, 1990:417–460.

19. Oermann CM, Stockrider MM, Giles D, et al. Comparison of high-frequency chest wall oscillation and oscillating positive expiratory pressure in the home management of cystic fibrosis: a pilot study. Pediatr Pulmonol 2001;32:372–377.

20. Cerny FJ. Relative effects of chest physiotherapy and exercise for in-hospital care of cystic fibrosis. Phys Ther 1989;69:633–639.

21. Oldenberg FA, Dolovich MB, Montgomery JM, et al. Effects of postural drainage, exercise and cough on mucus clearance in chronic bronchitis. Am Rev Respir Dis 1979;120:739–745.

22. Rossman CM, Waldes R, Sampson D, et al. Effect of physical therapy on the removal of mucus in patients with cystic fibrosis. Am Rev Respir Dis 1982;126:131–135.

23. Bilton D, Dodd ME, Abbot JV, et al. The benefits of exercise combined with physiotherapy in the treatment of adults with cystic fibrosis. Respir Med 1992;86:507–511.

24. Lannefors L, Wollmer P. Mucus clearance with three chest physiotherapy regimes in cystic fibrosis: a comparison between postural drainage, PEP and physical exercise. Eur Respir J 1992;5:748–753.

25. Desmond KJ, Schwenk WF, Thomas E, et al. Immediate and long-term effects of chest physiotherapy in patients with cystic fibrosis. J Pediatr 1983;103:538–542.

26. McIlwaine PM, Wong LT, Peacock D, et al. Long-term comparative trial of conventional postural drainage and percussion versus positive expiratory pressure physiotherapy in the treatment of cystic fibrosis. J Pediatr 1997;131:570–574.

27. Reisman JJ, Rivington-Lae B, Corey M, et al. Role of conventional physiotherapy in cystic fibrosis. J Pediatr 1988;113:632–636.

28. Eigen H, Rosenstein BJ, Fitzimmons S, et al. A multicenter study of alternate-day prednisone therapy in patients with cystic fibrosis. Cystic Fibrosis Foundation Prednisone Trial Group. J Pediatr 1995;126:515–523.

29. Balfour-Lynn IM, Klein NJ, Dinwiddie R. Randomised controlled trial of inhaled corticosteroids (fluticasone propionate) in cystic fibrosis. Arch Dis Child 1997;77:124–130.

30. Nikolaizik WH, Schoni MH. Pilot study to assess the effect of inhaled corticosteroids on lung function in patients with cystic fibrosis. J Pediatr 1996;128:271–274.

31. Auerbach HS, Williams M, Kirkpatrick JA, et al. Alternate-day prednisone reduces morbidity and improves pulmonary function in cystic fibrosis. Lancet 1985;28:686–688.

32. Konstan MW, Vargo KM, Davis PB. Ibuprofen attenuates the inflammatory response to *Pseudomonas aeruginosa* in a rat model of chronic pulmonary infection. Implications for antiinflammatory therapy in cystic fibrosis. Am Rev Respir Dis 1990;141:186–192.

33. Konstan MW, Byard PJ, Hoppel CL, et al. Effect of high-dose ibuprofen in patients with cystic fibrosis. N Engl J Med 1995;332:848–854.

34. Cerny FJ, Burton HW. Exercise Physiology for Health Care Professionals. Champaign, IL: Human Kinetics, 2001.

35. Shuleva KM, Hunter GR, Hester DJ, et al. Exercise oxygen uptake in 3- through 6-year-old children. Pediatr Exerc Sci 1990;2:130–139.

36. Danner F, Noland M, McFadden M. Description of the physical activity of young children using movement sensor and observation methods. Pediatr Exerc Sci 1991;3:11–20.

37. Godfrey S. Exercise Testing in Children. Applications in Health and Disease. Philadelphia: WB Saunders, 1974.
38. Dolan P, Cerny F. Oxygen uptake kinetics at onset of exercise in cystic fibrosis. [Abstract] Med Sci Sports Exerc 1983;15:138.
39. Nery LE, Wasserman K, Frender W, et al. Ventilatory and gas exchange kinetics during exercise in chronic airways obstruction. J Appl Physiol 1982;53:1594–1602.
40. Nixon PA, Joswiak ML, Fricker FJ. A six-minute walk test for assessing exercise tolerance in severely ill children. J Pediatr 1996;129:362–366.
41. Bradley J, Howard J, Wallace E, et al. Reliability, repeatability, and sensitivity of the modified shuttle test in adult cystic fibrosis. Chest 2000;117:1666–1671.
42. Cropp GJA. The exercise bronchoprovocation test: standardization of procedures and evaluation of response. J Allergy Clin Immunol 1979;64:627–633.
43. Cerny FJ, Cropp GJA, Bye MR. Hospital therapy improves exercise tolerance and lung function in cystic fibrosis. Am Rev Respir Dis 1984;138:261–265.
44. Lebeque P, Lapierre J-G, Lamarre A, et al. Diffusion capacity and oxygen desaturation effects on exercise in patients with cystic fibrosis. Chest 1987;91:693–697.
45. Coates AL, Desmond K, Asher MI, et al. The effect of digoxin on exercise capacity and exercise cardiac function in cystic fibrosis. Chest 1982;82:543–547.
46. Coates A, Boyce P, Muller D, et al. The role of nutritional status, airway obstruction, hypoxia and abnormalities in serum lipid composition in limiting exercise tolerance in children with cystic fibrosis. Acta Paediatr Scand 1980;69:353–358.
47. Marcotte JE, Grisdale RK, Levinson H, et al. Multiple factors limit exercise capacity in cystic fibrosis. Pediatr Pulmonol 1986;2:274–281.
48. Godfrey S, Mearns M. Pulmonary function and response to exercise in cystic fibrosis. Arch Dis Child 1971;46:144–151.
49. Keens T, Krastia JR, Wannamaker EM, et al. Ventilatory muscle endurance training in normal subjects and patients with cystic fibrosis. Am Rev Respir Dis 1977;116:853–860.
50. Orenstein D, Franklin BA, Doershuk CF, et al. Exercise conditioning and cardiopulmonary fitness in cystic fibrosis. Chest 1981;80:392–398.
51. Holzer FJ, Schnall R, Landau LI. The effect of a home exercise programme in children with cystic fibrosis and asthma. Aust Paediatr J 1984;20:297–302.
52. Strauss GD, Osher A, Wang C-I, et al. Variable weight training in cystic fibrosis. Chest 1987;92:273–276.
53. Prasad A, Cerny F. Factors that influence adherence to exercise and their effectiveness: application to cystic fibrosis. Pediatr Pulmonol 2002;34:66–72.
54. American College of Sports Medicine. Guidelines for Graded Exercise Testing and Exercise Prescription. 4th ed. Philadelphia: Lea & Febiger, 1990.
55. Zach MS, Oberwaldner B, Hausler F. Cystic fibrosis: physical exercise versus chest physiotherapy. Arch Dis Child 1982;57:587–589.
56. Zach MS, Purrer B, Oberwaldner B. Effect of swimming on forced expiration and sputum clearance in cystic fibrosis. Lancet 1981;2:1201–1203.
57. Asher M, Pardy R, Coates A, et al. The effects of inspiratory muscle training in patients with cystic fibrosis. Am Rev Respir Dis 1982;126:855–859.
58. O'Neill PA, Dodds M, Phillips B, et al. Regular exercise and reduction of breathlessness in patients with cystic fibrosis. Br J Dis Chest 1987;81:62–69.
59. Hebstreit A, Kersting U, Basler B, et al. Exercise inhibits epithelial sodium channels in patients with cystic fibrosis. Am J Respir Crit Care Med 2001;164:443–446.
60. Andreasson B, Jonson B, Kornfalt R, et al. Long-term effects of physical exercise on working capacity and pulmonary function in cystic fibrosis. Acta Paediatr Scand 1987;76:70–75.
61. Blomquist M, Freyschuss U, Wiman L-G, et al. Physical activity and self treatment in cystic fibrosis. Arch Dis Child 1986;61:362–367.
62. Edlund LD, French RW, Herbst JJ, et al. Effects of a swimming program on children with cystic fibrosis. Am J Dis Child 1986;140:80–83.
63. Stanghelle JK, Skyberg D. Cystic fibrosis patients running a marathon race. Int J Sports Med 1988;9 (suppl):37–40.
64. Stanghelle JK, Hjeltnes N, Bangstad H, et al. Effect of daily short bouts of trampoline exercise during 8 weeks on the pulmonary function and the maximal oxygen uptake of children with cystic fibrosis. Int J Sports Med 1988;9(suppl):32–36.

RELATED WEB SITES

The Cystic Fibrosis Foundation
www.cff.org

Cystic Fibrosis Information
www.cysticfibrosis.com

Cystic-L, Cystic Fibrosus Information and Support
www.cystic-l.org

Cardiovascular Conditions

18

Coronary Heart Disease

William L. Haskell and J. Larry Durstine

Coronary heart disease (CHD) is primarily the result of advanced coronary atherosclerosis and thrombosis, the causes of which have not been definitively established. During the past four decades, however, significant advances have been made in the earlier detection, prevention, and treatment of CHD. Contributing to these advances has been the use of exercise testing for the functional assessment, diagnosis, prognosis, and clinical management of patients with CHD and the use of exercise training for primary and secondary prevention and cardiac rehabilitation.

The recommendations provided in this chapter are general principles related to the design and conduct of testing protocols and training programs for patients with CHD. The characteristics of the exercise plan for a specific patient should be determined by the patient's physician or the cardiac rehabilitation team. The interaction of various circumstances that influence exercise program details requires that each plan be individualized and then be revamped as patient status changes. As with all cardiovascular therapies, no absolute assurance regarding benefit or safety can be ascribed to exercise testing or training for all patients.

Causes, Prevention, and Therapy

CHD continues to be the most frequent cause of death in economically developed Western countries and is rapidly becoming the major cause of death in developing and undeveloped countries (1). Currently in the United States, one third of all deaths are attributed to CHD, with approximately 681,000 deaths in 2000 (2). Fatality rates remain low under the age of 35 years then increase exponentially until age 85, with men experiencing higher mortality rates until age 75. The total number of deaths due to CHD in 2000 was similar in men (50.6%) and women (49.4%) (2). While mortality rates have decreased in the United States, 47% of persons who experience CHD in a given year will die from it, and 50% of men and 64% of women who die suddenly of CHD have no previous symptoms of their disease (2).

There are some indications that changes in health-related habits (especially in cigarette smoking, eating habits, and possibly physical activity) between 1970 and 2000 have contributed to the decline in CHD mortality, as well as a number of advances in medical therapy (3). Recognized improvements in therapy include more widespread control of hypercholesterolemia and hypertension, increased availability of emergency cardiac care (cardiopulmonary resuscitation [CPR] and coronary care units), the use of more effective antianginal and antiarrhythmic medications, and recently, judicious use of coronary artery bypass graft (CABG) surgery, percutaneous coronary interventions, and the use of coronary stents (4). Headed in the

285

opposite direction has been the prevalence of obesity and type 2 diabetes mellitus (3). Since this decrease in CHD mortality rate has occurred among men and women of all ages and most ethnicities, attribution of this decline to any single health habit change or therapy is highly speculative.

During the past few decades, it has become apparent that a person's risk of developing clinical complications from CHD is determined by interactions among a variety of environmental and hereditary factors. For a small percentage of the population, a high-risk genetic profile (e.g., low-density-lipoprotein cholesterol [LDL]-C receptor deficiency) is the major determinant of early-onset CHD. However, if heredity were the major determinant of CHD risk, then mortality rates would not change rapidly as they did in the United States during the 20th century. Similarly, we would not see a rapid increase in CHD risk when a low-risk population adopts the culture of a high-risk population (1). For most persons, environmental exposure or lifestyle is the major determinant of their CHD risk. The enormous difference in CHD risk observed between selected cultures throughout the world is more a function of how people interact with their environment than their selection of parents (3). Given a low- CHD-risk lifestyle, "bad genes" frequently will not be expressed and cause clinical CHD until very late in life or never, i.e., most "bad genes" usually act only in "bad" or high-risk environments. This does not mean that heredity is unimportant or that gene therapy cannot become a useful CHD management tool. It does mean that there are great opportunities to substantially reduce clinical CHD events by effective and sustained lifestyle modification.

CLINICAL CARDIAC EVENTS

Many clinical cardiac events, including myocardial infarction (MI), cardiac arrest, and unstable angina pectoris, occur when there is erosion or rupture of an atherosclerotic plaque, releasing platelet aggregation factors into the coronary artery lumen and stimulating the formation of a blood clot that can rapidly occlude the artery (5). These so-called culprit lesions that erode or rupture tend to be early lipid-filled plaques rather than more advanced complex lesions. Thus, prevention of clinical cardiac events may be achieved by reducing

new lesion formation, stabilizing existing lesions, reducing the rate of existing lesion growth or progression, decreasing lesion size or regression, and reducing platelet aggregation or increasing fibrinolysis.

PREVENTION AND THERAPY

Most preventive and therapeutic measures for CHD focus on maintaining or reestablishing a balance between myocardial oxygen supply and demand so that oxygen supply exceeds both immediate and long-term demands under a variety of situations. Because this balance can be upset by decreasing supply or increasing demand, maintenance or restoration of this balance may be achieved by increasing supply or decreasing demand. Myocardial oxygen supply can be influenced by decreasing the rate with which coronary atherosclerosis develops or its possible regression, formation of collateral coronary arteries, enlargement of the diameter of major coronary vessels, redistribution of coronary blood flow, and improved functioning of the clotting or fibrinolytic system. Myocardial oxygen demand can be decreased by reducing heart rate (HR), intramyocardial tension (indirectly indicated by systolic blood pressure [SBP]), myocardial contractility, and possibly ventricular volume.

The lifestyle measures most likely to increase or maintain myocardial oxygen supply include stop cigarette smoking; treat hypertension and hyperlipidemia by medication; reduce dietary saturated fat, cholesterol, and salt; maintain optimal body weight (calorie restriction and exercise); and exercise to modify lipoprotein and carbohydrate metabolism and platelet aggregation. Exercise training, hypertension control, weight loss, smoking cessation, and stress management can all contribute to reducing myocardial oxygen demand. Because most of these risk factors appear to have a synergistic effect in causing or accelerating the development of atherosclerosis, a multiple risk-factor reduction approach is strongly advocated, especially when designing programs for individuals at high risk or individuals known to have CHD (6–8).

Medical treatment for CHD is primarily focused on reducing myocardial oxygen demand by decreasing HR, BP, or myocardial contractility (use of nitroglycerin, β-blockers, or calcium antagonists).

Currently, there is no conclusive evidence regarding these drugs' effects on increasing myocardial oxygen delivery by decreasing coronary vascular resistance. However, a combination of drug therapies has shown improved vital organ blood flow in animals (9). Antiarrhythmic therapy frequently is used to treat patients, but evidence of its benefit in reducing new events has been difficult to obtain, except in patients who also have clinically significant left ventricular dysfunction. CABG surgery and percutaneous transluminal coronary angioplasty (PTCA) with coronary stenting now are the primary means to increase myocardial blood flow and hence oxygen supply (10). Improved functional capacity, clinical status, and longevity have been reported for subsets of patients with multivessel coronary disease or its equivalent who have undergone CABG surgery (11,12). Longitudinal studies show that PTCA relieves symptoms and increases functional capacity, while having mortality rates and arterial wall integrity similar to those of CABG surgery (13).

Cardiovascular Adjustment to Exercise

The exercise capacity of patients relatively soon after MI and CABG surgery is determined by the same parameters as in healthy individuals or other cardiac patients: genetic endowment, gender, age, physical training status, and the amount of myocardial dysfunction (either permanent or transient) that occurs with exercise. As well, their circulatory control mechanisms during exercise are similar to those of other patients. The magnitude of their functional impairment depends on the amount and location of myocardial damage due to MI, as well as the nature of the blood supply to the remaining viable myocardium. The other consideration is the time since MI, because exercise tolerance is decreased until significant myocardial healing occurs. Definitive data are lacking on this issue, but in patients <70 years old with medically uncomplicated MI, limitation of exercise tolerance due to healing is no longer observed after 8 to 12 weeks after MI (14). Peak HR 3 weeks after MI usually does not exceed 135 beats·min^{-1}, and HR at any given level of submaximal PO is decreased in patients 6 weeks after MI (15).

The capacity of the oxygen transport system is generally considered the limiting factor in large muscle dynamic (aerobic) exercise—that used for most exercise tolerance testing and training of patients with CHD. If the capacity of one or more components of the oxygen transport system becomes significantly limited due to disease, exercise tolerance declines. Oxygen transport can be described by a rearranged Fick equation: oxygen uptake ($\dot{V}O_2$) = (HR × stroke volume [SV]) × total arteriovenous oxygen difference or AVD-O$_2$. AVD-O$_2$ is determined by the distribution of arterial blood and local tissue factors influencing oxygen extraction. In healthy adults of similar age and gender, most of the variation in $\dot{V}O_{2max}$ is due to differences in SV at maximal exercise. At a given age, maximal HR and AVD-O$_2$ are similar. The inability to have SV continue to increase with exercise is not due to limitations in coronary blood flow, but more likely results from reduced left ventricular filling time at a high HR and/or the inability to further increase ventricular emptying because of increased "afterload" with rising systemic arterial pressure.

RESPONSE TO DYNAMIC EXERCISE

Patients with documented CHD may respond quite normally to dynamic exercise, or they might exhibit marked abnormalities due to myocardial ischemia, nonreversible myocardial necrosis, or injury to the conduction system. The magnitude of impaired cardiovascular adjustment to exercise will depend on disease severity. While the exercise capacity of some patients is indistinguishable from that of healthy subjects, most display diminished work tolerance that is due to diminished peak SV or HR, whereas AVD-O$_2$ is usually within normal limits. The arterial BP response at submaximal and maximal exercise can be elevated, normal, or diminished, the last being especially critical in patients with myocardial ischemia and impaired left ventricular function. The impaired left ventricular response to exercise can be due to either permanent myocardial lesions (scarring and fibrosis), which can increase compliance and produce akinetic or dyskinetic contraction patterns, or reversible ischemia. This transient ischemia is produced by increased myocardial oxygen requirements associated with increased HR, ventricular wall tension, and contractility.

Patients with normal hemodynamic function at rest can demonstrate an abnormal hemodynamic status during exercise, with evidence of diminished work tolerance without transient ischemia. Such responses are due to poor left ventricular compliance or abnormal contraction patterns and may become apparent only with increases in left ventricular work. More frequently, however, major decrements in work capacity in patients with normal hemodynamics at rest are due to effort-induced ischemia. In patients with normal resting hemodynamics, the cardiac output ($\dot{Q}$) for any given submaximal power output (PO) is usually within the normal range, as is AVD-O_2. On the other hand, this normal $\dot{Q}$ may be achieved by a lower SV and a higher HR. As left ventricular impairment increases (due to either fixed or transient abnormalities), increased HR does not fully compensate for the further decrease in SV, so that $\dot{Q}$ for a given PO decreases and a widening of the AVD-O_2 delivers the needed oxygen.

Because coronary reserve is not markedly impaired until atherosclerosis reduces the cross-sectional area of the coronary artery lumen by at least 70%, most patients with lesser narrowing do not demonstrate exercise-induced cardiac abnormalities. In fact, some patients with >70% narrowing of one or more arteries have normal responses. Average work capacity declines progressively with the degree of narrowing and number of major vessels involved, but the magnitude of physical impairment cannot be used to accurately predict the extent of anatomic involvement in an individual patient (16). If the pathophysiologic aspects are kept in mind, then this relative lack of correlation between coronary anatomy and exercise performance or hemodynamic responses is not surprising. In one patient with a critical lesion of a single coronary artery, work tolerance may be very low, with angina pectoris precipitated by mild effort. In contrast, another patient with double- or triple-vessel disease but with well-developed collateral vessels may be free of angina, arrhythmias, or left ventricular dysfunction at relatively high PO. Even though average or representative values are usually lower than those of age-matched counterparts, substantial variation exists, and the tolerance of any one patient cannot be estimated accurately from clinical data. The New York Heart Association's (NYHA) functional classification of patients with heart disease can be

related to exercise tolerance (expressed as $\dot{V}O_{2peak}$) obtained by exercise testing. Class I patients with no symptoms have a $\dot{V}O_{2peak}$ above 6 METs. Class II patients with symptoms during ordinary physical activity have a $\dot{V}O_{2peak}$ of 4 to 6 METs. Class III patients (symptoms with less than ordinary physical activity) have a 2- to 4- MET capacity. Class IV patients with symptoms at rest have a $\dot{V}O_{2peak}$ of <2 METs (17).

In addition to decreasing exercise tolerance, CHD appears to reduce the speed with which the patient can make circulatory adjustments to exercise. In patients with either poor left ventricular function or cardiac acceleration, the time required for $\dot{Q}$ and its components to meet the demands for a given exercise intensity is increased (18). The magnitude of this delayed response is probably related to the magnitude of left ventricular involvement and should be considered in exercise test protocol selection and design of the warm-up component of training.

Exercise-Induced Ischemia

Patients with increasing ischemia usually terminate exercise because they cannot transport sufficient oxygen to the working myocardium and the working muscles; the latter is often limiting in healthy persons. Increasing ischemia usually results in a diminished SV response (an increase instead of a decrease in end-systolic volume and a decrease in left ventricular ejection fraction); a more rapid increase in HR (but lower peak HR); an earlier widening of the AVD-O_2; and a subnormal rise in SBP, with the possibility of no increase or even a precipitous decline. Such abnormal responses can occur without such objective indicators of ischemia as angina pectoris or ST-segment displacement on the electrocardiogram (ECG). Decreased ventricular function may even occur without evidence of myocardial perfusion abnormalities, as assessed by thallium-201 imaging.

The onset of detectable ischemia (angina or ST-segment depression) occurs at a relatively constant threshold of myocardial work for an individual patient. This threshold can be best defined noninvasively by the HR × SBP product (rate-pressure product [RPP]). In the clinically stable patient, angina or ST depression occurs at a similar RPP during repeated bouts of exercise days or even months apart (19). Even when the RPP at a specific exercise PO is altered by adding static arm exercise, cigarette smoking, reduced environmental temperature, or food ingestion, the threshold for ischemia remains relatively constant (20,21). This close relationship between the onset of angina and RPP indicates that such determinants of myocardial oxygen demand as ventricular volume and contractility vary in proportion to the RPP, both in healthy subjects and in patients with CHD. In situations in which left ventricular volume differs from that occurring during upright dynamic leg exercise, however, the RPP threshold for ischemia may change. During supine exercise, left ventricular end-diastolic volume (EDV) is increased because of elevated central blood volume, and the onset of ischemia occurs at a lower RPP (22). The lower threshold might also result from a decrease in myocardial flow due to the effect of increased myocardial tension on the blood flow to small intramural vessels. The opposite reaction occurs with dynamic arm exercise, in which SV and left ventricular EDV (and possibly left ventricular end-diastolic pressure [EDP]) are lower at the same RPP, and the anginal threshold therefore tends to be somewhat higher (23).

RESPONSES TO STATIC EXERCISE

Static or isometric exercise primarily produces a pressure load on the myocardium, in contrast to the predominantly volume load elicited by large muscle dynamic exercise. A vigorous (>25% of maximal) static contraction of even a relatively small muscle mass in normal subjects produces a significant rise in HR, $\dot{Q}$, and systemic arterial pressures (systolic, diastolic, and mean) with minimal or no change in SV or total peripheral resistance. With the rise in arterial pressure, there normally is only a small rise in left ventricular EDP and a significant rise in left stroke work index. In patients with abnormal ventricular function at rest or with poor tolerance during dynamic exercise (NYHA classes II and III), sustained static exercise produces a significant rise in left ventricular EDP, no increase or even a decrease in SV, and only a small increase in left ventricular stroke work (24). Thus, in patients with poor dynamic exercise tolerance, the left ventricle has scant physiologic capacity to increase its output during static exercise, and a sustained contraction may produce myocardial ischemia, left ventricular failure, or

complex ventricular arrhythmias. In these patients, systemic arterial pressure rises normally with static exercise because of the increased peripheral arterial tone produced by a powerful activation of the adrenergic nervous system. Patients with relatively good dynamic exercise capacity (>6 METs) tolerate static exercise quite well. Because the increase in HR with static exercise is only about 50% (25–35 beats·min^{-1}) of that noted during symptom-limited cycle ergometer or treadmill testing (50–80 beats·min^{-1}) and the SBP increase is similar with the two types of exercise, the increase in myocardial oxygen demand is less for isometric exercise. Also, there is some evidence that the rise in diastolic pressure with static exercise increases diastolic filling of the coronary arteries; this occurrence actually results in a higher RPP threshold for ischemia (25).

The incorporation of static activity during dynamic exercise favorably modifies the myocardial oxygen supply/demand relationship in patients with CHD. Ischemic ECG responses attained during dynamic exercises were attenuated when dynamic and isometric exercises were combined and performed at the same RPP values that elicited significant ST-segment depression during dynamic exercise (26). These results have changed the previous cautious attitude held toward the inclusion of strength training in cardiac rehabilitation (27,28).

Benefits of Exercise Training

Participation in a program of endurance-type training generally improves the clinical status and exercise capacity of patients with CHD. For persons with exertional ischemia, the intensity needed to precipitate chest pain or ST-segment depression increases, and less antianginal medication may be required. These improvements appear to be due more to a reduction in myocardial work and oxygen demand at rest and submaximal exercise than to any substantial increase in myocardial oxygen supply. Reduced myocardial oxygen demand results primarily from decreases in HR, with possibly some drop in systemic arterial BP. The decrease in RPP is greatest during submaximal exercise with trained limbs, suggesting that the site of this important training effect is mainly the muscles used during training (29,30). Alterations in the metabolic capacity of skeletal muscle probably make a major contribution to the quite rapid decrease in HR and increase in AVD-O_2 that occur during submaximal exercise soon after the training begins. A slight reduction in $\dot{Q}$ during submaximal exercise after training is associated with a decrease in blood flow to working muscles and a small increase in flow to nonexercising tissue (31,32).

In contrast to the substantial data demonstrating a reduction in myocardial oxygen demand with training, there is still a limited amount of evidence that a significant increase in myocardial perfusion or oxygen supply occurs routinely in response to exercise training. Recently, it was demonstrated that training increases perfusion time for a given HR, suggesting that myocardial oxygen supply can be increased (33). So far, it has not been possible to systematically demonstrate in humans that training increases oxygen delivery to myocardial tissue by delaying the rate of atherosclerotic progression or by stimulating coronary collateral vascularization (34,35). Myocardial perfusion at rest and exercise has been studied using thallium-201 imaging before and after training in patients with established CHD. Even though a few patients show some improvement in perfusion with training, most test results have been negative (36). An exception to these observations that exercise training has little or no effect on increasing coronary artery dilation capacity and blood flow has been the findings by Hambrecht and colleagues (37,38). They demonstrated that CHD patients randomized to a 4-week endurance-exercise training program significantly increased endothelial-mediated vasodilation of the coronary arteries as well as coronary blood flow reserve. The increased dilating capacity of the coronary arteries appears to be due to increased nitric oxide synthase activity (38).

Exercise training above a moderate level favorably alters both lipoprotein (e.g., modest declines in LDL-C and increases in HDL-C) and carbohydrate metabolism and thus would seem to have the potential to modify the course of coronary atherosclerosis (39,40). Human studies directly addressing this issue are limited to the use of repeat coronary arteriography, which has low subject acceptance because of its invasive nature. Nevertheless, studies have shown encouraging associations between training and physiologic and metabolic adaptations (41–43). New procedures for image enhancement with computerized edge detection and volume calculations now make the study of progression or regression more feasible (6,44). The previous finding by researchers conducting animal studies that training might enhance coronary artery collateral development has not been seen in humans, possibly because of difficulties in measurement methodology. In four studies in which training periods lasted from 15 weeks to 1 year, no evidence of collateral development was seen. Direct measurement of coronary sinus blood flow during rest and exercise yields no evidence that maximal coronary blood flow or coronary blood flow at the onset of angina significantly increases as a result of training (35,45). In some cases, angina-limited exercise tolerance was increased by more than 35%, with no evidence of any improvement in coronary blood flow. Increases in angina threshold associated with short-term or low-intensity training are probably due to a decrease in HR, an increase in pain tolerance, or patient confidence after training or repeat testing (46).

As training increases in intensity, duration, or both, more general or central circulatory effects begin to occur, e.g., reductions in HR and sometimes BP at rest, and reductions in HR during exercise when using nontrained limbs. At this point, there often is an increase in SV at rest and during submaximal exercise (53). Some evidence indicates that longer, more vigorous training can increase the RPP at which ischemic ST-segment depression occurs (34,48). These changes are probably associated with alterations in central nervous system control of the myocardium or with enhanced intrinsic myocardial function. It is unlikely that increases in blood volume or red blood cell mass contribute much to these changes.

The rate and magnitude of hemodynamic and metabolic improvement due to training in patients with CHD appear to be a function of the viability of the myocardium and the characteristics of the exercise regimen. Ambulatory patients with severely compromised ventricular function and exercise-induced myocardial ischemia prior to training may have already used much of their adaptive capacity (e.g., widening of the AVD-O_2 and shunting of blood to working tissues) and therefore have minimal potential for improvement. In these instances, improvements seen with training may be due to corrected impaired vasodilatation (49). Some of these patients, however, do surprisingly well with training and show improvement in exercise capacity with no change in ventricular function (50,51). The occurrence of angina pectoris does not necessarily diminish a patient's potential for improved clinical status, because many angina patients improve exercise tolerance and symptom relief with appropriate programs. Even with long-term training (>26 weeks), however, the exercise capacity of patients is lower than that of age-matched normal individuals.

The cardiac function of some CHD patients will not improve with training. Myocardial damage (necrosis, dyskinesis, and ischemia) may minimize the potential for improvement or the progression of coronary atherosclerosis (despite concerned medical treatment) may negate or override any achievable training benefit. When the clinical status and exercise tolerance level of a patient continue to deteriorate despite adherence to an appropriate training program, alternate forms of medical or surgical therapy should be considered.

Aside from improvement in functional capacity and clinical status, training has been promoted to accelerate the return to work after MI or surgery, to improve psychologic status, and to reduce the occurrence of reinfarction and death. The improved functional status of many patients due to exercise probably increases their job potential and productivity, but the specific benefits attributable to training are not proven because of the numerous social and economic factors influencing an individual's return to work. A more-rapid return to work has been reported for patients who participate in work evaluation soon after hospitalization for MI (52). Improved self-confidence, the patient's age, and the physician's view on the extent to which the patient is vocationally disabled can contribute greatly to increased self-care or work potential (53).

Comprehensive cardiac rehabilitation appears to reduce the mortality rate due to reinfarction by 20 to 25%; the role that exercise alone plays in improving prognosis is not well established (54–56). A meta-analysis was used to evaluate 10 clinical trials in which patients after hospitalization for MI were randomized to exercise-based cardiac rehabilitation or usual care (55). Participation in these programs resulted in ~25% lower CHD or all-cause death rates but no difference in nonfatal MI. A similar analysis using the results from 22 cardiac rehabilitation studies found similar results (54). The power

of the individual studies to demonstrate a training benefit has been curtailed by a substantially lower than expected mortality rate in the usual-care patients, an inadequate sample size, and a relatively short period of follow-up (54,55,57).

Exercise Testing Considerations

Results from exercise tests of CHD patients can be used to objectively quantify the functional or clinical significance of disease; aid in determining appropriate therapy; contribute to the prognosis of new clinical events; help evaluate the effectiveness of various treatment regimens; promote patient confidence by providing reassurance that routine activities can be undertaken safely; and establish the appropriateness of performing specific job-related, leisure-time, or physical conditioning activities. Exercise testing, with one or more of these objectives as the primary indication, is routinely performed on chronic, stable, asymptomatic patients; those with exercise-induced ischemia; patients with known or suspected left ventricular dysfunction at rest or with exercise; and patients in the process of recovering from acute MI, CABG, or PTCA. The discussion in this section is limited to special considerations required in the exercise testing of patients with CHD for the primary purpose of prescribing exercise. Guidelines for exercise testing patients have been updated by the American Heart Association, American College of Cardiology, and the Canadian Association of Cardiac Rehabilitation (58–60).

The special considerations required for safe and effective exercise testing of CHD patients primarily emphasize (*a*) excluding patients for medical reasons that might put them at undue risk; (*b*) selecting an appropriate test protocol consistent with the likelihood of a restricted capacity; and (*c*) monitoring the patient to detect those abnormalities that provide information on the functional significance of the disease or, more importantly, are contraindications to further exercise. In many cases, no one single protocol has been demonstrated to be safer, elicit more precise or valid information, or be more cost-effective or acceptable to the patient, because tradeoffs exist between one procedure and another.

PATIENT EVALUATION AND CONTRAINDICATION TO TESTING

Immediately before testing, every patient with CHD should have a cardiovascular assessment, including medical history, laboratory tests, physical examination by a qualified physician, and a resting 12-lead ECG. Guidelines for such evaluations have been provided by the American Heart Association and the American College of Sports Medicine (58,28). Conditions generally considered contraindications to testing are included in Table 18-1. In special cases, these conditions may not be absolute contraindications, but special attention should at least be paid. For example, in testing the efficacy of a new antiarrhythmic drug, patients with more-frequent ventricular arrhythmias might be tested under close medical monitoring and safety considerations. Written informed consent with enough information to ensure that patients know and understand the purpose and risks associated with the test should be obtained before all testing is begun. Informed consent is especially important when the patient's clinical status significantly increases the risk of exertion-induced complications. Finally, patients should be given explicit instructions prior to testing to increase validity and data accuracy.

PROTOCOL SELECTION

Protocol selection should consider the purpose of the test, the specific outcomes desired, and the individual being tested. The general principles and guidelines for testing patients with CHD to assess the integrity of their oxygen transport system are similar to those described for healthy adults in Chapter 1. Special considerations concern the initial exercise intensity and the rate at which intensity is increased during the test; the need for closer and more frequent monitoring of the ECG, BP, and symptoms during exercise and recovery; the value of multiple-lead ECG recordings; and a longer post-exercise recovery period before the patient is discharged from the facility.

The use of motor-driven treadmills or cycle ergometers is preferred because exercises involving these devices maximally stress the cardiovascular system (instead of being limited by local muscle factors), require little special skill, can be calibrated,

TABLE 18-1 CONTRAINDICATIONS TO EXERCISE TESTING

Absolute contraindications
1. A recent significant change in the resting ECG suggesting significant ischemia, recent myocardial infarction, or other acute cardiac event
2. Recent complicated myocardial infarction
3. Unstable angina
4. Uncontrolled cardiac arrhythmias causing symptoms or hemodynamic compromise
5. Uncontrolled atrial dysrhythmias that compromise cardiac function
6. Third-degree A-V block
7. Acute congestive heart failure
8. Severe symptomatic aortic stenosis
9. Suspected or known dissecting aneurysm
10. Acute myocarditis or pericarditis
11. Thrombophlebitis or intracardiac thrombi
12. Acute pulmonary embolus or pulmonary infarction
13. Acute infection
14. Significant emotional distress (psychosis)

Relative contraindications
1. Resting diastolic blood pressure >120 mm Hg or resting systolic blood pressure >200 mm Hg
2. Moderate stenotic valvular heart disease
3. Left main coronary stenosis
4. Tachy- or bradyarrhythmias
5. High-degree A-V block
6. Known electrolyte abnormalities (hypokalemia, hypomagnesemia)
7. Fixed-rate pacemaker (rarely used)
8. Frequent or complex ventricular ectopy
9. Ventricular aneurysm
10. Cardiomyopathy, including hypertrophic cardiomyopathy and other forms of outflow obstruction
11. Uncontrolled metabolic disease (e.g., diabetes, thyrotoxicosis or myxedema)
12. Chronic infectious disease (e.g., mononucleosis, hepatitis, HIV-AIDS)
13. Neuromuscular, musculoskeletal, or rheumatoid disorders that are exacerbated by exercise
14. Advanced or complicated pregnancy

Adapted from American College of Sports Medicine. Guidelines for Exercise Testing and Exercise Prescription. 6th ed. Philadelphia: Lippincott Williams & Wilkins, 2000.

and exhibit relatively little interindividual variation in biomechanical efficiency. For patients with poor leg strength (especially those who have restricted their exercise for some time, older patients, and those with low total body weight), the treadmill is preferred. Because $\dot{V}O_2$ is usually not measured but is estimated from PO, the exercise device *must* be accurately calibrated. Further, because the treadmill provides a more common form of physiologic stress, the patient is more likely to attain a higher $\dot{V}O_2$ and peak HR than during the cycle ergometer test.

Before testing, many patients will have a limited exercise capacity and, even more important, the exercise capacity of some patients will be totally unpredictable (61). Thus, select a test protocol in which the initial exercise intensity is low and the increase in intensity is gradual, e.g., begin at 2 to 3 METs, with intensity not to increase more than 1 MET per minute. For patients with poor exercise tolerance, intensity should be increased by 1 MET every 2 or 3 min. Gradual increases in intensity are recommended because of the slower rate of cardiovascular adjustment in these patients. If intensity is increased by more than 2 to 3 METs every 3 min for patients with poor left ventricular function, the measured $\dot{V}O_2$ drops below the value estimated from previously reported data. This reduced rate of cardiovascular adjustment can result in overestimation of exercise tolerance. Ideally, increments in PO should be chosen so that the total test time is 8 to 12 min.

For screening asymptomatic subjects, single-lead monitoring may be optimal considering cost and the frequency of false-positive results. As CHD severity increases, however, using additional leads provides more information about the status of the myocardium because they may pick up ischemia otherwise not detected and aid in the detection and interpretation of cardiac dysrhythmias or altered electrical conduction. The use of 3 to 6 leads provides most of the information contained in as many as 12 to 14 leads but has the advantage of simplicity and lack of problems with lead adjustment (62). The capability to continuously observe the ECG on a monitor should be required because it is possible to identify a sudden change in ECG rhythm, HR, and ischemia (ST-segment displacement). The ECG should be recorded prior to increasing the PO, at times of major ECG abnormalities, at peak exercise, at the end of recovery, and possibly at the end of each minute of exercise. The major concern is not to miss data that may have clinical relevance.

The inability of a CHD patient to increase or maintain SBP during increasing exercise is a good indication of LV dysfunction or failure. Close, accurate monitoring of BP is therefore important. BP should be recorded in the last 20 to 30 sec of each PO; if 3-min stages are used, BP should be recorded in the last 20 to 30 sec of the first minute at each PO. Measurements should be made by using a high-quality stethoscope and mercury manometer. Most automatic or semiautomatic BP machines with good accuracy and reliability currently are too expensive for routine clinical use. Accurate BP recording during exercise, especially on the treadmill, requires careful execution and experience.

TEST TERMINATION CONSIDERATIONS

Except for special circumstances (e.g., very soon after acute MI), a general consensus now exists that symptom-limited or clinical maximal exercise testing is preferred to submaximal testing for assessing the cardiovascular response of patients with CHD. Symptom-limited testing is particularly valuable when the primary reason for the test is determining exercise capacity. With healthy individuals, responses to submaximal exercise can be used to predict exercise capacity (usually expressed as estimated $\dot{V}O_{2max}$) with a fair degree of accuracy. These predictions assume that the subject has a maximal HR somewhat close to the average for his or her age. For patients with CHD, this is not the case because their maximal or peak HR cannot be accurately estimated from age, clinical information, or submaximal exercise data. When a patient is tested, it is not possible to predict when an abnormality will develop that will contraindicate further exercise. The maximal or peak HR achieved by patients during testing usually is lower than that of their age-matched, healthy counterparts. Just as important, the variation in peak HR for patients at a given age is large. The usual standard deviation for peak HR in healthy adults at a given age is 9 to 11 beats·min^{-1}, whereas that for CHD patients is more than twice that amount.

The "clinical maximal" concept of exercise test termination seems the most appropriate for patients with CHD. This concept is based on the premise that patients should continue to exercise until they need to stop due to fatigue or until signs or symptoms develop that, given the reasons for testing and the testing environment, indicate that further exercise is not warranted. The specific signs or symptoms that make up the clinical indication for stopping vary with the clinical status of the patient, the primary reason for conducting the test, and the general test environment. For example, more conservative criteria are used early after an MI when the myocardium is still healing; in patients with known LV dysfunction who may develop congestive failure with exercise; or for patients with known ventricular irritability but for whom some objective measure of exercise tolerance is desired. If the primary reason for testing is to clear a patient for high-level exercise or for return to a demanding occupation (especially if a sudden cardiovascular complication would put other people in danger), then a more aggressive attitude regarding criteria for terminating the test should be used. Unless absolute contraindications to exercise occur first, patients should be pushed to levels of myocardial work above that they would be expected to reach in the activity for which they are being cleared. The more experienced the testing personnel and the more comprehensive the capability for immediate emergency medical care, the more liberal should be the criteria for test termination. Testing conducted in a major medical center may use criteria considered inappropriate for use in a private physician's office or a community exercise facility.

The same basic principle used to terminate maximal testing of healthy adults applies to symptom-limited testing of patients with CHD. The patient should be stopped when significant fatigue occurs or if signs or symptoms develop that indicate the patient's exercise tolerance level has been reached or exceeded. Continuing exercise at this point would not provide additional useful information and, more importantly, might rapidly lead to significant medical complications. Reasons for terminating a test specific to CHD manifestations include indications of increasing left ventricular failure, myocardial ischemia, myocardial irritability, orthostatic BP drop of >20 mm Hg, or intraventricular conduction abnormalities. Specific signs or symptoms that should be special considerations or indications for stopping the test are listed in Table 18-2. This list includes most of the common reasons for stopping symptom-limited tests in patients with CHD.

TABLE 18-2 INDICATIONS FOR STOPPING AN EXERCISE TEST

Symptoms
  New-onset anginal chest pain
  Increased angina to grade 3 as estimated by patient, with or without ECG changes
  Light-headedness or fainting
  Severe dyspnea
  Severe fatigue or muscle pain
  Nausea or vomiting
Clinical signs
  Pallor, cyanosis, cold moist skin
  Staggering gait, ataxia
  Confusion in response to inquiries or blank stare
Electrocardiographic signs
ST displacement (elevation or depression) or horizontal or descending type more than 0.3 mV above or below that of the resting tracing
Conduction disturbance other than first-degree A-V block (prolonged P-R interval)
Ventricular arrhythmias
  Ventricular tachycardia
  Ventricular fibrillation
  Ventricular premature beats with a frequency of 35% of beats lasting more than 30 sec
Supraventricular arrhythmias
  Atrial fibrillation occurring with exercise
  Supraventricular tachycardia occurring with exercise
Blood pressure abnormalities
  Fall in SBP with increase in workload of 10 mm Hg or more below any previously recorded blood pressure, with other symptoms or signs, especially a low HR
Rise in systolic blood pressure above 250 mm Hg or diastolic pressure above 120 mm Hg
Patient indicates desire to stop test
Failure of ECG or blood pressure monitoring systems

Adapted from Flecher GF, Balady GJ, Amsterdam EA, et al. American Heart Association: exercise standards for testing and training: a statement for healthcare professionals. Circulation 2001;104: 1694–1740.

TOTAL PATIENT MONITORING

The application of "total patient monitoring" should be emphasized during testing. There is a tendency to focus on the ST-segment or angina pectoris and to ignore other important signs or symptoms that indicate impending problems or aid in understanding the patient's limitations. For example, close monitoring for the development of undue fatigue, dyspnea, or systolic hypotension in patients with known or highly suspect LV dysfunction may give the first major clue that their exercise tolerance level has been reached. During testing, the patient's appearance should be observed (gait, skin color and temperature, and breathing rate), verbal communication should be maintained (pain, fatigue, and dyspnea), and the ECG and BP should be monitored. Rated perceived exertion (RPE) scales provide a useful adjunct to HR as a guide for pain and fatigue during exercise (63). Failure to incorporate these comprehensive approaches to patient monitoring within the testing protocol reduces the clinical value of the results and increases the risk of an exercise-related complication. The importance of this approach increases with the severity of the illness. The excellent safety record during testing of patients with CHD in many medical facilities over the past three decades can be attributed, in part, to implementation of comprehensive patient monitoring.

With tests of patients with known CHD, results are not used to diagnose CHD but primarily for determining the functional significance of the disease. Test interpretation will focus on how much exercise the patient can perform (watts, treadmill speed and grade, and METs), what limited the patient's capacity to perform the test (reasons for termination), and the occurrence of symptoms (pain and dyspnea) or signs (ECG and SBP) indicating an abnormal response. Strong indicators of severe CHD include very poor exercise tolerance (≤ 4 METs), significant myocardial ischemia (grade 3+ angina or ST-segment depression of ≥ 0.2 mV) at low POs or low HR, and an inadequate SBP response. The clinical significance of exercise-induced ventricular arrhythmias is not well established, but they are prognostic of new cardiac events in patients with poor left ventricular function. The prevalence of exercise-induced ventricular arrhythmias increases after CABG, but the occurrence of ventricular arrhythmias does not indicate an increased risk of cardiac death (64). Nevertheless, until additional data are collected and guidelines are revised, complex ventricular arrhythmias are considered potentially hazardous events, and patients should be informed about how to avoid them, since documented cases of sudden death have occurred in patients with ventricular tachycardia or ventricular fibrillation during exercise (65). The severity of myocardial damage (both necrosis and transient ischemia) re-

sulting from CHD is related inversely to exercise capacity, PO, or HR at the onset of ischemia or to a hypotensive pressure response. Combinations of these abnormalities increase the likelihood that multivessel disease exists and that substantial myocardium is necrotic or becomes dyskinetic during exercise.

DRUG EFFECTS ON RESPONSES TO EXERCISE

Several categories of drugs influence exercise test results because they produce abnormal ST responses that are not due to myocardial ischemia. Among the drugs that may affect the ECG response are digitalis preparations, sympathetic nervous system blocking agents (β-blockers, guanethidine, and methyldopa), diuretics, and nitroglycerin compounds. Other drugs known to alter the HR or ECG response are quinidine, procainamide, atropine sulfate, phenothiazine derivatives, and lithium. Diuretics may reduce serum potassium levels and cause abnormal ST-T changes or ventricular dysrhythmias during exercise.

If a patient has ST changes while receiving digitalis, the ECG cannot be interpreted. If documentation of ischemia is important, the test should be repeated after withdrawing the drug for at least 3 weeks. If a patient receiving digitalis has a normal ST response during the test, the result can be considered negative. β-Adrenergic blocking agents cause a reduction in resting and exercise HR. However, peak HR during testing can still be used to establish guidelines for training intensity. Estimated maximal HR based on age cannot be used. Information on the intensity or HR at the onset of symptoms or signs of myocardial ischemia or ventricular dysfunction is of clinical value. Significant attenuation of the HR response may be seen in patients taking other drugs affecting the sympathetic nervous system (e.g., methyldopa and guanethidine).

If one of the major reasons for an exercise test is to establish the appropriate intensity for training, the patient should continue the regimen of medication that will be followed during training. Withholding medications on the day of testing can significantly change a patient's symptom-free exercise tolerance as well as the relationship between

HR and total body or myocardial oxygen demand. These differences in exercise response can negate using test data to establish the correct training regimen. For example, if a patient is tested while all medications are withheld and then returns to using a β-blocker, it is likely that the training HR will be too high and will place the patient at undue risk. Please see reference 28 for more detailed information on the effects of various drugs on the exercise response during exercise testing and training of patients with CHD.

EXERCISE TRAINING CONSIDERATIONS

All ambulatory CHD patients should have an activity plan that includes both the proscription and prescription of exercise. Ideally, all patients will undergo a clinical evaluation with a symptom-limited exercise test to determine the severity of disease and to establish risk stratification for future cardiac events (Table 18-3). This evaluation should determine the amount of ischemic myocardium, the impairment of ventricular function, and the frequency and severity of various signs or symptoms, including silent and symptomatic ischemia, dysrhythmias, abnormal BP, and the heart's responses to exercise and fatigue. The special considerations advised for formulating and executing exercise programs for patients with CHD (beyond those recommended for healthy middle-aged and older adults) are needed because of the increased risk that exercise may precipitate cardiovascular complications. Of all non-traumatic sudden deaths during vigorous exercise in individuals over age 35 years, >85% occur in those with severe CHD (66). Based on information collected primarily in medically supervised exercise programs for cardiac patients, cardiac arrest is the most frequent major cardiovascular complication during exercise, whereas acute MI is relatively rare (67,68).

EXERCISE SELECTION

Most health and performance benefits for patients produced by training result from performing large muscle, dynamic activities frequently referred to as aerobic or endurance-type exercises. Activities such as walking, hiking, jogging, running, cycling, swim-

TABLE 18-3 LOW, INTERMEDIATE, AND HIGH RISK CLASSIFICATIONS

Low-risk patients
    Following uncomplicated myocardial infarction or bypass surgery by day 4
    Functional capacity of >8 METS[a] on 3-week exercise test
    Asymptomatic at rest with exercise capacity adequate for most vocational and recreational activities
    No ischemia, left ventricular dysfunction, or dysrhythmias
    Men <45 years, women <55 years
Intermediate-risk patients
    Functional capacity of <8 METs on 3-week exercise test
    Poor ventricular function (LVEF <30%)
    Shock or congestive heart failure during recent myocardial infarction (<6 months)
    Inability to self-monitor HR
    Failure to comply with exercise prescription
    Exercise-induced ischemia or <0.2 mV
    Men >45 years, women >55 years
High-risk patients
    Left ventricular failure
    Resting complex ventricular dysrhythmias (Lown grade IV and V)
    Premature ventricular contractions appearing or increasing with exercise
    Exertional hypotension at low workload (decrease in SBP of >15 mm Hg)
    Recent myocardial infarction (<6 months) complicated by serious ventricular dysrhythmias
    Exercise-induced ischemia of >0.2 mV
    Survivors of cardiac arrest

From Heath and Public Policy Committee, American College of Physicians; cardiac rehabilitation services. Ann Intern Med 1988; 15:671–673.
  [a]1 MET is considered the equivalent of a VO_2 of 3.5 mL·kg^{-1}·min^{-1}

ming, selected calisthenics, and active sports all can produce endurance-training effects. Decisions as to the most appropriate activities should be based on the patient's clinical status, exercise tolerance, interests, skills, location of facilities, and the availability of supervised exercise programs. During the early convalescent period after MI or surgery, stationary equipment (e.g., cycle ergometers, treadmills, and rowing machines) is useful.

For patients who perform heavy-resistance exercise with the arms during employment or leisure time, a special program of arm endurance and strength training should be considered. Because the stress placed on the myocardium by this type of exercise is primarily determined by the percentage of maximal strength at which a muscle must perform, an increase in strength will reduce myocardial work for any given amount of exercise. Patients (including those with angina pectoris) can safely increase arm endurance capacity during supervised arm-training programs or standard programs that contain an arm component (58). Program guidelines have been established for resistance training by low-risk patients (Table 18-3) whose program objectives include a significant increase in muscle strength (58–60,69).

ESTABLISHING EXERCISE INTENSITY

A major goal of the exercise prescription is to establish an appropriate intensity for each patient. The basic premise is that exercise should be intense enough to produce improvements in performance and health status but not so vigorous as to produce undue fatigue or precipitate cardiovascular complications. The necessary stimulus for producing changes in hemodynamic and metabolic function by endurance training appears to be an increase in energy expenditure above some threshold (best expressed as a percentage of functional capacity) and performed for an extended period. The nature and magnitude of the training effects depend on the total amount of energy expended above this threshold, with variations produced by different combinations of intensity, frequency, and duration.

Because HR increases proportionately with increases in total body energy expenditure and with increases in myocardial work during large-muscle dynamic exercise, HR is the single best guide of intensity for cardiac patients. If the target HR range concept is used properly, then the lower HR (70% of peak exercise test HR or the HR at 60% of exercise capacity) represents the "stimulus threshold," and the upper HR (usually 85% of peak exercise test HR or at 80% of exercise capacity) represents the "safety threshold" (Fig. 18-1). The more medically complicated the patient, the greater the emphasis on establishing a proper safety threshold.

The basic assumption in using exercise test results to determine training intensity for CHD patients is that the peak myocardial work during training should always be lower than that achieved during the exercise test when contraindications to

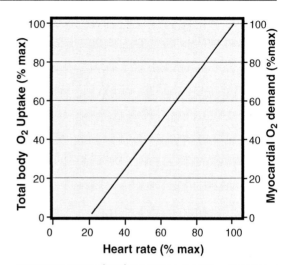

FIGURE 18-1 Use of HR for exercise prescription. Near-linear relationship of HR to total body oxygen uptake and myocardial oxygen demand during large muscle dynamic exercise (all variables expressed as a percentage of their maximal value for a specific individual). An increase in total body oxygen uptake is the necessary stimulus for cardiovascular conditioning; myocardial oxygen demand is the major limiting factor for exercise in patients with significant coronary heart disease. (Reprinted from Haskell W. Design of a cardiac conditioning program. In: Wenger NK, ed. Exercise and the Heart, Philadelphia: FA Davis, 1978:98.)

unmonitored exercise occurred. For the patient who performs a symptom-limited exercise test free of abnormalities, percentage of peak HR is an appropriate value to use, similar to the approach used with healthy adults. When abnormalities that occur during testing are associated with a significant risk of cardiovascular complications, the intensity at the onset of these abnormalities should then be used. For example, if a patient reports chest pain at a HR of 135 beats·min^{-1} but the test is not stopped because of grade 3+ angina pectoris until a HR of 144 beats·min^{-1} is achieved, a HR of 135 and the accompanying exercise are used to establish the training intensity. In this case, 70 to 85% of 135 (95–115 beats·min^{-1}) could be used as the training HR range. Another approach would be to subtract about 10 beats from the HR of 135 beats·min^{-1} and use that value as the high target HR. The lower target HR would be reduced to 15 to 20 beats, giving a training HR range of about 115 to 125 beats·min^{-1}. Similar approaches can be used when other contraindications to unmonitored exercise occur during testing (e.g., ST changes, ventricular arrhythmias, or an inadequate BP response).

Another way to establish exercise intensity is to use the RPE scale (63). Because RPE responses to graded exercise correlate highly with such cardiorespiratory and metabolic variables as $\dot{V}O_2$ and HR, this scale provides a valid and reliable indicator for the level of physical exertion during steady-state exercise. When the RPE scale is used, the fairly light (numerical value of 12) and somewhat hard (numerical value of 15) portion of the scale encompasses the range that most cardiac patients use during an exercise training session.

Because the likelihood of developing cardiovascular or orthopedic complications during exercise increases with intensity, high-risk patients should reduce intensity and increase duration or frequency to attain adequate exercise. Patients with poor exercise capacity (functional capacity of ≤ 5 METs) may be encouraged to exercise at lower intensities (40–50% instead of 60–85% for healthy adults) but for longer periods (walking for 1 h) or more frequently (once or twice daily). After hospitalization for MI, such low-level exercises as walking significantly improve functional capacity, with greater increases seen in patients without angina. As with healthy adults, patients should try to increase their exercise capacity so that they can exercise at an energy expenditure of as much as 300 kcal per session. Many patients will not be able to reach this level and will need individualized goals based on their own exercise tolerance. In these cases, 1600 kcal per week at moderate intensity is adequate to obtain significant benefits for CHD patients (70).

Completing a maximal or a symptom-limited exercise test before prescribing an exercise program may not always be feasible. In these cases, establishing suitable intensity levels is increasingly being assessed by RPE. Exercise programs for patients without preliminary testing should be implemented conservatively with close medical surveillance and continuous ECG monitoring, if feasible. The patient should be observed for signs and symptoms of exercise intolerance, and BP measurements should be obtained regularly. Patient questionnaires designed to estimate activity status and functional capacity (e.g., Duke Activity Status Index or Veterans Specific Activity Questionnaire) are also useful

(71,72). Initial intensities usually range from 2 to 3 METS or 20 to 30 beats·min^{-1} above standing rest HR (73). This can be gradually increased by 0.5 to 1 MET using the RPE.

Caution regarding environmental conditions during exercise is needed, especially for individuals who are symptomatic at a low exercise intensity. Whenever environmental stress may be added to the myocardial demands of exercise, the use of an appropriate target HR and RPE will greatly help the patient to maintain the proper exercise intensity. Readers should refer to Chapter 7 for detailed information on the effects of heat, cold, altitude, and pollution.

MEDICAL SUPERVISION

A major consideration of substantial clinical and economic significance in exercising patients with CHD is the extent of medical monitoring or supervision provided. Some general recommendations can be provided, but additional objective information is needed on the benefits, risks, and costs of various approaches before mandatory requirements or criteria are established. Situations in which patients are at high risk for fatal cardiovascular complications precipitated by exercise (Table 18-3) require close medical supervision, and continuous ECG monitoring may be needed. Such intensive supervision is suggested for patients with poor functional capacity (<8 METs); indications of left ventricular dysfunction (inadequate SBP response and decreased left ventricular ejection fraction [LVEF]); myocardial ischemia (angina or ST depression >0.2 mV); or complex ventricular dysrhythmias during exercise testing in those who plan to exercise above 50 to 60% of their symptom or sign-free exercise tolerance. Exercise performed at lower intensities, even within several weeks after an MI, may be at an acceptably low risk, such that direct medical supervision is not required (even though desirable). Such exercise, if performed regularly, may provide significant beneficial effects.

Patients at low risk (Table 18-3) and who have a symptom-free exercise capacity (>7 METs) require substantially less medical supervision during exercise training, even when exercising at 60 or 75% of their tolerance (as defined by the recent exercise test). After instruction and practice with regard to following an exercise prescription properly, high-capacity and low-risk patients may be encouraged to train without direct medical supervision in a community-based adult fitness program or on their own, using individually prescribed programs (67).

Detailed guidelines for supervising cardiac exercise programs have been published by the American Heart Association, the American College of Sports Medicine, and the American Association of Cardiovascular and Pulmonary Rehabilitation (27,28,58). These guidelines generally recommend the attendance of a physician or cardiovascular nurse at all exercise sessions conducted during the first 12 weeks of rehabilitation or as long as patients exhibit cardiac abnormalities associated with increased risk. This supervision should include emergency CPR equipment and a comprehensive emergency plan. Well-trained medical personnel can effectively resuscitate patients after cardiac arrest during supervised exercise, which is the most persuasive argument for recommending medical supervision (67). Use of lower-intensity exercise may significantly reduce the risk of major complications in patients with good function so that expensive medical monitoring can be restricted to those at highest risk.

EXERCISE DURING CONVALESCENCE

Patients frequently enter into medically supervised training programs during their hospitalization for acute MI or immediately after discharge from the hospital. These are low-level programs in which passive and active calisthenics are performed while sitting and standing, along with walking, slow stair climbing, and stationary cycling. Low-level treadmill testing is performed at or soon after hospital discharge to determine the appropriateness of a low-level exercise program. Testing is performed up to an HR of 110 to 130 beats·min^{-1}, an increase in HR of 20 beats·min^{-1}, or a workload of 5 METs. The general principles of exercise prescription and training apply to these patients, with special emphasis placed on low-intensity dynamic exercise, intermittent work bouts, and conservative criteria for exercise termination.

When a medically supervised exercise program is not available or feasible, patients with uncomplicated histories should be given a plan of unsupervised, low-intensity exercise during early posthospitalization. Individualized to a patient's clinical status, this plan should focus on walking or low-intensity stationary cycling, easy calisthenics, light household chores or recreational activities, and low-level, job-related tasks for patients who have returned to work (74). High-intensity exercise of any type, heavy resistance activities, and competitive situations should be avoided.

Each exercise plan should be in writing and include (*a*) characteristics of the exercise, (*b*) specific instructions on how to perform these exercises, and (*c*) how to monitor responses. All too frequently, such instructions are given verbally and are not specific enough for the patient to be confident of what to do and what to avoid. For unsupervised exercise, the patient should be provided a written prescription containing specific information on how to carry out an exercise plan.

If the patient has performed an exercise test recently, an exercise prescription using the target HR concept can be provided. If no contraindications to exercise exist, patients are given a target HR range that is approximately 15 to 30 beats below the peak HR achieved during the test. For the patient who does not perform an exercise test during the early convalescent period, exercise recommendations are based on clinical judgment, considering current clinical status, duration of convalescence, previous exercise habits, and age. All such patients should be given a conservative exercise plan in which the intensity is kept low and the duration and frequency are gradually increased. It is generally recommended that patients participate in activities requiring an increase in HR of no more than 30 or 40 beats·min^{-1} above resting or not above 110 to 120 beats·min^{-1} (lower if the patient is receiving such medications as β-blockers) or have an energy requirement of <4 to 6 METs. Activities of the proper type but too intense for patients during early convalescence include jogging, running, hiking in hills or mountains, and most active sports or games (e.g., basketball, handball, squash, and singles tennis). Activities of the wrong type include any heavy resistance or isometric exercise. Because their intensity can be easily controlled, walking, stationary cycling, and low-level bench stepping are useful conditioning activities. Walking can be performed when weather, daylight, and terrain permit.

Stationary cycling or bench stepping can be done when it is necessary or advisable to exercise indoors.

EXERCISE AFTER CONVALESCENCE

After patients have completed early convalescence (i.e., 12–16 weeks after MI or surgery) and have been performing a low-level exercise program on a reasonably regular basis, they may be ready for, and interested in, additional physical activities, especially some of higher intensity. If possible, patients should perform an exercise test to evaluate exercise capacity. The results of this test, along with data from the medical history and physical examination, should form the basis for an updated exercise plan. If the decision is made to increase intensity to the level of jogging or running, attempts should be made to enter a supervised program, preferably one with medical monitoring.

The exercise plan for patients not in a supervised program should keep intensity at 60 to 75% of the peak HR determined during the most recent exercise test and should emphasize a longer exercise session duration (30–60 min) and increased frequency (four or five times per week, instead of three or four times). They should have a prolonged warm-up period (10 min) at the beginning of each exercise session and a cool-down period (5–10 min) at the end. To control exercise intensity accurately, brisk walking, intermittent walking and jogging, continuous jogging, stationary cycling, or regular bicycle riding should be the primary activities. Such vigorous or competitive sports or games as handball or singles tennis should be delayed until patients increase their exercise capacity and are cleared after performing a maximal, multistage exercise test.

The same considerations for prescribing unsupervised exercise during the early convalescence phase still apply. As the patient's cardiovascular capacity increases, there is a need to learn to recognize early signs of overexertion, chronic fatigue, and orthopedic problems. The patient needs to know when not to exercise, when to slow down, and when to stop. As exercise capacity increases with training, a decision is needed regarding the level of exercise capacity that should serve as a goal. No specific answer to this question is applicable to all individuals, because each patient's potential depends on disease magnitude, age, gender, previous exercise habits, and heredity. The best guide to achieve and main-

tain the maximal health benefits from an exercise program is to exercise regularly (three to five times per week) for approximately 30 min at 60 to 80% of the maximal symptom-free HR. Exercise capacity can be maintained by regular participation at the lower limits of this recommendation.

EXERCISE AFTER CABG SURGERY

Although CABG surgery effectively increases the functional potential of many patients, too many of them remain unnecessarily incapacitated after surgery because of restrictive medical management. Limited activity before and after surgery results in substantial deconditioning, along with increased risk of pulmonary and thromboembolic complications. Overly conservative exercise advice compounds these problems and increases the depression and loss of self-confidence frequently experienced by these patients. Patients often confuse postoperative chest wall pain with angina and are hesitant to exercise because of fear they will injure their legs at the site of saphenous vein removal. If angina or other cardiac disease symptoms are not relieved by surgery, patients can become anxious and depressed regarding their prognosis and may be difficult to motivate regarding exercise.

The potential benefits of training for the post-surgery patient are similar to those for other CHD patients, i.e., improved functional capacity, clinical status, and possibly prognosis (75). The general principles of exercise prescription and training are also similar, but some specific consideration must be given to exercise of the chest wall and legs. In addition to slow walking, calisthenics designed to increase the strength and flexibility of the pectoral and leg muscles should be performed. Special exercises to improve chest wall function include deep breathing, shoulder shrugs and adduction, arm circles and lifts, trunk twisters, and wall pushups. These activities should begin within 5 days after surgery and continue in the hospital and then out of hospital in a manner similar to that recommended for post-MI patients.

Summary

- The impact of CHD on the functional capacity and the safety of exercise varies substantially among patients, ranging from no effects to major limitations. The magnitude of these effects for most patients cannot be accurately predicted from data collected at rest.

- Multistage, symptom-limited exercise testing using a motor-driven treadmill or cycle ergometer is the most accurate and reliable approach to determine the functional capacity and establish the intensity component of an exercise plan for patients with CHD.
- The concept of "total patient monitoring" should be used to maximize the information obtained from exercise testing. Monitoring should include continuous multilead ECG; BP; RPE; symptoms and signs of myocardial ischemia (chest or left arm pressure or pain); left ventricular dysfunction (lightheadedness or dizziness and blanching, clammy and/or cooling skin); or near-maximal effort (shortness of breath or dyspnea, unable to maintain work output).
- CHD is a chronic process, and the progression of disease can rapidly change the functional capacity of selected patients. Patients should be taught the signs and symptoms of myocardial ischemia and myocardial dysfunction during exertion and proper actions to reduce the risk of sudden cardiac death.
- All patients with CHD who are ambulatory should be given an exercise plan based on a clinical evaluation, ideally including an exercise test. The plan should be in writing and include both exercise proscription and prescription.

REFERENCES

1. Yusuf S, Reddy S, Ounpuu S, et al. Global burden of cardiovascular diseases: Part I: General considerations, the epidemiologic transition, risk factors, and impact of urbanization. Circulation 2001;104:2746–2753.
2. American Heart Association. Heart Disease and Stroke Statistics—2003 Update. Dallas: American Heart Association, 2002.
3. Cooper R, Cutler J, Desvigne-Nickens P, et al. Trends and disparities in coronary heart disease, stroke, and other cardiovascular diseases in the United States. Circulation 2000;102:3137–3147.
4. Detre K, Holubkov R. Coronary revascularization on balance: Robert L. Frye lecture. Mayo Clin Proc 2001;77–82.
5. Libby P. Current concepts of the pathogenesis of the acute coronary syndromes. Circulation 2001;104:365–372.
6. Haskell WL, Alderman EL, Fair JM, et al. Effects of intensive multiple risk factor reduction on coronary atherosclerosis and clinical cardiac events in men and women with coronary artery disease. Circulation 1994;93:975–990.
7. Gordon NF, English CD, Contractor AS, et al. Effectiveness of three models for comprehensive cardiovascular risk reduction. Am J Cardiol 2002;89:1263–1268.
8. Sdringola S, Nakagawa K, Nakagawa Y, et al. Combined intense lifestyle and pharmacologic lipid treatment further reduce coronary events and myocardial perfusion abnormalities compared with usual-care cholesterol-lowering drugs in coronary heart disease. J Am Coll Cardiol 2003:41:263–272.
9. Lurie K, Voelickel WG, Iskos DN, et al. Combination drug therapy with vasopressin, adrenaline (epinephrine) and nitroglycerin improves vital organ blood flow in a porcine model of ventricular fibrillation. Resuscitation 2002:54:187–194.
10. Poyen V, Silvestri M, Labrunie P, et al. Indications for coronary angioplasty and stenting in 2003: what is left to surgery? J Cardiovasc Surg 2003;44:307–312.
11. Lawrie GM, Morris GC, Howell JF, et al. The results of coronary bypass more than five years after operation in 434 patients: clinical, exercise treadmill and angiographic correlations. Am J Cardiol 1977;40:665–672.
12. Hedback B, Perk J, Hornblad M, et al. Cardiac rehabilitation after coronary artery bypass surgery: 10-year results on mortality, morbidity and readmissions to hospital. Cardiovasc Risk 2001;8:153–158.
13. van Domburg RT, Foley DP, Breeman A, et al. Coronary artery bypass graft surgery and percutaneous transluminal coronary angioplasty. Twenty-year clinical outcome. Eur Heart J 2002;23:543–549.
14. Savin W, Haskell W, Houston-Miller N, et al. Improvement in aerobic capacity soon after myocardial infarction. J Cardiac Rehabil 1981;1:337–342.
15. Wohl AJ, Lewis HR, Bampbell W, et al. Cardiovascular function during early recovery from acute myocardial infarction. Circulation 1977;56:931–937.
16. Fisher L, Kennedy JW, Chaitman BJ, et al. Diagnostic quantification of CASS (coronary artery surgery study): clinical and exercise test results of coronary artery disease. A multivariate approach. Circulation 1981;63:987–1000.

17. Naughton J, Haider R. Methods of exercise testing. In: Naughton J, Hellerstein HK, Mohler IC, eds. Exercise Testing and Exercise Training in Coronary Heart Disease. New York: Academic Press, 1973:79–91.

18. Auchincloss JH, Gilbert R, Koppinger M, et al. One- and three-minute exercise response in coronary artery disease. J Appl Physiol 1979;46:1132–1137.

19. Bartel AG, Behar V, Peter RH, et al. Graded exercise tests in angiographically documented coronary artery disease. Circulation 1974;49:348–356.

20. Aronow W, Goldsmith JR, Keld JC, et al. Effect of smoking cigarettes on cardiovascular hemodynamics. Arch Environ Health 1974;28:330–332.

21. Hung J, McKillip J, Savin W, et al. Comparison of cardiovascular response to combined static-dynamic effort, postprandial dynamic effort and dynamic effort alone in patients with chronic ischemic heart disease. Circulation 1982;65:1411–1416.

22. Thadani V, West RO, Mathew TM, et al. Hemodynamics at rest and during supine and sitting bicycle exercise in patients with coronary artery disease. Am J Cardiol 1977;39:776–783.

23. Clausen JP, Trap-Jensen J. Heart rate and arterial blood pressure during exercise in patients with angina pectoris. Circulation 1976;53:436–442.

24. Kivowitz C, Parmely WW, Donoso R, et al. Effects of isometric exercise on cardiac performance: the grip test. Circulation, 1971;44:994–1002.

25. Kerber RE, Miller R, Najjar S. Myocardial ischemia effects of isometric, dynamic and combined exercise in coronary artery disease. Chest 1975;67:388–394.

26. Bertagnoli K, Hanson P, Ward A, et al. Attenuation of exercise-induced ST depression during combined isometric and dynamic exercise in coronary artery disease. Am J Cardiol 1990;65:314–317.

27. American Association of Cardiovascular and Pulmonary Rehabilitation. Guidelines for Cardiac Rehabilitation and Secondary Prevention Programs. 3rd ed. Champaign, IL: Human Kinetics, 1999.

28. American College of Sports Medicine. Guidelines for Exercise Testing and Exercise Prescription. 6th ed. Philadelphia: Lippincott Williams & Wilkins, 2000.

29. Thompson P, Cullinane E, Lazarus B, et al. Effect of exercise training on the untrained limb exercise performance of men with angina pectoris. Am J Cardiol 1981;48:844–850.

30. Ben-Ari E, Kellermann JJ, Rothbaum DA. Effects of prolonged intensive versus moderate leg training on the untrained arm exercise response in angina pectoris. Am J Cardiol 1987;59:231–234.

31. Clausen JP, Trap-Jensen J. Effects of training on the distribution of cardiac output in patients with coronary heart disease. Circulation 1970:42:611–618.

32. Panigrahi G, Pedersen A, Boudoulas H. Effects of physical training on exercise hemodynamics in patients with stable coronary artery disease. The use of impedance cardiography. J Med 1983;14:363–373.

33. Cinquegrana G, Spinelli L, D'Aniello L, et al. Exercise training improves diastolic perfusion time in patients with coronary artery disease. Heart Dis 2002;4:13–17.

34. Franklin BA. Exercise training and coronary collateral circulation. Med Sci Sports Exerc 1991;23:648–653.

35. Ferguson RJ, Petitclerc R, Choquette G, et al. Effect of exercise training on treadmill exercise capacity, collateral circulation and progression of coronary disease. Am J Cardiol 1974;34:764–769.

36. Todd IC, Ballantyne D. Antianginal efficacy of exercise training: a comparison with beta blockade. Br Heart J 1990;64:14–19.

37. Hambrecht R, Wolff A, Gielen S, et al. Effect of exercise on coronary endothelial function in patients with coronary artery disease. N Engl J Med 2000;342:454–460.

38. Hambrecht R, Adams V, Erbs S, et al. Regular physical activity improves endothelial function in patients with coronary artery disease by increasing phosphorylation of endothelial nitric oxide synthase. Circulation 2003;107:3152–3158.

39. Hagberg JM. Physiologic adaptations to prolonged high-intensity exercise training in patients with coronary artery disease. Med Sci Sports Exerc 1991;23:661–667.

40. Van Dam RM, Schuit AJ, Feskens EJ, et al. Physical activity and glucose tolerance in elderly men: the Zutphen Elderly Study. Med Sci Sports Exerc 2002;34:1132–1136.

41. Perk J, Veress G. Cardiac rehabilitation: applying exercise physiology in clinical practice. Eur J Appl Physiol 2000;83:457–462.

42. Haskell WL. J. B. Wolffe memorial lecture. Health consequences of physical activity: understanding and challenges regarding dose-response. Med Sci Sports Exerc 1994;26:649–660.

43. LaMonte MJ, Durstine JL, Yanowitz FG, et al. Cardiorespiratory fitness and C-reactive protein among a tri-ethnic sample of women. Circulation 2002;106:403–406.

44. Galassi AR, Foti R, Azzarelli S, et al. Usefulness of exercise tomographic myocardial perfusion imaging for detection of restenosis after coronary stent implantation. Am J Cardiol 2000;85:1362–1364.

45. Tomanek RJ. Exercise-induced coronary angiogenesis: a review. Med Sci Sports Exerc 1994;26:1245–1251.

46. Payne TJ, Johnson CA, Penzien DB, et al. Chest pain self-management training for patients with coronary artery disease. J Psychosom Res 1994;38:409–418.

47. Hambrecht R, Gielen S, Linke A, et al. Effects of exercise training on left ventricular function and peripheral resistance in patients with chronic heart failure: a randomized trial. JAMA 2000;283:3095–3101.

48. Ehsani A, Heath GW, Hagberg JM, et al. Effects of 12 months of intense exercise training on ischemic ST-segment depression in patients with coronary artery disease. Circulation 1981;64:1116–1124.

49. Jetté M, Heller R, Landry F, et al. Randomized 4-week exercise program in patients with impaired left ventricular function. Circulation 1991;84:1561–1567.

50. Hedback B, Perk J. Can high-risk patients after myocardial infarction participate in comprehensive cardiac rehabilitation? Scand J Rehabil Med 1990;22:15–20.

51. Keteyian SJ, Duscha BD, Brawner CA, et al. Differential effects of exercise training in men and women with chronic heart failure. Am Heart J 2003;145:912–918.

52. Mital A, Shrey DE, Govindaraju M, et al. Accelerating the return to work (RTW) chances of coronary heart disease (CHD) patients: part 1—development and validation of a training programme. Disabil Rehabil 2000;22:604–610.

53. Mittag O, Kolenda KD, Nordman KJ, et al. Return to work after myocardial infraction/coronary artery bypass grafting: patients' and physicians' initial viewpoints and outcome 12 months later. Soc Sci Med 2001;52:1441–1450.

54. O'Connor GT, Buring JE, Yusuf S, et al. An overview of randomized trials of rehabilitation with exercise after myocardial infarction. Circulation 1989;80:234–244.

55. Oldridge NB, Guyatt GH, Fischer MB, et al. Cardiac rehabilitation after myocardial infarction: combined experience of randomized clinical trials. JAMA 1988;260:945–950.

56. Oldridge NB. Cardiac rehabilitation and risk factor management after myocardial infarction. Clinical and economic evaluation. Wien Klin Wochenschr Suppl 1997;2:6–16.

57. Dorn J, Naughton J, Imamura D, et al. Correlates of compliance in a randomized exercise trial in myocardial infarction patients. Med Sci Sports Exerc 2001;33:1081–1089.

58. Flecher GF, Balady GJ, Amsterdam EA, et al. American Heart Association exercise standards for testing and training: a statement for healthcare professionals. Circulation 2001;104:1694–1740.

59. Gibbons R, Balady GJ, Bricker T, et al. ACC/AHA 2002 guidelines update for exercise testing: summary article. Circulation 2002;106:1883–1892.

60. Canadian Association of Cardiac Rehabilitation. Canadian Guidelines for Cardiac Rehabilitation and Cardiovascular Disease Prevention. Winnipeg: Canadian Association of Cardiac Rehabilitation, 1999.

61. Haskell WL, Savin W, Oldridge N, et al. Factors influencing estimated oxygen uptake during exercise testing soon after myocardial infarction. Am J Cardiol 1982;50:299–304.

62. Chaitman BR, Waters DD, Bourassa MG, et al. The importance of clinical subsets in interpreting maximal treadmill exercise test results: the role of multiple lead ECG systems. Circulation 1979;59:560–570.

63. Borg G. Borg's Perceived Exertion and Pain Scales. Champaign, IL: Human Kinetics, 1998.

64. Yli-Mayry S, Huikuri HV, Korhonen UR, et al. Prevalence and prognostic significance of exercised-induced ventricular arrhythmias after coronary artery bypass grafting. Am J Cardiol 1990;66:1451–1454.

65. Mathes P. The effect of coronary revascularization on exercise-induced ventricular arrhythmias. Eur Heart J 1987;8(suppl):79–81.

66. Vuori I, Makarainen M, Jaaselainen A. Sudden death and physical activity. Cardiology 1978;63:287–304.

67. Thompson PD. The benefits and risks of exercise training in patients with chronic coronary artery disease. JAMA 1988;259:1537–1540.

68. Van Camp SP, Peterson RA. Cardiovascular complications of outpatient cardiac rehabilitation programs. JAMA 1986;256:1160–1163.

69. Franklin BA, Bonzheim K, Gordon S, et al. Resistance training in cardiac rehabilitation. J Cardiopulm Rehabil 1991;11:99–107.

70. Leon AS. Physical activity levels and coronary heart disease. Analysis of epidemiologic and supporting studies. Med Clin North Am 1985;69:3–20.

71. Hlatky MA, Boineau RE, Higginbotham MB, et al. A brief self-administered questionnaire to determine functional capacity (the Duke Activity Status Index). Am J Cardiol 1989;64:651–654.

72. Myers JD, Herbert W, Ribisl P, et al. A nomogram to predict exercise capacity from a specific activity questionnaire and clinical data. Am J Cardiol 1994;23:591–599.

73. American College of Sports Medicine. Exercise

Management for Persons with Chronic Diseases and Disabilities. 2nd ed. Champaign, IL: Human Kinetics, 2003.

74. Juneau M, Rogers F, Taylor CB, et al. Effectiveness of self-monitored, home-based moderate-intensity exercise training in middle-aged men and women. Am J Cardiol 1987;60:66–70.

75. Hedback B, Perk J, Engvall J, et al. Cardiac rehabilitation after coronary artery bypass grafting: Effects on exercise performance and risk factors. Arch Phys Med Rehabil 1990;71:1069–1073.

RELATED WEB SITES

Centers for Disease Control and Prevention—Physical Activity and Health: A Report of the Surgeon General
www.cdc.gov/nccdphp/sgr/sgr.htm

National Heart, Lung, and Blood Institute
www.nhlbi.nih.gov

American Heart Association
www.americanheart.org

American College of Sports Medicine
www.acsm.org

19

Hypertension

James S. Skinner

Hypertension (HTN) is the leading cardiovascular disease in industrial societies. It commonly begins at a young age, occurring in 5 to 10% of persons aged 20 to 30 years. The incidence increases with age, such that 20 to 25% of middle-aged adults and 50 to 60% of adults over age 65 have elevated blood pressure (BP). Sustained HTN is associated with a higher risk of stroke, myocardial infarction, kidney disorders, and heart failure.

Primary and Secondary Hypertension

Arterial HTN is a symptom, not a disease. In 5 to 10% of those with HTN, elevated BP is the result of some identifiable cause; this is designated secondary HTN. Most persons who are hypertensive (90–95%) have what is designated primary or essential HTN because there are no known or evident causes.

In adults, HTN has been defined as a systolic BP (SBP) of ≥140 mm Hg and/or a diastolic BP (DBP) of ≥90 mm Hg. According to the World Health Organization (WHO) (1), there are several stages of HTN: stage I (SBP 140–159 or DBP 90–99 mm Hg), stage II (SBP 160–179 or DBP 100–109 mm Hg), and stage III (SBP ≥180 or DBP ≥110 mm Hg). When SBP and DBP are in different categories, the higher category is used to classify HTN.

Recently, another classification (prehypertension) has been added that is associated with an SBP of 120–139 or a DBP of 80–89 mm Hg (2). This high-normal category was added to emphasize the need and importance of preventing HTN.

Essential HTN is the result of a number of genetic and environmental factors and their interactions. Heritability estimates of resting BP range from 25% in family studies to 70% in twin studies (3). Other primary risk factors include age, body mass (especially excess body fat), excessive sodium intake, increased alcohol intake, and inactivity. A family history of HTN increases the probability of developing HTN. Men develop HTN earlier than women and blacks have a higher incidence of HTN than whites or Asians.

Course of the Disease

When untreated, essential HTN is a long-term, chronic disorder that becomes progressively worse, affecting various target organs and eventually leading to irreparable damage to those organs. Recent evidence (4) suggests that persons who are normotensive at age 55 have a 90% risk of becoming hypertensive in their lifetime. The probability that persons with high-normal DBP (85–89 mm Hg) will develop diastolic HTN (>95 mmHg) is two times the risk in those with normal DBP (5).

Hemodynamics at Rest

Various BP control mechanisms are involved in the cause and pathophysiology of HTN. The relationship between BP, flow, and resistance is a simple and direct one, i.e., BP = cardiac output ($\dot{Q}$)× systemic vascular resistance (SVR). Anything that increases flow ($\dot{Q}$ = heart rate [HR] × stroke volume [SV]) will affect SBP more, while an increase in peripheral resistance has more effect on DBP. While the relationships among the variables that influence are simple, the mechanisms that control them are more complex.

Characteristic hemodynamic patterns vary with the stage or severity of HTN. The early phase of mild or borderline HTN (WHO stage 1) is often characterized by a higher resting HR and $\dot{Q}$, with or without an increased SV. There are no objective signs of organ damage at this stage.

Over time, there may be a gradual drop in $\dot{Q}$ and a continuous rise in SVR (6). By the time HTN becomes established (WHO stage 2), $\dot{Q}$, HR, and SV are normal, but SVR is elevated. At this stage, there is evidence of one or more of the following: an enlarged heart, narrowing of the arteries in the eye, and high levels of urinary protein.

With severe or advanced HTN (WHO stage 3), there is a further increase in SVR and a below-normal $\dot{Q}$ that is mainly due to a drop in SV resulting from the higher afterload on the heart. Importantly, there are signs and symptoms of damage to the heart, brain, eyes, and kidneys.

As stated by Sannerstedt (7), these are group patterns and individuals can vary greatly. As a result, there is overlap among the various stages, and this variation should be considered when treating patients with HTN.

Treating Hypertension

There are two general types of treatment for HTN, namely, lifestyle modifications and medications.

LIFESTYLE MODIFICATIONS

Included among the lifestyle modifications are losing weight (especially body fat), reducing intake of alcohol, exercising regularly, changing the diet (reducing salt intake and maintaining adequate levels of dietary potassium, magnesium, and calcium), and stopping the use of tobacco. The Joint National Committee on Prevention, Detection, Evaluation, and Treatment of High Blood Pressure (2) recommends modifying lifestyle as the first step for persons with mild to moderate HTN. If this fails to reduce BP after 3 to 6 months, then medications are usually prescribed. Persons who have higher BP levels also should consider lifestyle modifications, but they should not delay the use of medications, especially if they have damaged target organs or diabetes.

MEDICATIONS

Based on the hemodynamic patterns of each stage of HTN mentioned above, the medications of choice for each stage are evident. Table 19-1 lists various classes of drugs and their effects on different hemodynamic variables.

Because stage 1 is associated with a normal SVR but an elevated $\dot{Q}$, medications often prescribed first are the β-adrenoceptor blockers (β-blockers). These β-blockers decrease $\dot{Q}$ by reducing resting HR and by inhibiting its rise with stress or exercise. As well, they lower the force of contraction by the ventricles, thus reducing SV. Calcium-channel (Ca^{2+}) blockers also decrease $\dot{Q}$ by blocking the rise in contraction force of the ventricles. Another

TABLE 19-1   CLASSES OF MEDICATIONS FOR HYPERTENSION AND THEIR EFFECTS ON HEMODYNAMIC VARIABLES ASSOCIATED WITH BLOOD PRESSURE

Class of Medication	Effect on Hemodynamic Variable				
	HR	SV	SVR	SBP	DBP
β-Blockers	—	—	+/−	—	0/−
Vasodilators	+/0	—	—	—	—
Ca^{2+}-blockers	+/−	0	—	0/−	—
ACE inhibitors	0	0	—	—	—
Diuretics	0	—	—	—	—

HR, heart rate; SV, stroke volume; SVR, systemic vascular resistance; SBP, systolic blood pressure; DBP, diastolic blood pressure; −, decrease; 0, no change; +, increase.

Note: More than one symbol indicates different responses associated with different medications within the class.

medication that is prescribed early in treatment is a diuretic, which increases urination to reduce plasma and extracellular volumes, thus reducing SV and Q.

For the more advanced stages of HTN, emphasis is placed on reducing SVR. Drugs used to decrease SVR include α_1-receptor blockers (α_1-blockers), which dilate the arteries and two other drugs which block or reduce the ability of arterial smooth muscles to contract, namely, angiotensin-converting enzyme (ACE) inhibitors, which block the formation of angiotensin II from the kidneys, and Ca^{2+}-channel blockers. Some patients with HTN also have coronary artery disease (CAD) and take nitrates, which have a vasodilating effect. With more severe cases of HTN, combination therapy using several or all of these drugs is prescribed to lower BP and reduce the burden on the heart and other organs.

Ability to Exercise

As reviewed by Sannerstedt (7), the ability to exercise is not affected in persons with mild, borderline HTN. As the severity of HTN increases, however, the ability to exercise drops; this is especially the case when there is damage to the heart and other organs (8).

Effects of Exercise on BP

DYNAMIC EXERCISE

In persons with normal BP levels, Q rises during progressively increasing exercise intensities as a result of higher HR, SV, and force of cardiac contraction. Blood flow to working muscle is augmented by local vasodilation, while blood flow to nonworking muscle and visceral organs is diminished by sympathetic vasoconstriction. The net result is a rise in SBP with little change in DBP and a decrease in SVR.

In mild-to-moderate hypertension, Q increases normally but SBP, DBP, and SVR are higher at all levels of exercise compared with levels seen in normotensive subjects. In patients with severe hypertension, Q is lower than in age-matched controls because of a decreased SV associated with the higher afterload on the heart, while SBP, DBP and SVR are markedly increased.

STATIC OR ISOMETRIC EXERCISE

The normal response to isometric exercise is a rise in both SBP and DBP, commonly referred to as a *pressor response*. The pressor response is mediated by reflex increases in Q with little change in SVR. The magnitude of the BP rise is proportional to the combined size of muscle mass and the percentage of maximal effort used to perform the isometric contraction.

The increase in BP during isometric exercise may or may not be mediated by an increase in Q in individuals with HTN. Rather, the pressor response is mainly associated with an increase in SVR. This has been attributed to the inability to increase Q because of left ventricular hypertrophy or a blunted β-adrenergic reactivity and predominance of α-adrenergic reactivity.

The reactions to static exercise of patients with uncomplicated HTN (WHO stages 1 and 2) are similar to those of normotensive persons (7). At all levels of dynamic and isometric exercise, SBP and DBP are much higher in patients with HTN. However, the relative increase in BP from resting values is similar to that seen in those with normal BP, suggesting that BP is "reset" and maintained at higher levels throughout the spectrum of activity from rest to peak exercise.

Static exercise may put a greater strain on the vascular system than dynamic exercise. However, isometric exercise is generally done for a shorter time, BP drops immediately after the contraction, and BP will be at its resting level within 15 to 30 seconds.

Effects of Medications on Exercise Responses

The fact that HTN patients take medication(s) to lower BP should not stop them from exercising. However, some medications can affect their ability to exercise. For a good overview of medications to prescribe for patients with HTN who want to be quite active and perform in sports, the reader is referred to the review by Swain and Kaplan (9).

DYNAMIC EXERCISE

With β-blockers, resting and exercise HR, $\dot{Q}$, and SBP are lower. Because of the lower $\dot{Q}$, there is a drop in muscle blood flow and a reduced ability to exercise. As a result, some patients will feel sluggish and have difficulty climbing stairs. There is also some evidence (10) that β-blockers may compromise the ability to regulate body temperature; this would not be a problem unless one does prolonged exercise in a warm and especially humid environment. Interestingly, the use of a β-blocker may help patients with CAD and angina to exercise at higher levels because the drug reduces the work of the heart, which is a major limiting factor in their ability to exercise.

Diuretics cause increased urination and can lead to dehydration and a loss of certain electrolytes. Of particular concern is the loss of potassium, which can produce an irregular heart rhythm and muscle fatigue. Unless potassium is low, however, diuretics have few effects on the ability to exercise.

ACE inhibitors, Ca^{2+}-channel blockers and α-blockers do not appear to have any adverse effect on the ability to exercise (9). Nevertheless, if persons taking these vasodilators stop too fast after exercise, blood could pool in the lower extremities and they could feel lightheaded and, in rare cases, faint. Orthostatic hypotension may also occur after prolonged exercise in the heat.

STATIC EXERCISE

As mentioned above, the usual response to static exercise is a rise in SBP and DBP, mainly owing to an increase in $\dot{Q}$, and little change in SVR. Vasodilators (ACE inhibitors, Ca^{2+}-channel blockers and α-blockers) have little effect on this pattern of BP response. After treating patients with mild-to-moderate HTN with a β-blocker, however, Garavaglia et al. (11) found an exaggerated increase in SVR and less increase in $\dot{Q}$.

Exercise Testing

The American College of Sports Medicine (ACSM) guidelines for graded exercise testing (12) should be followed when testing persons with HTN, but with more attention given to the resting BP and the responses during exercise. A preliminary exercise test is strongly recommended for those with a resting BP above 140/90 mm Hg before they become more active. However, an exercise test is contraindicated with a resting SBP of >200 mm Hg or a resting DBP of >110 mm Hg, and an exercise test should be terminated with an SBP >260 mm Hg or a DBP >115 mm Hg (12).

If one of the reasons for an exercise test is to prescribe exercise, then patients with HTN should be tested while taking their usual medications. This is especially the case if they take a β-blocker, which lowers HR. If possible, the testing and the training should be done at the same time interval after taking the drug, and testing should be repeated if the type or amount of β-blocker changes (13).

Several precautions should be mentioned in interpreting electrocardiographic (ECG) data obtained from HTN patients during an exercise test. Many HTN patients take diuretics, which can lower the potassium level, resulting in spurious ST-segmental depression (14). As well, some HTN patients may have ECG evidence of left ventricular hypertrophy, which could make a diagnosis of myocardial ischemia more difficult (15).

There is evidence that the risk for developing HTN is two to four times greater in persons who have normal BP at rest but have an exaggerated increase during exercise (16). This hypertensive response is defined as an SBP of >220 mm Hg, a rise in DBP of >10 mm Hg, or a DBP of >90 mm Hg (17). Because of a number of limitations in the research on this question, as well as the costs involved, the ACSM does not recommend exercise testing for the sole purpose of predicting future HTN (16). However, if an exercise test is given for other reasons, then BP measurements may provide useful information about future risk.

Effects of Training

Exercise is an integral part of programs for modifying lifestyle to prevent, treat, and control HTN. As stated in the ACSM Position Stand on Exercise and Hypertension (16), "exercise programs that primarily involve endurance activity prevent the development of HTN and lower blood pressure (BP) in adults with normal BP and those with HTN."

After conducting a meta-analysis of studies on 1284 patients with HTN, Hagberg et al. (18) found that aerobic exercise training lowered BP in most patients with HTN. For example, SBP was reduced 11 mm Hg (76% of the patients had a significant drop), and DBP was reduced 8 mm Hg (81% had a significant drop). They concluded that women tended to have a greater drop in SBP and DBP than men. They also concluded that middle-aged patients (41–60 years old) had a larger drop in SBP than did the younger and older patients; there was a similar drop in DBP at all ages. Because of the low numbers of young and old patients, however, they urge caution when interpreting these findings.

Hagberg et al. (18) also found that significant reductions in SBP and DBP occurred during the first 10 weeks of aerobic exercise training. While there were no further reductions in DBP after 20 weeks or more, there was a greater drop in SBP with programs lasting more than 20 weeks.

As would be expected, the drop in BP with endurance-exercise training is less pronounced in persons with normal pressures than in patients with HTN, i.e., normal pressures are reduced but are still normal (19). A meta-analysis by Kelley et al. (20). found that aerobic exercise reduced BP by 4 to 5% in those with HTN compared with 1 to 2% in those with normal BP. Among HTN patients, Sannerstedt (7) stated that those with mild, borderline HTN and especially those with a high resting HR and $\dot{Q}$ (WHO stage 1) tend to improve more than those with established HTN (stage 2) in whom the main problem is an elevated SVR. There are few data on patients with severe, advanced HTN (stage 3), but Sannerstedt (7) estimates that it is unlikely there will be much change in BP in patients whose organs are damaged.

Because many HTN patients are overweight, one goal of treatment programs is to reduce body mass to improve general health and possibly to lower BP. The question remains, however, whether weight loss by itself will affect BP. The results of the meta-analysis by Hagberg et al. (18) found no relation between the change in body weight and the reduction in SBP ($r = 0.11$) or in DBP ($r = 0.07$). After a 9-month program for HTN patients, Dengel et al. (21) found similar BP reductions whether body weight loss was due to exercise, diet, or diet plus exercise, i.e., the effects were not additive.

When looking at the effect of exercise intensity on BP response to training, Hagberg et al. (18) concluded that the decrease in SBP was 11.1 mm Hg (79% had a drop) when training intensity was <70% $\dot{V}O_{2max}$ compared with a reduction of 7.6 mm Hg (75% had a drop) when intensity was >70% $\dot{V}O_{2max}$. The authors did not state whether this difference in BP reduction was significant. For DBP, the corresponding reductions were 7.6 and 6.7 mm Hg, respectively, with 81% of both groups having a decrease.

Fagard (19) did a meta-analysis of 44 randomized controlled trials on healthy persons with normal BP and those with HTN aged 21 to 79 years and reached a different conclusion. He found that the differences in BP changes after training were not related to frequency, duration, intensity, or total volume of training. Figures 19-1 and 19-2 demonstrate the lack of a clear difference in effect relative to exercise intensity in either normotensive or hypertensive subjects. He did find some suggestive evidence that exercising 7 days per week reduced BP more than 3 days per week, but there was no difference between 3 and 5 days per week.

Ishikawa-Takata et al. (22) studied 207 persons with stage 1 and 2 HTN who exercised at an intensity of about 50% $\dot{V}O_{2max}$ for 8 weeks. They classified the subjects by the time spent exercising per week (30–60, 61–90, 91–120, and >120 min per week). All four groups had significant reductions in resting BP. Although there were similar decreases in DBP in all groups, the decrease in SBP was less for the group exercising 30–60 min per week than in the groups who exercised longer. Given that the patients were not randomly assigned to a group, these results should be viewed with some caution. Nevertheless, they suggest that exercising for as little as 60–90 min per week is sufficient to reduce BP.

The evidence regarding the effects of resistance training (RT) on resting BP is less consistent. However, RT is not contraindicated for patients with mild, uncomplicated HTN (stages 1 and 2) (13). Fagard and Tipton (23) reviewed the evidence as of 1994 and concluded that the only studies on RT that showed a reduction in BP were those that combined RT with cardiovascular exercise; studies using RT alone did not lower BP. A meta-analysis done by Kelley and Kelley in 2000 (24) on randomized control trials did not agree. That analysis concluded

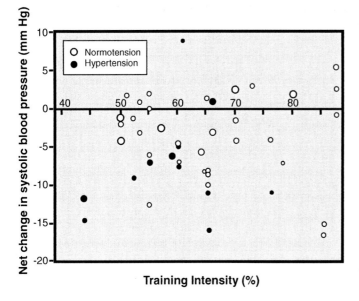

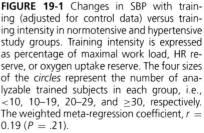

FIGURE 19-1 Changes in SBP with training (adjusted for control data) versus training intensity in normotensive and hypertensive study groups. Training intensity is expressed as percentage of maximal work load, HR reserve, or oxygen uptake reserve. The four sizes of the *circles* represent the number of analyzable trained subjects in each group, i.e., <10, 10–19, 20–29, and ≥30, respectively. The weighted meta-regression coefficient, $r = 0.19$ ($P = .21$).

that there were modest but significant reductions of 3 mm Hg for both SBP and DBP (2 and 4%, respectively). While this drop may seem insignificant, a reduction in BP of 3% is associated with a decrease in CAD of 5 to 9%, a decrease in stroke of 8 to 14%, and a drop in all-cause mortality of 4% (25).

One mechanism whereby RT may influence BP is by its attenuation of the pressor response. As mentioned before, the rise in BP with static exercise is associated with the muscle mass involved and the percentage of the maximal force of those muscles. If there is an increase in the maximal force of a muscle group, then any given weight lifted becomes a

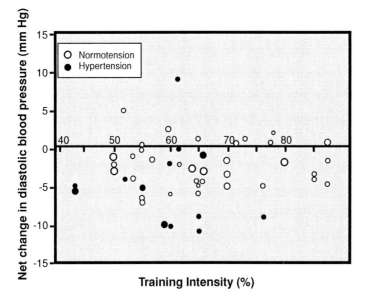

FIGURE 19-2 Changes in DBP with training (adjusted for control data) versus training intensity in normotensive and hypertensive study groups. Training intensity is expressed as percentage of maximal work load, HR reserve, or oxygen uptake reserve. The four sizes of the *circles* represent the number of analyzable trained subjects in each group, i.e., <10, 10–19, 20–29, and ≥30, respectively. The weighted meta-regression coefficient, $r = 0.01$ ($P = .93$).

lower percentage of that higher maximum. Thus, there will be a lower HR and a lower SBP, resulting in less work done by the heart, as estimated by the rate–pressure product (HR × SBP).

Exercise Prescription

The general ACSM guidelines for healthy adults (12) also apply to those with HTN, particularly those in stages 1 and 2. On the other hand, Sannerstedt (7) does not recommend RT for patients with stage 3 HTN, in which the SVR is elevated and there might be damage to some organs. Thus, endurance exercise with large muscles done 3 to 5 days per week and 20 to 60 min per day is appropriate; research findings (19) suggest that 3 days per week is the minimum for an effective program.

The question of exercise intensity is less clear. Several reviews differ on the effect of different intensities on BP. Hagberg et al. (18) suggest that an intensity $<70\%$ $\dot{V}O_{2max}$ may be more beneficial than an intensity $>70\%$ $\dot{V}O_{2max}$, while Fagard (19) found no difference among the different intensities. Regardless, it seems clear that it is easier for most patients to begin and continue exercising at low-to-moderate intensities, e.g., 50 to 70%. Given that higher intensities may not produce greater benefits and are associated with a greater risk of musculoskeletal injuries and cardiovascular problems, it is also prudent to exercise at low-to-moderate intensities.

Although RT may be effective in lowering BP, it should not be the only or the main form of exercise. A position stand of the American Heart Association (26) that was endorsed by the ACSM recommends mild-to-moderate RT to improve muscular strength and endurance, to prevent and manage a variety of chronic medical conditions, to modify CAD risk factors, and to enhance psychologic well-being.

An RT program that emphasizes muscle endurance more than strength is appropriate. Light weight-training (30–50% of maximal force) and/or circuit training with light loads and many repetitions are good examples. If there are any concerns about a given patient, then the BP should be measured after lifting weights. If there is an excessive rise in BP, especially DBP, then the exercise should be discontinued or the weight reduced until there is no longer a rise in DBP.

Summary

- Hypertension (HTN) affects or will affect many persons over their lives.
- Untreated, this condition becomes progressively worse. With adequate treatment, however, BP can be reduced to acceptable levels.
- Lifestyle modifications and medications are the main types of treatment.
- The ability to exercise is not affected in those with uncomplicated HTN. On the other hand, some medications can affect their ability to exercise.
- Regular endurance training and probably resistance training will reduce BP in persons with normal BP levels and in patients with HTN.
- The general ACSM guidelines for graded exercise testing and exercise prescription are appropriate for those with mild-to-moderate, uncomplicated HTN. Modifications may be needed if the condition worsens.
- Exercise is an integral part of any program for treating HTN. However, education, counseling, behavioral modification, and medications are also important.

REFERENCES

1. World Health Organization-International Society of Hypertension. 2003 World Health Organization (WHO)/International Society of Hypertension (ISH) statement on the management of hypertension. J Hypertens 2003;21:1983–1992.
2. Chobanian AV, Bakris GL, Black HR, et al. and the National High Blood Pressure Program Coordinating Committee. The seventh report of the Joint National Committee on Prevention, Detection, Evaluation, and Treatment of High Blood Pressure. The JNC 7 report. Hypertension 2003;42:1206–1252.
3. Williams RR, Hunt SC, Hasstedt SJ, et al. Are there interactions and relations between genetic and environmental factors predisposing to high blood pressure? Hypertension 1991;18:129–137.
4. Vasan RS, Beiser A, Seshadri S, et al. Residual lifetime risk for developing hypertension in middle-aged women and men: the Framingham Heart Study. JAMA 2002;287:1003–1010.

5. Leitschuh M, Cupples LA, Kannel W, et al. High-normal blood pressure progression to hypertension in the Framingham Heart Study. Hypertension 1991;17:22–27.

6. Lund-Johansen P. Age, hemodynamics and exercise in essential hypertension: difference between β-blockers and dihydropyridine calcium antagonists. J Cardiovasc Pharmacol 1989;14(suppl 10):S7–13.

7. Sannerstedt R. Hypertension. In: Skinner JS, ed. Exercise Testing and Exercise Prescription for Special Cases. 2nd ed. Philadelphia: Lea & Febiger, 1993:275–289.

8. Bahler RC, Gatzoylis K. Exercise performance in patients with hypertension. Relation to electrocardiographic criteria for left ventricular hypertrophy. J Electrocardiol 1990;23:41–48.

9. Swain R, Kaplan B. Treating hypertension in active patients: which agents work best with exercise? Physician Sportsmed 1997;25:1–13.

10. Gordon NF, Duncan JJ. Effect of beta-blockers on exercise physiology: implications for exercise training. Med Sci Sports 1991;23:668–676.

11. Garavaglia GE, Messerli FH, Schmieder RE, et al. Antihypertensive therapy and cardiovascular reactivity during isometric stress. J Hum Hypertens 1988;2:247–251.

12. American College of Sports Medicine. ACSM's Guidelines for Exercise Testing and Prescription. 6th ed. Baltimore: Lippincott Williams & Wilkins, 2000.

13. Gordon NF, Scott CB. Exercise and mild essential hypertension. Primary Care 1991;18:683–694.

14. Georgopoulos AJ, Proudfit WL, Page IH. Effect of exercise on electrocardiogram of patients with low serum potassium. Circulation 1961;23:567–572.

15. Hanson P, Ward A, Painter P. Exercise training for special patient populations. J Cardiopulm Rehabil 1986;6:104–112.

16. Pescatello LS, Franklin BA, Fagard R, et al. American College of Sports Medicine position stand. Exercise and hypertension. Med Sci Sports Exerc 2004;36:533–553.

17. American College of Sports Medicine. ACSM's Resource Manual for Guidelines for Exercise Testing and Prescription. 3rd ed. Baltimore: Lippincott Williams & Wilkins, 1998.

18. Hagberg JM, Park JJ, Brown MD. The role of exercise training in the treatment of hypertension. An update. Sports Med 2000;30:193–206.

19. Fagard RH. Exercise characteristics and the blood pressure response to dynamic physical training. Med Sci Sports Exerc 2001;33(6 Suppl):S484–492.

20. Kelley GA, Kelley KA, Tran ZV. Aerobic exercise and resting blood pressure: a meta-analytic review of randomized, controlled trials. Prev Cardiol 2001;4:73–80.

21. Dengel DR, Galecki AT, Hagberg JM, et al. The independent and combined effects of weight loss and aerobic exercise on blood pressure and oral glucose tolerance in older men. Am J Hypertens 1998;11:1405–1412.

22. Ishikawa-Takata K, Ohta T, Tanaka H. How much exercise is required to reduce blood pressure in essential hypertensives: a dose-response study. Am J Hypertens 2003;16:629–633.

23. Fagard RH, Tipton CM. Physical activity, fitness and hypertension. In: Bouchard C, Shephard RJ, Stephens T, eds. Physical Activity, Fitness and Health. Champaign, IL: Human Kinetics, 1994:633–655.

24. Kelley GA, Kelley KS. Progressive resistance exercise and resting blood pressure: a meta-analysis of randomized controlled trials. Hypertension 2000;35:838–843.

25. Whelton PK, He J, Appel LJ, et al. Primary prevention of hypertension: clinical and public health advisory from the National High Blood Pressure Education Program. JAMA 2002;288:1882–1888.

26. Pollock ML, Franklin BA, Gary J, et al. Resistance exercise in individuals with and without cardiovascular disease: benefits, rationale, safety, and prescription: an advisory from the Committee on Exercise, Rehabilitation, and Prevention, Council on Clinical Cardiology, American Heart Association. Circulation 2000;101:828–833.

RELATED WEB SITES

Centers for Disease Control and Prevention—Physical Activity and Health: A Report of the Surgeon General
www.cdc.gov/nccdphp/sgr/sgr.htm

National Heart, Lung, and Blood Institute
www.nhlbi.nih.gov

American Heart Association
www.americanheart.org

American College of Sports Medicine
www.acsm.org

Peripheral Arterial Occlusive Disease

Andrew W. Gardner and James S. Skinner

20

Atherosclerotic cardiovascular disease is the most significant health problem in the United States, as heart and cerebrovascular diseases were the first and fourth leading causes of death in 1990, respectively (1). Atherosclerosis in the arteries of the lower extremities (peripheral vascular disease) is also an important medical concern because there is a high risk that concomitant coronary and cerebral artery disease are present (2) and because ischemic pain in the leg musculature severely limits daily physical activities that can be performed. One of the more common forms of peripheral vascular disease is peripheral arterial occlusive disease (PAOD), which results from atherosclerosis of the arteries of the lower extremities.

Although much of the literature on PAOD has come from the disciplines of vascular surgery and medicine, the field of exercise physiology is growing in importance because of the need to rehabilitate this patient population with a program of regular exercise. The synergistic collaboration among these disciplines is particularly important for the clinical management of PAOD patients because the primary goal for the vascular specialist is to improve circulation and limb viability, while the primary concern of the exercise specialist is to help the patient regain lost function.

Description of the Disease

DEFINITION OF PAOD

PAOD occurs from lesions that develop in the abdominal aorta, and the iliac, femoral, popliteal, and tibial arteries. Consequently, blood flow distal to the arterial lesions is reduced, which ultimately has a negative impact on ambulation and functional independence of elderly patients with PAOD. The hallmark clinical measure for detecting PAOD is the ankle/brachial index (ABI), which is the ratio of systolic blood pressure (SBP) measured at the ankle and at the arm (3). In PAOD patients, the reduction in leg blood flow results in a low ankle pressure and a low ABI value. The prevalence of PAOD depends highly on the exact ABI cut-point used to detect inadequate peripheral circulation. Based on the literature, an abnormal ABI ranges from <0.80 to <0.97 (4–7), with a value of ≤0.90 generally considered the best reference standard (8). ABI values above 0.90 are considered within the normal range. The prevalence of PAOD is 10% in the general population above 55 years of age when an ABI value of ≤0.90 is used to define PAOD (8).

CLASSIFICATION OF PAOD

In the early stages of PAOD, reduced blood flow does not result in any noticeable symptoms; this is defined as stage I (asymptomatic PAOD) according to the widely accepted Fontaine classification system (Table 20-1) (9). As PAOD progresses, ischemic pain in the leg musculature occurs when patients walk and is classified as stage II (intermittent claudication). Stage II patients can be further classified as having mild intermittent claudication (pain-free walking distance >200 meters) or severe intermittent claudication (pain-free walking distance <200 meters). In more advanced stages of disease, blood flow is reduced to such an extent that pain is experienced even while at rest (stage III, rest pain). Further progression of the disease leads to ischemic ulcerations on the lower extremities and gangrene (stage IV, gangrene/tissue loss). Patients with stage III or stage IV PAOD have critical leg ischemia in which the ischemic process endangers part or all of the lower extremity. These patients usually are candidates for aggressive intervention such as surgery and are clinically managed by vascular surgeons.

Clinicians and exercise specialists clearly have their greatest impact on the clinical management of mildly affected patients with stage I and stage II PAOD. They also have an impact with revascularized patients who typically have significant hemodynamic improvements but who may remain functionally dependent because of the extreme deconditioning process that occurs with critical leg ischemia. These patients usually are good candidates for more conservative treatments such as exercise rehabilitation and/or medication therapy. If asymptomatic PAOD patients (stage I) can be identified, they probably are ideal candidates for exercise rehabilitation because the atherosclerotic process has not advanced enough to interfere with the ability to exercise. The focus of the remainder of this chapter centers on the evaluation and treatment of patients with Fontaine stage I and stage II PAOD.

Risk Factors for PAOD

Risk factors for PAOD are typical of those for coronary artery disease, including cigarette smoking, race (non-Caucasian), diabetes, age, elevated SBP, low levels of high-density lipoprotein cholesterol (HDL-C), and high total cholesterol level and body mass index (BMI) (10–12). In addition, properties of blood rheology and coagulation play a role in the development of PAOD. Increased blood viscosity and plasma fibrinogen are associated with the clinical course of PAOD (13), as well as with higher risks of coronary artery disease and recurrent myocardial infarction (14,15). Elevated levels of plasminogen activator inhibitor-1 activity and tissue plasminogen activator antigen also are related to the progression and complications of atherosclerosis (16–19). Finally, preliminary evidence shows that physical inactivity is independently associated with a lower ABI in persons who have ABI values in the normal range (20), supporting the notion that activity level may be a factor contributing to the development of PAOD (21).

Effects of PAOD on the Body

The presence of PAOD is associated with a poor prognosis of long-term survival (22–27), primarily because of increased risk of myocardial infarction and stroke. Compared with subjects without PAOD, the relative risk for all-cause mortality associated with PAOD ranges between 1.8 and 3.1 (24–26), indicating that the mortality rate is 80 to 210% higher in patients with abnormally low ABI values of ≤ 0.85 (24) or ≤ 0.90 (25,26). McKenna et al. (24) report 5-year survival estimates for PAOD patients and non-PAOD controls of 63 and 90%, respectively, while the 10-year survival was 46 and 77%. Vogt et al. (26) report even lower 10-year survival estimates of 39 and 35% for older men and women with PAOD, respectively.

Stage	Symptoms
TABLE 20-1	**FONTAINE CLASSIFICATION OF PERIPHERAL ARTERIAL OCCLUSIVE DISEASE**
Stage	Symptoms
I	Asymptomatic
II	Intermittent claudication
IIa	Pain-free, claudication walking >200 m
IIb	Pain-free, claudication walking <200 m
III	Rest pain
IV	Gangrene, tissue loss

The prognosis of PAOD patients worsens as the severity of PAOD increases (22–26). For example, patients with ABI values of ≤0.30 had a relative risk of death of 1.8 compared with the risk of patients with ABI values between 0.50 and 0.91 (23), and patients with ABI values of ≤0.40 had a 3.35 relative risk for mortality compared with that of patients with ABI values above 0.85 (24). Additionally, the cardiovascular mortality in symptomatic PAOD patients (Fontaine stages II, III, and IV) was 11 times higher than in non-PAOD controls (28), while the mortality rate in asymptomatic PAOD patients (Fontaine stage I) was 5 times higher.

The relationship between the presence and severity of PAOD with subsequent mortality is stronger than in many other medical conditions known to reduce survival. The adjusted relative risk for mortality associated with PAOD (2.36) was higher than the risk of diabetes (1.64) or stroke (1.88) and was similar to that for congestive heart failure (2.38) (24). However, PAOD patients with severe disease (ABI ≤0.30) had a greater relative risk than congestive heart failure patients (23). These data suggest that PAOD is of substantial medical concern and that, once identified, patients with PAOD should undergo interventions designed to improve their cardiovascular disease risk factor profile and to increase their functional capacity, to prevent complications from the disease.

Effects of PAOD on the Ability to Exercise

The primary effect of PAOD on short-term exercise is the development of claudication pain in the ischemic leg musculature during exercise because of insufficient arterial blood flow. When patients cease exercising, claudication pain gradually dissipates because the metabolic demand of the resting leg muscles no longer exceeds the capacity of the impaired blood flow to deliver the necessary amount of oxygen. After several minutes of rest, the perfusion of the leg musculature returns to baseline, and metabolic waste products within the musculature (e.g., lactic acid) are cleared. At this point, the patient may proceed to exercise free of pain for several minutes until ischemia once again occurs in the leg musculature. This cycle of repeated exercise

and rest periods is the reason why the symptom of PAOD is called intermittent claudication.

The rate of development of claudication pain during exercise varies greatly among patients, as some experience pain much sooner than others. The two primary factors that determine the rate of development of leg muscular ischemia and claudication pain is the intensity at which exercise is performed and the severity of PAOD. Consequently, claudication pain may occur quite rapidly in severely diseased patients who walk uphill, whereas pain development will be much slower in mildly diseased patients who walk on level ground (if it occurs at all).

Short-Term Effects of Exercise on PAOD

During ambulation, vasodilation occurs in the working lower extremity musculature. This vasodilation decreases the muscular vascular resistance, shunting the already compromised lower extremity blood flow in PAOD patients into the working muscles and away from cutaneous tissue and distal regions of the leg. However, the increased muscular blood flow is inadequate to meet the energy demands of the muscle, resulting in ischemic claudication pain in muscles distal to the arterial lesions. Claudication pain gradually increases during exercise until patients reach their maximal tolerable pain level, at which point exercise must be discontinued.

Circulatory impairment in PAOD patients is most evident immediately following exercise by measuring ankle SBP and ABI (3,6,7). Vasodilation in the leg musculature during and immediately following exercise causes the ankle SBP and ABI to decrease from their preexercise baseline values. As the vasodilatory stimulus gradually subsides during recovery, peripheral circulation is restored toward baseline, manifested by increases in ankle SBP and ABI.

Exercise Testing

As a result of insufficient blood flow to the lower extremities, claudication and peripheral hemodynamic measurements obtained from an exercise test are the primary criteria to assess the effectiveness of an exercise program (29). Given that claudication pain is experienced primarily during ambulation, treadmill testing is considered the gold-standard mode of exercise to assess claudication because it closely mimics "real-life" conditions, and it primarily stresses the affected calf musculature. Cycle ergometry may be an alternative exercise testing mode, but its usefulness is limited because the quadriceps muscles are primarily active rather than the calf musculature. Consequently, those with arterial lesions distal to the quadriceps muscles may be able to cycle without experiencing claudication pain.

Selecting an appropriate treadmill test to evaluate claudication is another important consideration. The two types of tests being used today are the progressive (P) multistage tests and single-stage (S) tests. Although both are used, the P test has several key advantages. By using a test with small increases in grade (i.e., exercise intensity), claudication distances of patients can be stratified according to disease severity better than when using an S test. Furthermore, P treadmill protocols that use a constant walking speed of 2 mph and gradual increases in grade of either 2.0 or 3.5% with each stage are highly reproducible (30,31). Gardner et al. had 10 patients walk to maximal claudication pain twice a month for 4 months (30). Patients walked at 1.5 mph up a 7.5% grade (S test) and at 2 mph on a 0% grade, increasing by 2% every 2 min (P test). Distance walked to the onset of claudication pain (CPD) and maximal walking distance (MWD) were recorded. Intraclass correlation coefficients (r) of CPD and MWD during the S tests were 0.53 and 0.55, respectively. In contrast, the respective r values during the P tests were 0.89 and 0.93. It was concluded that the severity of PAOD is better assessed by P treadmill tests because clinical measurements are more reliable during exercise and recovery.

The use of handrail support during the treadmill test should be avoided or at least minimized. The reason for this is that handrail support reduces the energy cost of walking and may decrease reproducibility unless the same pressure is applied to the handrails over repeated tests (32). Gardner et al. studied the effect of handrail support on claudication and hemodynamic responses and on their reproducibility during S (2 mph, 12% grade) and P

(2 mph, 0% grade with 2% increase every 2 min) treadmill protocols (32). Ten patients with stable PAOD performed both protocols three times, separated by 1 week, with and without handrail support. CPD and MWD were significantly longer ($P < .05$) when handrail support was permitted. CPD and MWD also increased ($P < .05$) over repeated tests. No increase was noted over the tests without support. Importantly, no patient had difficulty walking without support. Thus, handrail support may be an unnecessary safety precaution for most PAOD patients, and its use should not be encouraged unless balance cannot otherwise be maintained.

As mentioned above, the specific variables that are measured to assess the functional severity of PAOD include the distances (or times) to onset of claudication pain (CPD or CPT) and to maximal claudication pain (MWD or MWT). Peripheral hemodynamic measurements are obtained in conjunction with claudication measurements to provide a more objective assessment of disease severity. The most accepted variable is the ankle SBP measured before and after the treadmill test, which is needed to calculate ABI.

The primary objective of a treadmill test for patients with PAOD is to obtain reliable measures of (*a*) the rate of claudication pain development, (*b*) the peripheral hemodynamic responses to exercise, and (*c*) the presence of coexisting coronary heart disease. To assist the patient in evaluating claudication pain during the treadmill test, a pain scale is frequently used (0 = no pain, 1 = onset of pain, 2 = moderate pain, 3 = intense pain, and 4 = maximal pain) (33). Using this pain scale helps patients identify how their claudication pain progresses during the treadmill test. Typical distances to onset of pain and to maximal pain are approximately 170 m and 360 m, respectively (33). Circulatory inadequacy in the lower extremities with exercise can also be quantified accurately with treadmill testing by measuring the decrease in ABI from baseline (30). Gas exchange measures during the treadmill test show that PAOD patients with intermittent claudication have peak oxygen intake ($\dot{V}O_2$) values in the range of 12 to 15 mL·kg^{-1}·min^{-1} (31), which is approximately 50% of that seen in age-matched controls. Favorable changes following a program of exercise rehabilitation should include greater walking distances covered before the onset of pain and maximal claudication pain, an increase in peak VO_2, and possibly a blunted drop in ABI and a faster recovery of ABI to the resting baseline value.

Claudication pain and ABI are the most common measurements obtained because prior research has primarily taken a vascular perspective on this population. However, further research contributions concerning improved function of PAOD patients following exercise rehabilitation may be best accomplished by taking a more gerontological perspective which goes beyond the measurement of claudication distances and ABI. Because the typical profile of a PAOD patient is that of an elderly person with chronic ambulatory disability, the decline in physical functioning with aging may be accelerated in this population due to extreme deconditioning brought about by the disease process. Consequently, performance on a 6-minute walk test, as well as measures of gait, walking economy, balance, flexibility, and lower extremity strength, probably will be worse in PAOD patients than in age-matched controls; these variables may improve with a program of exercise rehabilitation. To date, however, information on these measures and whether they change with exercise rehabilitation in the PAOD population is sparse (34).

In addition to the above-mentioned laboratory measures of physical function, assessing the impact that ambulatory and functional limitations have on routine activities performed in the community setting may provide a truer measure of disability. The free-living daily physical activity measured by an accelerometer is one such measure because it quantifies the amount of movement done over an extended period of time. Free-living daily physical activity, as measured by an accelerometer, is approximately 33% lower in PAOD patients than in non-PAOD subjects of similar age. Activity progressively decreases in claudicants with worsening disease severity as measured by ABI (35). Furthermore, cigarette smoking (which is common in the PAOD population) decreases free-living daily physical activity by an additional 30% (36). Thus, PAOD patients with intermittent claudication are at the extreme low end of the physical activity spectrum.

Paterson et al. found that daily activities of independent living require a VO_2 of about $15 \text{ mL·kg}^{-1}\cdot\text{min}^{-1}$ (37). Given that this is at or above the peak VO_2 of 12 to 15 $\text{mL·kg}^{-1}\cdot\text{min}^{-1}$ for many PAOD patients (31) and that walking 2 to 3 mph requires a VO_2 of 8.9 to 11.6 $\text{mL·kg}^{-1}\cdot\text{min}^{-1}$, clearly PAOD patients are working close to their maximum when walking and when doing many activities of daily living. Therefore, it is not surprising that they are often fatigued and want to stop. However, by stopping, they become more deconditioned, and many activities of daily living become even more difficult to do.

It is not clear whether the typical improvements in claudication distances following exercise rehabilitation translate into increases in free-living daily physical activity in the community setting. Further research is needed to examine this issue, as well as to determine if functional improvements are related to enhanced quality of life in this elderly, disabled population.

Exercise Prescription

The primary objective of an exercise program for PAOD patients who are limited by intermittent claudication is to improve CPD and MWD. A meta-analysis found that the average increase in CPD was 179% following exercise rehabilitation, and the average increase in MWD was 122% (38). Exercise rehabilitation programs using treadmill walking were most effective in lengthening these distances. Although exercise rehabilitation effectively lengthens claudication distances, considerable variability exists. For example, CPD increased between 72 and 746%, and MWD increased between 61 and 739% (38). Differences in the components of exercise programs (e.g., intensity, duration, and frequency of exercise sessions) may largely account for these widely divergent responses.

The following recommendations for prescribing exercise are based on the results of a meta-analysis (38) that examined the most important factors of an exercise rehabilitation program to improve claudication distances in PAOD patients with intermittent claudication. In this meta-analysis, the following six components of an exercise rehabilitation program were compared to identify which were most important for eliciting optimal improvements in claudication pain distances: (*a*) frequency of exercise (sessions per week), (*b*) duration of exercise (minutes per session), (c) mode of exercise (walking vs. a combination of exercises), (*d*) length of the program (weeks), (*e*) claudication pain endpoint used in the program (onset of pain vs. near maximal pain), and (*f*) level of supervision (supervised vs. supervised plus home-based exercise). All of the exercise rehabilitation components had a significant effect on the magnitude of change in the claudication distances, except for the level of supervision. For example, programs that exercised patients to near-maximal claudication pain were more effective than programs that exercised patients to only the onset of pain. Additionally, programs consisting of longer exercise duration, higher frequency, greater program length, and walking as the only mode of exercise were more effective than programs consisting of shorter exercise duration, lower frequency, shorter program length, and having patients train by a variety of exercise modes. The addition of home exercise to supplement the amount of exercise performed in a supervised setting did not result in additional ambulatory benefit.

Of the five components that had an effect on the change in claudication distances, multivariate analyses found only three that had independent effects. These components were the claudication pain endpoint used in the program, length of the program, and mode of exercise (38). The combination of these components explained nearly 90% of the variance in the increase in walking distances following exercise rehabilitation. Although duration and frequency of exercise sessions are not independent predictors of the change in claudication pain times, programs should have patients walk for at least 30 min per session and for at least three sessions per week, as these amounts were more beneficial than programs using a shorter exercise duration and a lower frequency.

Finally, the appropriate exercise intensity to use during training is not known at this time because no study has addressed this issue. There is a common misconception that walking beyond the onset of pain to near maximal pain is an increase in intensity when, in fact, it is merely an increase in duration. The rate of work performed while walking, regardless of the duration, is the important consideration when setting the appropriate exercise intensity. Since heart rate (HR) is commonly used to adjust exercise intensity, a conservative recommendation for claudicants who are beginning a rehabilitation program is to walk at an appropriate speed and grade on a treadmill to elicit an intensity of approximately 50% of their HR reserve. They

TABLE 20-2 RECOMMENDED EXERCISE PROGRAM FOR PATIENTS WITH PERIPHERAL ARTERIAL OCCLUSIVE DISEASE	
Exercise Component	**Comment**
Frequency	3 exercise sessions per week
Intensity	Progression from 50% of peak exercise capacity to 80% by the end of the program
Duration	Progression from 15 min of exercise per session to more than 30 min by the end of the program
Mode	Weight bearing (e.g., walking, stair climbing); non-weight-bearing tasks (e.g., bicycling) may be used for warming up and cooling down
Type of exercise	Intermittent walking to near maximal claudication pain
Program length	At least 6 months

should gradually increase the intensity to 70 to 80% by completion of the program. Recommendations for an exercise program for patients with PAOD are summarized in Table 20-2.

Effects of Training on PAOD

IMPROVEMENTS IN CLAUDICATION MEASUREMENTS

Significant improvements in claudication pain occur following exercise rehabilitation. For example, a meta-analysis (38) demonstrated that in 21 exercise rehabilitation studies (39–59) conducted between 1966 and 1993, the average CPD increased 179%, from 126 ± 57 m (mean $\pm$ standard deviation) to 351 ± 189 m following rehabilitation. The average MWD increased 122%, from 326 ± 148 m to 723 ± 592 m.

IMPROVEMENTS IN RISK FACTORS

Exercise training has a beneficial effect in reducing blood viscosity and red cell aggregation in PAOD patients (39), as well as improving the fibrinolytic profile in young and old healthy subjects (60), patients who have experienced myocardial infarction (61), and patients with type II diabetes (62). Thus, exercise rehabilitation may improve clinical outcomes of PAOD patients by altering more traditionally accepted risk factors (e.g., blood lipids, blood pressure, obesity) as well as measures of blood rheology and coagulation. Furthermore, exercise rehabilitation is the method of choice to improve functional outcomes in PAOD patients who have ambulatory disability due to intermittent claudication (38).

POTENTIAL MECHANISMS FOR THE IMPROVEMENT IN CLAUDICATION MEASUREMENTS

Numerous mechanisms have been proposed to explain the improvement in CPD and MWD following exercise rehabilitation. These mechanisms primarily center on hemodynamic and enzymatic adaptations within the exercising musculature of the symptomatic leg(s). Specifically, these mechanisms include increased blood flow (40,49,58,63) to the exercising leg musculature; a more favorable redistribution of blood flow (59,64); greater use of oxygen (65) because of a higher concentration of oxidative enzymes (43); improved hemorheologic properties of the blood (39); decreased reliance upon anaerobic metabolism (57,65); and an improvement in the efficiency of walking (66,67). It may be that no one particular mechanism is primarily responsible for the improvement in claudication pain symptoms with exercise rehabilitation. Rather, a combination of changes in these factors may contribute to improved walking distances. Improvements in psychosocial attitude due to accomplishments that are achieved during exercise rehabilitation may further enhance this effect.

To address the peripheral hemodynamic mechanism, a number of studies have assessed ABI and calf blood flow both before and after a program of exercise. On average, calf blood flow under resting and maximal conditions increases by approximately 19% (43–46,49,50,52–54,59,65,68–71), and ABI increases by approximately 7% (47,51–54, 57,63,64,70–72) following exercise rehabilitation. Only a few studies have examined the change in redistribution of peripheral blood flow, blood viscosity, leg arteriovenous oxygen difference, concentration of oxidative enzymes, and efficiency of walking. Consequently, the changes in these variables

following exercise rehabilitation are not well established in PAOD patients. Since the magnitude of change in calf blood flow and ABI does not approach that of the changes in CPD (179%) and MWD (122%) (38), either small changes in peripheral blood flow yield exponential improvements in claudication pain symptoms or the other mechanisms mentioned above also contribute to the improved outcome.

Summary

PAOD is a significant health concern in the elderly population that will continue to increase in future years. Conservative management of patients with asymptomatic PAOD and of patients with intermittent claudication is recommended to modify risk factors and improve ambulatory ability. Patients with more severe PAOD typically require revascularization of the lower extremities. Exercise rehabilitation is a highly effective, conservative treatment to improve ambulation in patients with intermittent claudication. To date, the primary focus of attention on the benefits of exercise rehabilitation has centered on the CPD and MWD during a treadmill test. Future research should focus on the improvement in other functional outcomes commonly reported in the geriatric literature that may be more representative of everyday activities, such as submaximal exercise performance, walking economy, balance, flexibility, and lower-extremity strength. Until these measures are obtained, the full benefit of exercise rehabilitation for PAOD patients remains unclear.

REFERENCES

1. U.S. Health trends. J NIH Res 1992;4:95.
2. Kannel WB. Some lessons in cardiovascular epidemiology from Framingham. Am J Cardiol 1976;37:269–282.
3. Carter SA. Clinical measurement of systolic pressures in limbs with arterial occlusive disease. JAMA 1969;207:1869–1874.
4. Criqui MH, Fronek A, Barrett-Connor E, et al. The prevalence of peripheral arterial disease in a defined population. Circulation 1985;71:516–521.
5. Hiatt WR, Marshall JA, Baxter J, et al. Diagnostic methods for peripheral arterial disease in the San Luis Valley Diabetes Study. J Clin Epidemiol 1990;43:597–606.

6. Carter SA. Indirect systolic pressures and pulse waves in arterial occlusive disease of the lower extremities. Circulation 1968;37:624–637.

7. Ouriel K, McDonnell AE, Metz CE, et al. A critical evaluation of stress testing in the diagnosis of peripheral vascular disease. Surgery 1982;91:686–693.

8. Weitz JI, Byrne J, Clagett P, et al. Diagnosis and treatment of chronic arterial insufficiency of the lower extremities: A critical review. Circulation 1996;94:3026–3049.

9. Pentecost MJ, Criqui MH, Dorros G, et al. Guidelines for peripheral percutaneous transluminal angioplasty of the abdominal aorta and lower extremity vessels. Circulation 1994;89:511–531.

10. Newman AB, Sutton-Tyrell K, Rutan GH, et al. Lower extremity arterial disease in elderly subjects with systolic hypertension. J Clin Epidemiol 1991;1:15–20.

11. Newman AB, Siscovick DS, Manolio TA, et al. Ankle-arm index as a marker of atherosclerosis in the cardiovascular health study. Circulation 1993;88:837–845.

12. Newman AB, Sutton-Tyrell K, Kuller LH: Lower-extremity arterial disease in older hypertensive adults. Arterioscl Thromb 1993;13:555–562.

13. Dormandy JA, Hoare E, Khattab AH, et al. Prognostic significance of rheological and biochemical findings in patients with intermittent claudication. Br Med J 1973;4:581–583.

14. Kannel WB, Wolf PA, Castelli WP, et al. Fibrinogen and risk of cardiovascular disease: the Framingham Study. JAMA 1987;258:1183–1186.

15. Benderly M, Graff E, Reicher-Reiss H, et al. Fibrinogen is a predictor of mortality in coronary heart disease patients. Arterioscl Thromb Vasc Biol 1996;16:351–356.

16. Hamsten A, Wiman B, DeFaire U, et al. Increased plasma levels of a rapid inhibitor of tissue plasminogen activator in young survivors of myocardial infarction. N Engl J Med 1985;313:1557–1563.

17. Huber K, Jorg M, Probst P, et al. A decrease in plasminogen activator inhibitor 1 activity is associated with a significantly reduced risk for coronary restenosis. Thromb Haemost 1992;67:209–213.

18. Jansson JH, Nilsson TK, Olofsson BO. Tissue plasminogen activator and other risk factors as predictors of cardiovascular events in patients with severe angina pectoris. Eur Heart J 1991;12:157–161.

19. Lindgren A, Lindoff C, Norrving B, et al. Tissue plasminogen activator and plasminogen activator inhibitor-1 in stroke patients. Stroke 1996;27:1066–1071.

20. Gardner AW, Sieminski DJ, Montgomery PS. Physical activity is related to ankle/brachial index in subjects without peripheral arterial occlusive disease. Angiology 1997;48:883–891.

21. Housley E, Leng GC, Donnan PT, et al. Physical activity and risk of peripheral arterial disease in the general population: Edinburgh Artery Study. J Epidemiol Community Health 1993;47:475–480.

22. Howell MA, Colgan MP, Seeger RW, et al. Relationship of severity of lower limb peripheral vascular disease to mortality and morbidity: a six-year follow-up study. J Vasc Surg 1989;9:691–697.

23. McGrae-McDermott M, Feinglass J, Slavensky R, et al. The ankle-brachial index as a predictor of survival in patients with peripheral vascular disease. J Gen Intern Med 1994;9:445–449.

24. McKenna M, Wolfson S, Kuller L. The ratio of ankle and arm arterial pressure as an independent predictor of mortality. Atherosclerosis 1991;87:119–128.

25. Vogt MT, Cauley JA, Newman AB, et al. Decreased ankle/arm blood pressure index and mortality in elderly women. JAMA 1993;270:465–469.

26. Vogt MT, McKenna M, Anderson SJ, et al. The relationship between ankle-arm index and mortality in older men and women. J Am Geriatr Soc 1993;41:523–530.

27. Vogt MT, Wolfson SK, Kuller LH. Segmental arterial disease in the lower extremities: Correlates of disease and relationship to mortality. J Clin Epidemiol 1993;46:1267–1276.

28. Criqui MH, Langer RD, Fronek A, et al. Mortality over a period of 10 years in patients with peripheral arterial disease. N Engl J Med 1992;326:381–386.

29. Hiatt WR, Hirsch AT, Regensteiner JG, et al. Clinical trials for claudication: assessment of exercise performance, functional status, and clinical end points. Circulation 1995;92:614–621.

30. Gardner AW, Skinner JS, Cantwell BW, et al. Progressive versus single-stage treadmill tests for evaluation of claudication. Med Sci Sports Exerc 1991;23:402–408.

31. Hiatt WR, Nawaz D, Regensteiner JG, et al. The evaluation of exercise performance in patients with peripheral vascular disease. J Cardiopulm Rehabil 1988;12:525–532.

32. Gardner AW, Skinner JS, Smith LK. Effects of handrail support on claudication and hemodynamic responses to single-stage and progressive treadmill protocols in peripheral vascular occlusive disease. Am J Cardiol 1991;68:99–105.

33. Gardner AW, Ricci MR, Pilcher DB,, et al. Practical equations to predict claudication pain distances from a graded treadmill test. Vasc Med 1996;1:91–96.

34. Montgomery PS, Gardner AW. The clinical utility of a 6-minute walk test in peripheral arterial occlusive disease patients. J Am Geriatr Soc 1998;46:706–711.

35. Sieminski DJ, Gardner AW. The relationship between daily physical activity and the severity of

peripheral arterial occlusive disease. Vasc Med 1997; 2:286–291.

36. Gardner AW, Sieminski DJ, Killewich LA. The effect of cigarette smoking on free-living daily physical activity in older claudication patients. Angiology 1997;48:947–955.

37. Paterson DH, Cunningham DA, Koval JJ, et al. Aerobic fitness in a population of independently living men and women aged 55–65 years. Med Sci Sports Exerc 1999;31:1813–1820.

38. Gardner AW, Poehlman ET. Exercise rehabilitation programs for the treatment of claudication pain: A meta-analysis. JAMA 1995;274:975–980.

39. Ernst EEW, Matrai A. Intermittent claudication, exercise, and blood rheology. Circulation 1987;76: 1110–1114.

40. Alpert JS, Larsen A, Lassen NA. Exercise and intermittent claudication: Blood flow in the calf muscle during walking studied by the Xenon-133 clearance method. Circulation 1969;39:353–359.

41. Carter SA, Hamel ER, Paterson JM, et al. Walking ability and ankle systolic pressures: Observations in patients with intermittent claudication in a short-term walking exercise program. J Vasc Surg 1989;10:642–649.

42. Clifford PC, Davies PW, Hayne JA, et al. Intermittent claudication: is a supervised exercise class worth while? Br Med J 1980;281:1503–1505.

43. Dahllof AG, Björntorp P, Holm J, et al. Metabolic activity of skeletal muscle in patients with peripheral arterial insufficiency: effect of physical training. Eur J Clin Invest 1974;4:9–15.

44. Dahllof AG, Holm J, Schersten T, et al. Peripheral arterial insufficiency: effect of physical training on walking tolerance, calf blood flow, and blood flow resistance. Scand J Rehab Med 1976;8: 19–26.

45. Ekroth R, Dahllof AG, Gundevall B, et al. Physical training of patients with intermittent claudication: indications, methods, and results. Surgery 1978;84:640–643.

46. Ericsson B, Haeger K, Lindell SE. Effect of physical training on intermittent claudication. Angiology 1970;21:188–192.

47. Feinberg RL, Gregory RT, Wheeler JR, et al. The ischemic window: a method for the objective quantitation of the training effect in exercise therapy for intermittent claudication. J Vasc Surg 1992;16: 244–250.

48. Holm J, Dahllof AG, Björntorp P, et al. Enzyme studies in muscles of patients with intermittent claudication: effect of training. Scand J Clin Lab Invest (suppl 128) 1973;31:201–205.

49. Jonason T, Ringqvist I. Effect of training on the post-exercise ankle blood pressure reaction in patients with intermittent claudication. Clin Physiol 1987;7: 63–69.

50. Larsen OA, Lassen NA. Effect of daily muscular exercise in patients with intermittent claudication. Lancet 1966;2:1093–1096.

51. Lepantalo M, Sundberg S, Gordin A. The effects of physical training and flunarizine on walking capacity in intermittent claudication. Scand J Rehab Med 1984;16:159–162.

52. Lundgren F, Dahllof AG, Schersten T, et al. Muscle enzyme adaptation in patients with peripheral arterial insufficiency: spontaneous adaptation, effect of different treatments and consequences on walking performance. Clin Sci 1989;77:485–493.

53. Mannarino E, Pasqualini L, Menna M, et al. Effects of physical training on peripheral vascular disease: a controlled study. Angiology 1989;40:5–10.

54. Mannarino E, Pasqualini L, Innocente S, et al. Physical training and antiplatelet treatment in stage II peripheral arterial occlusive disease: alone or combined? Angiology 1991;42:513–521.

55. Rosetzsky A, Struckmann J, Mathiesen FR. Minimal walking distance following exercise treatment in patients with arterial occlusive disease. Ann Chir Gynecol 1985;74:261–264.

56. Rosfors S, Bygdeman S, Arnetz BB, et al. Longterm neuroendocrine and metabolic effects of physical training in intermittent claudication. Scand J Rehab Med 1989;21:7–11.

57. Ruell PA, Imperial ES, Bonar FJ, et al. Intermittent claudication: the effect of physical training on walking tolerance and venous lactate concentration. Eur J Appl Physiol 1984;52:420–425.

58. Skinner JS, Strandness DE Jr. Exercise and intermittent claudication: II. Effect of physical training. Circulation 1967;36:23–29.

59. Zetterquist S. The effect of active training on the nutritive blood flow in exercising ischemic legs. Scand J Lab Invest 1970; 25:101–111.

60. Stratton JR, Chandler WL, Schwartz RS, et al. Effects of physical conditioning on fibrinolytic variables and fibrinogen in young and old healthy adults. Circulation 1991;83:1692–1697.

61. Estelles A, Aznar J, Tormo G, et al. Influence of a rehabilitation sports programme on the fibrinolytic activity of patients after myocardial infarction. Thromb Res 1989;55:203–212.

62. Schneider SH, Kim HC, Khachadurian AK, et al. Impaired fibrinolytic response to exercise in type II diabetes: effects of exercise and physical training. Metabolism 1988;37:924–929.

63. Hall JA, Barnard RJ. The effects of an intensive 26–day program of diet and exercise on patients with peripheral vascular disease. J Cardiac Rehabil 1982;2:569–574.

64. Jonason T, Ringqvist I. Prediction of the effect of training on the walking tolerance in patients with intermittent claudication. Scand J Rehabil Med 1987;19:47–50.

65. Sorlie D, Myhre K. Effects of physical training in intermittent claudication. Scand J Clin Lab Invest 1978;38:217–222.

66. Ernst E. Physical exercise for peripheral vascular disease: a review. Vasa 1987;16:227–231.

67. Womack CJ, Sieminski DJ, Katzel LI, et al. Improved walking economy in patients with peripheral arterial occlusive disease. Med Sci Sports Exerc 1997;29:1286–1290.

68. Jonason T, Ringqvist I, Oman-Rydberg A. Home-training of patients with intermittent claudication. Scand J Rehabil Med 1981;13:137–141.

69. Fitzgerald DE, Keates JS, MacMillan D. Angiographic and plethysmographic assessment of graduated physical exercise in the treatment of chronic occlusive arterial disease of the leg. Angiology 1971;22:99–106.

70. Hiatt WR, Regensteiner JG, Hargarten ME, et al. Benefit of exercise conditioning for patients with peripheral arterial disease. Circulation 1990;81:602–609.

71. Lundgren F, Dahllof AG, Lundholm K, et al. Intermittent claudication—surgical reconstruction or physical training? A prospective randomized trial of treatment efficiency. Ann Surg 1989;209:346–355.

72. Williams LR, Ekers MA, Collins PS, et al. Vascular rehabilitation: benefits of a structured exercise/risk modification program. J Vasc Surg 1991;14:320–326.

RELATED WEB SITES
Vascular Disease

Society for Vascular Medicine and Biology
www.svmb.org

American College of Angiology
www.collegeofangiology.org

American Association for Vascular Surgery and the Society for Vascular Surgery
www.vascularweb.org

Cardiovascular Issues

American Heart Association
www.americanheart.org

Exercise Rehabilitation and Exercise Testing Patients with Intermittent Claudication

American College of Sports Medicine
www.acsm.org

American Association of Cardiovascular and Pulmonary Rehabilitation
www.aacvpr.org

General Information Relevant to Aging

Gerontological Society of America
www.geron.org

21

Heart Failure

Robert S. McKelvie

Description

Heart failure (HF) is a syndrome resulting from multiple different causes, the most common of which are coronary artery disease and hypertension. However, HF can result from a number of other causes including diabetes mellitus and valvular heart disease, as well as other less common causes (1). The symptomatic findings consist predominantly of shortness of breath and fatigue. Physical findings may consist of edema, crackles on chest examination, and elevated jugular venous pressure. Based on symptoms, patients are often classified into one of four New York Heart Association functional classes (NYHA FC). Class I represents asymptomatic individuals; class II patients are symptomatic during usual exertion; class III patients are symptomatic during less than usual activities; and class IV patients are symptomatic during minimal activity or even at rest.

The incidence of HF is 1/1000 men a year and 0.4/1000 women a year for individuals less than 65 years old, increasing to 11/1000 men a year and 5/1000 women a year for those over 65 years of age (1). Under 65 years of age, the prevalence of HF is 1/1000 men and 1/1000 women; over 65 years, it is 40/1000 men and 30/1000 women (1). The prognosis of HF is poor, with 5-year mortality ranging from 26 to 75% (1). Up to 16% of persons are readmitted with HF within 6 months of the first admission (1).

Over the years, pharmacologic therapy for HF has improved dramatically, and a number of the agents presently used affect the overall clinical outcome of these patients significantly (1). The angiotensin-converting enzyme inhibitor class of drugs was the first found to reduce clinical events convincingly (1). Since then, β-blockers have also been found to reduce clinical event rates convincingly, while spironolactone has benefit in reducing clinical events in NYHA FC III–IV patients (1). Digoxin also reduces hospitalizations (1). Therefore, there are now therapies available that not only improve symptoms but also reduce the risk of experiencing a clinical event.

Effects of Heart Failure on the Body and Ability to Exercise

HF patients exhibit no relation between left ventricular ejection fraction (LVEF) and peak exercise performance (2–6). Furthermore, peak oxygen uptake ($\dot{V}O_{2peak}$) is not related to the change in LVEF from rest to peak exercise (2,4). The degree of right ventricular dysfunction at rest may predict exercise performance, because a relation was found between peak exercise performance and right ventricular EF at rest in one study (7). However, other studies (4,8) have found no such relation.

Maskin et al. (9) found that short-term infusion of dobutamine improved exercise cardiac output (Q̇), but this was not associated with increased exercise performance. In another study (10), the response to short- and long-term (3 months) administration of cilazapril was compared in patients with congestive HF. Short-term administration of cilazapril improved central hemodynamic variables during exercise but not exercise performance, whereas long-term administration produced a further slight improvement in central hemodynamic variables and a significant increase in $\dot{V}O_{2peak}$.

These studies suggest that the reduction in exercise capacity experienced by patients with HF may be influenced more significantly by factors other than poor ventricular function. In the last few years, a theory has been proposed that implicates abnormalities of the skeletal muscles as being responsible in part for the clinical presentation and progression of HF in these patients (11). Skeletal muscle ergoreceptors are sensitive to, and monitor, the metabolic state of skeletal muscle and send information back to the brain that results in increased ventilation and a sympathetic outflow that produces vasoconstriction in distant nonexercising vascular beds, with consequent effects on blood pressure and possibly a small increase in heart rate (HR). Ergoreceptors have the properties necessary to link the skeletal muscle abnormality to the fatigue, dyspnea, hyperpnea, and sympathoexcitation characteristic of HF. In this hypothesis, another cycle of deterioration is proposed similar to those of the neuroendocrine activation theory of HF. Reduced left ventricular function sets in motion a series of metabolic events that lead to wasting of skeletal muscles and resultant abnormalities of muscle metabolism and function. In response to early metabolic changes in exercising muscle, an exaggerated ergoreflex activation occurs that the patient perceives as both muscle fatigue and dyspnea. This reflex also leads to excessive sympathetic vasoconstrictive drive to nonexercising beds and an excessive ventilatory response. The theory suggests that improvement of the exercise response will be delayed after instituting treatment to correct the hemodynamics until the skeletal muscle abnormalities have been resolved. This theory suggests that specifi-

cally improving skeletal muscle function (e.g., by exercise training) should also improve functional capacity.

HF patients have been found to have lower maximal muscle strength than healthy subjects (12,13), although not in all studies (14). This difference probably relates to patient selection, because those in the study by Lipkin et al. (12) and Buller et al. (13) had severe HF, whereas those in the study by Minotti et al. (14) had a wider range of clinical HF. However, studies have consistently demonstrated that the development of fatigue for a given power output is greater in HF patients than among healthy subjects (12–14). These findings have led to the suggestion that skeletal muscle abnormalities may contribute to the decline of functional capacity observed in HF patients.

SKELETAL MUSCLE ATROPHY

Skeletal muscle atrophy is often observed in HF patients and can occur early in the course of the disease (12,15). Muscle atrophy may be related to diminished physical activity or circulating cytokine levels (16). Gas exchange measurements during exercise in healthy subjects tend to support the hypothesis that a decreased muscle mass may partially contribute to the impairment of exercise capacity (8). The gas-exchange pattern in healthy subjects differs in relation to the amount of muscle mass used to perform exercise (e.g., treadmill exercise vs. one-leg exercise). A healthy subject cycling using one leg had a gas-exchange pattern that was similar to that of a patient with mild HF, suggesting that muscle atrophy may be partly responsible for the impaired exercise capacity (8). Mancini et al. (15) assessed muscle mass in relation to exercise performance in 62 patients in NYHA FC I–IV with an average EF of $23 \pm 12\%$. They found significant positive linear correlations between $\dot{V}O_{2peak}$ and midarm circumference, muscle circumference, muscle area, skeletal muscle mass, and creatinine/height index. This suggests that muscle atrophy contributes to effort intolerance. However, when the power output is matched for the difference in work capacity or for muscle cross-sectional area, the abnormal muscle metabolism persists, suggesting that there are qualitative changes in skeletal muscle of HF patients (15,17).

ABNORMALITIES OF SKELETAL MUSCLE BLOOD FLOW

Studies dating back to the 1930s (18) have suggested impaired blood flow to the skeletal muscles in HF patients; this has been confirmed in both human and animal studies (19). A number of potential mechanisms underlie the reduction in vasodilatory capacity, including a reduction in endothelium-derived relaxing factor, salt retention, and increases in various vasoconstrictive neurohormones such as endothelin, norepinephrine, renin, angiotensin II, and vasopressin (22–25). There is evidence from human and animal studies (20) that exercise training may improve skeletal muscle blood flow. The improved skeletal muscle blood flow during exercise is not related to improved central hemodynamic variables, occurs gradually after several weeks of training, and appears to be related to improvements in exercise capacity (10,26).

ABNORMALITIES OF SKELETAL MUSCLE METABOLISM

Reduced skeletal muscle blood flow is not the only factor responsible for the impaired exercise performance of HF patients. An abnormality in intrinsic skeletal muscle performance may also contribute (14).

Muscle metabolism has been examined using phosphorus-31 magnetic resonance imaging (MRI) studies. Wilson et al. (27) used phosphorous-31 MRI to examine forearm muscle metabolism during exercise in nine HF patients and eight age-matched control subjects. Exercise resulted in a pronounced increase in the inorganic phosphate/phosphocreatine ratio (Pi/CP) and a pronounced decrease in pH in HF patients, whereas the control group had only a moderate increase in Pi/CP and a minimal decrease in pH. Massie et al. (17) performed a similar study that examined changes in forearm skeletal muscle metabolism in 11 HF patients and 7 age-matched controls. In their study, the increase in Pi/CP and decrease in pH in forearm skeletal muscle during exercise were similar to the changes observed by Wilson et al. (27). The pronounced increase in Pi/CP and decrease in pH could reflect a loss of muscle mass rather than an intrinsic muscle abnormality, but this possibility was excluded by a study (17) that found a lower CP

and pH at submaximal loads in HF patients than in control subjects (17). Massie et al. (28) studied nine HF patients and nine control subjects who performed repetitive finger flexion at submaximal workloads while blood flow to exercising muscle was totally occluded. The HF patients continued to have a greater decline in CP and pH during exercise than control subjects, consistent with a primary abnormality of muscle metabolism. Therefore, the data would support a primary abnormality of muscle metabolism as the reason for impaired exercise performance rather than muscle atrophy or alterations in skeletal muscle blood flow.

Some studies (29–31) in HF patients have examined muscle metabolism during calf muscle (a weight-bearing muscle) exercise and found abnormalities similar to those in the forearm. The results from those studies would support the conclusion that there is an intrinsic abnormality in skeletal muscle metabolic function in HF patients.

The mechanism by which these metabolic changes impair exercise performance is unknown. It may be that the early increase in Pi and decrease in pH are responsible for producing premature fatigue in HF patients. This is supported by studies of skinned muscle fiber and isolated muscle preparations suggesting that the increase in Pi or H_2PO_4 interferes with muscle contraction. In human studies, there is a close relation between the increase in H_2PO_4 and the decline in the force of maximal voluntary contraction during exercise.

HISTOLOGIC AND BIOCHEMICAL ABNORMALITIES OF SKELETAL MUSCLE

Lipkin et al. (12) noted a predominance of type II (fast-twitch) muscle fibers in HF patients. Mancini et al. (32) compared results from 22 HF patients and 8 normal subjects. The patients were found to have smaller areas of type IIa and IIb fibers, a significant increase in the percentage of type IIb fibers, and lower 3-hydroxyacyl-coenzyme A dehydrogenase activity. Citrate synthase (CS) activity was normal, indicating normal oxidative enzyme levels, as were phosphofructokinase (PFK) levels, suggesting maintenance of glycolytic enzymes. Sullivan et al. (33) examined 11 patients with long-standing HF and 9 normal subjects and found significantly lower concentrations of the mitochondrial enzymes succinate dehydrogenase (SDH) and CS in the HF patients. They also found lower 3-hydroxacyl-coenzyme A-dehydrogenase and glycogen content, a reduced percentage of type I (slow-twitch) and a higher percentage of type IIb fibers (although the cross-sectional area of these fibers was lower). Patients with HF had fewer capillaries per fiber, but the ratio of capillaries to cross-sectional fiber area did not differ between the two groups. Drexler et al. (34) examined the mitochondria in 57 HF patients and 18 healthy control subjects. They found a significant 20% reduction in mitochondrial volume density and surface density of mitochondrial cristae in HF patients. Cytochrome oxidase activity in mitochondria was significantly lower, and fiber-type distribution shifted to type II. Mitochondrial volume density and surface density of mitochondrial cristae were significantly related to $\dot{V}O_{2peak}$ and to $\dot{V}O_2$ at the anaerobic threshold. The mitochondrial volume density was inversely related to the duration of HF. In a subgroup of patients who underwent repeat biopsies at 4 months, a relation was found between the change in mitochondrial volume density and the change in $\dot{V}O_{2peak}$.

Exercise Testing

Exercise testing has been performed using either a cycle ergometer or a treadmill, and the accepted contraindications to exercise testing also apply for the HF population. Incremental or ramp protocols have been used in this population, and generally the increments in power output are relatively low, and each stage is relatively prolonged (35,36). Respiratory gas-exchange measurements are often used when testing these patients; however, this is not an absolute requirement when performing the test. Without respiratory gas-exchange measurements, an accurate assessment of $\dot{V}O_{2peak}$ cannot be obtained from the prediction equations for $\dot{V}O_{2peak}$ for either the cycle ergometer or the treadmill. Properly supervised exercise testing of HF patients has been found safe (35,38).

Exercise testing is used to set the exercise prescription for patients entering into exercise-training programs (39) as well as to monitor change in functional capacity following training or alterations in drug therapy. The measured $\dot{V}O_{2peak}$, obtained from a cardiopulmonary exercise test is a descriptive indicator with both prognostic power and decisional implications. $\dot{V}O_{2peak}$ is a continuous variable that has been categorized by many investigators for practical purposes. Patients with a $\dot{V}O_{2peak}$ of 10 ml·kg^{-1}·min^{-1} have been found to have the worst prognosis, while those with a $\dot{V}O_{2peak}$ > 18 mL·kg^{-1}·min^{-1} have been found to be low risk and are expected to do well with drug therapy (35). Some (40) but not all (35, 41) studies have found that a $\dot{V}O_{2peak}$ of 14 mL·kg^{-1}·min^{-1} is a prognostic and decisional value that defines patients at greater risk, thus indicating the need for heart transplantation. Therefore, cardiopulmonary exercise testing is now used to further define the prognosis and to help decide the best management of HF patients.

Exercise Prescription

No standardized guidelines for exercise training of HF patients have been established, although some recommendations have been made (39) based on the results of previous studies or on experience from rehabilitation of coronary patients without HF and modified for the HF population (39,42). Recommendations for exercise training should be based on measurements obtained during exercise testing, the patient's response to exercise, and consideration of the patient's status including medication, risk factor profile, behavioral characteristics, personal goals, and exercise preferences. These should be based on the underlying pathophysiology found in HF patients. Accordingly, the documented pathophysiology would support the use of an exercise-training program designed to improve their aerobic and strength capacities.

ELIGIBILITY AND PATIENT EVALUATION

Published studies of exercise training for HF patients have all enrolled patients with stable chronic HF (37,39,42). None of these studies has randomized patients with unstable HF, and there are very few data on patients with NYHA FC IV symptoms

(43). Eligible patients are essentially those with stable NYHA FC II–III symptoms. Patients with NYHA FC IV symptoms who are carefully selected and properly motivated could also be considered eligible for training. However, these individuals must be free of symptoms of dyspnea at rest and require a great deal of supervision during exercise (39). No minimal LVEF is required to be eligible for exercise training, as the published reports have trained stable patients with LVEFs as low as 5 to 9% (39,42). Although the benefits of training do not appear to depend on the cause of HF, specific contraindications would include obstructive valvular disease (especially aortic stenosis) or active myocarditis (either viral or autoimmune). There are few data about exercise training HF patients with significant regurgitant valvular disease. If at all possible, significant valvular heart disease should be surgically corrected first. Following this, the patient could be considered for exercise training, even if left ventricular dysfunction remains severe. Studies of exercise training with HF patients have generally excluded individuals with evidence of ventricular tachycardia or other serious ventricular arrhythmias on exercise (39,42). Thus, patients with serious exercise-induced ventricular arrhythmias should not be advised to exercise train until they have been properly investigated and treated. Other common abnormalities such as angina, silent myocardial ischemia, marked hypotension, and atrial arrhythmias should be thoroughly evaluated prior to initiating an exercise-training program.

All patients should be carefully reviewed by a cardiologist prior to initiating an exercise program. This evaluation would include a history and physical examination to identify cardiac and noncardiac problems that may potentially limit participation in an exercise program (e.g., anemia, peripheral vascular disease, reversible airways disease). Blood tests (e.g., electrolytes, renal function) and an exercise test, preferably a cardiopulmonary exercise test, also should be performed.

AEROBIC-EXERCISE TRAINING

Aerobic exercise has been most commonly used in studies examining the effects of exercise training in patients (42,43). There has been extensive variability in the types of exercise programs used, ranging from 11 min per day of calisthenics and stationary running to jogging, calisthenics, and cycling 55 min in the morning, with 30 to 60 min of walking in the afternoon at 70 to 80% of peak HR 5 days per week (42,43). Although walking, jogging, cycling, swimming, rowing, and calisthenics have been applied in previous studies and clinical practice, HF patients may be more limited in the types of activities they can perform.

Cycle ergometer exercise training allows exercising at very low power outputs, the power outputs can be applied in a reproducible fashion, and the patient's weight is supported by the cycle. These features make cycle ergometry training generally a favorable type of aerobic exercise, especially for patients with severe exercise intolerance or other comorbidities (e.g., obesity, orthopedic, neurologic, and/or age-related limitations for other types of exercise). However, directly applying indoor cycle ergometry training to outdoor cycling is not possible because of environmental factors influencing cardiovascular stress (e.g., wind, slopes). Even outdoor cycling at a very slow speed (12 km·h^{-1}) requires a $\dot{V}O_2$ of almost 1.0 L·min^{-1}, corresponding to 50 to 60 W (44). Thus, outdoor cycling could be recommended for only a relatively small group of long-term clinically stable patients with a documented high exercise capacity. Jogging is not advisable for any except the most stable and physically fit patients. This is because even jogging at a slow pace requires a $\dot{V}O_2$ of approximately 1.2 L·min^{-1}, which represents a relatively high demand for most patients. However, walking offers a form of activity that can be tolerated by a wide range of HF patients because the required $\dot{V}O_2$ of walking, in most cases, is well tolerated.

There are at least three different approaches to determine the intensity of exercise (39); these include % $\dot{V}O_{2peak}$, % peak HR, and ratings of perceived exertion (RPEs). Many of the published studies have used % $\dot{V}O_{2peak}$ to set the exercise intensity (42,43). Intensities of 40 to 80% $\dot{V}O_{2peak}$ have been used successfully, indicating that patients with a low exercise tolerance respond to a low exercise intensity (42,43). As intensity and duration of exercise are closely interrelated in terms of expected training benefit, it is reasonable to increase the duration of training or frequency of training for individuals working at very low intensities. HR is used as a guide for exercise intensity because of the relatively linear relationship between HR and $\dot{V}O_2$ (44). In previous studies, either 60 to 80% of HR reserve or 60 to 80% of the predetermined peak HR have been used to set exercise intensity. Using the Borg scale, RPE has been found to relate to $\dot{V}O_2$. Training intensities of 40 to 80% of $\dot{V}O_{2peak}$ have been demonstrated in healthy subjects to correlate positively with RPEs of 12 to 15 (light–moderate/heavy) using the 6–20 Borg scale (44). In HF patients, Borg scale ratings of <13 (somewhat hard) have been reported to be well tolerated and successfully applied (45). However, the Borg scale should not be used to set the exercise intensity but should be considered mainly an adjunct to training intensity determined by the % $\dot{V}O_{2peak}$ or HR response. The RPE determined during cardiopulmonary exercise testing may not translate consistently to the same intensity as that during exercise training. Furthermore, a certain percentage of HF patients cannot use the Borg scale reliably. As ratings of fatigue and dyspnea are often perceived differently during exercise, both symptoms should be monitored.

As stated above, intensity and duration of exercise are closely interrelated, and frequency of training is related to both of the factors. Therefore, these factors can be altered to optimize training programs so the patient is exposed to an adequate training stimulus without experiencing intolerable symptoms of fatigue or other discomforts. Thus, the duration and frequency of training for a patient depend on the baseline clinical and functional status. The general principles of exercise prescription with regards to duration and frequency can be applied to HF patients (39,44). Stable HF patients with a functional capacity below 3 METS (approximating 25–40 W) benefit from short daily exercise sessions of 5 to 10 min each. Patients with a functional capacity of 3 to 5 METS (approximating 40–80 W) can usually tolerate one to two sessions per day of 15 min each. For patients with a functional capacity above 5 METS, three to five sessions per week lasting 20 to 30 min a session are recommended.

The rate of progression of the exercise-training prescription must be specific to the individual patient. Progression rate depends on the baseline functional capacity, clinical status, individual adaptability to a training program, comorbidities, and (biological) age of the patient. There are three stages of progression: (*a*) initial; (*b*) improvement; and (*c*) maintenance. In general, the progression of exercise training should be in the order of duration, then frequency, and finally intensity. For the initial stage, intensity should be kept at a low level (e.g., 40–50% $\dot{V}O_{2peak}$) until an exercise duration of 10–15 min is achieved. Duration and frequency of exercise training are increased according to symptoms and clinical status. During the improvement stage, an increase in exercise intensity is the primary goal, with patients progressing from 40% $\dot{V}O_{2peak}$ to 80% $\dot{V}O_{2peak}$, as tolerated. The prolongation of a session to 15 to 20 min or even up to 30 min if tolerated is a secondary goal of this stage. Repeat exercise testing is used to evaluate whether the patient is ready for an increase in training intensity. The maintenance stage usually begins after the first 6 months of training (44). Individually tailored training allows clinically stable patients to maintain their exercise capacity and/or slow down or delay the muscle wasting and loss of aerobic capacity typical of progressive HF. The effects of exercise training are lost after only 3 weeks of inactivity in HF patients (46). These findings emphasize the need for including long-term exercise training into their management.

RESISTANCE-EXERCISE TRAINING

Although muscle strength is an independent predictor of exercise capacity in HF patients (47), aerobic-exercise programs have been used almost exclusively to train them (42,43). Furthermore, activities of daily living require a combination of endurance and strength. Aerobic-exercise training does not specifically improve muscle strength, and because it is performed in a continuous fashion, this form of training may not be well tolerated by all HF patients. Although the rationale exists to support the use of other forms of exercise training targeted at improving strength and endurance, the evidence to date, although promising, is limited in support of these alternative programs.

Resistance weight-lifting training, which specifically improves muscle strength and submaximal exercise endurance, is now routinely used for patients with coronary artery disease (CAD)(48) but has not been used as routinely in HF patients because of concerns about the hemodynamic responses.

The general protocol used for CAD patients is circuit resistance training, during which the patient performs a number of exercises designed to train different muscle groups. The intensity is set at 40 to 70% of one repetition maximum (1RM), which is the amount of weight a person can lift one time through a full range of motion. Individuals typically start at 40%, and intensity is increased over a number of weeks to 70%. Each exercise consists of 10 (usually arm exercises) to 15 (usually leg exercises) repetitions. When the patient first starts resistance training, the complete set of exercises is performed once. As fitness improves, the patient will perform three sets of each exercise. The patient uses a single limb to perform each exercise and is encouraged to take a short break (minimum 1–2 min) between each exercise.

Studies of exercise programs that have included resistance training have demonstrated improvements in aerobic capacity and strength in CAD patients (48). Although there has been some concern about applying resistance training to HF patients, recent studies suggest this should not be the case (49,50). One recent study compared the hemodynamic responses to cycling and leg press resistance exercise in HF patients (49). Blood pressures were measured with an intraarterial catheter and cardiac volumes were measured using echocardiography during both types of exercise. The patients randomly performed cycling at 70% of peak power output and leg press at 70% of 1 RM. Cycling resulted in greater HR and rate-pressure product responses than leg press exercise, with no difference between the two types of exercise for end-diastolic or end-systolic volumes. Another study examined rhythmic double leg press exercise at loads of 60 and 80% of 1RM using interval modes with 60-sec work phases of 12 repetitions each and 120-sec rest phases (50). While performing this type of exercise, HF patients responded with increased left ventricular stroke work index and decreased systemic vascular resistance. Thus, the data suggest that resistance exercise would be an acceptable method to train HF patients.

Previous studies have documented that the amount of cardiovascular stress during resistance exercise depends on the muscle mass (single-leg vs. double-leg exercise) involved in performing the activity (48). One of the main potential advantages to resistance exercise training is that it can be performed in a segmental fashion (51). Individual muscle groups can be targeted, which would permit adequate perfusion of the exercising muscle without placing excessive demands on the cardiovascular system. Furthermore, this approach would permit patients to train at an adequate intensity and thus obtain maximum benefit from the sessions. In fact, because resistance training can be performed in a segmental fashion, it may be valuable in patients with more advanced states of HF. For these very debilitated patients with substantial loss of skeletal muscle mass, resistance training that aims to rebuild muscle mass may be an important step before initiating a program of aerobic-exercise training. Once muscle strength has improved from resistance training, it would be feasible to add an aerobic component. However, experience with this form of training is relatively limited in HF patients, and more experience in larger patient populations is needed before a general recommendation can be provided.

INTERVAL EXERCISE TRAINING

A number of studies have demonstrated that the intensity of exercise training has the most pronounced effect on a subject's exercise capacity (52). Therefore, another potential way to improve exercise is to use intense exercise stimuli applied during short phases that are repeated in sequence. Interval exercise training is based on this principle.

Interval exercise training can be performed with either the cycle ergometer or treadmill. The best-established mode for HF patients is the cycle ergometer (53). To set the exercise prescription, patients first perform a steep ramp test on the cycle ergometer to determine maximum short-time exercise capacity (MSEC) (53). For the steep ramp test, patients start with unloaded pedaling for 3 min, after which power output is increased 25 W every 10 sec. Many patients achieve a peak power output of 150 to 200 W (53). The peak power output achieved on the steep ramp test is much greater than that found when patients perform an ordinary ramp test with power output increases of 12.5 W per min. In clinical practice, the interval cycling usually consists of work phases of 30 sec and recovery phases of 60 sec (53). The usual intensity for the work phase of training is 50%

MSEC. During the recovery phase, patients pedal at 0 or 10 W. Other combinations of work/recovery phases of 15 sec/60 sec and 10 sec/60 sec with 70 and 80% of MSEC, respectively, can also be used by HF patients (54). During the first three work phases of training, power output is successively increased to reach the final level in the fourth work phase. Depending on the work/recovery interval, about 10 to 12 work phases are performed per session.

The response of the cardiovascular system to different modes of interval training has been compared with the response observed during submaximal exercise at 75% $\dot{V}O_{2peak}$ determined from an ordinary ramp exercise test (54). In this study, patients performed interval exercise at 50% MSEC with 30/60-sec work/recovery phases, at 70% MSEC with 15/60-sec phases, and at 80% MSEC with 10/60-sec phases. The metabolic and cardiac responses of the three interval exercises were compared with the responses during exercise at 75% $\dot{V}O_{2peak}$ determined from an ordinary ramp exercise test. For the three modes of interval exercise, mean $\dot{V}O_2$ ranged from 754 to 803 mL·min^{-1}, mean HR from 78 to 86 bpm, mean systolic blood pressure from 122 to 136 mm Hg, mean lactate from 1.10 to 1.41 mM, and mean RPE from 9.3 to 12.4. Although interval training allowed patients to work at a much greater power output (range of 71–111 W) than exercise at 75% $\dot{V}O_{2peak}$ (53 W), the clinical responses to interval training were no different from those observed with aerobic training. Although power output is markedly higher during interval training, LVEF has been shown to increase significantly and by the same magnitude as observed during steady-state exercise. Furthermore, HR and mean arterial blood pressure were similar to those seen with steady-state exercise, while blood lactate was significantly higher during interval exercise (55). These data suggest that interval training results in a greater exercise stimulus for the peripheral skeletal muscles with no greater stress on the heart than is observed with steady-state cycle ergometer exercise.

Although cycle ergometer training is preferred for applying interval training, this method can also be applied on a treadmill. In this case, a practical way is to chose work and recovery phases of 60 sec each. During work phases, walking speed is adjusted to the HR tolerated by the patient during interval cycle ergometer training. During recovery phases, walking speed should be as slow as possible (56).

Interval exercise would appear to be an acceptable method of training HF patients. However, as with resistance training, experience with this form of training is relatively limited, and more experience in larger patient populations is needed before a more general recommendation can be provided.

Effects of Exercise Training in Heart Failure Patients

Mechanisms responsible for an increase in $\dot{V}O_{2peak}$ following exercise training are multifactorial and involve both central and peripheral factors.

CARDIAC FUNCTION

Improvement in maximal $\dot{Q}$ has been found in some but not all studies examining the effects of exercise training. When observed, the increase in $\dot{Q}$ is associated with a modest 4 to 8% increase in peak HR (57–61) and a modest increase in stroke volume that may be due to left ventricular dilation (62). Improved diastolic filling rate has also been observed, which is significantly correlated with an increased cardiac index at peak exercise (63). Improved myocardial thallium uptake and left ventricular response to low-dose dobutamine infusion has been found following exercise training, suggesting improved myocardial perfusion and function (64). However, improved myocardial function has not been found in all studies, as other reports have found unchanged left ventricular contractility after exercise training both at rest and during exercise (60,65,66). Furthermore, there has been no effect observed on LVEF following exercise training. There had been some concern based on an early study (67) that exercise training might adversely affect cardiac function. These concerns have been alleviated by more recent studies demonstrating that regular exercise training did not have significant adverse effects on left ventricular volumes or wall thickness or result in thinning of the infarcted area (60,65). Importantly, data from a study examining the effects of exercise training in post-myocardial-infarction patients with left ventricular dysfunction found the training attenuated the unfavorable effects of left ventricular remodeling (66).

SKELETAL MUSCLE BLOOD FLOW

Evidence from human and animal studies suggests that exercise training may improve skeletal muscle blood flow (20). Hornig et al. (68) demonstrated that following 4 weeks of daily handgrip training, flow-dependent dilation was restored. Furthermore, 6 weeks after cessation of handgrip training, the response was again impaired. In another study, leg blood flow was examined following 6 months of exercise training (57). The patients in the exercise training group had a 28% increase in peak leg blood flow response. Katz et al. (69) examined endothelium-dependent and -independent vasodilation in skeletal muscle resistance vessels following 8 weeks of handgrip exercise. After training, vasodilatory responses to acetylcholine (endothelium-dependent vasodilation) increased significantly compared with pretraining values, while the vasodilatory responses to nitroglycerine (endothelium-independent vasodilation) did not change. Hambrecht et al. (70) compared the vasodilatory response in 20 HF patients prospectively randomized to either 6 months of exercise training (10 patients) or usual care (10 patients). Exercise training did not result in changes in nitroglycerin-induced endothelium-independent vasodilation. There was a significant 203% increase in femoral artery blood flow in response to acetylcholine infusion (endothelium-dependent vasodilation), and the inhibiting effect of N^G-monomethyl-L-arginine increased by 174% following exercise training. The increase in $\dot{V}O_{2peak}$ was significantly correlated with the endothelium-dependent change in peripheral blood flow. Thus, the increase in peak leg blood flow is likely due to enhanced endothelium-dependent vasodilation (68–70) and contributes to the improvement in leg $\dot{V}O_2$ that is observed with training HF patients (57).

SKELETAL MUSCLE METABOLISM AND HISTOLOGY

Studies have demonstrated that regular training results in changes in skeletal muscle metabolism and histology. Minotti et al. (71) studied HF patients who performed single-arm training for 28 days. Although no change was observed in the size of the trained forearm flexor muscle, a two- to threefold increase in endurance associated with a slower increase in Pi and a decline in CP with a decrease in Pi/CP versus power output slope was observed, indicating improved oxidative metabolism. Adamopoulos et al. (31) examined the metabolic changes in the gastrocnemius muscle after 8 weeks of home-based cycle exercise training. There was improved plantar-flexion exercise tolerance that was associated with reduced CP depletion, less ADP used during exercise, and an increased CP resynthesis rate during recovery. These changes suggest that exercise training improves the impaired oxidative capacity of skeletal muscle found in HF patients. Sullivan et al. (20) also found that exercise training HF patients resulted in lessening the metabolic abnormalities observed before training. A study by Hambrecht et al. (57) examined the change in total volume density of mitochondria (Vvm-total) and volume density of cytochrome C oxidase-positive mitochondria (Vvm-cox+) in 22 HF patients. There was a significant 41% increase in Vvm-cox+ and a significant 19% increase in Vvm-total in the 12 exercise-trained patients, with no significant changes in the 10 physically inactive patients. Furthermore, the change in Vvm-cox+ after endurance training was significantly correlated with changes in $\dot{V}O_{2peak}$. Additionally, a reshift in the ratio type I fibers/type II fibers was observed from 48:52% at baseline to 52:48% after exercise training (72).

CLINICAL OUTCOMES

The accumulated data demonstrating beneficial changes in skeletal muscle function and cardiac function following exercise training suggest that there should be associated improvements in functional capacity and quality of life for HF patients. A number of uncontrolled or nonrandomized studies and randomized controlled studies have assessed the effects of exercise training on exercise performance and quality of life (42,43,73). Generally, the uncontrolled or nonrandomized studies have demonstrated improvements in peak exercise performance. As well, measures of quality of life or well-being have improved. Interestingly, a study by Wilson et al. (74) demonstrated that not all patients benefit from exercise training. They recruited 32 patients into a 12-week exercise-training program at 60 to 70% of maximal HR three times per week. There were 21 patients with a normal $\dot{Q}$ response, and 9 of these responded to training (defined as an increase of >10% in $\dot{V}O_{2peak}$ and the anaerobic threshold). Eleven patients had a reduced $\dot{Q}$ response to exercise, and only one of these patients responded to the exercise training. The results of this study suggest that the level of circulatory dysfunction may influence the response to exercise training.

The randomized controlled trials have generally demonstrated improved $\dot{V}O_{2peak}$ and quality of life or well-being following exercise training (43,73). However, these studies have generally had only small numbers of patients. More recently, papers have been published with larger numbers achieved through either prospective randomization of patients or pooling of data from other studies in an overview type of analysis. The European Heart Failure Training Group has published a pooled analysis of the data from a number of smaller studies that they performed examining the effects of exercise training (75). A total of 134 patients had been studied in randomized controlled trials of exercise training. The results demonstrated a significant training effect, with a 13% increase in $\dot{V}O_{2peak}$ and 17% increase in exercise duration. There also was significant improvement reported for NYHA FC.

A study by Belardinelli et al. (36) examined 99 patients with NYHA FC II–IV symptoms; 50 patients were randomized to the exercise group at the hospital gymnasium under the supervision of a cardiologist and 49 to the no-exercise control group. Exercise training continued for 1 year. $\dot{V}O_{2peak}$ increased by 18% by the 2-month follow-up. Although it remained increased at 1 year, no further increase occurred with further training above the $\dot{V}O_{2peak}$ measured at 2 months. Quality of life improved along with the thallium activity score. Exercise training was also associated with lower mortality (9 vs. 20, for those with training and those

without, respectively; relative risk 0.37, $P = .01$) and hospital readmissions for heart failure (5 vs. 14; relative risk 0.29, $P = .02$). However, these data must be interpreted cautiously, as the numbers are small. Although they are promising and support the hypothesis that exercise training will reduce clinical events, confirmation is required from a large clinical trial powered to examine the effects of exercise training on clinical outcomes. In fact, a large clinical trial (HF ACTION) to be performed in the USA and Canada (funded by the NIH) that examines the effects of exercise training on mortality and morbidity in NYHA FC II–IV patients started randomizing patients early in 2003.

The Exercise Rehabilitation Trial (EXERT) examined 181 patients with NYHA FC I–III symptoms, ejection fraction of <0.40, and 6-min walk distance of <500 m (37). Patients were randomized to receive either usual medical care plus 3 months of supervised exercise training in a rehabilitation program, followed by 9 months of home-based exercise training or just usual medical care. After 3 months of exercise training, there was a significant 10% increase in $\dot{V}O_{2peak}$, with a 14% increase after 12 months of training. No significant changes were observed in cardiac function, nor were there any significant differences observed in mortality, hospitalization for HF, or worsening HF. Adherence to exercise was good during the supervised training but was reduced during home-based training. Therefore, patients show significant improvement in functional capacity in a supervised setting, but it seems to be more difficult for them to remain compliant when they are in a home-based program with less supervision. Thus, the findings from this study suggest that most patients with HF will require close follow-up in supervised programs in the long term to encourage compliance with exercise training.

Summary

- HF is a common syndrome that affects approximately 1-2% of the population.
- Mortality and morbidity rates remain unacceptably high, despite the pharmacological therapies available to treat these patients.
- Peripheral factors (to some extent unrelated to the decline in cardiac function) may be importantly

responsible for the reduction of exercise capacity and symptoms described by these patients.

- The skeletal muscle hypothesis of HF outlines how, after the initial development of cardiac dysfunction, skeletal muscle abnormalities may result in progression of cardiac dysfunction and worsening symptoms of HF.
- Exercise training can improve symptoms and increase exercise capacity.
- Training techniques are similar to those employed for patients without HF, including resistance training or interval training.
- Compliance to long-term training will be an important issue and efforts will need to be directed towards encouraging compliance.
- Although there are no well-established techniques to encourage compliance in these patients, one potential method would be to have them exercise in supervised settings for a period of 3 to 6 months before entering a home-based phase. During the home-based program, they would continue to come to rehabilitation 1 to 2 times per month for follow-up visits.
- All HF patients should be advised about physical activity and encouraged to remain as fit as possible.
- Ideally, training should be initiated in the setting of a supervised exercise training program. However, if this is not possible, then explicit recommendations with appropriate follow-up should be provided so these patients can exercise using a home-based program.

REFERENCES

1. McKelvie RS. Clinical evidence. Heart Failure 2001; 5:43–62.
2. Higginbotham MB, Morris KG, Conn EH, et al. Determinants of variable exercise performance among patients with severe left ventricular dysfunction. Am J Cardiol 1983;51:52–56.
3. Franciosa JA, Park JA, Levine TB. Lack of correlation between exercise capacity and indices of resting left ventricular performance in heart failure. Am J Cardiol 1981;47:33–39.
4. Salachcic J, Massie BM, Kramer BL, et al. Correlates and prognostic implications of exercise capacity in chronic congestive heart failure. Am J Cardiol 1985;55:1037–1042.
5. Port S, McEwan P, Cobb FR, et al. Influence of resting ventricular function on left ventricular response to exercise in patients with coronary artery disease. Circulation 1981;63:856–863.
6. Liang C, Stewart D, LeJemtel TH, et al. Characteristics of peak aerobic capacity in symptomatic and asymptomatic subjects with left ventricular dysfunction. Am J Cardiol 1992;69:1207–1211.
7. Baker BJ, Wilen MM, Boyd CM, et al. Relation of right ventricular ejection fraction to exercise capacity in chronic left ventricular failure. Am J Cardiol 1984;54:596–599.
8. Buller NB, Poole-Wilson PA. Extra polluted maximum oxygen consumption: a new method for the objective analysis of respiratory gas exchange during exercise. Br Heart J 1988;59:212–217.
9. Maskin CS, Forman R, Sonneblick EH, et al. Failure of dobutamine to increase exercise capacity despite hemodynamic improvement in severe congestive heart failure. Am J Cardiol 1983;51:177–182.
10. Drexler H, Banhardt U, Meinertz T, et al. Contrasting peripheral short-term and long-term effects of converting enzyme inhibition in patients with congestive heart failure. A double-blind, placebo-controlled trial. Circulation 1989;79:491–502.
11. Piepoli M, Clark AL, Volterrani M, et al. Contribution of muscle afferents to the hemodynamic, autonomic, and ventilatory responses to exercise in patients with chronic heart failure. Effects of physical training. Circulation 1996;1996:940–952.
12. Lipkin DP, Jones DA, Round JM, et al. Abnormalities of skeletal muscle in patients with chronic congestive heart failure. Int J Cardiol 1988;18:187–195.
13. Buller NP, Jones D, Poole-Wilson PA. Direct measurement of skeletal muscle fatigue in patients with chronic heart failure. Br Heart J 1991;65:20–24.
14. Minotti JR, Christoph I, Oka R, et al. Impaired skeletal muscle function in patients with congestive heart failure. Relationship to systemic exercise performance. J Clin Invest 1991;88:2077–2082.
15. Mancini D, Walter G, Reichek N, et al. Contribution of skeletal muscle atrophy to exercise intolerance and altered muscle metabolism in heart failure. Circulation 1992;85:1364–1373.
16. Levine B, Kalian J, Mayer L, et al. Elevated levels of tumor necrosis factor in severe chronic heart failure. N Engl J Med. 1990;323:236–244.
17. Massie B, Conway M, Yonge R, et al. Skeletal muscle metabolism in patients with congestive heart failure: relation to clinical severity and blood flow. Circulation 1987;76:1009–1019.
18. Weiss S, Ellis LB. Oxygen utilization and lactic acid production in the extremities during rest and exercise. Arch Intern Med 1935;55:665–680.
19. Zelis R, Longhurst J, Capone RJ, et al. A comparison of regional blood flow and oxygen utilization during dynamic forearm exercise in normal subjects

and patients with congestive heart failure. Circulation 1974;50:137–143.

20. Sullivan MJ, Higginbotham MB, Cobb F. Exercise training in patients with severe left ventricular dysfunction: hemodynamic and metabolic effects. Circulation 1988;78:506–515.

21. Reading JL, Goodman JM, Plyley MJ, et al. Vascular conductance and aerobic power in sedentary and active subjects and heart failure patients. J Appl Physiol 1993;74:567–573.

22. Lucher TF, Noll G. Endothelium-dependent vasomotion in aging, hypertension, and heart failure. Circulation 1993;87(suppl VII):VII-97–VII-103.

23. Sinoway L, Minotti J, Musch T, et al. Enhanced metabolic vasodilation secondary to diuretic therapy in decompensated congestive heart failure secondary to coronary artery disease. Am J Cardiol 1987;60:107–111.

24. Francis GS, Goldsmith SR, Levine TB, et al. The neurohormonal axis in congestive heart failure. Ann Intern Med 1984;101:370–377.

25. Ferguson DW, Berg WJ, Sander JS, et al. Sympathoinhibitory responses to digitalis glycoside in heart failure patients. Direct evidence from sympathetic neural recordings. Circulation 1989;80:65–77.

26. Sinoway LI, Minotti JR, Davis D, et al. Delayed reversal of impaired vasodilation in congestive heart failure after heart transplantation. Am J Cardiol 1988;61:1076–1079.

27. Wilson JR, Fink L, Maris J, et al. Evaluation of energy metabolism in skeletal muscle of patients with heart failure with gated phosphorus-31 nuclear magnetic resonance. Circulation 1985;71:57–62.

28. Massie B, Conway M, Rajagopalan B, et al. Skeletal muscle metabolism during exercise under ischemic conditions in congestive heart failure. Evidence for abnormalities unrelated to blood flow. Circulation 1988;78:320–326.

29. Mancini DM, Ferraro N, Tuchler M, et al. Detection of abnormal calf muscle metabolism in patients with heart failure using phosphorus-31 nuclear magnetic resonance. Am J Cardiol 1988;62:1234–1240.

30. Arnolda L, Conway M, Dolecki M, et al. Skeletal muscle metabolism in heart failure: a 31P nuclear magnetic resonance spectroscopy study of leg muscle. Clin Sci (Colch) 1990;79:583–589.

31. Adamopoulos S, Coats AJ, Brunotte F, et al. Physical training improves skeletal muscle metabolism in patients with chronic heart failure. J Am Coll Cardiol 1993;21:1101–1106.

32. Mancini D, Coyle E, Coggan A, et al. Contribution of intrinsic skeletal muscle changes to 31P NMR skeletal muscle metabolic abnormalities in patients with chronic heart failure. Circulation 1989;62:1338–1346.

33. Sullivan MJ, Green HJ, Cobb FR. Skeletal muscle biochemistry and histology in ambulatory patients with long-term heart failure. Circulation 1990;81:518–527.

34. Drexler H, Riede U, Munzel T, et al. Alterations of skeletal muscle in chronic heart failure. Circulation 1992;85:1751–1759.

35. Opasich C, Pinna DG, Bobbio M, et al. Peak exercise oxygen consumption in chronic heart failure: toward efficient use in the individual patient. J Am Coll Cardiol 1998;31:766–775.

36. Belardinelli R, Georgiou D, Cianci G, et al. Randomized, controlled trial of long-term moderate exercise training in chronic heart failure. Effects on functional capacity, quality of life, and clinical outcome. Circulation 1999;99:1173–1182.

37. McKelvie RS, Teo KK, Roberts R, et al. Effects of exercise training in patients with heart failure: the Exercise Rehabilitation Trial (EXERT). Am Heart J. 2002;144:23–30.

38. Tristani FE, Hughes CV, Archibald DG, et al. Safety of graded symptom-limited exercise testing in patients with congestive heart failure. Circulation 1987;(suppl VI):VI-54–VI-58.

39. Gianuzzi P, Tavazzi L, Meyer K, et al. Recommendations for exercising training in chronic heart failure patients. Eur Heart J 2001;22:125–135.

40. Pina IL. Optimal candidates for heart transplantation: is 14 the magic number? J Am Coll Cardiol 1995;25:1143–1153.

41. Kao W, Winkel EM, Johnson MR, et al. Role of maximal oxygen consumption in establishment of heart transplant candidacy for heart failure patients with intermediate exercise tolerance. Am J Cardiol 1997;79:1124–1127.

42. McKelvie RS, Teo KK, McCartney N, et al. Effects of exercise training in patients with congestive heart failure: a critical review. J Am Coll Cardiol 1995;25:789–796.

43. Lloyd-Williams F, Mair FS, Leitner M. Exercise training and heart failure: a systematic review of current evidence. Br J Gen Pract 2002;52:47–55.

44. American College of Sports Medicine. ACSM's Guidelines for Exercise Testing and Prescription. Baltimore: Williams & Wilkins, 1995.

45. Keteyian SJ, Levine AB, Brawner CA, et al. Exercise training in patients with heart failure. A randomized controlled trial. Ann Intern Med 1996;124:1051–1057.

46. Meyer K, Schwaibold M, Westbrook S, et al. Effects of short-term exercise training and activity restriction on functional capacity in patients with

severe chronic congestive heart failure. Am J Cardiol 1996;78:1017–1022.

47. Volterrani M, Clark AL, Ludman PF, et al. Predictors of exercise capacity in chronic heart failure. Eur Heart J 1994;15:801–809.

48. McCartney N. Acute responses to resistance training and safety. Med Sci Sports Exerc 1999;31:31–37.

49. McKelvie RS, McCartney N, Tomlinson CW, et al. Comparison of hemodynamic responses to cycling and resistance exercise in congestive heart failure secondary to ischemic cardiomyopathy. Am J Cardiol 1995;76:977–979.

50. Meyer K, Hajric R, Westbrook S, et al. Hemodynamic responses during leg press exercise in patients with chronic congestive heart failure. Am J Cardiol 1999;83:1537–1543.

51. Douard H, Thiaudiere E, Broustet JP. Value of segmental rehabilitation in patients with chronic heart failure. Heart Failure 1997;13:77–82.

52. Fox EL, Bartels RL, Billings CE, et al. Frequency and duration of interval training programs and changes in aerobic power. J Appl Physiol 1975;38:481–484.

53. Meyer K, Roskamm H. What is the best training method for improving aerobic capacity in chronic heart failure patients? Heart Failure 1997;Summer:83–91.

54. Meyer K, Samek L, Schwaberger G, et al. Physical responses to different modes of interval exercise in patients with chronic heart failure—application to exercise training. Eur Heart J 1996;17:1040–1047.

55. Meyer K, Foster C, Georgakopoulos N, et al. Comparison of left ventricular function during interval versus steady-state exercise training in patients with chronic congestive heart failure. Am J Cardiol 1998;82:1382–1387.

56. Meyer K, Schwaibold M, Westbrook S, et al. Effects of exercise training and activity restriction on 6-minute walking test performance in patients with chronic heart failure. Am Heart J 1997;133:447–453.

57. Hambrecht R, Niebauer J, Fiehn E, et al. Physical training in patients with stable chronic heart failure: effects on cardiorespiratory fitness and ultrastructural abnormalities of leg muscles. J Am Coll Cardiol 1995;25:1239–1249.

58. Belardinelli R, Georgiou D, Scocco V, et al. Low intensity exercise training in patients with chronic heart failure. Heart Failure 1995;26:975–982.

59. Dubach P, Meyers J, Dziekan G, et al. Effect of high intensity exercise training on central hemodynamic responses to exercise in man with reduced left ven-

tricular function. J Am Coll Cardiol 1997;29:1591–1598.

60. Dubach P, Myers J, Dziekan G, et al. Effect of exercise training on myocardial remodeling in patients with reduced left ventricular function after myocardial infarction: application of magnetic resonance imaging. Circulation 1997;95:2060–2067.

61. Kiilavuory K, Sovijarvi A, Navery H, et al. Effect of physical training on exercise capacity and gas exchange in patients with chronic heart failure. Chest 1999;110:985–991.

62. Demopoulos L, Bijou R, Fergus I, et al. Exercise training in patients with severe congestive heart failure: enhancing peak aerobic capacity while minimizing the increase in ventricular wall stress. J Am Coll Cardiol 1997;29:597–603.

63. Belardinelli R, Georgiou D, Cianci G, et al. Effects of exercise training on left ventricular filling at rest and during exercise in patients with ischemic cardiomyopathy and severe left ventricular systolic dysfunction. Am Heart J 1996;132:61–70.

64. Belardinelli R, Georgiou D, Ginzton L, et al. Effects of moderate exercise training on thallium uptake and contractile response to low dose dobutamine of dysfunction myocardium in patients with ischemic cardiomyopathy. Circulation 1998;97:553–561.

65. Giannuzzi P, Tavazzi L, Temporelli PL, et al. Long-term physical training and left ventricular remodeling after anterior myocardial infarction: results of the Exercise in Anterior Myocardial Infarction (EAMI) Study Group. J Am Coll Cardiol 1993;22:1821–1829.

66. Giannuzzi P, Temporelli PL, Corra' U, et al. Attenuation of unfavorable remodeling by exercise training in postinfarction patients with left ventricular dysfunction: results of the exercise in left ventricular dysfunction (ELVD) trial. Circulation 1997;96:1790–1797.

67. Jugdutt BI, Michorowski BL, Kappagoda CT. Exercise training after anterior Q wave myocardial infarction: importance of regional function and topography. J Am Coll Cardiol 1988;12:362–372.

68. Hornig B, Maier V, Drexler H. Physical training improves endothelial function in patients with chronic heart failure. Circulation 1996;93:210–214.

69. Katz A, Yuen J, Bijou R. Training improves endothelial-dependent vasodilation in resistance vessels of patients with heart failure. J Appl Physiol 1997;82:1488–1492.

70. Hambrecht R, Fiehn E, Weigl C, et al. Regular physical exercise corrects endothelial dysfunction and

improves exercise capacity in patients with chronic heart failure. Circulation 1998;98:2709–2715.

71. Minotti JR, Johnson EC, Hudson TL, et al. Skeletal muscle response to exercise training in congestive heart failure. J Clin Invest 1990;86:751–758.

72. Hambrecht R, Fiehn E, Jiangtao Y, et al. Effects of endurance training on mitochondrial ultra structure and fiber type distribution in skeletal muscle of patients with stable chronic heart failure. J Am Coll Cardiol 1997;29:1067–1073.

73. Coats AJ. Exercise and heart failure. Cardiol Clin 2001;19:517–524.

74. Wilson JR, Groves J, Rayos G. Circulatory status and response to cardiac rehabilitation in patients with heart failure. Circulation 1996;94:1567–1572.

75. European Heart Failure Training Group. Experience from controlled trials of physical training in chronic heart failure. Protocol and patient factors in effectiveness in the improvement in exercise tolerance. Eur Heart J 1998;19:466–475.

RELATED WEB SITES

American College of Cardiology
www.acc.org

Canadian CHF Clinics Network
www.cchfcn.org/english/index.htm

Canadian Association of Cardiac Rehabilitation
www.cacr.ca

American Heart Association
www.americanheart.org

Journal of the European Society of Cardiology
www.eurheartj.com

American Association of Cardiovascular and Pulmonary Rehabilitation
www.aacvpr.org

22

Heart Disease in Children

Reginald L. Washington

Cardiac Anomalies in Children

INCIDENCE

Congenital heart disease is the most common congenital defect, occurring in approximately 0.8% of all live births. The high incidence of congenital heart disease makes it likely that clinicians and exercise specialists will evaluate, treat, and make exercise recommendations regarding congenital heart disease patients during their years of practice. Many patients will have undergone surgical repair or cardiac catheterization intervention for their structural defect. Health care providers need to know the more common cardiac defects, their treatment, residual defects, and postintervention complications (surgical or following an interventional cardiac catheterization) to better advise and treat these patients. Most congenital heart disease patients will be followed by a pediatric or adult cardiologist, but often these patients will not have had a recent evaluation.

Advances in pediatric cardiothoracic surgery have allowed a change from predominantly palliative types of cardiac surgery to complete repairs. There have also been improvements in the medical managements of patients with a resultant decrease in the morbidity and mortality associated with surgery. Survival rates of children with complex congenital heart disease are increasing, as is their lifespan. Therefore, it is now likely that general pediatricians, family practitioners, or internal medicine physicians will see patients with repaired cardiac disease during their careers.

Regular exercise benefits patients with congenital heart disease. Individuals involved in regular exercise have an improved sense of well-being, increased exercise tolerance, and possibly fewer illnesses. These results are even more important in this patient group, since they may have limited exercise tolerance and may not tolerate frequent illnesses. Also, the psychologic benefits of exercise may assist in long-term patient care.

The diagnosis of congenital heart disease is made in the first few years of life, making the likelihood of a school-aged child with significant undiagnosed cardiac disease unlikely. However, there have been several well-published sudden deaths in young athletes, increasing the level of concern that a significant cardiac defect may have been missed.

Preparticipation Physical Examination

Guidelines for sports participation have been published in the past for competitive athletes with congenital heart disease (1–3). These guidelines were developed because of the well-publicized deaths

337

among high school, college, and professional athletes and the identification of congenital heart disease patients as a high-risk group.

Children with congenital heart disease are, in general, at low risk for sudden death during exercise. There are a few exceptions to this generalization, including such defects as severe aortic valve stenosis, hypertrophic cardiomyopathy, coronary artery anomalies, long Q-T interval syndromes, Marfan syndrome, and myocarditis (4,5). The risk for patients who have undergone complete surgical repairs is not as well documented, and no widely accepted guidelines in this category of patients are available.

Evaluation

HISTORY

The cardiac history should be thorough. Standard questionnaires are available but may not adequately cover the cardiovascular system in potential athletes who have had congenital heart disease. The past medical history for cardiac patients should cover the type of cardiac defect; surgical or other interventions that have occurred; and results of the latest complete evaluation (cardiac catheterization, echocardiograms, exercise stress tests, etc.).

Current health status history should include questions regarding (*a*) presence of chest pain or discomfort during or after exercise; (*b*) a history of presyncope or syncope with or without exercise; (*c*) excessive or unexplained fatigue, shortness of breath, or decreased exercise tolerance; (*d*) history of current or past cardiac murmurs; (*e*) history of systemic hypertension; and (*f*) the presence of palpitations or irregular heart beats.

The athletes and their parents should address the family history carefully, because children often are not aware of a family history of heart disease in older relatives. Questions should include, but not be limited to, heart disease in family members less than 55 years of age and should include such disorders as hypertension, long Q-T interval syndrome, congenital deafness, sudden or unexpected deaths with or without exercise, cardiomyopathy or other chronic cardiac disabilities, presyncope or syncope, use of pacemakers, history of Marfan syndrome, or elevated lipid levels in younger relatives. Any of these could be a clue to the risk of a cardiac complication in the young athlete.

PHYSICAL EXAMINATION

A complete physical examination of the cardiovascular system should include inspection, palpation, auscultation, and percussion. Blood pressure should be determined in the right arm and the leg if there is a discrepancy in pulses. If the patient is cyanotic, oxygen saturations should be measured at rest and during exercise using pulse oximetry. Careful auscultation should occur in a quiet room so that soft murmurs are readily appreciated. The patient should be examined in the supine and sitting positions. While heart murmurs are commonly heard in up to 85% of young athletes, most of these murmurs are considered functional or innocent. Once detected, however, the examiner should ask the following questions: (*a*) is the murmur functional or organic? (*b*) if the murmur is organic, should participation in physical activity be limited? and (*c*) what type of evaluation should be completed before participation in physical activity is allowed?

LABORATORY STUDIES

Individuals with known cardiac disease or who have heart disease suspected after the history and physical examination may require additional testing prior to clearance for sports participation. These studies often include a chest x-ray, a 12-lead resting electrocardiogram (ECG), an echocardiogram, an exercise stress test with or without collection of expiratory gases, and often a referral to a pediatric or adult cardiologist who specializes in congenital heart defects. These more sophisticated evaluations should be conducted by someone experienced in treating congenital heart defects so that unnecessary studies are not ordered.

Classification of Sports and Physical Activity

Sports and physical activity may be classified according to the type and intensity of exercise performed and according to the danger of body collision (1). There are two general types of exercise: static

TABLE 22-1 SPORTS CLASSIFICATION BY INTENSITY			
High-to-Moderate Intensity		**High-to-Moderate Static Intensity**	**Low Dynamic and Low Intensity**
Boxing	Badminton	Archery	Bowling
Crew/rowing	Baseball	Auto racing	Cricket
Cross-country skiing	Basketball	Diving	Curling
Cycling	Field hockey	Equestrian	Golf
Downhill skiing	Lacrosse	Field events (jumping)	Riflery
Fencing	Orienteering	Field events (throwing)	
Football	Ping-pong	Gymnastics	
Ice hockey	Race walking	Karate or judo	
Rugby	Racquetball	Motorcycling	
Running (sprint)	Soccer	Rodeo	
Speed skating	Squash	Sailing	
Water polo	Swimming	Ski jumping	
Wrestling	Tennis	Water skiing	
	Volleyball	Weight lifting	

From Maron BJ, Mitchell JH. 26th Bethesda conference: Recommendations for determining eligibility for competition in athletes with cardiovascular abnormalities. J Am Coll Cardiol 1994;24:846–899.

(isometric) and dynamic (isotonic). In addition, sports may be characterized by their intensity into low-, medium-, and high-intensity activities (Table 22-1).

Dynamic exercise involves changes in muscle length and joint movement with rhythmic contractions that develop a relatively smaller force, whereas static exercise involves development of a relatively larger force with little or no change in muscle length or joint movement. These two types of exercise should be thought of as the two extremes of a continuum, with most physical activity having both static and dynamic demands (1).

Dynamic exercise performed with a large muscle mass causes a marked increase in oxygen intake ($\dot{V}O_2$) and cardiac output. There is an increase in systolic blood pressure (SBP), while diastolic blood pressure (DBP) and mean pressures remain relatively constant, and peripheral vascular resistance decreases. On the other hand, static exercise, which usually involves a much smaller muscle mass than dynamic exercise, causes a small increase in $\dot{V}O_2$ and cardiac output. There is a marked increase in SBP, DBP, and mean arterial pressure. Peripheral vascular resistance increases only slightly. During dynamic exercise, there is an increase in stroke volume and small changes in mean arterial pressure, whereas the stroke volume changes little during static exercise with an increase in mean arterial pressure. Thus,

dynamic exercise may be thought of as primarily causing a volume load and static exercise as producing a pressure load on the left ventricle.

The difficulty with classification schemes is that they do not consider training programs required for each of the specific sports, i.e., these might require a different type and increased intensity of exercise, thereby increasing the risk. Athletes should have individualized training regimens, acknowledging the static and dynamic characteristics of their individual sport (1).

Specific Congenital Heart Defects

ATRIAL SEPTAL DEFECT

Atrial septal defect (ASD) is a frequent cardiac disorder, occurring as an isolated defect in about 5 to 8% of all congenital heart disease patients. ASDs are characterized by a direct communication between the right and left atria, allowing blood to shunt from one side to the other, depending upon the pressures in each chamber. The size of the defect can vary along with the location in the atrial septum. Depending on this location, defects are classified as primum, secundum, sinus venosus, or coronary sinus ASDs.

ASDs can be divided also into small, medium, and large, based on the size of the defect and the shunting across it. Smaller defects do not cause right ventricular dilatation. Moderate or large ASDs will cause right ventricular volume overload with right ventricular dilatation. In the presence of a large left-to-right shunt, changes can occur in the pulmonary vasculature, leading to elevated pulmonary vascular resistance and resultant pulmonary hypertension. The incidence of elevated pulmonary vascular resistance increases with the age of the patient if no surgery is performed.

Other complications associated with ASDs are paradoxical embolism caused by a thrombus from the right side of the heart or venous system crossing the atrial defect and embolizing (paradoxically) to the arterial system. This is the cause of some "cryptogenic" strokes.

The exercise capacity of children before surgical repair is slightly lower than normal. The limiting factor for the working capacity appears to be the degree of pulmonary hypertension and not merely the size of the shunt. Patients with normal pulmonary artery pressures have nearly normal working capacities, even with a moderate-to-large left-to-right shunt (6,7). There also is a significant correlation with exercise capacity and the level of habitual physical activity prior to surgical repair (7,8). When the exercise capacity is compared in the same patient preoperatively and postoperatively, there is very little improvement (6,9).

When children who have undergone surgical repair of ASDs are compared with healthy controls, the classical physical fitness parameters between the two groups are generally identical, including maximal exercise performance. The ASD repair group, however, reaches an ventilatory anaerobic threshold at a lower exercise intensity and as a group has a lower peak heart rate (HR) (10,11). These differences do not appear to be clinically significant. One study did demonstrate a significant increase in supraventricular and ventricular arrhythmias in the postoperative group, but these were not felt to be clinically significant (11).

Patients with small ASDs who do not have pulmonary hypertension may participate in any and all sports and activities. If pulmonary hypertension is present, the patient should be restricted to low-intensity activities and sports. If there is a marked elevation in right-sided heart pressures (right atrium or right ventricle), the patient should not participate in any competitive sports (1).

Evaluation of athletes and active patients after the closure of an ASD should include a complete history, physical examination, chest x-ray, and 12-lead ECG. The history should review the possibility that the athlete or active patient has had dysrhythmias in the past (palpitations, racing HR, presyncope, or syncope). If cardiomegaly is present on the chest x-ray, an echocardiogram should be evaluated to assess the possibility of residual shunting or right ventricular hypertension and/or pulmonary hypertension. Following repair of an ASD, the patient should not participate in any competitive or collision sports for 6 months.

In summary, children with ASDs have a slightly reduced exercise capacity. Pulmonary hypertension, although more frequently observed in adults, limits exercise performance. Surgical correction of the ASD will not dramatically improve exercise capacity in children. After surgical correction, exercise capacity is normal or slightly reduced. Impaired chronotropism and lack of habitual physical activity may possibly influence exercise capacity negatively.

VENTRICULAR SEPTAL DEFECT

Ventricular septal defect (VSD) is the most common congenital heart disease, accounting for 15 to 20% of all congenital heart disease. A VSD is a direct communication between the right and left ventricles of the heart. Blood usually shunts from the higher-pressure left ventricle to the lower-pressure right ventricle. A small VSD may have a loud cardiac murmur on examination but rarely produces symptoms or cardiac chamber enlargement. Moderate-to-large VSDs allow a large volume of blood to flow from the left ventricle to the right ventricle, producing dilatation of the left ventricle and the left atrium from the increased pulmonary venous return.

VSDs also vary in location and may require closure because of the potential negative effects on the aortic valve rather than the degree of shunting. Aortic insufficiency is an indication for surgical closure of these types of defects. Small VSDs diagnosed in infancy often close spontaneously and have no hemodynamic significance. Defects that are still present by the time the child reaches 5 to 6 years of age are not likely to close spontaneously.

Most studies that evaluate the exercise capacity of patients who have undergone surgical closure of VSDs were carried out in an era when (*a*) early surgical closure was not performed and (*b*) the physical activity of these patients was restricted by their health care providers. These studies did demonstrate a decrease in exercise capacity and often an increase in exercise ability following surgical repair as long as no pulmonary hypertension was present (12).

A study that looked at the long-term outcome of patients with VSDs considered too small to require surgical closure in childhood demonstrated a mean exercise capacity that was 92% of expected; 87% of these patients had no arrhythmias on Holter monitoring. It was concluded that the outcome in this well-selected group of patients was good and that there were no symptoms related to the VSD (13).

Studies that have evaluated the exercise capacity of patients who have undergone early surgical repair of their VSDs in the "modern era" have demonstrated improvement in maximal VO_2 and ventilatory anaerobic threshold as well as a decrease or absence of pulmonary hypertension (12,14). The degree of habitual physical activity following surgery is also a key factor in determining the exercise capacity of these children following their surgical repair.

Postoperatively, these patients may have residual defects and also may experience a variety of dysrhythmias. Right bundle-branch block is a frequent finding, but it usually has little, if any, clinical significance. This finding is becoming rarer, as the surgical closure of the VSD is now usually performed via an atrial approach across the tricuspid valve, as opposed to approaches that involve a right ventriculotomy. Some patients (3–14%) develop late postoperative abnormalities, including mild mitral regurgitation, subvalve aortic stenosis, or progressive aortic insufficiency. If any of these defects are moderate or severe, they may interfere with the hemodynamic performance of the heart and thus limit the exercise capacity of these children.

After a surgical repair, patients should not participate in activities for 6 months. After 6 months, they should be thoroughly evaluated for residual defects and symptoms. If there are no residual defects, no symptoms, and no evidence of pulmonary hypertension or dysrhythmias, they may participate in all sports and activities. If there is a moderate-sized residual defect (with a heart murmur), participation should be limited to low-intensity sports and activities. It is rarely necessary to restrict patients with a repaired VSD from recreational sports, however (1).

In summary, VSDs that have been closed in older children often have residual findings that limit their exercise capacity. On the other hand, early surgical closure will perhaps limit these residual findings, so that these children will enjoy normal exercise capacity. Studies are ongoing to evaluate the validity of this theory.

PULMONARY STENOSIS

Pulmonary valve stenosis accounts for 8 to 12% of all congenital heart disease and is usually tolerated well by children. The stenosis may be valvular, subvalvular, or supravalvular; this discussion is limited to valvular pulmonary stenosis (PS).

Most patients with mild-to-moderate PS are asymptomatic. PS involves a fixed obstruction to the right ventricular outflow. There is increased right ventricular systolic pressure and increased myocardial oxygen demand at rest. In mild PS (gradients of <50 or 60 mm Hg), exercise tolerance is normal. Exercise tolerance is usually decreased with moderate or severe disease (gradient of >50 or 60 mm Hg). Myocardial oxygen demand of the right ventricle is determined by the right ventricular systolic pressure, mass, and HR. During exercise, coronary blood flow may not meet the metabolic demand, resulting in right ventricular ischemia, dysfunction, and ultimately fibrosis.

Postoperatively, working capacity and endurance time are usually decreased, whereas the HR response to exercise is normal. This decreased exercise tolerance is probably due to reduced stroke volume and cardiac output. In severe stenosis, there is a low resting stroke volume and no increase in stroke volume during exercise.

Exercise tolerance in children and adults with mild valvular PS is nearly normal but is diminished in those with moderate and severe stenosis, indicating an impaired ability to sustain adequate cardiac output. Following relief of stenosis, cardiac performance improves in children but remains abnormal in adults (15). This appears to be related to postoperative resolution of the right ventricular hypertrophy in children, whereas myocardial fibrosis may explain the lack of improvement in adults.

Following a percutaneous repair of PS, patients may participate in any and all sports and activities 1 month following the procedure. If a surgical approach was used, the patient should wait 3 months. If there is a persistent gradient exceeding a peak of 50 mm Hg, patients should be evaluated by a pediatric cardiologist who will usually do an ECG and an echocardiogram to evaluate not only the degree of stenosis but also the right ventricular function and degree of pulmonary insufficiency, if any. If the gradient is >50, these patients should refrain from vigorous competitive sports (1). Patients who continue with high gradients across the valve are at increased risk for sudden death with exercise (15–17).

CONGENITAL VALVULAR AORTIC STENOSIS

Congenital aortic stenosis is often identified in early childhood and accounts for 3 to 6% of all congenital heart disease. Patients with mild-or-moderate aortic stenosis are often asymptomatic but may have some exercise intolerance or exertional chest pain. The stenosis is classified as mild, moderate, or severe on the basis of the peak gradient: mild is <20 mm Hg; moderate, 21 to 49 mm Hg; and severe, >50 mm Hg. Because aortic stenosis often progresses, patients with this disorder require regular follow-up and evaluation by a cardiologist knowledgeable about the diagnosis.

The increased stroke volume with exercise and fixed aortic obstruction results in increased left ventricular pressure and an increased aortic valve gradient. Patients with severe disease or with symptoms such as dizziness or lightheadedness related to the stenosis are at increased risk for sudden death (16,18).

An ST depression of ≥2 mm during exercise testing is usually associated with an aortic valve gradient of >50 mm Hg. An exercise profile of ST depression of ≥2 mm, a blunted or declining exercise SBP, and reduced working capacity are signs of severe obstruction, resulting in subendocardial ischemia and serious left ventricular impairment. These exercise responses may occur in some patients whose physical examination does not suggest a severe obstruc-

tion (19). One study performed prospective exercise tests using patients with isolated, severe aortic stenosis and found that the 6% of patients who exhibited symptoms later experienced sudden death. The study concluded that exercise testing is safe in this patient population and may be prognostic in predicting sudden death in asymptomatic patients (20).

Some patients with aortic stenosis and aortic insufficiency undergo a Ross procedure, during which the pulmonary root and valve are harvested and transferred to the aortic position and a homograft valve is placed in the pulmonary position. In addition, the coronary arteries are implanted into the pulmonary autograft. This procedure is more common in children than in adults, and better results seem to be obtained in the pediatric population.

Advantages of this repair compared with repair with prosthetic valves include the avoidance of anticoagulation and valve growth with the patient. There seems to be a long-term durability of the pulmonary valve in the aortic position. Postoperative complications include aortic insufficiency, stenosis of the homograft in the pulmonary position, and deterioration of the neoaortic valve. There is concern that the degree of insufficiency or regurgitation may progress with exercise. After the Ross procedure, patients have valve competence and transaortic gradients similar to those seen in controls at baseline and with exercise. Some patients following a Ross procedure often have significantly higher baseline pressures. Exercise-induced dysrhythmias may occur during exercise as well (21). The most common dysrhythmias include premature ventricular contractions.

Following repair, assessment for residual narrowing or stenosis and the presence of aortic valve insufficiency should be made. This will include a thorough history and physical examination (for the presence of murmurs signifying stenosis or insufficiency) as well as an echocardiogram. Exercise stress testing may be considered to see if subjects can increase their SBP during exercise, as well as to see if exercise can be performed without evidence of ischemia. Patients with residual stenosis should be restricted from vigorous static or isometric activities. Patients with mild or moderate aortic insufficiency, with normal or only mildly increased left ventricular size, may participate in all activities and sports, except vigorous static sports. If a patient has dysrhythmias with activity, an evaluation by a pediatric cardiologist is warranted (1).

COARCTATION OF THE AORTA

Coarctation of the aorta is a narrowing of the aorta at the level of the juxtaductal or juxtaligamental area that is located between the distal transverse aortic arch and the proximal descending thoracic aorta. It occurs as an isolated defect in 8 to 10% of all congenital heart disease. Elevated blood pressure occurs in the arms with a lower blood pressure in the legs. Normally, the blood pressure in the lower extremities is 10 to 20 mm Hg higher than it is in the upper extremities because of amplification of the pulse wave as it travels toward the peripheral arteries. In the presence of a coarctation, physical examination reveals a discrepancy between the upper and lower extremity pulses and an arm-to-leg blood pressure difference. Patients may also be hypertensive in their right arms (precoarctation). These differences in blood pressure are exaggerated during exercise.

Correction of the coarctation is performed percutaneously in the cardiac catheterization laboratory using a balloon, or the correction may be performed surgically. Repair is usually considered adequate if a residual gradient between the upper and lower extremity blood pressures is less than 20 mm Hg. Problems encountered following a repair include residual stenosis, left ventricular hypertrophy, systemic hypertension, or a residual obstruction that is only evident with exercise.

Traditionally, exercise stress testing was essential in the management of children and adults who had a coarctation repair (a) to evaluate the hemodynamic success of the repair, (b) to provide objective information for individual recommendations of physical activity, and (c) to determine if residual hypertension should be treated with medication or repaired by further surgery or balloon angioplasty (22).

A recent study has suggested that in the postoperative patient, a positive arm-to-leg exercise gradient partially represents a physiologic circulatory adaptation to ergometry and is, therefore, not appropriate to evaluate residual narrowing. Exercise-induced hypertension of the arms late after coarctation repair may be caused by impaired arterial reactivity that results from structural or functional abnormalities or both. This study suggests that

other diagnostic modalities such as echocardiography should be used to evaluate residual coarctation that may be present (23). Patients who have had coarctation repairs also commonly manifest excessive reliance on anaerobic metabolism during exercise. This phenomenon may result in persistent blood flow abnormalities across the aortic arch during exercise, which may be present even after apparently successful surgery (24).

Evaluation after repair should include a history and physical examination, as well as careful measurement of blood pressures in both arms and one leg. Exercise stress testing is often used to reveal a gradient across the area of repair. If this gradient is >20 mm Hg or if the patient has decreased ventricular function (assessed by echocardiogram) or exercise-induced systemic hypertension, the patient should be restricted to lower-intensity activities and should refrain from high static activities. Collision sports should be restricted for 1 year following surgery (1).

TETRALOGY OF FALLOT

Tetralogy of Fallot is defined by four abnormalities: (a) a large nonrestrictive ventricular septal defect, (b) aortic override of the VSD, (c) infundibular pulmonary stenosis, and (d) right ventricular hypertrophy. Tetralogy of Fallot occurs in about 6% of congenital heart disease and is the most common form of cyanotic cardiac disease. Complete repair of this defect is usually performed in the first year of life.

Repair of tetralogy of Fallot includes closure of the VSD and opening up of the right ventricular outflow tract. The latter often requires a transannular pulmonary incision and placement of a pericardial patch on the right ventricular outflow tract. In addition, there is commonly a need to augment the main and branch pulmonary arteries by placing patch material in these locations. Postoperative complications include residual VSDs, residual right ventricular outflow tract obstruction, pulmonary artery stenosis, dysrhythmias of either atrial or ventricular origin, conduction problems (most commonly right bundle-branch block or complete atrioventricular [AV] block), and ventricular dysfunction.

Following intracardiac repair, 80 to 85% of patients have normal working capacity with exercise testing. Decreased exercise capacity is related to the degree of pulmonary insufficiency and the presence of abnormal right ventricular function. Patients with severe pulmonary insufficiency often show an increased exercise capacity following placement of a valve conduit in the right ventricular outflow tract (25).

The HR response to exercise is decreased at maximal and submaximal levels of exercise and may be secondary to sinus node dysfunction. After complete repair, the cardiac output is normal at rest and may be normal in response to exercise (26–28).

Patients with mild pulmonary insufficiency and mild residual right ventricular outflow tract obstruction have no functional limitations. Ventricular dysrhythmias occur in up to 73% of patients after repair in some studies and are related to the outcome of surgery and length of time since repair (29). A Holter unit should be used to monitor HR because cardiac dysrhythmias are frequent after tetralogy of Fallot repair. Most of these patients, however, will be asymptomatic.

Patients should be evaluated with a thorough history, physical examination, echocardiogram, and an exercise stress test prior to participation in activities and competitive sports. Those with a significant residual defect (significant stenosis, residual shunts, or pulmonary insufficiency) should be restricted until fully evaluated. Those with residual pulmonary outflow gradients of <40 mm Hg who are asymptomatic may participate fully in all activities and sports. Small residual VSDs do not necessitate restriction of activities. Often the ventricular function is mildly depressed. If this is the case, patients should be restricted from vigorous static activities. Patients who have had repair of tetralogy of Fallot often exhibit progression of these residual defects. Therefore, they should be evaluated every year while participating in competitive sports (1).

TRANSPOSITION OF THE GREAT ARTERIES

Transposition of the great arteries occurs in about 5% of all patients with congenital heart disease. In this defect, the aorta (which should arise posteriorly from the left ventricle) arises anteriorly from the right ventricle and the pulmonary artery (which should arise anteriorly from the right ventricle) arises posteriorly from the left ventricle. This results in a parallel circuit instead of circulation in a series. Patients with transposition of the great arteries

have surgery early in life with either a baffling in the atria (Mustard or Senning procedure) or an arterial switch operation.

The arterial switch operation is most commonly used at present. Surgery involves transecting the great arteries above the valve annulus and anastomosing them to the proximal end of the other great artery. The coronary arteries must also be transferred. There is a risk that the coronaries can be kinked or become stenotic after reimplantation. Coronary stenosis may occur as a long-term complication and appears to occur more frequently when the pattern of the coronary arteries is complicated or if there is an associated single coronary artery. Other postoperative complications include narrowing of the pulmonary artery at the anastomotic site in 5 to 10% of patients, complete heart block in 5 to 10% of patients, and aortic regurgitation as a late development in up to 20% of patients.

During exercise testing, these individuals generally have normal $\dot{V}O_2$ but may experience ST-T wave changes that are usually of no clinical significance. These patients rarely have coronary artery ischemia (30–32).

Patients who have had an atrial baffle procedure (Mustard or Senning operation) continue to use the anatomic right ventricle as the systemic ventricle. The pulmonary venous drainage is baffled to the systemic right ventricle and the systemic venous drainage is baffled to the left ventricle. This procedure allows the unoxygenated blood to be pumped out to the pulmonary artery by the left ventricle and the oxygenated blood to be pumped out of the aorta by the right ventricle. Complications associated with these procedures include baffle obstruction, dilatation or poor function of the right ventricle, pulmonary stenosis, tricuspid insufficiency (which is the systemic AV valve), and significant atrial or ventricular dysrhythmias. The functional reserve and durability of the right ventricle is intrinsically lower than that of the left ventricle. Changes resulting from exercise in a systemic right ventricle, which must support the peripheral blood flow and blood pressure, are unknown. Changes in the left ventricle with exercise training include increased muscle mass and enlargement of the chamber for an increased stroke volume. It is not known if these changes will occur in the right ventricle, which now functions as a systemic ventricle, in those patients who have undergone an atrial baffle repair.

Patients with atrial baffle procedure often are asymptomatic when performing usual levels of activity, generally lead normal lives, and participate in most school activities (33). Nevertheless, over half of patients who have undergone an atrial baffle will exhibit important abnormalities during exercise tests. They demonstrate decreased cardiac output and decreased exercise performance secondary to a limited stroke volume and a blunted peak HR response. They also have decreased peak $\dot{V}O_2$ ($\dot{V}O_{2peak}$) and an abnormal ventilatory anaerobic threshold. They also fatigue sooner than control subjects. Work performance is approximately 70 to 80% of normal, and the maximal HR is 75 to 85% of normal. Approximately 70% have a low resting HR. Sinus rhythm is present in only 77% of these patients at 5 years and 40% at 20 years after repair. The systemic ventricular function is abnormal in 60% of patients, and 84% have abnormal right (systemic) ventricular function. Baffle obstruction occurs in 10 to 20% of patients, and pulmonary venous obstruction is present in approximately 5% of patients (34–37).

Patients should have a thorough history, physical examination, chest x-ray, ECG, Holter monitor (to evaluate 24-h HR and rhythm), echocardiogram, and exercise stress test prior to participating in competitive sports. Patients who have a normal heart size, no residual defects, normal ventricular function, no dysrhythmias, and a normal exercise study may participate in all sports except very high static activities. If patients have residual defects, their activities may be restricted as directed by their pediatric cardiologist (1).

THE FONTAN OPERATION (SINGLE VENTRICLE, TRICUSPID ATRESIA, HYPOPLASTIC LEFT HEART)

Patients with a single ventricle vary according to their underlying cardiac defect, including, but not limited to, a hypoplastic left heart syndrome, tricuspid atresia, and pulmonary atresia with intact ventricular septum. The emphasis of surgery for these disorders now is a staged approach, reaching a Fontan operation at completion. Patients with this anatomy frequently have previous shunts to increase the pulmonary blood flow prior to the completion of their Fontan procedure.

The Fontan procedure attempts to separate oxygenated blood from the unoxygenated blood by a combination of operations. This is accomplished by attaching the superior vena cava to the right pulmonary artery and baffling or shunting the inferior vena cava blood to the pulmonary arteries directly. This procedure shunts venous blood directly to the pulmonary arteries without the benefit of pulsatile flow provided by the beating heart. Oxygenated blood returns to the heart via the pulmonary veins and is pumped by the single ventricle to the body via the aorta. A fenestration or a hole may be made in the baffle or shunt, allowing blood to flow from the venous circuit to the systemic circuit, resulting in a right-to-left shunt. These patients are often cyanotic, especially during exercise.

The exercise tolerance of patients with single ventricles is lower than that of patients with structurally normal hearts. Right-to-left intracardiac shunting and chronotropic insufficiency contribute to the lower exercise tolerance. Exercise requiring high static loads may also be poorly tolerated as a result of the anatomy of the underlying ventricle. If this ventricle is an anatomic right ventricle, patients have a fixed stroke volume and can increase cardiac output only by increasing HR during exercise. Following the Fontan procedure, there is increased risk of atrial dysrhythmias because of the extensive atrial surgery involved in the repair. Other postoperative complications include poor ventricular function, baffle or shunt obstruction, and the development of pulmonary arteriovenous fistula, which cause increasing cyanosis.

During exercise testing, these patients have decreased peak HR, decreased $\dot{V}O_{2peak}$, decreased stroke index, abnormal ventilatory anaerobic thresholds, and increased anaerobic metabolism during peak exercise (38–39). Some of these parameters may improve with training (40). Patients with single ventricle anatomy should refrain from competitive athletics and most high static activities (1).

Guidelines for Pediatric Exercise Testing

Exercise testing of children differs from adult exercise testing in many ways beyond the technical issues related to the test performance that were addressed in the guidelines published by the American Heart Association (41). The precise role of exercise testing in patient evaluation or long-term management of the cardiac patient varies depending upon the indication for the study and the information being sought. Exercise testing, however, is often essential to diagnose and to direct treatment in a wide variety of clinical problems. The staff of the pediatric exercise laboratory should be aware of the expected findings in patients with congenital heart disease, as well as the appropriate indications for terminating a test.

Patients with severe valvular aortic stenosis may develop ischemic ST changes or a decreased blood pressure response to exercise. Patients with coarctation of the aorta may develop severe hypertension and a diminished work capacity. Patients with unrepaired cyanotic heart disease may experience profound desaturation and ischemia during exercise. They rarely experience neurologic changes. Patients who have undergone corrective surgery may develop significant dysrhythmias requiring termination of the test. In general, however, exercise stress testing is a safe method to evaluate the exercise capacity and tolerance of patients with congenital heart disease (41).

General Considerations for Prescribing Exercise

All patients, regardless of their cardiac diagnosis and previous treatment, must be as active as possible. This is especially important because treatment of these patients is improving, and they are living longer than ever before. Their activity, however, must be safe. Before designing an exercise program for these patients, the health care provider (physician, exercise specialist, health center director) must have a basic knowledge of the patient's diagnosis and previous treatment.

Adhering to the information presented in this chapter, further diagnostic tests may be required before initiating an exercise program. This often requires obtaining medical records to acquire a complete understanding of the previous congenital heart disease. Specific recommendations regarding sports or activity participation by any patient with congenital heart disease are necessary. Recommended sports or activities should be discussed with both patient and parents and should include

interests outside traditional athletics. The expectations and interests of the family and patient must be considered along with the expected clinical course of the disease and any limitations that the disease may impose. For example, it would be inappropriate for someone with moderate or severe valvular aortic stenosis to become interested in sports requiring isometric activity (wrestling, weight lifting, football, etc.). These patients, however, should be encouraged to participate in certain aerobic activities such as running. In contrast, patients with mild congenital heart disease or with a good surgical repair should be reassured and encouraged to lead fully normal lives with physical activities.

Summary

- All children, including those with congenital heart disease, need to be active.
- This activity must be safe.
- All children with congenital heart disease (repaired or unrepaired) must be evaluated to define the limits of safe activity.
- This evaluation may require referral to a specialist familiar with congenital heart defects.
- This evaluation should be repeated periodically to ensure the ongoing safety of the activity.

REFERENCES

1. Maron BJ, Mitchell JH. 26th Bethesda conference: Recommendations for determining eligibility for competition in athletes with cardiovascular abnormalities. J Am Coll Cardiol 1994;24:846–899.
2. Kaplan S, Perloff JK. Exercise and athletics before and after cardiac surgery or interventional catheterization. In: Perloff JK, Child JS, eds. Congenital Heart Disease in Adults. Philadelphia: WB Saunders. 1991:189–199.
3. Liberthson RR. Arrhythmias in the athlete with congenital heart disease: guidelines for participation. Annu Rev Med 1999;50:441–452.
4. Virmani R, Burke AP, Farb A, et al. Causes of sudden death in young and middle-aged competitive athletes. Cardiol Clin 1997;15:439–466.
5. Liberthson RR. Sudden death from cardiac causes in children and young adults. N Engl J Med 1996;334:1039–1044.
6. Duffie ER, Adams FH. The use of the working capacity test in the evaluation of children with congenital heart disease. Pediatrics 1963;32:757–768.

7. Frick M, Punsar S, Somer T. The spectrum of cardiac capacity in patients with nonobstructive congenital heart disease. Am J Cardiol 1966;17:20–26.

8. Reybrouck T, Weymans M, Stijns H, et al. Ventilatory anaerobic threshold for evaluating exercise performance in children with congenital left-to-right intracardiac shunt. Pediatr Cardiol 1986;7:19–24.

9. Petersson PO. Atrial septal defect of secundum type, clinical findings before and after operation. Acta Paediatr Scand 1967;174:19–27.

10. Rosenthal M, Redington A, Bush A. Cardiopulmonary physiology after surgical closure of asymptomatic secundum atrial septal defects in childhood. Exercise performance is unaffected by age at repair. Eur Heart J 1997;18:1816–1822.

11. Meijboom F, Hess J, Szatmari A, et al. Long-term followup 9 to 20 years after surgical closure of atrial septal defects at a young age. Am J Cardiol 1993;72:1431–1434.

12. Wolfe RR, Bartle L, Daberkow E, et al. Exercise responses in ventricular septal defect. Prog Pediatr Cardiol 1993;2:24–29.

13. Gabriel HM, Heger M, Innerhofer P, et al. Long-term outcome of patients with ventricular septal defect considered not to require surgical closure during childhood. J Am Coll Cardiol 2002;39:1066–1071.

14. Meijboom F, Szatmari A, Utens E. Long-term followup after surgical closure of ventricular septal defect in infancy and childhood. J Am Coll Cardiol 1994;24:1358–1364.

15. Steinberger J, Moller JH. Exercise testing in children with pulmonary valve stenosis. Pediatr Cardiol 1999;20:27–31.

16. Reybrouck T, Rogers R, Weymans M, et al. Serial cardiorespiratory exercise testing in patients with congenital heart disease. Eur J Pediatr 1995;154:801–806.

17. Krabill KA, Wang Y, Enzig S, et al. Rest and exercise hemodynamics in pulmonary stenosis: comparison of children and adults. Am J Cardiol 1985;56:360–365.

18. Atwood JE, Kawanishi S, Myers J, et al. Exercise testing in patients with aortic stenosis. Chest 1988;93:1083–1087.

19. James FW. Exercise response in aortic stenosis. Prog Pediatr Cardiol 1993;2:1–7.

20. Amato MC, Moffa PJ, Werner KE, et al. Treatment decision in asymptomatic aortic valve stenosis: role of exercise testing. Heart 2001;86:381–386.

21. Phillips JR, Daniels CJ, Orsinelli DA, et al. Valvular hemodynamics and arrhythmias with exercise following the Ross procedure. Am Coll Cardiol 2001;87:577–583.

22. Rocchini AS. Exercise evaluation after repair of coarctation of the aorta. Prog Pediatr Cardiol 1993;2:14–19.

23. Guenthard J, Wyler F. Exercise-induced hypertension in the arms due to impaired arterial reactivity after successful coarctation resection. Am J Cardiol 1995;75:814–817.

24. Rhodes J, Geggel RL, Marx GR, et al. Excessive anaerobic metabolism during exercise after repair of aortic coarctation. J Pediatr 1997;131:210–214.

25. Eyskens B, Reybrouck T, Bogaert J, et al. Homograft insertion for pulmonary regurgitation after repair of tetralogy of Fallot improves cardiorespiratory exercise performance. Am J Cardiol 2000;85:221–225.

26. Wessel HU, Paul MH. Exercise studies in tetralogy of Fallot: a review. Pediatr Cardiol 1999;20:39–47.

27. Mulla N, Simpson P, Sullivan NM, et al. Determinants of aerobic capacity during exercise following a complete repair of tetralogy of Fallot with a transannular patch. Pediatr Cardiol 1997;18:350–356.

28. Tomassoni TL, Galioto FM, Vaccaro P. Cardiopulmonary exercise testing in children following surgery for tetralogy of Fallot. Am J Dis Child 1991;145:1290–1293.

29. Ross-Hesselink J, Perlroth MG, McGahie J, et al. Atrial arrhythmias in adults after repair of tetralogy of Fallot. Correlations with clinical, exercise, and echocardiographic findings. Circulation 1995;91:2214–2219.

30. Mahle WT, McBride MG, Paridon SM. Exercise performance after arterial switch operation for d-transposition of the great arteries. Am J Cardiol 2001;87:753–758.

31. von Bernuth G. Twenty-five years after the first arterial switch procedure: midterm results. Thorac Cardiovasc Surg 2000;48:228–232.

32. Massin M, Hovels-Gurich H, Dabritz S, et al. Results of the Bruce treadmill test in children after arterial switch operation for simple transposition of the great arteries. Am J Cardiol 1998;81:56–60.

33. Paul MH, Wessel HU. Exercise studies in patients with transposition of great arteries after atrial repair operations (Mustard/Senning): a review. Pediatr Cardiol 1999;20:49–55.

34. Hechter SJ, Webb G, Fredriksen PM. Cardiopulmonary exercise performance in adult survivors of the Mustard procedure. Cardiol Young 2001;11:407–414.

35. Singh TP, Wolfe RR, Sullivan NM, et al. Assessment of progressive changes in exercise performance in patients with a systemic right ventricle following an atrial switch repair. Pediatr Cardiol 2001;22:210–214.

36. Douard H, Labbe L, Barat JL, et al. Cardiorespiratory response to exercise after venous switch operation for transposition of the great arteries. Chest 1997;111:23–29.

37. Reybrouck T, Gewillig M, Dumoulin M, et al. Cardiorespiratory exercise performance after Senning operation for transposition of the great arteries. Br Heart J 1993;20:175–179.

38. Durongpisitkul K, Driscoll DJ, Mahoney DW, et al. Cardiorespiratory response to exercise after modified Fontan operation: determinants of performance. J Am Coll Cardiol 1997;29:785–790.

39. Driscoll DJ, Durongpisitkul K. Exercise testing after the Fontan operation. Pediatr Cardiol 1999;20: 57–59.

40. Minamisawa S, Nakazawa M, Momma K, et al. Effective aerobic training on exercise performance in patients after a Fontan operation. Am J Cardiol 2001;88:695–698.

41. Washington RL, Bricker T, Alpert BS. Guidelines for exercise testing in the pediatric age group. Circulation 1994;90:2166–2179.

Other Conditions

23

End-Stage Renal Disease

Patricia L. Painter

Chronic renal failure (CRF) results from structural renal damage and progressively diminished renal function. Once initiated, the disease typically progresses to end-stage renal disease (ESRD), in which there is inadequate or nonexistent kidney function, requiring some form of renal replacement therapy such as dialysis or transplantation. In recent years, there were nearly 120,000 patients treated with dialysis in the United States. Another 9000 received kidney transplants (1,2).

The initial damage to the kidney may be the result of long-standing hypertension, vascular changes associated with diabetes mellitus, autoimmune processes, chronic infection, congenital abnormalities, or other unknown causes. Although the rate of progression to end-stage varies, the biochemical, endocrine, and metabolic disorders associated with decreased renal function are similar, regardless of the initial cause of dysfunction. Progressive renal failure results in the loss of both excretory and regulatory functions of the kidney. The gradual deterioration of function is monitored clinically by serum levels of blood urea nitrogen (BUN) and creatinine. The inability to excrete substances results in a condition known as uremia, which is characterized by fatigue, nausea, malaise, anorexia, and subtle neurologic symptoms. Uremia secondarily impairs the function of other metabolic and organ systems.

Treatment of progressive renal failure consists of medical management (with aggressive dietary protein restriction) until serum creatinine clearance is <5 mL·min^{-1}, at which time some form of renal replacement therapy is required—either dialysis or transplantation.

There are two forms of dialysis available to patients with CRF. Hemodialysis is the most common form, with approximately 79% of all patients treated in a clinical center or at home. This is a process of ultrafiltration (fluid removal) and clearance of excess toxic solutes from the blood. It necessitates the placement of an arteriovenous (a-v) fistula in the arm or leg, from which the blood is removed from the body at a rate of 200 to 300 mL·min^{-1} (the total amount of blood extracorporeal at one time never exceeds 500 mL). The blood is passed through a dialyzing chamber, across a semipermeable membrane that separates the blood from a dialysis fluid. The osmotic gradient and osmolar concentration of this dialysis fluid is controlled to draw specific molecular weight substances and excess fluids from the blood. The blood is then returned to the body through the a-v fistula. The hemodialysis treatment requires between 2.5 and 4 hours to complete and must be done three times per week. Side effects of the treatment may include fatigue, hypertension, cramping, and general malaise (3). Hemodialysis therapy requires such additional therapeutic measures as anticoagulants, replacement of vitamins and other required substances that may be removed by dialysis, and administration of human recombinant erythropoietin to increase red blood cell production.

Another form of dialysis, which is used by approximately 14% of patients with CRF, is peritoneal dialysis (3). This therapy uses the peritoneal membranes for ultrafiltration of fluids and clearance of toxic substances by introduction of a dialysis fluid into the peritoneal cavity through a permanent catheter placed in the abdominal wall. This fluid is introduced over a 12-hour period by a machine that cycles the fluid continuously (continuous cycling peritoneal dialysis) or manually through 2-L bags, which are changed every 4 hours during the day by the patient (continuous ambulatory peritoneal dialysis).

Although dialysis therapy is life sustaining, patients still experience significant clinical problems including renal osteodystrophy with significant orthopedic concerns, decreased growth, muscle weakness and cramping, peripheral neuropathy, hypertension, accelerated atherosclerosis, anemia, and a wide variety of electrolyte imbalances and hormonal/metabolic derangements. Cardiovascular dysfunction in dialysis patients is common and is secondary to several factors: such hemodynamic factors as pressure and volume overload; such metabolic factors as acidosis, anemia, electrolyte abnormalities, abnormal lipid metabolism, and uremic toxins; and such pathologic factors as coronary artery disease, infectious endocarditis, left ventricular hypertrophy, pericardial disease, and myocardial calcification. Any or all of these may be present and result in electrocardiographic (ECG) abnormalities, cardiomegaly, congestive heart failure, and/or dysrhythmias. Additionally, patients and their families must face significant psychosocial issues as part of dealing with a chronic, life-threatening disease and dependence on the health care community and a machine for maintenance of life (3).

Renal transplantation has become the treatment of choice for most patients with ESRD. Approximately 28% of all patients receive transplants. Kidneys are obtained from either a living relative (family member) or a cadaver (2). Patients with severe cardiac, cerebrovascular, or pulmonary disease and neoplasia are not considered appropriate candidates for transplant. Extensive immunologic

studies are performed on recipients and donors to minimize the immunologic response to the transplanted kidney that results in rejection of the organ. When an appropriate immunologic match is found, it is placed in the extrailiac position, attached to the iliac artery. Following the transplant, patients must take immunosuppressive medications, which typically include prednisone and cyclosporine, although the combinations and dosages may vary between centers. Most metabolic, endocrine, and biochemical derangements of uremia are corrected following transplantation. Complications following kidney transplantation are primarily related to immunosuppressive therapy, with infection and side effects of the medications becoming problematic for many patients.

Transplant recipients are at a higher risk for developing cardiovascular disease than the general population (4–6). This risk is associated independently with cumulative dosage of prednisone, lipid abnormalities, hypertension, and smoking (7). Weight gain is a significant problem following transplantation and may result from one or a combination of factors: increased appetite secondary to prednisone, removal of restrictions in the diet, and food tasting better. Long-term corticosteroid therapy may result in osteonecrosis, particularly affecting the hip, knee, and shoulder joints. Although psychosocial issues may be less evident following transplantation, the stress of uncertainty of rejection is consistently present. Additionally, patients experience financial stresses associated with employment and medical insurance payment of medications.

Functional Status

The functional status of patients with ESRD is severely reduced. Gutman et al. reported that of 2481 dialysis patients interviewed, only 50% of the nondiabetic population and 23% of the diabetic patients were capable of physical activity beyond caring for themselves (8). Significant efforts have been made by many researchers to assess and document functional status in ESRD patients (9–13). Data from questionnaires and interviews show that significant numbers of patients report limitations in various physical tasks. In a population of 430 dialysis patients aged 56 ± 14 years, 36% could not perform routine living chores without assistance. Only 32% participated in any activities outside of their dialysis regimen. Of the diabetic subgroup in this study, 68% were limited in all activities to their residence because of physical debilitation (10). Kutner et al. (12–14) report that older adults on chronic dialysis were significantly more immobile on a daily basis and reported significantly more difficulty in bathing, climbing stairs, walking several blocks, and performing heavy household chores than a similar-aged group of persons without renal disease.

Patients with ESRD treated with dialysis have very low self-reported levels of physical functioning (i.e., as measured by questionnaires such as the SF-36) (15–18). The levels reported are similar to those reported by patients with congestive heart failure and with chronic obstructive pulmonary disease (19,20).

EXERCISE CAPACITY

Cardiorespiratory fitness levels in patients treated with dialysis are reported to be low (Fig. 23-1). Studies of the direct measurement of maximal aerobic power ($\dot{V}O_{2peak}$) report values only half of those expected for normal subjects of the same age. $\dot{V}O_{2peak}$ values reported are those in "the best" (i.e., no other coexisting medical conditions), thus

those unable to perform such testing are even lower. $\dot{V}O_{2peak}$ in hemodialysis patients range from 15.3 to 21.0 $mL \cdot kg^{-1} \cdot min^{-1}$ (21–37). Patients treated with peritoneal dialysis do not differ significantly from hemodialysis patients (25,32,38,39), with average $\dot{V}O_{2peak}$ levels of 21.1 $mL \cdot kg^{-1} \cdot min^{-1}$. Exercise capacity may be even lower in patients with other coexisting medical problems, who are more representative of the general dialysis populations (25,40).

One of the major limiting factors to exercise in ESRD may be anemia. Correction of the anemia of CRF with human recombinant erythropoietin (EPO) has resulted in significant increases in exercise capacity (about 17%), but even with correction of the anemia, $\dot{V}O_{2peak}$ levels remain low (17.6 $mL \cdot kg^{-1} \cdot min^{-1}$) (21,34,35,41).

Other conditions that may limit exercise capacity in dialysis patients include autonomic dysfunction, which may limit the increase in heart rate (HR) during exercise; cardiovascular dysfunction, which may limit the stroke volume increase during exercise; and abnormal peripheral metabolism and/or skeletal muscle function. Thus, both central and peripheral limitations may exist (25,33,42,43).

Diesel et al. reported a more significant relationship between isokinetic muscle strength and $\dot{V}O_{2peak}$ than between $\dot{V}O_{2peak}$ and such oxygen transport factors as hemoglobin and hematocrit

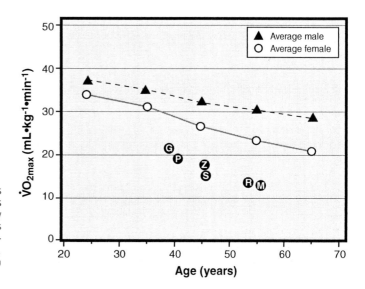

FIGURE 23-1 Reported $\dot{V}O_{2peak}$ values ($mL \cdot kg^{-1} \cdot min^{-1}$) of hemodialysis patients compared with values for normal sedentary males and females. Sedentary normal levels are as reported by the American Heart Association. G, Goldberg et al.; P, Painter et al; Z, Zabetakis et al.; S, Shalom et al.; R, Robertson et al.; M, Moore et al.

(23). This and several other reports of abnormal skeletal muscle structure and function (26,30,44,45) suggest that peripheral mechanisms are most important to exercise limitations in this patient group and are consistent with subjective reports of patients who experience significant muscle weakness with minimal activity.

The low exercise capacity is demonstrated in physical performance tests. In a study that included many patients who could not perform maximal exercise testing, Painter et al. (16,17) showed that dialysis patients have much lower scores than age-predicted values on a standard test of gait speed (64% of age-predicted values) and sit-to-stand test (24% of age-predicted values). At least part of the exercise limitation may be physical inactivity, because few patients receive counseling or encouragement to participate in exercise training. We found that only 8% of our in-center hemodialysis patients participated in a regular exercise program at home that involved activities other than necessary daily tasks (unpublished data). Measurement of physical activity in dialysis patients using accelerometers showed that they were significantly less active than age-matched controls (46).

Exercise capacity increases dramatically following successful kidney transplantation (47,48). The removal of the uremic state may in some way remove some of the physiologic limitations to exercise mentioned above in dialysis patients, because transplantation corrects most metabolic, endocrine, and biochemical derangements. The initial increases in exercise capacity may be related only to the physiologic improvements resulting from transplantation, because reportedly physical activity levels do not increase spontaneously. Gallagher (47) reported initial increases in exercise capacity soon after transplantation but no further increases over the next 6 months. Similarly, patient participation in regular physical activity did not increase.

Patients who are physically active following transplantation can achieve normal (or higher) levels of $\dot{V}O_{2peak}$. In a cross-sectional study of participants in the 1996 U.S. Transplant Games, kidney transplant recipients who reported participation in regular physical activity had $\dot{V}O_{2peak}$ levels that averaged 102% of age-predicted values; inactive recipients averaged 86% of age-predicted values (49). The values for the inactive transplant recipients were similar to those reported for well-trained dialysis patients.

Exercise-Training Effects

Exercise conditioning programs consistently increase exercise capacity in hemodialysis patients (Fig. 23-2). Increases in $\dot{V}O_{2peak}$ between 2 and 42% (average of 16.4% across studies) have been reported following training programs lasting 3 to 12 months (21,26,30,31,34,36,37,50,51). Patients with other coexisting medical problems may

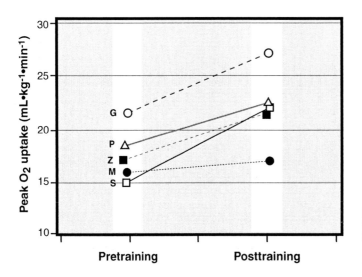

FIGURE 23-2 Changes in $\dot{V}O_{2peak}$ ($mL \cdot kg^{-1} \cdot min^{-1}$) with exercise training in hemodialysis patients. G, Goldberg et al.; P, Painter et al.; Z, Zabetakis et al.; S, Shalom et al.; M, Moore et al.

exhibit less improvement in peak exercise capacity. Improvement on physical performance tests was also reported following exercise training in the Renal Exercise Demonstration Project (16,17). This project also showed significant improvements in self-reported functioning on the SF-36 questionnaire.

Cardiovascular risk factors may improve after exercise training in this patient group, including improved lipid profiles (decreased triglycerides and [very-low-density lipoprotein] VLDL-cholesterol plus increased [high-density lipoprotein] HDL-cholesterol) (50); improved glucose metabolism (decreased fasting insulin with improved insulin binding and glucose disappearance rates) (50); and improved blood pressure (31,52).

Renal transplant recipients respond to exercise training with increased $\dot{V}O_{2peak}$ (53–55). Exercise training increases skeletal muscle strength in these patients, which is important, because prednisone therapy results in significant muscle weakness (e.g., renal transplant patients have quadriceps strength values that average only 70% of normal sedentary levels (56). Transplant recipients have been shown to normalize muscle strength through resistance training (56). No studies of the effects of exercise training on cardiovascular risk factors in transplant recipients have been reported.

Exercise Testing Considerations

The use of exercise testing in patients with ESRD prior to starting an exercise program is difficult to assess (57). Assuming that the reasons for performing an exercise test prior to initiating exercise training are to define the degree of risk associated with increasing exercise intensity and to establish the ap-

propriate exercise intensity for exercise prescription, the dialysis patient presents some specific challenges to some basic principles of exercise testing for the following reasons (summarized in Table 23-1).

1. The peak exercise capacity in this patient group is very low and, in most cases, similar to the metabolic cost of activities of daily living. Thus, if patients do not present with symptoms during activities of daily living, predictably exercise testing may not provide more information about their cardiac status. Skeletal muscle fatigue limits exercise for most patients, which prevents them from attaining enough myocardial stress to induce electrocardiographic changes or symptoms, thereby limiting the diagnostic information obtained. In terms of exercise prescription, the results of an exercise test on one day may not apply on another day when the patient is fluid overloaded because of dietary indiscretion or volume depleted by aggressive dialysis treatment. The changing physiology of these patients poses problems in applying the test results to all possible days.

2. Most studies of dialysis patients report low peak exercise HRs, which average less than 75% of age-predicted levels. In a group of 337 patients tested on the cycle ergometer, the average was 70% of age-predicted levels. This is well below the 85% of age-predicted levels needed to ensure adequate myocardial stress diagnostic reliability of the test. It has been suggested that muscle contractile function limits power generation, thus limiting heart rate response (58). Whether the limited heart rate response is due to autonomic neuropathy, uremic neuropathy, and/or peripheral limitations, the exercise ECG is an unreliable diagnostic criterion for coronary artery disease.

3. Most patients on hemodialysis exhibit abnormal resting ECGs, which may affect the interpretation of ischemia during exercise. Conditions (e.g., long-standing left-ventricular hypertrophy, electrolyte abnormalities, and digitalis preparations) may be present and result in exercise ECGs that are uninterpretable for ischemia. Dysrhythmias noted at rest or during exercise may actually be related to the electrolyte and/or acid–base status of the patient at that time; this could change after a dialysis treatment and might not result from underlying cardiac pathology.

TABLE 23-1   FACTORS THAT MAY COMPLICATE ECG INTERPRETATION IN RENAL DIALYSIS PATIENTS

Long-standing left ventricular hypertrophy
Electrolyte abnormalities
Attenuated heart rate responses to exercise (maximal heart rates of <85% of age-predicted values)
Peripheral limitations to exercise
Very low peak exercise capacity
Medications (e.g., digitalis preparations)

---

4. Blood pressure responses to exercise may also be affected by the changing physiologic status: *(a)* the fluid status of the patient may fluctuate dramatically, depending on compliance with dietary and fluid recommendations as well as on fluid removal during dialysis, and *(b)* antihypertensive therapy may include a prescription of medication to be taken at or above a given systolic pressure or a prescription to skip a dose before dialysis to avoid dialysis-related hypotension and/or removal of the medication by dialysis. In our experience, only 36% of 337 patients had resting systolic pressures below 140 mm Hg (59). The average increase in systolic pressure was 22 mm Hg/metabolic equivalent (MET). This excessive blood pressure response to very low level exercise is typical and illustrates the difficulty in regulating blood pressure in these patients.

Patients tolerate symptom-limited exercise testing well. The most common reason for stopping tests is leg (skeletal muscle) fatigue; the second is abnormal hypertensive responses to the exercise.

Obviously, the requirement for exercise testing prior to initiating exercise training is the decision of the medical director of the dialysis or transplant unit and/or of the exercise therapy program. However, such a requirement presents a significant barrier to beginning an exercise training program that will be of very low level intensity and may be costly and not useful for diagnostic purposes (57). For evaluation of benefits resulting from exercise training, this author recommends use of standard physical performance tests such as gait speed, sit-to-stand tests, and stair climbing (40).

1. Timing of the test. Most patients feel best and are more "normal" physiologically on a nondialysis day. Testing immediately prior to dialysis may result in more frequent dysrhythmias, more symptoms of shortness of breath, and lower exercise tolerance because of excess fluid and electrolyte elevations. Testing immediately following dialysis has been done without problems by some (36), but our experience has been a high incidence of symptomatic postexercise hypotension. This was probably due to volume depletion from dialysis, with maximal vasoconstrictive compensation for maintenance of blood pressure. When exercise was applied and the vasodilation occurred, the patient was unable to compensate further to maintain pressure. When using testing to evaluate effects of training, one must perform the tests at the same time in relation to the dialysis treatment.

2. The test protocol. If exercise testing is performed, the test should start at a very low exercise intensity (probably 1.5 METs) and increase very gradually with 0.5 METs per stage. This protocol allows more stages and more physiologic measurements. It also encourages patients psychologically and allows progress at a reasonable pace. Patient experience with the Bruce protocol are typically negative and discouraging—they cannot stay with the protocol for any length of time because of the inappropriate starting levels and large increments in intensity per stage.

3. Type of testing. Because leg fatigue is the primary endpoint, treadmill exercise may be most appropriate because of the localized leg fatigue associated with cycle ergometry. However, for patients who have bone or joint discomfort with weight-bearing activities, cycle ergometry may be more appropriate. Again, physical performance testing is preferred to facilitate low-level fitness levels and ensure that most patients will be able to perform the testing.

4. Physiologic measurements. Standard physiologic measurements should be made during exercise testing. In light of the changing physiologic condition of these patients, the use of a rating of perceived exertion (RPE) scale is also highly recommended and should be fully explained to the patient, with the goal of understanding how this measure can be an important guide for regulating exercise training intensity.

Standard practice for exercise testing should be applied to renal transplant recipients. The only modifications in exercise protocol would be in the case of patients with orthopedic limitations, for whom non-weight-bearing exercise testing should be used (e.g., cycle ergometry).

Exercise Prescription

Exercise training for patients treated with dialysis will be very low level and should progress gradually according to individual tolerances. The exercise training should begin as soon as the patient is stabilized on dialysis. Following transplantation, exercise training should begin as soon as clinically appropriate (within 1 week) after surgery to ensure that the patient and family consider regular exercise an integral part of the transplant therapy. The following are specific considerations.

TYPE OF PROGRAM

Hemodialysis patients have a high prevalence of cardiac risk factors, and the prevalence of cardiac disease is also high. Thus, according to available guidelines, they should probably exercise in a supervised setting with personnel trained to respond to a medical emergency. However, there may be problems in recommending such an approach in this population. First, very few such programs are available and Medicare (which covers 80% of their medical costs) does not cover supervised exercise training. Thus, the cost of participation in a cardiac rehabilitation program will be prohibitive for most patients. Second, considering the amount of time devoted to their disease and treatment (at least 3 hours per treatment, 3 days per week), it may be unreasonable to require patients to exercise in a supervised setting on 3 other days of the week. Third, considering the low peak exercise capacity, the level of prescribed exercise intensity will be very low, and the initial duration will be very limited, making the risk of the exercise program no more than that associated with the patient's daily activities. Thus, requiring the patient to participate in a supervised setting is unreasonable and will be unsuccessful.

An acceptable and highly recommended approach to exercise training for hemodialysis patients and one that alleviates many of these concerns is to have the patient use an exercise bicycle during the dialysis treatment (31). This involves no extra time, because patients are essentially a "captive audience," guaranteed to be there three times per week. It does not affect the dialysis treatment in any way, especially if performed within the first hour of treatment. The dialysis staff is prepared to respond to any emergency related to dialysis, which can include cardiac arrest, myocardial infarction, or other cardiovascular emergencies. Such a program is cost-effective in that the dialysis staff can be trained to set up the bicycle and help to motivate patients to participate and progress with their programs. Such a program does not necessarily incur additional costs, depending on the personnel involved. Exercise training during dialysis has been effective in increasing exercise capacity and modifying some cardiovascular risk factors (31). It has produced surprisingly high participation rates and was well accepted by patients and staff in a large multicenter clinical program.

If the dialysis clinic cannot provide the opportunity to exercise during treatment, home exercise (or at such community programs as the YMCA) must be encouraged (60). In this case, the following considerations are appropriate and are summarized in Table 23-2.

TIMING AND TYPE OF EXERCISE

Timing
Patients on hemodialysis may feel more like exercising on their nondialysis day. However, considering their low exercise capacity, patients should exercise daily, as tolerated. Patients treated with peritoneal dialysis may consider exercising during a dialysis "exchange" when the abdomen is empty of fluid. This may be more comfortable and may facilitate exercise at a higher intensity. Exercising "empty" may also reduce any risk of increased intraabdominal pressure causing leaks around the catheter.

Type
As discussed above, exercise training during the dialysis treatment can be performed only using a stationary cycle. Exercise off dialysis may incorporate any other mode of exercise. The only consideration would be for those with orthopedic problems to use a non-weight-bearing activity. Also, patients who are severely deconditioned may require muscle-strengthening exercises prior to being able to perform other activities for adequate conditioning.

Patients treated with peritoneal dialysis may participate in most activities; however, swimming will require special hygienic care of the catheter site (61). The dialysis staff should be consulted concerning this catheter care prior to starting a swimming program.

Transplant recipients should be very aware that activities that place significant stress on the joints (e.g., jogging) may cause problems secondary to prednisone use. Because only a few patients experience joint deterioration after transplant, jogging and such activities are not contraindicated, but the need for increased awareness of the body's response to exercise suggests that education on appropriate

TABLE 23-2 SPECIAL CONSIDERATIONS FOR EXERCISE PRESCRIPTION FOR EACH OF THE TREATMENT MODES OF END-STAGE RENAL DISEASE

Consideration	Hemodialysis	Peritoneal Dialysis	Transplant
Timing of exercise	Off-dialysis days During dialysis	During dialysis exchange	Start early posttransplant
Type of exercise			
Walking	No problems	No problems	No problems
Walk/jog	Bone/joint concerns Low exercise capacity	Bone/joint concerns Low exercise capacity	Bone/joint concerns
Stationary cycle	No problems	No problems	No problems
Swim	Low exercise capacity	Special catheter care Low exercise capacity	No concerns
Stair exercise	Low exercise capacity	Low exercise capacity	Recommended
Aerobics	Bone/joint concerns Low exercise capacity	Bone/joint concerns Low exercise capacity	Bone/joint concerns
Frequency	4–5 times/week	4–5 times/week	4–5 times/week
Duration			
Warm-up	3–5 min	3–5 min	3–5 min
Conditioning			
Initial	2–3 min/intervals	4–5 min/intervals	5–10 min/continuous
Goal	30 min/continuous	30 min/continuous	30 + min/continuous
Cool-down	5 min (longer during dialysis)	5 min	5 min
Intensity			
Warm-up	RPE 8–9	RPE 8–9	RPE 8–9
Conditioning	RPE 12–13	RPE 12–13	RPE 13–14(65–85% max HR)
Cool-down	RPE 8–9	RPE 8–9	RPE 8–9
Other considerations	Slow progression Realistic goals	Home program Weight control Slow progression Realistic goals	Strength training Weight control "Normal activities"

footwear and choice of exercise surfaces is essential. Strength training and/or stair exercise may also be important for patients following transplant, because the large muscle groups of the legs are most affected by the muscle-wasting properties of prednisone.

FREQUENCY, DURATION, AND INTENSITY OF EXERCISE

Frequency

Exercise should be performed 4 to 6 days per week, although exercise on dialysis days may be at a lower intensity. Most patients state that some type of physical activity every day helps prevent joint stiffness and bone pain. Initially after transplant, two sessions of exercise per day may be most appropriate to increase caloric expenditure. Leg muscle weakness may limit most patients in exercising continuously for enough time to counteract the increased caloric intake experienced after transplant.

Duration

Patients on dialysis typically have such a limited exercise capacity that interval exercise may have to be incorporated (work intervals of 2 min, followed by rest intervals of 1 min, and repeated as tolerated). The patient should then gradually increase the duration of the work intervals, working toward 30 min of continuous exercise.

Given that transplant patients typically are limited initially by leg muscle fatigue, exercise sessions starting with 5 min and progressing by 2 to 3 min each day (two sessions/day) are tolerated very well by most and ensure appropriate skeletal muscle adaptation to the increasing levels of exercise.

Intensity

Exercise intensity should be prescribed to dialysis patients with the RPE scale because of their abnormal HR responses to exercise. The relationship between the percentage of maximal HR and percentage of $\dot{V}O_{2peak}$ is 20% lower than in normal subjects(62). The changing fluid status of these patients may also change the HR response to exercise. If exercise is performed during the dialysis treatment, the very rapid changes in fluid may alter the HR responses, thus RPE prescription of intensity is recommended.

Autonomic dysfunction of uremia typically normalizes within 6 months of transplantation, making intensity prescription by HR appropriate at that time. Initially after transplant, however, medications are being adjusted, the patient is adjusting to a new physiology with the transplanted kidney, and it may be best to use RPE. This will accommodate the "ups and downs" experienced following transplantation and ensure that patients are "tuned in" to their bodies during the exercise session. Patients seem to understand the use of RPE and use it appropriately in most cases.

General Considerations

ESRD is a chronic condition that will result in death if some form of renal replacement therapy is not successfully and consistently implemented. Patients treated with dialysis are constantly confronted with their disease, which often results in significant psychologic adjustments. Thus, it is prudent to assess the psychologic status of the patient prior to initiating exercise training. For some, this intervention may definitely help in the adjustment, providing a way to make them feel "more normal." For others, however, the psychologic adjustment to chronic disease may be overwhelming, making participation in exercise training inappropriate and unreasonable until a later time.

Patients treated with dialysis are often fatigued and experience frequent hospitalizations, sometimes making it difficult for them to continue to progress with their exercise. They often find themselves "starting over." Encouragement and support from the health care staff is essential in this ongoing process. Patients may also change modalities of therapy. Some patients may choose or have

to change dialysis therapies secondary to infection or complications associated with the current treatment. Many dialysis patients (often the most healthy) will be called for transplantation. Some of these may experience rejection of the transplanted kidney, necessitating the return to dialysis to maintain life. Thus, the exercise prescription must be modified appropriately as the treatment changes.

After transplantation, patients may experience mild rejection episodes, which are often treated with medications that have adverse effects of varying severity. Patients often leave the hospital with the new kidney and progress extremely well with exercise, only to return for treatment of rejection. The medications cause the patient to have severe flulike symptoms that reduce energy levels significantly and last up to 6 to 8 weeks after the treatment. Patients must be encouraged to participate as tolerated and to progress gradually until the effects of the medications subside.

With any of these patients, one must be realistic about what benefits will be gained with exercise. Not all patients will increase their hematocrit or be able to control their blood pressure with regular exercise. However, data show that these positive benefits are possible and, therefore, worth seeking. The most certain result of regular exercise is increased functional capacity, making activities of daily living easier. Most patients experience feelings of increased energy (especially transplant recipients) with regular exercise and general feelings of well being. Exercise is an excellent way to focus attention and energy on health and away from disease. Exercise provides something patients *can* do and should be presented as a positive part of their medical therapy. For patients who depend on the medical community and a machine for their lives and who live with many restrictions, taking responsibility for their physical functioning may be the part of the treatment that has been missing.

Summary

- Patients with ESRD have extremely low exercise tolerance and require routine assessment of physical functioning and counseling for increasing physical activity.
- Exercise tolerance is limited by many factors associated with the disease and/or treatment that may

limit the levels achievable with exercise training. Thus, a goal of maintenance of functioning is a positive outcome from training, since most patients deteriorate over time to a point of physical disability.

- Standard exercise testing probably presents more of a barrier to initiating a program of exercise training and is limited in diagnostic utility. Standard tests of physical performance such as gait speed, sit-to-stand, and stair climbing are recommended to assess physical functioning and assess progress with exercise training.
- Patients with ESRD have changing medical status and often change treatment modes. Thus, continuous encouragement for physical activity is required when they experience medical setbacks.
- Dialysis staff and physicians should be educated about the importance of exercise for their patients and should consistently encourage patients to adopt and maintain a program of physical activity.

REFERENCES

1. United States Renal Data System. USRDS 1999 Annual Data Report. Bethesda, MD: National Institutes of Health, NIDDK, 1999.
2. United Network for Organ Sharing. UNOS Update 1996, Organ Procurement and Transplantation Network and Scientific Registry for Organ Transplantation, Richmond, VA, 1999.
3. Nissenson AR, Fine RN. Dialysis Therapy. 2nd ed. Philadelphia: Hanley & Belfus, 1993.
4. Kassiske BL. Risk factors for accelerated atherosclerosis in renal transplant recipients. Am J Med 1988;84:985–992.
5. Kassiske BL, Guijarro C, Massy ZA, et al. Cardiovascular disease after renal transplantation. J Am Soc Nephrol 1996;7:158–165.
6. Levey AS, Beto JA, Coronado BE, et al. Controlling the epidemic of cardiovascular disease in chronic renal disease: what do we know? what do we need to learn? where do we go from here? Am J Kidney Dis 1998;32:853–906.
7. Kassiske BL. Risk factors for cardiovascular disease after renal transplantation. Miner Electrolyte Metab 1993;19:186–195.
8. Gutman RA, Stead WW, Robinson RR. Physical activity and employment status of patients on maintenance dialysis. N Engl J Med 1981;304:309–313.
9. Ifudu O, Paul H, Mayers JD, et al. Pervasive failed rehabilitation in center-based maintenance hemodialysis patients. Am J Kidney Dis 1994;23:394–400.
10. Ifudu O, Mayers J, Matthew J, et al. Dismal rehabilitation in geriatric inner-city hemodialysis patients. JAMA 1994;271:29–33.
11. Kutner NG, Cardenas DD, Bower JD. Rehabilitation, aging, and chronic renal disease. Am J Phys Med Rehabil 1992;71:97–101.
12. Kutner NG, Brogan DJ. Assisted survival, aging, and rehabilitation needs: comparison of older adialysis and age-matched peers. Arch Phys Med Rehabil 1992;73:309–315.
13. Kutner NG, Zhang R, McClellan WM. Patient-reported quality of life early in dialysis treatment: effects associated with usual exercise activity. Nephrol Nurs J 2000;27:357–368.
14. Kutner N, Pianta T. Improving physical functioning in the dialysis patient: relevance of physical therapy. J Am Nephrol Nurse Assoc 1999;26:11–14.
15. DeOreo PB. Hemodialysis patient-assessed functional health status predicts continued survival, hospitalization and dialysis-attendance compliance. Am J Kidney Dis 1997;30:204–212.
16. Painter PL, Carlson L, Carey S, et al. Physical functioning and health related quality of life changes with exercise training in hemodialysis patients. Am J Kidney Dis 2000;35:482–492.
17. Painter PL, Carlson L, Carey S, et al. Low functioning patients improve with exercise training. Am J Kidney Dis 2000;36:600–608.
18. Braun-Curtin, R, Lowrie E, Deoreo P. Self-reported functional status: an important predictor of health outcomes among end-stage renal disease patients. Adv Renal Replacement Ther 1999;6:133–140.
19. Ware J. SF-36 Health Survey: Manual and Interpretation Guide. Boston: Health Institute, 1993.
20. Stewart AL, Greenfield R, Hays RD, et al. Functional status and well-being of patients with chronic conditions. JAMA 1989;262:907–913.
21. Akiba T, Matsui N, Shinohara S, et al. Effects of recombinant human erythropoietin and exercise training on exercise capacity in hemodialysis patients. Artif Organs 1995;19:1262–1268.
22. Barnea N, Drory Y, Iaina A, et al. Exercise tolerance in patients on chronic hemodialysis. Isr J Med Sci 1980;16:17–21.
23. Diesel W, Noakes TD, Swanepoel C, et al. Isokinetic muscle strength predicts maximum exercise tolerance in renal patients on chronic hemodialysis. Am J Kidney Dis 1990;16:109–114.
24. Goldberg AP, Hagberg JM, Delmez JA, et al. The metabolic and psychological effects of exercise training in hemodialysis patients. Am J Clin Nutr 1980;33:1620–1628.

25. Johansen KL. Physical functioning and exercise capacity in patients on dialysis. Adv Renal Replacement Ther 1999;6:141–148.

26. Kouidi E, Albani M, Natsis K, et al. The effects of exercise training on muscle atrophy in haemodialysis patients. Nephrol Dial Transplant 1998;13:685–699.

27. Lundin AP, Stein RA, Frank F. Cardiovascular status in long-term hemodialysis patients: an exercise and echocardiographic study. Nephron 1981;28:234–238.

28. Lundin AP, Ackerman MJ, Chesler RM, et al. Exercise in hemodialysis patients after treatment with recombinant human erythropoietin. Nephron 1991;58:315–319.

29. Moore GE, Brinker KR, Stray-Gundersen J, et al. Determinants of VO2peak in patients with end-stage renal disease: on and off dialysis. Med Sci Sports Exerc 1993;25:18–23.

30. Moore GE, Parsons DB, Painter PL, et al. Uremic myopathy limits aerobic capacity in hemodialysis patients. Am J Kidney Dis 1993;22:277–287.

31. Painter PL, Nelson-Worel JN, Hill MM, et al. Effects of exercise training during hemodialysis. Nephron 1986;43:87–92.

32. Painter PL, Messer-Rehak D, Hanson P, et al. Exercise capacity in hemodialysis, CAPD and renal transplant patients. Nephron 1986;42:47–51.

33. Painter P. The importance of exercise training in rehabilitation of patients with end stage renal disease. Am J Kidney Dis 1994;24(suppl 1):S2–S9.

34. Painter PL, Moore GE, Carlson L, et al. The effects of exercise training plus normalization of hematocrit on exercise capacity and health-related quality of life. Am J Kidney Dis 2002;39:257–265.

35. Robertson HT, Haley NR, Guthrie M. Recombinant erythropoietin improves exercise capacity in anemic hemodialysis patients. Am J Kidney Dis 1990;15:325–332.

36. Ross, DL, Grabeau GM, Smith S, et al. Efficacy of exercise for end-stage renal disease patients immediately following high-efficiency hemodialysis: a pilot study. Am J Nephrol 1989;9:376–383.

37. Shalom R, Blumenthal JA, Williams RS. Feasibility and benefits of exercise training in patients on maintenance dialysis. Kidney Int 1984;25:958–963.

38. Beasley RW, Smith A, Neale J. Exercise capacity in chronic renal failure patients managed by continuous ambulatory peritoneal dialysis. Aust NZ J Med 1986;16:5–10.

39. Lo C, Li L, Lo WK. Benefits of exercise training on continuous ambulatory peritoneal dialysis. [Abstract] Am J Kidney Dis 1998;32:1011–1018.

40. Painter PL, Stewart AL, Carey S. Physical functioning: definitions, measurement, and expectations. Adv Renal Replacement Ther 1999;6:110–123.

41. Mayer G, Thum J, Cada E, et al. Working capacity is increased following recombinant human erythropoietin treatment. Kidney Int 1988;34:525–528.

42. Painter PL, Moore GEM. The impact of recombinant human erythropoetin on exercise capacity in hemodialysis patients. Adv Renal Replacement Ther 1994;1:55–65.

43. Moore GE. Integrated gas exchange responses in chronic renal failure. In: Roca J, Rodriques-Roisin R, Wagner PD, eds. Pulmonary and Peripheral Gas Exchange in Health and Disease. New York: Marcel Dekker, 2000:649–684.

44. Moore GE, Bertocci LA, Painter PL. 31P-Magnetic resonance spectroscopy assessment of subnormal oxidative metabolism in skeletal muscle of renal failure patients. J Clin Invest 1993;91:420–424.

45. Diesel W, Emms M, Knight BK, et al. Morphologic features of the myopathy associated with chronic renal failure. Am J Kidney Dis 1993;22:677–684.

46. Johansen KL, Chertow GM, Ng AV, et al. physical activity levels in patients on hemodialysis and healthy controls. Kidney Int 2000;57:2564–2570.

47. Gallagher-LePak S. Functional capacity and activity levels before and after renal transplantation. Am Nephrol Nurs Assoc J 1991;18:378–382.

48. Painter P, Hanson P, Messer-Rehak D, et al. Exercise tolerance changes following renal transplantation. Am J Kidney Dis 1987;10:452–456.

49. Painter PL, Luetkemeier MJ, Dibble S, et al. Health related fitness and quality of life in organ transplant recipients. Transplantation 1997;64:1795–1800.

50. Goldberg, AP, Geltman EM, Hagberg JM, et al. Therapeutic benefits of exercise training for hemodialysis patients. Kidney Int 1983;S16:S303–S309.

51. Zabetakis PM, Gleim GW, Pasternak FL, et al. Long-duration submaximal exercise conditioning in hemodialysis patients. Clin Nephrol 1982;8:17–22.

52. Hagberg JM, Goldberg AP, Ehsani AA, et al. Exercise training improves hypertension in hemodialysis patients. Am J Nephrol 1983;3:209–212.

53. Kempeneers G, Myburgh KH, Wiggins T, et al. Skeletal muscle factors limiting exercise tolerance of renal transplant patients: effects of a graded exercise training program. Am J Kidney Dis 1990;14:57–65.

54. Miller TD, Squires RW, Gau GT, et al. Graded

exercise testing and training after renal transplantation: a preliminary study. Mayo Clin Proc 1987;62:773–777.

55. Painter PL, Tomlanovich SL, Hector LA, et al. A randomized trial of exercise training following renal transplantation. Transplantation 2002;74: 42–48.

56. Horber FF, Sheidegger JR, Grunig BE, et al. Evidence that prednisone-induced myopathy is-reversed by physical training. J Clin Endocrinol Metab 1985;61:83–88.

57. Copley JB, Lindberg JS. The risks of exercise. Adv Renal Replacement Ther 1999;6:165–171.

58. Painter P, Blagg C, Moore GE. Exercise for the Dialysis Patient: A Comprehensive Program. Madison, WI: Medical Education Institute, 1995.

59. Carey S, Painter P. An exercise program for CAPD patients. Nephrol News Issues 1997;June:15–18.

RELATED WEB SITES

Life Options Rehabilitation Program
www.lifeoptions.org

This web site has the document "Exercise for the Dialysis Patient: A Comprehensive Program," which can be downloaded and which is essential for anyone working with dialysis patients and exercise.

National Kidney Foundation
www.kidney.org

United Network for Organ Sharing
www.unos.org

Cancer

Kirstin Lane and Donald C. McKenzie

Cancer is not a single disease but rather a term that describes the uncontrolled proliferation of cells. When these cells multiply but do not invade other tissues, the cancer is termed *benign*. When the cells invade local tissues or migrate to other parts of the body, the cancer is *malignant*. The type of cancer depends on the cell line from which it originates. Cancer that develops in the endothelial cells that line many organs are carcinomas; cancer originating in connective tissue and bones, sarcomas; lymphomas develop in the tissues that are responsible for immune function; and the leukemias originate in the cells that develop into white blood cells. Given that cancer can develop from any cell line and involve every organ system, it is not surprising that the clinical presentation of patients with cancer can vary.

Therapeutic advances in the management of patients with cancer occur frequently. With improvements in the detection and treatment, the 5-year survival rate for all cancers now exceeds 60%. More and more patients are learning to *live with cancer;* it is a chronic disease.

Although structured exercise programs exist for patients with cardiac and pulmonary disease, this is generally not the case for the oncology patient. In fact, the usefulness of exercise as a therapeutic tool in these patients is only now being appreciated. Well-controlled studies on the effects of exercise on patients with malignant disease are being published, and clinical practice guidelines for the rehabilitation of these patients are imminent (1,2).

The treatment for cancer can involve surgery, chemotherapy, and radiation, and some treatment regimens may last up to 3 years. This treatment is often compounded by bed rest or reduced activity, which may result in significant deconditioning. Chemotherapy agents are not always selective, and normal tissues can be affected. In addition, the goal of tissue destruction has well-documented systemic side effects. Radiation is an effective adjunct in the treatment plan of many cancers, but it too has long-lasting effects on the tissues that it reaches. Therefore, the side effects can be localized to the tumor site(s) but often have systemic properties. Indeed, generalized fatigue is the commonest complaint among patients who are being treated for cancer or who have survived the disease.

Risk Factors

A number of risk factors are associated with the development of specific cancers. For the most part, these are well-known lifestyle issues such as tobacco use, poor diet, and lack of exercise (3). Genetic factors play a small (5–10%) role in the development of malignant disease (1). With the exception of genetic factors, these lifestyle issues are under control of the patient and are modifiable. Physical inactivity has surpassed all other risk factors as the commonest reason of all-cause mortality in men and women in North America. This represents a challenge to the primary care physician and exercise specialist, who can obviously play an important role in cancer prevention.

Immediate Effects of Cancer

The immediate effects of cancer on physical functioning depend on the type and stage of cancer and the resulting treatment. Local disease may have little impact on the performance of day-to-day activities. Indeed, some patients are not limited physically until their disease has progressed to an advanced stage. In contrast, patients whose presenting symptom is pain may be severely limited early in the disease process.

With reference to treatment, surgery can have both peripheral and central effects. Local excision may result in decreased strength, endurance, and range of motion of the affected limb, while surgery on specific organs may affect function of that physiologic system (e.g., surgery for lung cancer may compromise pulmonary function). Common side effects of chemotherapy include fatigue, nausea, vomiting, insomnia, weight gain, and anemia (4), while radiation therapy can result in fatigue and the potential for scar tissue formation in the irradiated area. The severity of fatigue limits physical activity in many cancer patients. Although it is important to rest and allow the body time to recover from the adjuvant therapy treatments, long-term reduction in physical activity can lead to a decline in aerobic fitness, a loss of lean body mass, and an increase in body fat (5). The potential long-term health consequences of poor aerobic fitness secondary to cancer include increased anxiety and depression, as well as a greater risk of coronary heart disease, hypertension, non-insulin-dependent diabetes mellitus, osteoporosis, and colon cancer (6). Thus, patients who have completed treatment for cancer will likely experience a decrease in lean body mass, aerobic fitness, muscular strength, muscular endurance, and flexibility and an increase in body fat. This decline in overall physical fitness could impede the ability of the cancer patient to carry out activities of normal daily living. The health benefits of regular physical activity are well documented. Prescribing exercise to cancer patients may help to counteract the adverse effects of treatment and improve quality of life.

Exercise Testing

Testing is an essential component in designing a safe and appropriate exercise program for the cancer patient, and an overview of exercise testing for individuals with cancer is presented in Table 24-1. It is not unreasonable to assess patients during all phases of their disease. Exercise testing prior to treatment helps to determine the individual's tolerance to exercise. The response of the cancer patient to a short-term bout of exercise is important clinical information. Exercise testing provides an appreciation of the functional capacity of the patient and is useful in determining the initial exercise prescription. An additional benefit of testing prior to treatment is that cancer patients may have other health conditions that would alter the exercise prescription or preclude them from exercising altogether.

Exercise testing during treatment allows quantification of changes in functional capacity as a result of surgery and/or adjuvant therapy, so that safe and appropriate modifications in the exercise program can be made. Cancer patients may experience a wide range of side effects due to adjuvant therapy that will influence their physical health. However, not all cancer patients show the same rate of change in functional capacity or the same degree of fatigue. Knowing how each cancer patient responds to adjuvant therapy allows development of individualized exercise programs to combat the effects of cancer treatment.

There are several reasons to continue with exercise testing after treatment has ended. First, regular testing in the posttreatment period allows evaluation of the efficacy of the exercise program. Each cancer patient recovers at a different rate. Therefore, one must continually adjust the exercise program to ensure that maximal health benefits are being achieved. Second, exercise testing during the posttreatment recovery period can help to establish when the cancer patient has the necessary physical abilities to perform tasks that are beyond those of

TABLE 24-1 OVERVIEW OF EXERCISE TESTING FOR THE CANCER PATIENT

Stage of Treatment	Purpose of Exercise Testing	Suggested Test Battery	Time of Testing
Pretreatment	• Determines the response of the patient to exercise • Identifies other health conditions that may alter the exercise prescription or preclude the individual from exercising altogether	*Comprehensive* fitness test • PAR Med-X • Medical history questionnaire • Body composition (height, weight, skinfolds, limb circumferences) • Aerobic fitness (functional capacity measures, symptom-limited maximal aerobic capacity test) • Pulmonary function assessment (as indicated) • Muscular strength/endurance • Flexibility • Quality of life questionnaires	• Immediately before the start of surgery and/or adjuvant therapy treatment
Treatment	• Quantifies changes in functional capacity and physical fitness as a result of the surgery and/or adjuvant therapy	*Modified* fitness test • PAR-Med-X • Body composition • Aerobic fitness (functional capacity measures) • Flexibility • Quality of life questionnaires	• Midpoint and at end of treatment phase
Posttreatment (1st year after treatment)	• Evaluates the efficacy of the prescribed exercise program • Monitors any potential side effects from treatment that may compromise health in the recovery period • Verifies when the individual has the necessary physical fitness to perform tasks that are beyond those of normal, daily living	Modified fitness test (see treatment period for suggested protocols) Comprehensive fitness test (see pre-treatment period for suggested protocols)	• ~8 weeks after the end of treatment • Regular intervals throughout the posttreatment period until functional capacity returns to pre-treatment levels or individual requests to perform comprehensive test battery • At least once during 1st year posttreatment or on request of cancer survivor
Posttreatment (>2 years after treatment)	• As above	Comprehensive fitness test Comprehensive or modified fitness test	• At least once per year depending on the patient's goals. The modified test battery may be substituted for the comprehensive test battery for other testing sessions throughout the year

normal daily living. This is important for those who may be returning to physically demanding occupations that require a minimum level of physical fitness to perform the job-related tasks safely. Many cancer patients want to participate in leisure time pursuits and/or athletic endeavors with vigor. Thus, one must determine when individuals with cancer can safely return to their occupation or previous exercise routine without exacerbating their medical condition or increasing the risk of injury or illness.

Exercise testing during and after treatment is necessary to identify potential side effects from cancer treatment that may compromise health in the posttreatment period. The effects of chemotherapy and radiation on work capacity are not well known, and there is little information, to date, on whether these effects are transient or permanent. Radiation therapy to the lung, for example, can cause pulmonary fibrosis. Patients receiving radiotherapy for breast cancer are at an increased risk of developing adhesive capsulitis of the shoulder. Therapy to the heart may result in cardiac dysfunction, and these patients should be monitored for signs of coronary heart disease and encouraged to reduce other risk factors (7). Other effects of treatment that may compromise physical functioning in the recovery period include decreased pulmonary function as a result of lung cancer (8), increased risk of osteoporosis due to chemical or surgical castration (9), increased body fat due to adjuvant chemotherapy (4,10), increased risk of cardiac events due to certain drugs used as part of a chemotherapy regime (11), an impaired oxygen-transport system (12), and reduced exercise tolerance (13). However, there is little information about whether these side effects are permanent, how long they may persist into the posttreatment period, or if they have a significant impact on functional capacity during this time.

EXERCISE TEST BATTERY

Because of the complexity of this disease and the different therapeutic modalities used in the treatment of cancer, it is impossible for a single test battery to be suitable for all cancer patients. The type and stage of cancer, stage of treatment (pretreatment, active treatment, posttreatment), concomitant health conditions, previous physical activity patterns, and goals of the individual will influence the protocols selected.

Before conducting any testing, as a minimum, a completed PARmed-X (Physical Activity Readiness Medical Examination; please see the CSEP web site listed at the end of the chapter) should be obtained from the treating physician. Information should be requested as necessary from the oncologist on the type and stage of cancer, prescribed course of treatment, and medications that could influence the testing. To gather comprehensive baseline data on the cancer patient, it is suggested that the pretreatment test battery include functional capacity measures, laboratory tests of physical fitness, and an assessment of quality of life. When choosing a mode for the exercise tests, consideration should be given to the limitations imposed by the type of cancer and the activity preferences of the individual. Flexibility is a key concept in the design of the testing program. Cancer affects each patient differently, and the exercise specialist must understand the need for individualized testing and programs.

During adjuvant therapy treatment, a comprehensive test battery may not be warranted because of the severity of the side effects associated with chemotherapy and radiation. Simple functional tests may provide useful information during this period. These tests can be repeated throughout the cancer treatment.

During the early stages of the posttreatment or recovery period, cancer patients may not have the endurance, strength, or desire to perform a comprehensive exercise test battery. Thus, the modified test battery should be used as the basis for the exercise prescription until functional capacity returns to prediagnosis levels. Once functional capacity is restored, the original test battery can be repeated. Changes in all areas of physical fitness can be documented, and an appropriate exercise prescription can be designed based on these data. If the cancer patient is highly motivated or is returning to a physically demanding occupation, then the pretreatment test battery can be performed as soon as the survivor feels able, so that physical work capacity can be fully assessed.

Regardless of the stage of treatment of the cancer patient, the ideal test battery should include measures of body composition, aerobic fitness, muscular strength and endurance, and flexibility. These measures assess the physical well being of the patient. Cancer has an enormous psychologic cost, and quality-of-life questionnaires should be administered to follow the mental health of these patients (2).

Assessing body composition before and after treatment helps to determine changes that may have occurred as a result of adjuvant therapy and may eventually impose a health risk. Women with breast cancer can gain 2.5 to 6.2 kg during chemotherapy, with most of this weight gain due to an increase in body fat (4,10). This is somewhat surprising considering the side effects of chemotherapy (i.e., nausea, vomiting and mucositis), and the exact mechanisms for the weight gain have yet to be determined. Not only does weight gain tend to be undesirable and have negative psychologic effects (14), but increased body fat may also predispose the cancer survivor to other well-documented medical problems.

Descriptive anthropometry should include height, weight, body mass index, and sum of skinfolds. If there is a risk of lymphedema, then limb circumferences should be monitored or arm volume determined using water displacement. A DEXA scan may be warranted for patients with cancers treated with androgen-deprivation therapy or surgical castration, which leaves the individual at a greater risk of osteoporosis. Daniell et al. (9) found that men who had androgen-deprivation therapy for prostate cancer had much faster femoral neck bone loss than normal men of similar age. Further, women who had bilateral oophorectomy had 20% trabecular bone loss in the first 18 months after surgery (15). Tracking changes in bone density can ensure that appropriate measures are taken to reduce complications of low bone density.

Assessing aerobic fitness before, during, and after treatment allows monitoring of the functional capacity of the cancer patient. Tests of aerobic fitness should include a submaximal test of functional capacity, such as the 12-min walk, that can be performed at all stages of the treatment process (16). As well, a symptom-limited, maximal aerobic assessment should be conducted, if possible, prior to treatment and in the posttreatment period. This testing provides objective documentation of aerobic capacity and helps identify medical problems that are evident only at higher workloads. Further, it has been suggested that because radiation toward the mediastinum may cause or accelerate coronary atherosclerosis (7), exercise electrocardiograms (ECGs) should be conducted at regular intervals in the posttreatment period as a precautionary measure. Pulmonary function assessment is also warranted for lung cancer patients and those who have had radiation therapy involving the lung region.

Muscular strength, muscular endurance, and flexibility should also be assessed before, during, and after treatment. Depending on the type of cancer, the resulting surgery can reduce muscular strength, endurance, and flexibility of an affected limb. Consequently, the cancer patient may have difficulty performing normal activities of daily living such as lifting groceries, getting out of the bathtub, or reaching for an item on an overhead shelf. Further, ~50% of persons with cancer have progressive loss of lean body mass (cachexia) (17). Monitoring changes in muscular strength and endurance can help to detect significant muscle wasting and assist in developing an appropriate resistance-training program to counteract these changes in lean mass.

CONTRAINDICATIONS TO TESTING

Cancer patients with a good prognosis, as well as most cancer survivors, can safely perform most exercise protocols. Maximal exercise testing may not be warranted for individuals with metastatic or advanced disease. Few studies suggest that exercise testing is justified for cancer patients in palliative care. While Porock et al. (18) reported that a low-intensity exercise program given to nine patients in palliative care did not worsen fatigue and did improve quality of life, maximal exercise testing of this population is not justified. However, a modified fitness test battery, as described above, may allow changes in functional capacity to be monitored. A thorough medical examination and chart review should be done prior to any maximal exercise testing of cancer patients to ensure that blood counts are at an acceptable level for low-to-moderate–intensity exercise. Further, cancer patients should not have fever, ataxia, or extreme fatigue that might preclude them from exercise altogether.

Exercise Prescription

Currently, there are no clear and established guidelines for exercise testing and prescription for patients being treated for, or recovering from, cancer. To date, only 26 studies investigating the efficacy of prescribing exercise to individuals with cancer have been published (Tables 24-2 and 24-3). Interpreting and comparing the findings is difficult because these studies are often limited by methodological issues such as self-reported exercise levels, incomplete data regarding training duration or intensity, small sample size, and/or failure to include a control group. Moreover, these investigations vary in

(*text continues on page 372*)

TABLE 24-2 SUMMARY OF RANDOMIZED CONTROLLED TRIALS EVALUATING EXERCISE PROGRAMS FOR CANCER PATIENTS DURING TREATMENT

| | | Exercise Prescription | | | | Results | | | |
Author	N	Intervention	Frequency (days/wk)	Intensity	Time	Psychologic	Functional	Fatigue	Other Notable Findings
Cunningham et al.[28]	T[a] = 20 C = 10	5-wk resistive exercise program during bone marrow transplantation	3 or 5	15 reps of 8 exercises	~30 min				T = results favored a muscle protein-sparing effect of exercise although there was no difference in protein-sparing between resistive exercise performed 3 days or 5 days/week
Dimeo et al.[21]	T = 27 C = 32	~2-wk interval exercise on a bed ergometer during HDC and PBSCT	7	50% HRR	30-min intervals 15 × 1 min: 1 min (passive rest)	T: ↓ psychological distress C: ↑somatic complaints		C: ↑	
Dimeo et al.[29]	T = 5	6-wk walking program during and after CT/RT	5	80% HR_{max}	15–30 min		T: ↑performance (treadmill test)		Pilot study: Exercise and resting ECG showed no pathologic changes of heart activity, functions, or dimensions
Dimeo et al.[20]	T = 33 C = 37	~2-wk interval exercise on a bed ergometer during HDC and PBSCT	7	50% HRR	30-min intervals 15 × 1 min: 1 min (passive rest)		T: ↑performance (treadmill test)		T: ↓hospitalization days, severity of diarrhea, severity of pain, duration of neutropenia
Mac Vicar & Winningham[30]	T = 10 C = 6	10-wk cycle ergometer program during CT	3	60–7–85% HR_{max}		T: ↑mood states	T: ↑functional capacity		

Study	N	Intervention	Frequency (d/wk)	Intensity	Duration				Comments
Mac Vicar et al.[31]	T = 18 C = 16 P = 11	T: 10-wk interval cycle ergometer program during CT P: 10-wk nonaerobic stretching and flexibility program	3	60–85% HRR	Not reported		T: ↑ functional capacity (symptom-limited, $\dot{V}O_{2max}$ test)		
Mock et al.[32]	T = 50[a] (22 low-walkers, 28 high-walkers)	4–6-month exercise program (self-selected exercises) during length of CT	~5–6	Self-paced	15–30 min continuous	High-walkers: ↓emotional distress ↑QOL	High-walkers ↑ 12-min walk	High-walkers:↓	Many control subjects kept exercising during CT so subjects were divided into low-walkers (<90 min/wk, <3 days) and high-walkers (>90 min/wk, >3 days)
Mock et al.[33]	T = 9 C = 5	4–6-month walking program during length of CT	4–5	Self-paced	10–45 min continuous	T: ↓SAS	T: ↑ 12-min walk		
Mock et al.[34]	T = 22 C = 24	6-wk walking program during RT	4–5	Self-paced	20–30 min continuous	T: ↓SAS	T: ↑ 12-min walk	T: ↓	
Na et al.[35]	T = 17 C = 18	2-wk training program (arm and bike ergometer) after surgery	2×/day, 5×/wk	60% HR$_{max}$	30 min continuous				T: Significant increase in natural killer cell activity
Porock et al.[18]	T = 9	4-wk individualized training program (self-selected exercises) during palliative care	Variable	Variable	Variable				Pilot study: Fatigue was not made worse and QOL showed improvement
Schwartz et al.[36c]	T = 61 (A = 37, N = 24)	8-wk training program (self-selected exercises) during CT	3–4	Self-paced	15–30 min continuous		A: ↑12-min walk	A: ↓	
Schwartz[23c]	T = 27 (A = 16, N = 11)	8-wk training program (self-selected exercises) during CT	3–4	Self-paced	15–30 min continuous	A: Less overall decline in QOL	A: ↑12-min walk		

(continued)

369

TABLE 24-2 SUMMARY OF RANDOMIZED CONTROLLED TRIALS EVALUATING EXERCISE PROGRAMS FOR CANCER PATIENTS DURING TREATMENT (Continued)

		Exercise Prescription				Results			
Author	N	Intervention	Frequency (Days/wk)	Intensity	Time	Psychologic	Functional	Fatigue	Other Notable Findings
Schwartz[23c]	T = 71 (A = 32 N = 29)	8-wk training program (self-selected exercises) during CT	~4	Self-paced	15–30 min continuous		A: ↑12 min walk		A: Maintained body weight during CT N: Gained an average of 3.2 kg
Schwartz[37c]	T = 27 (A = 16 N = 11)	8-wk training program (self-selected exercises) during CT	3–4	Self-paced	15–30 min continuous		A: ↑12-min walk		↑
Segal et al[38]	T[b] = 82 C = 41	26-wk walking program during CT	5	50–60% $\dot{V}O_{2max}$	Not reported	No change in QOL for any group T (self-directed): ↑SF-36	No change in any group (mCAFT)		
Shore & Sheppard[39]	T = 3	12-wk training program (self-selected exercises) during CT	3	70–85% HR_{max}	30 min continuous		No change in $\dot{V}O_{2max}$		Acute exercise response-leukocytosis and lymphocytosis (time course similar to normal children) T: No significant change in cell counts
Winningham et al[14]	T = 12 C = 12	10–12-wk interval training program on a cycle ergometer during CT	3	60–85% HR_{max}	20–30-min interval				T: Decrease in sum of skinfolds and %body fat; increase in lean mass

T, treatment group; C, control group; P, placebo exercise group; CT, chemotherapy; RT, radiotherapy; HRR, heart rate reserve; HDC, high-dose chemotherapy; PBSCT, peripheral blood stem cell transplantation; QOL, quality of life.
[a] 10 subjects performed resistive exercises on 3 days/week; 10 subjects performed exercises on 5 days/week.
[b] 40 subjects were in a self-directed exercise program; 42 subjects were in a supervised exercise program.
[c] At the end of the study, subjects who adhered to the exercise program (A) were compared with those who did not (N).

TABLE 24-3 SUMMARY OF RANDOMIZED CONTROLLED TRIALS EVALUATING EXERCISE PROGRAMS IN CANCER PATIENTS WHO HAVE COMPLETED TREATMENT

Author	N	Intervention	Exercise Prescription: Frequency (Days/wk)	Exercise Prescription: Intensity	Exercise Prescription: Time	Results: Psychologic	Results: Functional	Results: Other Notable Findings
Derman et al.[40]	T = 6 C = 6	12-wk program immediately after CT	Not reported	Not reported	Not reported			Skeletal muscle histology was not abnormal in either group
Dimeo et al.[41]	T = 20	6-wk treadmill program immediately after HDC and PBSCT	5	~ 80% HR$_{max}$	15–30 min		T: ↑Performance (treadmill test)	No control group
Dimeo et al.[20]	T = 16 C = 16	6-wk treadmill program immediately after HDC and PBSCT	5	~ 80% HR$_{max}$	15–30 min		T: ↑Performance (treadmill test)	T: ↑ hemoglobin concentration
Durak et al.[42]	T = 20	20-wk aerobic and weight training program ~14 months postdiagnosis	2	Variable	Aerobic: variable Strength: 2–3 sets of 6 exercises	T: ↑QOL	T: ↑muscle strength & endurance	No control group
Durak et al.[43]	T = 25	20-wk aerobic and weight training program ~3 years postdiagnosis	2	Not reported	Not reported	Carcinoma/ leukemia group only: ↑QOL	Carcinoma/ leukemia group only: ↑muscle strength; ↑time on aerobic machines	No control group
McTieran et al.[19]	T = 9	8-wk walking/ biking program 1–5 years posttreatment	6	70–80% HR$_{max}$	30–45 min continuous			Pilot project T: trend to lose weight (2.6 lb) and gain lean mass (2.3%)
Nieman et al.[44]	T = 6 C = 6	8-wk treadmill and resistance training program (7 exercises) 3 years posttreatment	3	Aerobic: 75% HR$_{max}$ Strength: 2 sets × 12 reps	Aerobic: 30 min continuous		T: ↑ 6-min walk	No difference in leg extension strength or NKCA activity after training
Segar et al.[45]	T[a] =16 C=8	10-wk training program (self-selected exercises) performed 3.5 years posttreatment	4	>60% HR$_{max}$	30–40 min continuous	T: ↓depression & anxiety; ↑self-esteem		C at cross-over demonstrated comparable decrease in depression and anxiety

T, treatment group; C, control group; CT, chemotherapy; RT, radiotherapy; HDC, high-dose chemotherapy; PBSCT, peripheral blood stem cell transplantation; QOL, quality of life; NKCA, natural killer cell cytotoxic activity.
[a]8 subjects were in an exercise program only, while 8 subjects were in a behavior-modification and exercise program.

the type of cancer, the stage of treatment, and the frequency, intensity, and duration of the exercise program. Consequently, it is difficult to develop precise exercise prescription guidelines for cancer patients.

Most research has focused either on early-stage cancer patients with a good prognosis during treatment (Table 24-2) or cancer survivors who have completed treatment (Table 24-3). Only one study, done by Porock et al. (18), examined the efficacy of prescribing exercise to cancer patients receiving palliative care.

Despite the limitations in the current investigations, the literature reveals some apparent trends. Regardless of the stage of treatment, most of the studies have demonstrated that an exercise program given to cancer patients with a good prognosis results in favorable changes in quality of life, fatigue levels, and functional status. Other positive results include a decrease in hospitalization days, severity of diarrhea, and pain and improvement in body composition (14,19) and an increase in hemoglobin (20,21). During adjuvant therapy, most investigators chose to prescribe a low-intensity ($\sim$60%

HR_{max} or self-paced) walking program performed 3 to 5 days per week. During the posttreatment recovery period, most studies were completed within $\sim$2 years of treatment and a moderate-intensity ($\sim$80% HR_{max}) program, performed 3 to 5 days per week was prescribed. Only two studies in the literature involved a resistance-training program as part of the exercise prescription.

Design of The Exercise Program

As with choosing exercise test protocols for the cancer patient, designing an exercise program must consider the type and stage of cancer, the stage of treatment, other concomitant medical conditions, previous physical activity patterns, and the goals of the individual. The 1998 ACSM guidelines represent an appropriate exercise prescription for most cancer survivors (22). However, a more conservative approach to the exercise program is better for most cancer patients who are still receiving therapy (Table 24-4).

TABLE 24-4 PRECAUTIONS AND CONTRAINDICATIONS TO EXERCISE FOR THE CANCER PATIENT

Complication	Recommendation
Anemia	Avoid maximal testing or intense physical activity with significant aerobic demands
Low WBC count	Avoid maximal tests; avoid situations with an increased risk of infection (swimming, crowded areas)
Low platelet count	Avoid tests or physical activity that increase the risk of trauma
Fever	Avoid physical activity until the cause of fever is determined
Dyspnea	Investigate cause; limit exercise intensity
Severe cachexia	Exercise should be low intensity and extremely conservative
Extreme fatigue/weakness	Initial exercise intensity should be low, but increase as tolerated; intermittent activities may be preferred to continuous exercise
Mouth sores/ulcerations	Avoid tests that require a mouthpiece (use a face mask for gas collection)
Severe nausea/vomiting	Avoid testing or physical activity until symptoms improve; initiate physical activity at a level that can be tolerated
Bone pain	Avoid high-impact testing or physical activity; swimming may be ideal
CNS abnormality or peripheral neuropathy	Avoid tests and physical activities that require balance and coordination
Poor functional status	Avoid maximal testing; exercise intensity should be low with extremely conservative increases made in intensity and duration

EARLY-STAGE CANCER PATIENTS DURING TREATMENT

The goal of the exercise program for cancer patients receiving treatment is to minimize the effects of cancer-related fatigue, increase the quality of life, and maintain or prevent a decline in functional capacity. Designing exercise programs for cancer patients receiving active treatment requires consideration of how the patient responds to the particular adjuvant therapy, when the side effects tend to peak, the prediagnosis physical activity patterns, and motivation to exercise. Rest days should be given when fatigue is greatest, usually 24 to 48 hours after each chemotherapy cycle (23) and 24 hours after radiation therapy. Regardless of whether the patient was active prior to diagnosis, a conservative approach to the exercise prescription is recommended. As reported in a retrospective survey by Schwartz (24), 76% of cancer survivors who were active prior to diagnosis had to decrease the intensity, frequency, or duration of exercise during treatment. These same respondents, however, still felt it important to maintain a low-to-moderate–intensity exercise program to combat cancer-related fatigue. In another retrospective study, Courneya and Friedenreich (25) found that exercise levels in colorectal cancer survivors decreased from diagnosis to treatment and increased posttreatment (but not to prediagnosis levels).

Table 24-5 outlines an exercise prescription recommendation appropriate for early-stage cancer patients. This recommendation is based on current research that showed that a low-to-moderate–intensity exercise program performed three to five days per week for 15 to 30 min can be tolerated by most cancer patients and can lead to favorable results. Because some medications may affect the normal heart rate response to exercise, Borg's rating of perceived exertion scale should be used to monitor intensity during adjuvant therapy. High-intensity exercise should be avoided until research can determine if there are immunosuppressive effects associated with this activity that might interfere with cancer treatment or the disease itself.

Most cancer patients would benefit from a walking program, as it relates to most activities of daily living, requires little equipment, and is safe for those with most types of cancer. Other modes of activity such as cycling or rowing are not contraindicated unless the person is suffering from central nervous system dysfunction due to the disease or treatment or cannot perform the activity because of the type of surgery.

TABLE 24-5   GENERAL EXERCISE RECOMMENDATIONS FOR OTHERWISE HEALTHY CANCER PATIENTS DURING TREATMENT

Component	Recommendation
Goal[a]	• Minimize the effects of cancer-related fatigue • Increase quality of life • Maintain or prevent a decline in functional capacity
Frequency	3–5 days per week; daily low-intensity exercise is not contraindicated
Intensity	Begin at a very low intensity and increase only after duration and frequency goals have been achieved; RPE ~11–14
Duration	15–30 min; those new to exercise or who are experiencing side effects due to treatment may benefit from intermittent rather than continuous exercise
Types	• Walking, cycling, swimming, rowing (any dynamic exercise involving large muscle groups that does not cause discomfort) • Strength training should accompany cardiovascular fitness; 2 sets of 10 repetitions of exercises for all major muscle groups, 2–3 sessions per week
Progression	Changes in the exercise prescription should first be made in the duration and frequency of exercise; progression may have to be slower than for other populations

[a] The goal may vary depending on the individual and the type of cancer.

Cancer patients who are new to exercise or who are having moderate-to-severe reactions to adjuvant therapy should try to accumulate the prescribed duration of exercise rather than perform it in a continuous manner. Several studies (20,21) used an interval training model, alternating low-intensity exercise (1 min) with rest (1 min) for a total of 30 min. These studies demonstrated improved quality of life and functional ability, as well as reduced fatigue, hospitalization days, and severity of diarrhea and pain. Not all cancer patients undergoing adjuvant therapy will report the same severity or timing of side effects. Thus, each exercise program must be individualized. Moreover, cancer patients (especially those who are new to exercise) may need counseling to help them make physical activity an enduring lifestyle change.

LATE-STAGE CANCER PATIENTS DURING TREATMENT

There is little information to determine if prescribing exercise to late-stage cancer patients with a poor prognosis is safe and will lead to positive physiologic and psychologic effects. As mentioned above, Porock et al. (18) conducted a pilot study looking at the efficacy of prescribing individualized, low-intensity exercise programs to nine patients in palliative care. These patients had various cancers (bowel, pancreas, melanoma, breast, and oral) and an estimated life expectancy of at least 1 month. The results indicated that these subjects did not experience increased fatigue as a result of the 4-week program. In fact, quality of life was improved. Caution should be used when prescribing exercise to late-stage cancer patients until further research can determine optimal doses for this patient population.

CANCER SURVIVORS

The goal of the exercise program in the posttreatment or recovery period is to increase functional capacity, improve or maintain healthy body weight, reduce the risk of other comorbidities secondary to cancer, and ensure that the cancer patient can return to a physically demanding occupation and/or leisure-time pursuit. Once functional status has returned to prediagnosis levels, the ACSM guidelines for prescribing exercise should be adequate for most cancer survivors. However, individually modified programs are still recommended, as the persistence and severity of side effects from adjuvant therapy into the posttreatment period will likely vary. Concomitant health conditions may also affect the exercise prescription. For example, those with a preexisting heart condition secondary to cancer may benefit more from a rehabilitation program targeted to heart patients.

RESISTANCE TRAINING

Little research has been conducted investigating the efficacy of prescribing resistance-training programs to cancer patients and cancer survivors. Because ~50% of cancer patients develop cachexia (17), resistance training would appear to be an appropriate countermeasure to reverse muscle wasting. Further, strength training would help to regain any losses in muscle strength or endurance due to surgery or inactivity. In other special populations, such as HIV patients and aging persons, resistance-training programs result in an anabolic effect (26). However, more research needs to be done on the effects of resistance training on the muscles of cancer patients to determine the dose-response relationship.

Benefits of Exercise Training

Many myths are associated with prescribing exercise to cancer patients (27). For example, there are clinical concerns regarding increased fatigue due to the cumulative effect of cancer treatment and physical activity; concerns regarding immunosuppression following intense exercise; heart failure due to the effects of exercise on a heart with compromised function following chemotherapy; and fracture of bone that has been weakened by disease, treatment, or prolonged inactivity. While studies completed to date have not dispelled all of the above concerns, research investigating the efficacy of prescribing low-to-moderate–intensity exercise to low-stage cancer patients with good prognosis has shown positive findings. Not only can exercise be tolerated, but it can also lead to positive physical and emotional changes without exacerbating pain, nausea, or fatigue. Specifically, regular exercise has improved quality of life, fatigue levels, and functional status; reduced hospitalization days, severity of diarrhea, and pain (20); improved body composition (14,19); and increased hemoglobin levels (20,21). Exercise has become an important therapeutic tool for the physician and exercise therapist.

REFERENCES

1. Courneya KS, MacKey JR, Quinney HA. Neoplasms. In: Myers J, Herbert WH, Humphrey RH, eds. ACSM's Resources for Clinical Exercise Physiology. Baltimore: Lippincott Williams & Wilkins, 2002:179–191.
2. Courneya KS, MacKey JR, McKenzie DC. Exercise for breast cancer survivors: research evidence and clinical guidelines. Physician Sports Med 2002; 8: 33–42.
3. Harvard Report on Cancer Prevention, vol 1: causes of human cancer. Cancer Causes Control 1996;7: S3–S59.
4. Demark-Wahnefried W, Peterson BL, Winer EP, et al. Changes in weight, body composition, and factors influencing energy balance among premenopausal breast cancer patients receiving adjuvant chemotherapy. J Clin Oncol 2001;19:2381–2389.
5. Greenleaf JE, Kozlowski S. Reduction in peak oxygen uptake after prolonged bed rest. Med Sci Sports Exerc 1982;14:477–480.
6. Surgeon General's report on physical activity and health. JAMA 1996;276:522.
7. Gustavsson A, Bendahl P, Cwikiel M, et al. No serious late cardiac effects after adjuvant radiotherapy following mastectomy in premenopausal women with early breast cancer. Int J Radiat Oncol Biol Phys 1999;43:745–754.
8. Miyazawa M, Haniuda M, Nishimura H, et al. Longterm effects of pulmonary resection on cardiopulmonary function. J Am Coll Surg 1999;189: 26–33.
9. Daniell HW, Dunn SR, Ferguson D, et al. Progressive osteoporosis during androgen deprivation therapy for prostate cancer. J Urol 2000;163:181–186.
10. Denmark-Wahnefried W, Winer EP, Rimer BK. Why women gain weight with adjuvant chemotherapy for breast cancer. J Clin Oncol 1993;11:1418–1429.
11. Meinardi MT, Gietema JA, van der Graaf W, et al. Cardiovascular morbidity in long-term survivors of metastatic testicular cancer. J Clin Oncol 2000;18:1725–1732.
12. Johnson D, Perrault H, Fournier A, et al. Cardiovascular responses to dynamic submaximal exercise in children previously treated with anthracycline D. Am Heart J 1997;133:169–173.
13. Nugent A, Steele IC, Carragher AM, et al. Effect of thoracotomy and lung resection on exercise capacity in patients with lung cancer. Thorax 1999;54:334–338.
14. Winningham ML, MacVicar MG, Bondoc M, et al. Effect of aerobic exercise on body weight and composition in patients with breast cancer on adjuvant chemotherapy. Oncol Nurs Forum 1989;16:683–689.
15. Cann CE, Genant HK, Ettinger B, et al. Spinal mineral loss in oophorectomized women. Determination by quantitative computerized tomography. JAMA 1980;244:2056–2059.
16. Cooper KH. A means of assessing maximal oxygen uptake. JAMA 1968;203:133–138.
17. Tisdale MJ. Biology of cachexia. J Natl Cancer Inst 1997;89:1763–1773.
18. Porock D, Kristjanson LJ, Tinnelly K, et al. An exercise intervention for advanced cancer patients experiencing fatigue: a pilot study.: J Palliat Care 2000;16:30–36.
19. McTiernan A, Ulrich C, Kumai C, et al. Anthropometric and hormone effects of an eight-week exercise-diet intervention in breast cancer patients: results of a pilot study. Cancer Epidemiol Biomarkers Prev 1998;7:477–481.
20. Dimeo FC, Fetscher S, Lange W, et al. Effects of aerobic exercise on the physical performance and incidence of treatment-related complications after high-dose chemotherapy. Blood 1997;90:3390–3394.
21. Dimeo FC, Stieglitz R, Novelli-Fischer U, et al. Effect of physical activity on the fatigue and psychological status of cancer patients during chemotherapy. Cancer 1999;85:2273–2277.
22. American College of Sports Medicine position stand: the recommended quantity and quality of exercise for developing and maintaining cardiorespiratory and muscular fitness and flexibility in healthy adults. Med Sci Sports Exerc 1998;30:975–991.
23. Schwartz AL. Daily fatigue patterns and effect of exercise in women with breast cancer. Cancer Pract 2000;8:16–24.
24. Schwartz AL. Patterns of exercise and fatigue in physically active cancer survivors. Oncol Nurs Forum 1998;25:485–491.
25. Courneya KS, Friedenreich CM. Relationship between exercise pattern across the cancer experience and current quality of life in colorectal cancer survivors. J Alternat Complement Med 1997;3: 215–226.
26. Al-Majid S, McCarthy DO. Cancer-induced fatigue and skeletal muscle wasting: the role of exercise. Biol Res Nurs 2001;2:186–197.
27. Courneya KS, Mackey JR, Jones LW. Coping with cancer: can exercise help? Physician Sports Med 2000;28:49–73.

28. Cunningham BA, Morris G, Cheney CL, et al. Effects of resistive exercise on skeletal muscle in marrow transplant recipients receiving total parenteral nutrition. J Parenter Enteral Nutr 1986;10:558–563.

29. Dimeo F, Rumberger BG, Keul J. Aerobic exercise as therapy for cancer fatigue. Med Sci Sports Exerc 1998;30:475–478.

30. MacVicar MG, Winningham ML. Response of cancer patients on chemotherapy to a supervised exercise program. Cancer Bull 1986;13:265–274.

31. MacVicar MG, Winningham ML, Nickel JL. Effect of aerobic interval training on cancer patients' functional capacity. Nurs Res 1989;38:348–351.

32. Mock V, Pickett M, Ropka ME, et al. Fatigue and quality of life outcomes of exercise during cancer treatment. Cancer Pract 2001;9:119–127.

33. Mock V, Burke MB, Sheehan P, et al. A nursing rehabilitation program for women with breast cancer receiving adjuvant chemotherapy. Oncol Nurs Forum 1994;21:899–907.

34. Mock V, Dow KH, Meares CJ, et al. Effects of exercise on fatigue, physical functioning, and emotional distress during radiation therapy for breast cancer. Oncol Nurs Forum 1997;24:991–1000.

35. Na YM, Kim MY, Kim YK, et al. Exercise therapy effect on natural killer cell cytotoxic activity in stomach cancer patients after curative surgery. Arch Phys Med Rehabil 2000;81:777–779.

36. Schwartz AL, Mori M, Gao R, et al. Exercise reduces daily fatigue in women with breast cancer receiving chemotherapy. Med Sci Sports Exerc 2001;33:718–723.

37. Schwartz AL. Fatigue mediates the effects of exercise on quality of life. Qual Life Res 1999;8:529–538.

38. Segal R, Evans W, Johnson D, et al. Structured exercise improves physical functioning in women with stages I and II breast cancer: results of a randomized controlled trial. J Clin Oncol 1999;19:657–665.

39. Shore S, Shephard RJ. Immune responses to exercise in children treated for cancer. J. Sports Med Phys Fitness 1999;39:240–243.

40. Derman WE, Coleman KL, Noakes TD. Effects of exercise training in patients with cancer who have undergone chemotherapy. Med Sci Sports Exerc 1999;31:S368 (abstr).

41. Dimeo F, Bertz H, Finke J, et al. An aerobic exercise program for patients with haematological malignancies after bone marrow transplantation. Bone Marrow Transplant 1996;18:1157–1160.

42. Durak EP, Lilly PC. The application of an exercise and wellness program for cancer patients: a preliminary outcomes report. J Strength Cond Res 1998;12:3–6.

43. Durak EP, Lilly PC, Hackworth JL. Physical and psychosocial responses to exercise in cancer patients: a two year follow-up survey with prostrate, leukemia, and general carcinoma. J Exp Phys Online 1999;2.

44. Nieman DC, Cook VD, Henson DA, et al. Moderate exercise training and natural killer cell cytotoxic activity in breast cancer patients. Int J Sports Med 1995;16:334–337.

45. Segar ML, Katch VL, Roth RS, et al. The effect of aerobic exercise on self-esteem and depressive and anxiety symptoms among breast cancer survivors. Oncol Nurs Forum 1998;25:107–113.

RELATED WEB SITES

American Cancer Society
www.cancer.org

Canadian Cancer Society
www.cancer.ca

National Cancer Institute of Canada
www.ncic.cancer.org

National Cancer Institute
www.nci.nih.gov

Canadian Breast Cancer Research Initiative
www.breast.cancer.ca

Canadian Society for Exercise Physiology (for PARmed-X forms)
www.csep.ca

25

Pregnancy

Larry A. Wolfe

Pregnancy is a complex biologic process that has profound effects on maternal anatomy, physiology, and responses to exercise. Pregnancy and lactation involve dynamic structural and functional adaptations that are driven by gestational hormones to accommodate the changing needs of the developing child. Physical conditioning may augment, diminish, or have no effect on the magnitude of gestational changes, depending on the specific variable concerned (1,2).

In designing exercise programs for pregnant women, the well-being of the fetus and the mother must be considered. That the increased demands of maternal exercise may result in competition between the mother and fetus for blood flow, substrate availability, and heat dissipation has been the basis of the traditional medical advice that pregnant women should rest. However, recent research indicates that healthy women experiencing normal pregnancies benefit from regular, appropriately prescribed exercise (1,3,4). Conversely, inactivity may increase the risk of excessive weight gain, gestational diabetes mellitus, preeclampsia, varicose veins, deep vein thrombosis, and poor psychologic adjustment to the physical changes of pregnancy (4).

The safety and efficacy of exercise during pregnancy depend on the relationships between exercise quantity and quality and the extent of maternal–fetal physiologic reserve. If exercise exceeds this reserve, then fetal development may be affected adversely. Conversely, if the level of exercise stress is insufficient, beneficial changes may not occur. Therefore, preparticipation health screening, individualized exercise prescription, and ongoing medical monitoring are essential to ensure exercise safety (4).

Anatomic and Physiologic Changes

Maternal systems respond to gestational hormones (3,5). These effects include changes in maternal anatomy and the control of metabolic and cardiopulmonary functions (Fig. 25-1).

BODY WEIGHT AND COMPOSITION

During the first two trimesters, higher circulating levels of estrogen and progesterone promote pancreatic β-cell hyperplasia and greater insulin sensitivity, resulting in augmented insulin secretion (6,7) and increased maternal adiposity. In late gestation, maternal adiposity tends to decrease in association with greater fetal energy needs and maternal insulin resistance (7).

Weight gain during pregnancy averages 12 kg. Of this, the fetus accounts for 3.5 kg, larger uterus 1.0 kg, larger breasts 1.5 kg, placenta 0.7 kg,

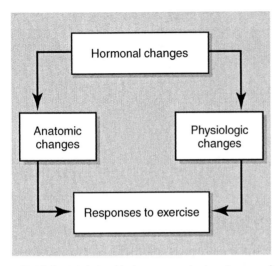

FIGURE 25-1 Relationship between endocrine changes of pregnancy, anatomic and physiologic changes of pregnancy and maternal responses to exercise. (Modified from Wolfe LA, Mottola MF. Aerobic exercise in pregnancy: an update. Can J Appl Physiol 1993;18:119–147, with permission.)

amniotic fluid 0.8 kg, maternal fluid gain 2.0 kg, and higher maternal fat 2.5 kg (7,8). Weight gain averages 1 to 3 kg in the first trimester, 6 to 8 kg in the second trimester and 3.5 to 4 kg in the third trimester, with a plateau near term (8). Weight gain of less than 1 kg per month during the last two trimesters is usually a cause for clinical concern.

MUSCULOSKELETAL SYSTEMS

The physical changes of pregnancy and associated weight gain alter balance, posture, and locomotion. The pregnant uterus weighs about 6 kg at term. Its development causes abdominal protrusion and upward displacement of the diaphragm, leading to compensatory increases in the anteroposterior and transverse diameters of the thoracic cage, as well as changes in spinal mechanics and pelvic rotation. Substernal angle and thoracic cage circumference also increase (9).

It is widely assumed that pregnancy displaces the line of gravity forward and causes exaggerated lumbar lordosis, forward flexion of the cervical spine, anterior pelvic tilt, and slumping shoulders. However, studies have shown that the lower back may actually flatten in many women (10). Regardless of the cause, about 50% of pregnant women report low-back pain (10–13).

Increased production of estrogens and relaxin leads to greater laxity of connective tissue, possibly predisposing pregnant women to joint and ligament damage and overuse orthopedic injury. Round and broad ligament strain and pubic joint pain are common. Diastasis recti, in which the rectus abdominis muscles split and the anterior uterine wall protrudes through the opening, is sometimes observed (14,15).

METABOLISM AND SUBSTRATE USE

Resting oxygen intake ($\dot{V}O_2$) gradually rises 20 to 30% (16–18) because of increased fat-free body mass resulting from fetal growth, the anatomic changes described above, and increased cardiac work and oxygen cost of breathing. As described above, more insulin is secreted in early gestation, causing greater carbohydrate use, increased lipogenesis, reduced lipolysis, and greater maternal adiposity. In late gestation, insulin resistance develops because of the influence of human chorionic somatomammotropin and other "antiinsulin" hormones, resulting in reduced carbohydrate use, more lipolysis, and reduced maternal fat stores (6,7). Because glucose is the primary fetal fuel and crosses the placenta by facilitated diffusion, the apparent purpose of such insulin resistance is to protect fetal glucose availability. If insulin resistance is excessive, gestational diabetes may develop. Fetal morbidity related to maternal diabetes can include macrosomia and neonatal hypoglycemia, hypocalcemia, hyperbilirubinemia, and respiratory distress (7).

CARDIOVASCULAR SYSTEM

Endocrine influences lead to important changes in cardiovascular function. Increased aldosterone secretion and associated sodium and water retention cause a gradual increase of 40 to 50% in blood volume (19,20). Because red cell volume increases to a lesser extent, hematocrit and hemoglobin concentration decrease, and a relative state of anemia ensues (21). The greater blood volume is preceded by vascular relaxation, enlargement of the pelvic veins, and greater venous capacitance mediated by gestational hormones (22). The heart also dilates as a result of the direct influence of estrogen and/or chronic hemodynamic loading related to increased blood volume and augmented venous return (23). Stroke volume (SV) increases as a result of a larger left ventricular end-diastolic volume and moderately improved contractility (23).

Resting heart rate (HR) rises 5 to 10 beats·min^{-1} during the first month of gestation, possibly because of human chorionic gonadotropin (hCG) (24). As pregnancy progresses, peripheral vascular resistance decreases because of the development of the vascular shunt caused by the growing uteroplacental unit and the vasodilating effects of reproductive hormones (20). Because hCG levels decline after early gestation, further progressive increases in resting HR are probably due to hemodynamic reflexes to maintain adequate blood pressure (BP) (20). Increases in resting cardiac output ($\dot{Q}$) tend to balance the reduction in peripheral vascular resistance during the first two trimesters so that systolic (SBP) and diastolic (DBP) pressures are maintained or only slightly lower than the nonpregnant values (25). In the third trimester, venous return is often reduced because of mechanical compression of the inferior vena cava by the gravid uterus. This effect is greatest in the supine posture, is least evident in the left lateral decubitus position, and is only partly compensated by increases in resting HR (26).

PULMONARY VENTILATION

Chest cage remodeling and upward displacement of the diaphragm change lung volumes and capacities, e.g., reduced residual volume, expiratory reserve volume, and functional residual capacity. However, inspiratory capacity increases, and vital capacity is not unchanged. Thus, total lung capacity is only moderately reduced, and resting pulmonary function is generally well preserved (9).

Apart from anatomic changes, the most important effect on the pulmonary system is increased ventilatory sensitivity, mediated by higher circulating progesterone levels, an estrogen-mediated increase in hypothalamic progesterone receptors, and perhaps other chemical factors (26). A lower response threshold and increased sensitivity to CO_2 result in a larger tidal volume and minute ventilation (16–18). With increased pulmonary ventilation, arterial PO_2 levels rise to about 100 mm Hg, and arterial PCO_2 levels drop to 30 to 32 mm Hg (27).

The resulting respiratory alkalosis is only partly compensated by excreting bicarbonate by the kidney; blood pH is about 7.46 (27,28). Augmented work of breathing related to more diaphragmatic work and greater use of accessory muscles of respiration is partly offset by decreased bronchial smooth muscle tone and reduced pulmonary resistance (26).

Maternal Adaptations to Acute Exercise

SUBMAXIMAL EXERCISE

Changes in energy requirement for submaximal exercise depend on whether the exercise is weight supported (e.g., stationary cycling, swimming) or weight dependent (e.g., walking, running). The net $\dot{V}O_2$ of weight-supported exercise is not changed significantly, whereas that of weight-dependent activities rises in proportion to gains in body weight (18,19,30). Thus, conventional equations to predict the energy cost of cycling and treadmill walking or running are probably valid during pregnancy, provided that revised estimates of resting $\dot{V}O_2$ are incorporated. The energy cost of activities requiring agility or body stabilization should be higher than that predicted from changes in body weight alone.

Changes in cardiopulmonary responses to standard steady-state exercise in the upright posture are in the same direction as those seen in the resting state, i.e., higher values for HR (18,23,31), SV (31,32), $\dot{Q}$ (31,32), tidal volume, minute ventilation ($\dot{V}_E$), and ventilatory equivalents for oxygen and carbon dioxide (18,28). Arterial PCO_2 and pH values are significantly lower than those seen in the nonpregnant state (28). SBP and DBP are usually unchanged or slightly reduced at any absolute submaximal $\dot{V}O_2$ (32). Despite changes in cardiopulmonary regulation, perception of exertion at any given submaximal power output is unchanged (18,33,34).

In late gestation, SV and $\dot{Q}$ during standard weight-supported exercise may be lower than values seen in early and midpregnancy (35). As in the resting state, this effect is most evident during supine exercise and is attributed to compression of the inferior vena cava by the gravid uterus (impeding venous return). Dyspnea is commonly experienced at rest and during exercise (36) and may result from altered perception of increased ventilatory demand (36,37).

RESPONSES TO BRIEF, STRENUOUS EXERCISE

Early research on $\dot{V}O_{2max}$ was limited because of ethical concerns for fetal well-being. However, recent studies support the concept that absolute $\dot{V}O_{2max}$ ($L \cdot min^{-1}$) is not greatly affected by pregnancy and may vary in accordance with changes in physical activity habits during the course of gestation (38–40). Values expressed as $mL \cdot kg^{-1} \cdot min^{-1}$ usually decline significantly because of maternal weight gain.

A few studies reported a lower maximal HR in late gestation (32,38,41), probably due to blunted sympathoadrenal responses to exercise (42,43). Because resting HR is also increased, there is a reduced maximal HR reserve (3,23,44; Fig. 25-2). One must consider these changes when submaximal tests to predict $\dot{V}O_{2max}$ are based heart rate versus power output/$\dot{V}O_2$ relationships (45,46).

Studies involving progressive maximal or near-maximal cycle ergometer testing support the concept that the $\dot{V}O_2$ at the ventilatory threshold (Tvent), and the point of respiratory compensation for metabolic acidosis (RC) are not changed by healthy human pregnancy (16,40,47). A recent study (40) also reported that the respiratory exchange ratio (RER) at peak exercise, peak postexercise blood lactate concentration, and excess postexercise oxygen consumption (EPOC) are all reduced with maximal cycle ergometer testing in late gestation. Other studies also report lower peak RER values or peak postexercise lactate concentrations in late gestation (37,38,48). Because a significant fall in maternal blood glucose during or following strenuous exercise in late gestation is also a common finding (42,49), it is hypothesized that the combined effects of reduced maternal liver glycogen stores (50) and blunted sympathoadrenal responses to strenuous exercise in late gestation lead to reduced availability of carbohydrate to contracting maternal skeletal muscle (16,40) and a lower ability to exercise anaerobically. Reduced glucose availability to the fetus from the maternal blood glucose pool might affect fetal growth if strenuous exercise is repeated regularly in late gestation (51).

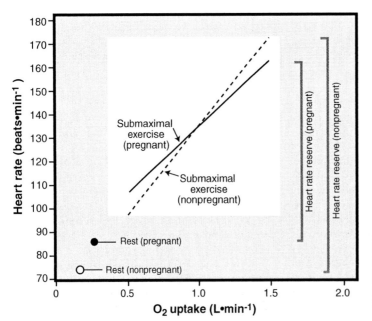

FIGURE 25-2 Pregnancy-induced changes in resting heart rate, heart rate responses to exercise, and maximal heart rate reserve. (Modified from Wolfe LA, Mottola MF. Aerobic exercise in pregnancy: an update. Can J Appl Physiol 1993;18:119–147, with permission.)

RESPONSES TO PROLONGED SUBMAXIMAL EXERCISE

A few studies have examined maternal metabolic and substrate responses to submaximal exercise of >30-min duration (42,52–54). An important common finding was a significant reduction in maternal blood glucose levels, which theoretically could lower glucose availability to the fetus (51). We have hypothesized that such reactions are the combined result of reduced liver glycogen stores (50) and blunted catecholamine-mediated glycogen breakdown during strenuous exercise (42,43). Whether these responses have any effect on fetal growth is not known, and the possibility that they could be modified by maternal physical conditioning must be examined (2).

STATIC AND HIGH-RESISTANCE EXERCISE

Studies report that maternal HR during heavy static exercise and weight training is higher than in the nonpregnant state (25,55); this probably reflects a higher resting HR, since exercise-induced increases in HR are unchanged. Maternal BP during heavy resistance exercise is similar to, or slightly lower than, that seen in the nonpregnant state, depending on gestational age. Values tend to be lower at midgestation and a bit higher near term.

Fetal Responses to Acute Maternal Exercise

The most important concerns for fetal well-being during acute maternal exercise are related to uteroplacental blood flow and oxygen delivery, heat dissipation, prevention of fetal hyperthermia, and availability of glucose for fetal metabolism(2). Data from exercising laboratory animals and limited human data suggest lower absolute uteroplacental blood flow during maternal exercise. The magnitude of this reduction is related directly to the exercise intensity and duration (56–58). Mechanisms that may compensate for this reduction and minimize fetal hypoxia include hemoconcentration of maternal blood during exercise, redistribution of uteroplacental blood flow to favor the cotyledons at the expense of myometrial flow (59–61), and

increased uteroplacental arteriovenous oxygen difference (62).

Concern has been expressed that fetal hyperthermia associated with increased maternal body temperature could cause fetal developmental defects (63). In particular, teratogenic effects have been reported relative to maternal fever (63,64) and chronic temperature stress in animals (65) during closure of the neural tube in early pregnancy, resulting in central nervous system defects. Maternal core temperature is the most important determinant of fetal temperature. At rest, fetal temperature is about 0.5°C higher than maternal core temperature (66,67). Thus, if maternal core temperature increases with intensive exercise, the fetus could, in theory, become hyperthermic. However, changes in the maternal system help to minimize exercise-induced increases in core temperature, including enhanced peripheral vasodilation, reduced sweating threshold, and increased ventilatory heat loss (49,68,69). We are unaware of any published reports of exercise-induced teratogenic effects in humans.

Glucose is the primary fuel for fetal metabolism, and its availability is critical for fetal well-being and growth (6,7). Carbohydrate use by skeletal muscle increases as a function of exercise intensity. Therefore, combined maternal–fetal demands during strenuous exercise in late gestation can lead to a postexercise fall in maternal blood glucose (17,42,44) and a transient reduction in fetal glucose uptake (51). It is not known if compensatory mechanisms exist.

Evaluating fetal oxygen supply, temperature, and carbohydrate metabolism is problematic in exercising human subjects. However, fetal HR (FHR) has been used as an index of fetal well-being because it is the primary determinant of fetal $\dot{Q}$ and because gross changes in FHR patterns are often associated with fetal distress (2). In particular, fetal bradycardia (FHR <120 beats·min^{-1} for >2 min) and other deceleratory patterns are common reactions to hypoxic stress. Fetal bradycardia is an early response to moderate hypoxia and appears to be a reflex response mediated by fetal arterial chemoreceptors to minimize fetal oxygen demand. Tachycardia (FHR >160 beats·min^{-1}) is observed during mild hypoxia or during recovery from hypoxia (2).

The normal response to aerobic exercise is a gradual increase in FHR, with a subsequent return to preexercise baseline by about 20 min after exercise (2,70–72). The magnitude of FHR acceleration appears to be related to exercise intensity and duration (70), but such factors as increased fetal temperature or state of wakefulness may also contribute (2). Fetal bradycardia is a sign of fetal hypoxic stress but is occasionally observed during or following exercise in healthy women with normal pregnancies (71,73,74). The likelihood of such reactions appears to increase as a function of exercise intensity and duration as well as maternal fitness (71,72). A recent study (75) found modest reductions in FHR variability and reduced reactivity (FHR acceleration in association with fetal movement) but no instances of bradycardia following brief maximal cycle ergometer testing of healthy fit women with normally grown fetuses in late gestation. However, Manders et al. (74) observed several instances of bradycardia and transient reductions in variability and reactivity in the fetuses of healthy women during a prolonged maximal treadmill test.

There is little information on fetal responses to heavy muscular conditioning exercise. Recently, we (55) examined the effects of different maternal postures (supine–30° tilt vs. sitting), muscle masses (handgrip vs. single-leg extension vs. double-leg extension), and contraction intensities (50 vs. 70 vs. 90% of 10 repetition maximum) on FHR responses to strength conditioning exercises in late gestation. FHR responses to all exercise conditions were minimal. Moderate fetal bradycardia was seen occasionally at rest, during, and following exercise in the supine–30° tilt position, suggesting that this posture should be avoided in late pregnancy.

Maternal Physical Conditioning Effects

In view of the profound changes in regulating metabolic and cardiorespiratory functions, it is logical to expect that maternal responses to physical conditioning differ. Unfortunately, controlled longitudinal physical-conditioning studies of pregnant women are still scarce. Nevertheless, existing published reports suggest the following:

- Both $\dot{V}O_{2max}(L·min^{-1})$ and the ventilatory anaerobic threshold are increased in previously inactive pregnant women (16,17,76,77).
- At rest and during mild steady-state exercise, the hemodynamic effects of pregnancy appear to dominate those of physical conditioning. HR is not significantly reduced and SV is not markedly increased at any given exercise power output (PO) after training (18,23,78).
- During moderate and heavy steady-state exercise, HR reduction at any given external PO in response to physical conditioning becomes more evident than during rest or mild exercise (18,23).
- Perception of effort at any given PO is reduced by physical conditioning. This effect becomes more evident as exercise intensity increases (33).
- Adiposity, as reflected by skinfold thicknesses, may not decrease as much in response to moderate aerobic conditioning during pregnancy (79).
- Ventilatory demand, respiratory perception of exertion, and carbohydrate use are reduced at any given submaximal exercise PO (16–18).

In summary, aerobic performance and cardiopulmonary reserve are enhanced by endurance-type physical conditioning in pregnancy. Thus, physically fit pregnant women may better satisfy fetal physiologic demands during exposure to metabolic, environmental, or physiologic stresses.

Physical Conditioning and Pregnancy Outcome and Early Postnatal Development

The effect of maternal physical conditioning and/or daily occupational work on birth weight and other aspects of fetal development and pregnancy outcome remains a subject of considerable controversy (2,80). It is well established that chronic heavy work coupled with inadequate nutrition can result in unacceptably low birth weight. On the other hand, lack of exercise and overnutrition may contribute to the development of excessive insulin resistance, gestational diabetes mellitus, and fetal macrosomia (birth weight >4 kg).

Early investigations (81) reported that recreational athletes who continued to exercise vigorously in the third trimester delivered lighter babies at an earlier gestational age than did controls who discontinued exercise in late gestation. Similar findings were reported later (82) in women who exercised vigorously. Subsequent studies (83) suggested that the lower birth weights of such women were primarily due to a lower neonatal fat mass and that other fetal growth variables were not significantly affected. Another study (84) reported that heavy physical conditioning during pregnancy results in a significant increase in birth weight. This could be attributed to a stimulatory effect of intermittent exposure of the fetoplacental unit to exercise-induced hypoxia in early gestation (85). Finally, studies of moderate aerobic fitness training have consistently reported no significant effect of such training on birth weight (86–88).

The information presented above supports a dose–response effect for the quantity and quality of maternal exercise (Fig. 25-3). Moderate-intensity conditioning has no significant effect on fetoplacental growth. Strenuous exercise within maternal and fetal adaptive reserve may stimulate fetal growth,

especially if exercise is initiated in early pregnancy. If exercise is beyond this adaptive capability, fetal growth and pregnancy outcome may be negatively affected. This hypothesis is consistent with recent findings (87) that exercise less than 1 day per week and 5 or more days per week were both associated with a lower than average birth weight (<15th percentile).

Preparticipation Medical Screening: Physical Activity Readiness Medical Examination for Pregnancy

Exercise prescription and monitoring during pregnancy requires expertise from the fields of obstetrics and exercise physiology and specialized knowledge on the interactive effects of pregnancy and exercise on maternal–fetal biologic and psychosocial functions. Thus, a team approach is

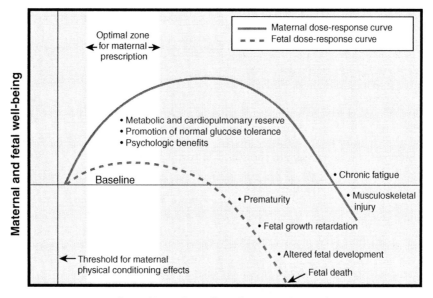

Quantity and quality of maternal exercise

FIGURE 25-3 Postulated dose–response relationship between quantity and quality of prenatal exercise with maternal and fetal well-being. (Wolfe LA, Brenner IKM, Mottola MF. Maternal exercise, fetal well-being and pregnancy outcome. Exerc Sport Sci Rev 1994;22:145–194, with permission.)

recommended in which the obstetrician or midwife provides initial medical clearance and ongoing monitoring of her health status and suggests general limits for the exercise regimen as gestation progresses. Ideally, a prenatal exercise instructor with a thorough knowledge of maternal–fetal exercise physiology would then formulate a specific exercise prescription. The woman's lifestyle and exercise preferences should be considered, and she should be actively involved in the day-to-day monitoring of her exercise program. Three-way communication of this nature is essential for safe and effective prenatal exercise programs.

Research has confirmed that a healthy woman experiencing a normal pregnancy can participate safely in a moderate conditioning program designed to improve or maintain aerobic and muscular fitness and to prepare for the stresses of childbirth (16–18,23,71,72). However, prenatal exercise may be unsafe if a normal level of physiologic reserve does not exist or if exercise exceeds existing adaptive reserve. Therefore, medical screening is an important first priority for all women who wish to start or continue a physical fitness program during pregnancy (4).

The *Physical Activity Readiness Medical Examination (PARmed-X for Pregnancy)* was formulated in our laboratory and revised and published in cooperation with the Canadian Society for Exercise Physiology and Health Canada in 1996. Further revisions were incorporated in 2002 (90). A companion booklet for pregnant women and prenatal fitness instructors is also available (91). The exercise participant completes sections A (basic contact information) and B (general health information; any signs and symptoms in the current pregnancy; recent activity habits; prenatal exercise intentions) and then asks her prenatal health care provider to complete section C. This section is a convenient checklist to indicate the presence or absence of well-accepted absolute and relative contraindications to prenatal exercise. If appropriate, the physician or midwife then provides initial medical clearance for exercise by completing the Health Evaluation Form. This form is then given to the participant for her prenatal exercise instructor.

An important feature of the *PARmed-X for Pregnancy* form is that recommendations for aerobic exercise and muscular conditioning are provided. Regular use will help to familiarize physicians and midwives with evidence-based practices for prenatal exercise prescription. General advice for active living, healthy eating and maintenance of a positive body image, prenatal exercise safety considerations, and reasons to consult a prenatal health care provider are also included (90,91).

Prescription of Exercise

Prenatal exercise classes usually involve muscular and aerobic conditioning, as well as appropriate warm-up and cool-down/relaxation periods (90–93). The muscular-conditioning phase incorporates specific strengthening exercises to prevent such conditions as diastasis recti, low-back pain, and urinary incontinence and also to strengthen muscles involved in the labor process (90–93). Aerobic conditioning increases cardiopulmonary adaptive reserve and may prevent maternal obesity (79,94). It may also help in preventing gestational diabetes (92,95–97) and preeclampsia (98,99).

AEROBIC CONDITIONING

Current evidence confirms that it is safe for healthy women experiencing normal pregnancies to begin a new exercise program at the start of the second trimester (16–18,23,71,72). Exercise intensity and duration can then increase during the course of the second trimester, when the discomforts of pregnancy and potential for conflicting demands of pregnancy and exercise are lowest. Because chronic exposure to high temperature may disrupt closure of the neural tube in early pregnancy (~4–5 weeks), it is prudent to avoid any increase in exercise quantity and quality during the first trimester. Similarly, exercise should not be increased in late gestation (after 28 weeks) when the potential for conflicting maternal and fetal demands during exercise are greatest. Exercise intensity and duration should be reduced or exercise should be canceled in late gestation if the individual feels fatigued.

Exercise Modality

Common sense dictates that pregnant women should not participate in aerobic games or activities that involve significant risk of traumatic injury

(4,90–92), as well as in those activities involving hyperbaric (e.g., scuba diving) or hyperthermic environmental stress (92,100,101). Because gestational hormones increase the laxity of connective tissue throughout the body, activities that emphasize weight-bearing or repeated bouncing movements (e.g., running, aerobic dance) may predispose the individual to musculoskeletal overuse injury. Conversely, the most desirable activities are those in which the body is partly supported or that minimize vertical displacement of the center of gravity. These include walking, upright leg cycling (16–18,25), arm ergometry (96,97), low-impact aerobics (52), and "aquafit" exercises (48,102,103). Exercise in the water is particularly appropriate because body weight is supported by the buoyant effect of water. Plasma volume expansion during immersion may help maintain uterine blood flow (48,102), and heat dissipation is facilitated if water temperature is less than skin temperature (104).

Exercise Intensity

Prescribing and monitoring exercise intensity is complicated by alterations in the control of both cardiovascular and pulmonary functions during pregnancy. As discussed above, resting HR rises throughout pregnancy, and maximal HR is reduced in late gestation (41,46). Thus, pregnant women have a reduced HR reserve (43,44; Fig. 25-2), and the use of conventional age-predicted HR target zones is less reliable. Revised age-related HR target zones for exercise are in the *PARmed-X for Pregnancy* (90). This is based on the idea that the width of HR target zone for a healthy nonpregnant woman (60–75% of maximal HR reserve) is approximately 20 beats·min^{-1}. To adjust for the lower maximal HR and HR reserve, the target zone for nonpregnant adults was reduced from 20 to 15 beats·min^{-1} by lowering the upper end of the zone by 5 beats·min^{-1} (90,91).

Since ratings of perceived exertion (RPEs) at any given external PO are not significantly affected by pregnancy or advancing gestational age (18,33,34), we have recommended that Borg's 15-point (6 to 20) RPE scale be used in conjunction with the revised HR target zone (90,91). In our experience, RPEs of 12 to 14 ("somewhat hard") are a suitable target intensity range for most exercising pregnant women (90,91). Use of the "talk test" (ability to

talk while exercising) is also recommended to avoid overexertion (90,91).

Exercise Duration

The interaction of intensity and duration of exercise is important because both factors contribute to reducing uterine blood flow and increasing maternal core and fetal temperatures (62). Assuming that exercise intensity is determined using the procedures outlined above, a minimal duration of 15 min per session is recommended to ensure an adequate conditioning stimulus (90,91). Previously sedentary women can then gradually increase exercise duration by 1 to 2 min per week during the second trimester to a maximum of 30 min per session (16–18,23).

Frequency of Exercise

Good agreement exists that aerobic conditioning should be done regularly, while allowing sufficient time for recovery between sessions (90–92). Initially, a previously inactive woman might exercise 3 days per week, with alternating days of exercise and rest. As exercise tolerance improves, this can be increased to 4 to 5 days per week, with no more than 2 consecutive days of strenuous aerobic exercise. A recent study (89) reported that an exercise frequency of 5 days or more per week was associated with a birth weight below the 15th percentile. Thus, pregnant women should not exercise 5 or more days per week on a consistent basis.

It is particularly important to avoid aerobic exercise in warm or humid environments. Because the effects of pregnancy on maternal thermoregulatory capacities are not fully understood (49,68,69), it is prudent to reduce exercise intensity and duration or to avoid exercise if ambient temperature and/or relative humidity are high. Women should drink water before and after aerobic exercise to ensure adequate hydration and normal thermoregulation. Finally, the use of fans during stationary activities will increase convective and evaporative heat loss.

In summary, these guidelines for aerobic exercise prescription are suitable for most healthy pregnant women. However, an individualized exercise prescription is strongly advised because optimal procedures vary depending on maternal age, occupation, socioeconomic factors, physical fitness, nutrition, and personal exercise goals. Attention to the safety of aerobic exercise is essential, and recommended safety precautions should be well known and implemented by the class leader and participants (90,91).

Warm-up and Cool-down

Warm-up before muscular and aerobic conditioning activities should include moderate range-of-motion exercises for all major joints, plus mild static stretching for all major muscle groups. Cool-down following aerobic exercise should be gradual, especially in late gestation when $\dot{Q}$, arterial BP, and splanchnic blood flow may fall precipitously with abrupt cessation of muscular contraction, because of impedance of venous return by the gravid uterus. Mild static stretching and relaxation exercises are recommended to conclude the exercise session (91).

MUSCULAR CONDITIONING

An overview of major exercise categories is provided in *PARmed-X for Pregnancy* (90), and specific exercises are described in detail in the companion booklet (91). Strengthening exercises during pregnancy should involve moderate resistance and the performance of several repetitions to achieve muscular fatigue. To prevent hypotension, pregnant women should avoid the Valsalva maneuver and should not exercise in the supine position. This is particularly important after the fourth month of gestation when the gravid uterus may impede venous return. Rapid changes of direction and bouncing movements should be avoided to prevent injury of joints and ligaments that are relaxed by the effects of gestational hormones. Abdominal conditioning exercises should be discontinued if diastasis recti develops.

Value of Prenatal Exercise to Prevent or Treat Maternal/Fetal Diseases

Gestational diabetes mellitus and preeclampsia are the two most prevalent maternal/fetal disease states. Existing epidemiologic evidence supports the concept that exercise may be useful for the primary prevention of gestational diabetes, especially in morbidly obese women (92,97). Evidence also supports the concept that exercise may be an important adjunctive therapy when glycemic control is not achieved by diet alone (92).

High levels of leisure-time physical activity are associated with a lower incidence of preeclampsia in nulliparous women (98), and a protective effect of exercise against preeclampsia has been hypothesized (99). Multicenter epidemiologic studies and mechanistic physiologic studies are both needed to establish the usefulness of exercise to prevent or treat gestational diabetes and preeclampsia and to establish guidelines for these two special populations.

Summary

- Pregnancy is an exceedingly complex biologic process that results in hormonally mediated changes in maternal anatomy and altered regulation of metabolic and cardiopulmonary functions. Adaptations to standard submaximal exercise include increases in HR, $\dot{Q}$, and ventilation.
- $\dot{V}O_{2max}$ during weight-supported exercise ($L \cdot min^{-1}$) is not greatly affected by pregnancy, but the capacity for weight-dependent exercise decreases as a function of gestational weight gain.
- Maternal responses to aerobic conditioning differ from those of nonpregnant women. Such women do not appear to develop bradycardia, and body fat stores may be protected because of hyperinsulinemia. Expected increases in submaximal exercise SV may be masked by gestational effects on blood volume and venous return. However, HR responses to heavy submaximal exercise are significantly reduced by aerobic conditioning, owing to a widened arteriovenous oxygen difference.
- Concerns for fetal well-being during acute maternal exercise center on the transient reduction in uterine blood flow, interruption of fetal glucose availability, and risk of fetal hyperthermia in early gestation. However, sufficient maternal–fetal physiologic reserve appears to exist in healthy, well-nourished women to accommodate maternal and fetal needs during moderate exercise.
- Physical conditioning programs for pregnant women usually include both muscular and aerobic conditioning. The purposes of the former include (*a*) promoting good posture; (*b*) preventing

diastasis recti, low-back pain, and urinary incontinence; and *(c)* strengthening specific muscle groups involved in the active stage of labor.

- The best time for previously sedentary women to begin a new aerobic conditioning regimen is during the second trimester, when the discomforts of pregnancy and risks to fetal well-being are lowest. Exercise intensity can be prescribed and monitored by the combined use of revised HR target zones and conventional perception of exertion scales. The "talk test" is also useful to prevent overexertion. Minimal and maximal recommended durations for aerobic exercise are 15 and 30 min, respectively. Pregnant women should exercise 3 to 4 days per week.

- Safety considerations for prenatal exercise include thorough medical screening and ongoing medical surveillance, avoidance of hyperbaric and hyperthermic environments, attention to adequate nutrition and hydration, individualized exercise prescription, and good communication between the exercising woman, her obstetrician, and the exercise instructor.

- Existing information suggests that fit, healthy women (athletes, military women, fire-fighters etc.) undergoing normal pregnancies can safely perform brief acute bouts of maximal or near-maximal exercise or moderate prolonged acute bouts of moderate-intensity exercise. However, more research is needed to determine whether or not high-intensity or prolonged exercise can be performed long term without affecting fetal growth and development.

- Existing information suggests that regular exercise is useful to prevent and/or treat gestational diabetes mellitus and preeclampsia.

Acknowledgments

The Exercise/Pregnancy Research Program at Queen's University has been supported by the Advisory Research Committee (Queen's University), Fitness Canada, the Canadian Fitness and Lifestyle Research Institute, the Ministry of Health (Ontario), the Ministry of Tourism and Recreation (Ontario), the Ontario Thoracic Society, the Ontario Thoracic Society (Block Term Grant Funding), Health and Welfare (Canada), NSERC (Canada), the U.S. Army Medical Research and Materiel Command (Contract #DAMD 17-96-C-6112), the Canadian Forces Personnel Support Agency, the William M. Spear Endowment Fund for Pulmonary Research at Queen's University, and the Garfield-Kelly Cardiovascular Research and Development Fund.

REFERENCES

1. Wolfe LA, Weissgerber TL. Clinical physiology of exercise in pregnancy: a literature review. J Obstet Gynaecol Can 2003;25:473–483.
2. Wolfe LA, Brenner IKM, Mottola MF. Maternal exercise, fetal well-being and pregnancy outcome. Exerc Sport Sci Rev 1994;22:145–194.
3. Wolfe LA, Mottola MF. Aerobic exercise in pregnancy: an update. Can J Appl Physiol 1993;18:119–147.
4. Davies GAL, Wolfe LA, Mottola MF, et al. Joint SOGC and CSEP clinical practice guideline. Exercise during pregnancy and postpartum. Can J Appl Physiol 2003;28:329–341 and J Obstet Gynaecol Can 2003;25:516–522.
5. Creasy RK, Resnick R, eds. Maternal-Fetal Medicine. Philadelphia: WB Saunders, 1998.
6. Catalano PM. Carbohydrate metabolism and gestational diabetes. Clin Obstet Gynecol 1994;37:25–38.
7. Boden G. Fuel metabolism in pregnancy and in gestational diabetes. Obstet Gynecol Clin North Am 1996;23:1–10.
8. Clark N. Shower your baby with good nutrition. Physician Sportsmed 1992;20:39,40,45.
9. Ratigan TR. Anatomic and physiologic changes of pregnancy: anesthetic considerations. J Am Assoc Nurse 1983;51:38–42.
10. Moore K, Dumas GA, Reid JG. Postural changes associated with pregnancy and their relationship with low-back pain. Clin Biomech 1990;5:169–174.
11. Fast A, Weiss L, Docummun EL, et al. Low-back pain in pregnancy. Abdominal muscles, sit-up performance, and back pain. Spine 1990;15:28–30.
12. Dumas GA, Reid JG, Wolfe LA, et al. Exercise, posture and back pain during pregnancy. Part 1. Exercise and posture. Clin Biomech 1995;10:98–103.
13. Dumas GA, Reid JG, Wolfe LA, et al. Exercise, posture and back pain during pregnancy. Part 2. Exercise and back pain. Clin Biomech 1995;10:104–109.
14. Boissonnault JS, Blaschak MJ. Incidence of diastasis recti abdominis during the childbearing year. Phys Ther 1988;68:1082–1086.
15. Gilleard WL, Brown JMM. Structure and function of the abdominal muscles in premigravid subjects during pregnancy and the immediate postbirth period. Phys Ther 1996;76:750–762.

16. Wolfe LA, Walker RMC, Bonen A, et al. Effects of pregnancy and chronic exercise on respiratory responses to graded exercise. J Appl Physiol 1994; 76:1928–1936.

17. Wolfe LA, Heenan AP, Bonen. Aerobic conditioning effects on substrate responses to graded cycling in pregnancy. Can J Physiol Pharm 2003;81:696–703.

18. Ohtake PJ, Wolfe LA. Physical conditioning attenuates respiratory responses to steady-state exercise in late gestation. Med Sci Sports Exerc 1998;30:17–27.

19. Longo LD. Maternal blood volume and cardiac output during pregnancy; a hypothesis of endocrinologic control. Am J Physiol 1983;245:R720–R729.

20. Duvekot JJ, Cheriex EC, Pieters FA, et al. Early pregnancy changes in hemodynamics and volume homeostasis are consecutive events triggered by a primary fall in systemic vascular tone. Am J Obstet Gynecol 1993;169:1382–1392.

21. Pivarnik JM, Mauer MB, Ayers NA. Effect of chronic exercise on blood volume expansion and hematologic indicies during pregnancy. Obstet Gynecol 1994;83:265–269.

22. Goodrich SM, Wood JE. Peripheral venous distensibility and velocity of venous blood flow during pregnancy or during oral contraceptive therapy. Am J Obstet Gynecol 1964;90:740–744.

23. Wolfe LA, Preston RJ, Burggraf GW, et al. Effects of pregnancy and chronic exercise on maternal cardiac structure and function. Can J Physiol Pharm 1999;77:909–917.

24. Clapp JF III. Maternal heart rate in pregnancy. Am J Obstet Gynecol 1985;152:659–660.

25. Lotgering FK, van den Berg A, Struijk PC, et al. Arterial pressure response to isometric exercise in pregnant women. Am J Obstet Gynecol 1992;166:538–542.

26. Wolfe LA, Kemp JG, Heenan AP, et al. Acid-base regulation and control of ventilation in human pregnancy. Can J Physiol Pharm 1998;76:815–827.

27. Templeton A, Kelman G R. Maternal blood gases. (PA_{O2}-Pa_{O2}), physiological shunt and VD/VT in normal pregnancy. Br J Anaesth 1976;48:1001–1004.

28. Heenan AP, Wolfe LA. Plasma acid-base regulation above and below ventilatory threshold in late gestation. J Appl Physiol 2000;88:149–157.

29. Artal R, Masaki DI, Khodiguian N, et al. Exercise prescription in pregnancy: weight-bearing versus non-weight-bearing exercise. Am J Obstet Gynecol 1989;161:1464–1469.

30. Clapp JF III. Oxygen consumption during treadmill exercise before, during and after pregnancy. Am J Obstet Gynecol 1989;161:1458–1464.

31. Pivarnik JM, Lee W, Clark SL, et al. Cardiac output responses of primigravid women during exercise determined by the direct Fick technique. Obstet Gynecol 1990;75:954–959.

32. Sady SP, Carpenter MW, Thompson PD, et al. Cardiovascular response to cycle exercise during and after pregnancy. J Appl Physiol 1989;66:336–341.

33. Ohtake PJ, Wolfe LA, Hall P, et al. Physical conditioning effects on exercise heart rate and perception of exertion in pregnancy. Can J Sport Sci 1988;13:71P (abstr).

34. Pivarnik JM, Lee W, Miller JF. Physiological and perceptual responses to cycle and treadmill exercise during pregnancy. Med Sci Sports Exerc 1991;23:470–475.

35. Ueland K, Novy MJ, Peterson EN, et al. Maternal cardiovascular dynamics. IV. The influence of gestational age on the maternal cardiovascular response to posture and exercise. Am J Obstet Gynecol 1969;104:856–864.

36. Garcia-Rio F, Pino JM, Gomez L, et al. Regulation of breathing and perception of dyspnea in healthy pregnant women. Chest 1996;110:446–453.

37. Field SK, Bell G, Cenaiko DF, et al. Relationship between inspiratory effort and breathlessness in pregnancy. J Appl Physiol 1991;71:1897–1902.

38. Lotgering FK, Van Doorne MB, Struijk PC, et al. Maximal aerobic exercise in pregnant women: heart rate, O_2 consumption, CO_2 production and ventilation. J Appl Physiol 1991;70:1016–1023.

39. Spinnewijn WEM, Wallenberg HCS, Struijk PC, et al. Peak ventilatory responses during cycling and swimming in pregnant and nonpregnant women. J Appl Physiol 1996;81:738–742.

40. Heenan AP, Wolfe LA, Davies GAL. Maximal exercise testing in late gestation: maternal responses. Obstet Gynecol 2001;97:127–134.

41. Artal R. Exercise and pregnancy. Clin Sports Med 1992;11:363–377.

42. Bonen A, Campagna P, Gilchrist L, et al. Substrate and endocrine responses during exercise at selected stages of pregnancy. J Appl Physiol 1992;73:134–142.

43. Avery ND, Wolfe LA, Amara CE, et al. Effects of human pregnancy on autonomic function above and below the ventilatory threshold. J Appl Physiol 2001;90:321–328.

44. Pivarnik JM, Stein AD, Rivera JW. Effect of pregnancy on heart rate/oxygen consumption calibration curves. Med Sci Sports Exerc 2002;34:750–755.

45. Sady SP, Carpenter MW, Sady MA, et al. Prediction of $\dot{V}O_{2max}$ during cycle exercise in pregnant women. J Appl Physiol 1988;65:657–661.

46. Lotgering FK, Struijk, PC, Van Doorne MB, et al. Errors in predicting maximal oxygen consumption in pregnant women. J Appl Physiol 1992;72:562–567.

47. Lotgering FK, Struijk PC, VanDoorne MB, et al. Anaerobic threshold and respiratory compensation in pregnant women. J Appl Physiol 1995;78:1772–1777.

48. McMurray RG, Katz VL, Berry MJ, et al. The effect of pregnancy on metabolic responses during rest, immersion and aerobic exercise in the water. Am J Obstet Gynecol 1988;158:481–486.

49. Clapp JF III, Wesley M, Sleamaker RH. Thermoregulatory and metabolic responses prior to and during pregnancy. Med Sci Sports Exerc 1987;19:124–130.

50. Mottola MF, Christopher PD. Effects of exercise on liver and skeletal muscle glycogen storage in pregnant rats. J Appl Physiol 1991;1015–1019.

51. Treadway JL, Young JC. Decreased glucose uptake in the fetus after maternal exercise. Med Sci Sports Exerc 1989;21:140–145.

52. McMurray RG, Hackney AC, Guion WK, et al. Metabolic and hormonal responses to low-impact aerobic dance during pregnancy. Med Sci Sports Exerc 1996;28:41–46.

53. Soultanakis HN, Artal R, Wiswell RA. Prolonged exercise in pregnancy: glucose homeostasis, ventilatory and cardiovascular responses. Semin Perinatol 1996;20:315–327.

54. Lotgering FK, Spinnewijn WEM, Struijk PC, et al. Respiratory and metabolic responses to endurance cycle exercise in pregnant and postpartum women. Int J Sports Med 1998;19:193–198.

55. Avery ND, Stocking KD, Tranmer JE, et al. Fetal responses to maternal strength conditioning exercises in late gestation. Can J Appl Physiol 1999;24:362–376.

56. Morris N, Osborn SB, Wright MP, et al. Effective uterine blood-flow during normal and pre-eclamptic pregnancies. Lancet 1956;2:481–484.

57. Lotgering FK, Gilbert RD, Longo LD. Exercise responses in pregnant sheep: oxygen consumption, uterine blood flow and blood volume. J Appl Physiol 1983;55:834–841.

58. Morrow RJ, Ritchie JWK, Bull SB. Fetal and maternal hemodynamic responses to exercise in pregnancy assessed by Doppler ultrasonography. Am J Obstet Gynecol 1989;160:138–140.

59. Curet LB, Orr JA, Rankin JHG. Effect of exercise on cardiac output and distribution of uterine blood flow in pregnant ewes. J Appl Physiol 1976;40:725–728.

60. Greiss FC Jr. Differential reactivity of the myoendometrial and placental vasculatures: adrenergic responses. Am J Obstet Gynecol 1972;112:20–30.

61. Hohimer AR, Bissonette JM, Metcalfe J, et al. Effect of exercise on uterine blood flow in the pregnant pygmy goat. Am J Physiol 1984;246:H207–H212.

62. Lotgering FK, Longo LD. Exercise and pregnancy—how much is too much? Contemp Obstet/Gynecol 1984;23:63–77.

63. Smith DW, Clarren SK, Harvey MAS. Hyperthermia as a possible teratogenic agent. Pediatrics 1978;92:878–883.

64. Pleet H, Graham JM, Smith DW. Central nervous system and facial defects associated with maternal hyperthermia at 4–15 weeks gestation. Pediatrics 1981;67:785–789.

65. Kilham L, Ferm VH. Exencephaly in fetal hamsters following exposure to hyperthermia. Teratology 1976;14:323–326.

66. Abrams R, Caton D, Clapp J, et al. Thermal and metabolic features of life in utero. Clin Obstet Gynecol 1970;13:459–564.

67. Lotgering FK, Gilbert RD, Longo LD. Exercise responses in pregnant sheep: blood gases, temperatures, and fetal cardiovascular system. J Appl Physiol 1983;55:842–850.

68. Jones RL, Bati JJ, Anderson, WM, et al. Thermoregulation during aerobic exercise in pregnancy. Obstet Gynecol 1985;65:340–345.

69. Clapp JF III. The changing thermal response to endurance exercise during pregnancy. Am J Obstet Gynecol 1991;165:1684–1689.

70. Clapp JF III, Little KD, Capeless EL. Fetal heart rate response to sustained recreational exercise. Am J Obstet Gynecol 1993;168:198–206.

71. Webb KA, Wolfe LA, McGrath MJ. Effects of acute and chronic maternal exercise on fetal heart rate. J Appl Physiol 1994;77:2207–2213.

72. Brenner IKM, Wolfe LA, Monga M, et al. Physical conditioning effects on fetal heart rate responses to graded maternal exercise. Med Sci Sports Exerc 1999;31:792–799.

73. Carpenter MW, Sady SP, Hoegsberg B. Fetal heart rate response to maternal exertion. JAMA 1988;259:3006–3009.

74. Manders MAM, Sonder GB, Mulder EJH, et al. The effects of maternal exercise on fetal heart rate and movement patterns. Early Hum Dev 1997;48:237–247.

75. MacPhail A, Davies GAL, Victory R, et al. Maximal exercise testing in late gestation: fetal responses. Obstet Gynecol 2000;96:565–570.

76. Wolfe LA, McAuley SE, McGrath MJ. Controlled randomized study of aerobic conditioning effects on metabolic responses to graded exercise in pregnancy. Med Sci Sports Exerc 1998;30:S24 (abstr).

77. McAuley SE, Wolfe LA, McGrath MJ. Controlled randomized study of aerobic conditioning effects on respiratory responses to graded exercise in pregnancy. Med Sci Sports Exerc 1998;30:S24 (abstr).

78. Morton, MJ, Paul MS, Compos GR. Exercise dynamics in late gestation: effects of physical training. Am J Obstet Gynecol 1985;152:91–97.

79. Greer FA, Wolfe LA. Chronic exercise effects on subcutaneous adiposity in pregnancy. Med Sci Sports Exerc 1994;25:S119 (abstr).

80. Pivarnik JM. Potential effects of physical activity on birth weight: brief review. Med Sci Sports Exerc 1998;30:400–406.

81. Clapp JF, Dickstein S. Endurance exercise and pregnancy outcome. Med Sci Sports Exerc 1984;16:556–562.

82. Bell RJ, Palma SM, Lumley JM. The effect of vigorous exercise during pregnancy on birth-weight. Aust NZ J Obstet Gynecol 1995;35:46–51.

83. Clapp JF III, Capeless EL. Neonatal morphometrics after endurance exercise during pregnancy. Am J Obstet Gynecol 1990;163:1805–1811.

84. Hatch MC, Shu X, McLean DE, et al. Maternal exercise during pregnancy, physical fitness, and fetal growth. Am J Epidemiol 1993;137:1105–1114.

85. Clapp JF III, Kim H, Burciu B, et al. Beginning regular exercise in early pregnancy: effect on fetoplacental growth. Am J Obstet Gynecol 2000;183:1484–1488.

86. Brenner IKM, Monga M, Webb KA, et al. Controlled prospective study of aerobic conditioning effects on pregnancy outcome. Med Sci Sports Exerc 1991;23:S169 (abstr).

87. Wolfe LA, Mottola MF, Bonen A, et al. Controlled randomized study of aerobic conditioning effects on neonatal morphometrics. Med Sci Sports Exerc 1999;31:S138 (abstr).

88. Lokey EA, Tran VE, Wells CL, et al. Effects of physical exercise on pregnancy outcomes: a meta-analytic review. Med Sci Sports Exerc 1991;23:1234–1239.

89. Campbell KM, Mottola MF. Recreational exercise and occupational activity during pregnancy and birthweight: a case-control study. Am J Obstet Gynecol 2001;184:403–408.

90. Canadian Society for Exercise Physiology (CSEP). Physical Activity Readiness Medical Examination for Pregnancy (PARmed-X for Pregnancy). Available from CSEP, 185 Sommerset St. W., Suite 202, Ottawa, ON K2P 0J2, Canada, 2002.

91. Canadian Society for Exercise Physiology (CSEP). (Kochan-Vintinner A, Wolfe LA, Mottola MF, eds.) Active Living during Pregnancy. Available from CSEP, 185 Somerset St. West, Suite 202, Ottawa K2P 0J2, Canada, 1999.

92. American College of Obstetricians and Gynecologists (ACOG). Exercise during Pregnancy and the Postnatal Period. ACOG committee opinion no. 267:1–3. Washington, DC: ACOG, 2002.

93. Harvey M-A. Pelvic floor exercises during and after pregnancy: a systematic review of their role in preventing pelvic floor dysfunction. J Obstet Gynaecol Can 2003;25:487–498.

94. Clapp FJ III, Little KD. Effects of recreational exercise on pregnancy weight gain and subcutaneous fat deposition. Med Sci Sports Exerc 1995:27:170–177.

95. Jovanovic-Peterson L, Durak EP, Peterson CM. Randomized trial of diet versus diet plus cardiovascular conditioning on glucose levels in gestational diabetes. Am J Obstet Gynecol 1989;161:415–419.

96. Jovanovic-Peterson L, Peterson CM. Exercise and the nutritional management of diabetes during pregnancy. Obstet Gynecol Clin North Am 1996;23:75–86.

97. Dye TD, Knox KL, Artal R, et al. Physical activity, obesity, and diabetes in pregnancy. Am J Epidemiol 1997;146:961–963.

98. Marcoux S, Brisson J, Fabia J. The effect of leisure time physical activity on the risk of pre-eclampsia and gestational hypertension. J Epidemiol Community Health 1989;43:147–152.

99. Yeo SA, Davidge ST. Possible beneficial effect of exercise, by reducing oxidative stress, on the incidence of preeclampsia. J Women's Health Gender-Based Med 2001;10:983–989.

100. Camporesi EM. Diving and pregnancy. Semin Perinatol 1996;20:292–302.

101. Artal R, Fortunato V, Welton A, et al. A comparison of cardiopulmonary adaptations to exercise in pregnancy at sea level and altitude. Am J Obstet Gynecol 1995;172:1170–1180.

102. Katz VL, McMurray RG, Berry MJ, et al. Fetal and uterine responses to immersion and exercise. Obstet Gynecol 1988;72:225–230.

103. McMurray RG, Hackney AC, Katz VL, et al. Pregnancy-induced changes in the maximal physiological responses during swimming. J Appl Physiol 1991;71:1454–1459.

104. Mottola MF, Fitzgerald HM, Wilson NC, et al. Effect of water temperature on exercise-induced

maternal hyperthermia on fetal development in rats. Int J Sports Med 1993;14:248–251.

RELATED WEB SITES/RESOURCES

Canadian Society for Exercise Physiology (CSEP)
www.csep.ca/forms.asp
Physical Activity Readiness Medical Examination for Pregnancy (PARmed-X for Pregnancy) (download free from site) or Active Living During Pregnancy. Physical Activity Guidelines for Mother and Baby © 1999 (cost: $11.95). Available online and/or available from CSEP, 185 Sommerset St. W., Suite 202, Ottawa, Ontario K2P 0J2, Canada. Tel. 1-877-651-3755; Fax: (613) 877-3755; E-mail: info@csep.ca.

Health Canada
www.hc-sc.gc.ca
Nutrition for a Healthy Pregnancy: National Guidelines for the Childbearing Years © 1999. Available from Health Canada, Minister of Public Works and Government Services Canada, Ottawa, Ontario, Canada or online.

The Society of Obstetricians and Gynaecologists of Canada
www.sogc.org/SOGCnet/sogc docs/common/guide/pdfs/ps129.pdf

Canadian Society for Exercise Physiology (CSEP)
www.csep.ca

Davies GAL, Wolfe LA, Mottola MF, MacKinnons C. Joint SOGC/CSEP clinical practice guideline. Exercise in pregnancy and the postpartum period. J Obstet Gynecol Can 2003;25:516–522 and J Appl Physiol 2003;28:329–341.

The Society of Obstetricians and Gynaecologists of Canada
www.sogc.org
Healthy Beginnings: Your Handbook for Pregnancy and Birth © 1998. Available online. Cost: $12.95.

26

Mental Retardation

Kenneth H. Pitetti and Bo Fernhall

Definition and Etiology

An individual is considered to have mental retardation (MR) based on the following three criteria: (a) intellectual functional level (IQ) below 70 to 75; (b) significant limitations in two or more adaptive skill areas; and (c) the condition existing since childhood (defined as age 18 or less) (1). Adaptive skills areas are skills needed to live, work, and play (i.e., recreational activities) in the community. They include communication, self-care, home living, social skills, leisure skills, health and safety skills, self-direction, functional academics (reading, writing, and basic math), and community use and work responsibility. Approximately 3% of the general population in the United States, or over 7.5 million individuals, have MR (2). MR is 10 times more common than cerebral palsy, is 28 times more prevalent than neural tube defects such as spina bifida, and affects 25 times as many persons as blindness (2). MR is present in all racial, ethnic, educational, and economic groups, and one of 10 American families is directly affected by this condition.

Approximately 87% of individuals with MR have mild MR and are only a little "slower" than average in learning new information and skills. For those with mild MR, their MR is often not readily apparent and may not be identified until they enter school. As adults, these individuals can lead independent lives in the community (i.e., be self-supporting). The remaining 13% of persons with MR have serious functional limitations and require more support systems.

MR can be caused by any condition that impairs development of the brain before birth, during birth, or in early childhood. Several hundred causes have been discovered, but the cause remains unknown in about one-third of the persons affected (1). The known causes of MR can be categorized as follows (1,2):

- **Genetic conditions:** abnormality of inherited genes (e.g., PKU and fragile X-syndrome), errors when chromosomes divide unevenly as in nondisjunction (e.g., Down syndrome), or genetic disruptions (i.e., deletions) caused by overexposure to x-rays during pregnancy
- **Problems during pregnancies:** use of alcohol (e.g., fetal alcohol syndrome), drugs, or tobacco by pregnant mothers; hydrocephalus; malnutrition; and infections such as toxoplasmosis, cytomegalovirus, rubella, and syphilis
- **Problems at birth:** prematurity and low birth weight, and oxygen deprivation during delivery
- **Problems after birth:** childhood diseases such as whooping cough, chicken pox, and measles that can lead to meningitis and encephalitis; accidents

such as a blow to the head or near drowning; and lead, mercury, and other environmental toxins that can cause damage to the brain
- **Poverty and cultural deprivation:** research strongly suggests that understimulation of children due to deprivation of common cultural and day-to-day experiences can cause MR

Diagnosis

The American Association on Mental Retardation's process for diagnosing and classifying a person as having MR contains three diagnostic steps. First, a qualified person (usually within a school system) gives one or more standardized intelligence tests and standardized adaptive skills tests on an individual basis. Second, the person's strengths and weaknesses are described across four dimensions: *(a)* intellectual and adaptive behavior skills; *(b)* psychologic/emotional considerations; *(c)* physical/health etiologic considerations; and *(d)* environmental considerations. Strengths and weaknesses within each of the four dimensions may be determined by formal testing, observations, interviewing key people in the individual's life, interviewing the individual, and interacting with the person in his or her daily life.

The third diagnostic step requires an interdisciplinary team to determine support needed across the four dimensions. There are four levels of support:

- **Intermittent:** support on an "as needed basis," required occasionally over a lifespan, but not on a continuous daily basis (e.g., finding a new job in the event of a job loss)
- **Limited:** support during a transition from school to work or in time-limited job training (i.e., support is limited to the time necessary to provide appropriate support or training)
- **Extensive:** assistance needed on a daily basis, at home or at work
- **Pervasive:** constant support that may include life-sustaining measures

Intermittent, limited, and extensive support may not be needed in all dimensions, but pervasive support would include all dimensions.

This chapter is limited to individuals with mild MR, with intermittent-to-extensive support across the four dimensions, since this describes the characteristics for most individuals with MR who reside in the community setting.

Cardiorespiratory Capacities

This section discusses the cardiorespiratory fitness of persons with MR with and without Down syndrome (DS). Since the cardiorespiratory responses to exercise of individuals with and without DS differ considerably, these groups are discussed separately (3–7).

INDIVIDUALS WITHOUT DOWN SYNDROME

Most laboratory-based studies of the cardiorespiratory capacities ($\dot{V}O_{2peak}$) of adults with MR but without DS have evaluated young adults (18–40 years). These studies reported mean cardiovascular fitness of young adults with MR ranging from low ($\dot{V}O_{2peak} = 30$ mL·kg^{-1}·min^{-1}) (5,6,8) to average (38–42 mL·kg^{-1}·min^{-1}) (8–11). Studies (5,8–13) including both men and women reported that women with MR demonstrated cardiovascular fitness levels 10 to 20% lower than those of their male peers, consistent with data on nondisabled individuals. Interestingly, in the largest study to date (276 adults with MR), the mean $\dot{V}O_{2peak}$ (males and females combined) of the group with MR was very close to an age- and gender-matched control group composed of nondisabled individuals (33.8 vs. 35.5 mL·kg^{-1}·min^{-1}, respectively) (14). Most participants with MR in these studies (5,8–14) lived in a community setting either with caregivers or in group homes, and their activity level was considered sedentary. However, Frey et al. (13) reported a mean $\dot{V}O_{2peak}$ of 56 mL·kg^{-1}·min^{-1}) for 9 trained runners with MR. Thus, based on laboratory studies, adults with MR without DS exhibit low-to-normal levels of aerobic power, but well-trained individuals with MR may have high $\dot{V}O_{2peak}$ values.

Recent studies on laboratory-based cardiovascular capacities of children and adolescents with MR but without DS report values similar to those discussed above for young adults with MR. These studies reported $\dot{V}O_{2peak}$ values below or close to those of their nondisabled peers. Fernhall, Pitetti, and colleagues have reported low mean $\dot{V}O_{2peak}$ values for male (32–36 mL·kg^{-1}·min^{-1}) and female (26–35 mL·kg^{-1}·min^{-1}) children and adolescents with MR (15–17). In another study (18), Fernhall, Pitetti and colleagues reported mean cardiovascular fitness levels for combined male and female children and adolescents with MR that were well within the normal range (39.4–46.0 mL·kg^{-1}·min^{-1}) of their nondisabled peers. Teo-Koh and McCubbin (19) also reported mean $\dot{V}O_{2peak}$ values of children and adolescents with MR that were well within the normal range (41 mL·kg^{-1}·min^{-1}). Another study by Pitetti et al. (20) reported high values for boys with MR (46 mL·kg^{-1}·min^{-1}) but relatively low values for girls with MR (31 mL·kg^{-1}·min^{-1}). In this study (20), the $\dot{V}O_{2peak}$ levels of the males with MR did not differ from those of their nondisabled peers, but the females with MR had significantly lower $\dot{V}O_{2peak}$ values than females without MR. Thus, male children and adolescents with MR have either low or close to expected levels of $\dot{V}O_{2peak}$, whereas females tend to have lower than expected $\dot{V}O_{2peak}$ values.

Both adults and children with MR without DS have lower peak minute ventilation (V_{Epeak}, L·min^{-1}) at maximal exercise than their peers without MR. It is unclear if the low V_{Epeak} is a limitation to exercise or just a function of their sedentary status and low $\dot{V}O_{2peak}$ values. Peak ventilation in well-trained individuals with MR is at expected levels (13) and $\dot{V}O_{2peak}$ of those individuals with low aerobic power is comparable to that seen in other sedentary populations with low aerobic power (21). Thus, it appears that V_{Epeak} is appropriate for the $\dot{V}O_{2peak}$ achieved in persons with MR. Furthermore, peak respiratory exchange ratios (RER_{peak}) are within normal limits, and most individuals with MR (without DS) can achieve an RER_{peak} of 1.1 or above (5,14).

Adults with MR typically have lower than expected maximal/peak heart rate (HR_{peak}) (5); a recent study showed that individuals with MR without DS typically exhibit an HR_{peak} 15 beats per minute (bpm) lower. Thus, the commonly used formula of 220 – age does not work for this population (14). Children with MR also exhibit a slightly reduced maximal/peak HR, but usually only 5 to 9 bpm lower (17,18,22). The reason for the lower than predicted maximal/peak heart rate in individuals with MR is not known at this time.

INDIVIDUALS WITH DOWN SYNDROME

DS is one of the major known causes of MR in the United States (3). Several physiologic alterations associated with DS place these individuals at greater disadvantage concerning physical capacities than their peers with MR but without DS (4). Some of these physiologic alterations that affect exercise capacity are congenital heart defects, pulmonary hypoplasia, skeletal muscle hypotonia, and atlantoaxial instability. Although it is beyond the scope of this chapter to identify all of the specific physiologic alterations associated with DS, recent research has clearly established that persons with DS have worse physical fitness profiles than their peers with MR but without DS (5–7).

Laboratory-based studies of $\dot{V}O_{2peak}$ of young adults (mean ages 18–30 years) with DS consistently report low values, with most studies reporting mean $\dot{V}O_{2peak}$ values averaging only 25 mL·kg^{-1}·min^{-1} (5,23–26). In addition, comparative studies have reported that the cardiovascular capacities of adults with DS are lower than those of their peers with MR but without DS (5,24). Pitetti et al. (24) compared two groups of 16 young adults (12 males and 4 females) with and without DS and reported that the mean $\dot{V}O_{2peak}$ was 31% lower (24.6 vs. 35.6 mL·kg^{-1}·min^{-1}) than that of their peers without DS. Fernhall et al. (5) complemented and extended these findings (24) by comparing 47 young adults (31 males and 16 females) with DS to 64 young adults (35 males and 29 females) without DS and reported that the mean $\dot{V}O_{2peak}$ for the group with DS was significantly lower than that of their non-DS peers (25.1 vs. 30.6 mL·kg^{-1}·min^{-1}). In both studies (5,24), $\dot{V}O_{2peak}$ for the females with DS was 9 to 20% lower than that of their male peers.

One study (26) reported close to normal $\dot{V}O_{2peak}$ values in individuals with DS who trained 5 hours per week. These individuals had a mean $\dot{V}O_{2peak}$ of 34.3 mL·kg^{-1}·min^{-1}, compared with 27.4 mL·kg^{-1}·min^{-1} for a sedentary, age-matched group of persons with DS. However, the reported

$\dot{V}O_{2peak}$ of the training group in this study (26) would still be considered low compared with values from nondisabled adults in their mid-20s with a similar training volume.

Adolescents (23,25) and children with DS (27) exhibit $\dot{V}O_{2peak}$ values similar to those of adults with DS. Based on the results of these studies, it appears that the cardiovascular fitness of children, adolescents, and young adults with DS is lower than both that of their nondisabled peers and that of their peers with MR but without DS.

Like their peers without DS, individuals with DS exhibit a low V_{Epeak} (5,14). However, their V_{Epeak} is appropriate for their $\dot{V}O_{2peak}$ and comparable to values seen in other populations with similar aerobic power. Their RER_{peak} is typically lower (6,14,27), averaging between 1.05 and 1.1 (5,14,23–25). These lower RER_{peak} values are not related to poor effort (6), but reflect true maximal effort of individuals with DS.

The HR_{peak} of individuals with DS is substantially reduced (5,14,23,25,26). The HR_{peak} is typically between 150 and 175 bpm (regardless of age) and averages around 30 bpm below expected values (14). The mechanism behind this poor chronotropic response is unknown, but it is not a function of poor motivation or effort (6).

Possible Contributing Factors to Low Aerobic Power in Individuals with MR

MOTIVATION AND TASK UNDERSTANDING

During the 1970s and 1980s, some of the commonly cited causes of poor cardiovascular test results of persons with MR, with and without DS were poor motivation and task understanding (11,28,29). It was generally thought that because of their below-normal IQ and associated behavioral problems, persons with MR *(a)* would have difficulty understanding the concept of "giving your best" during exercise testing and *(b)* are not motivated to perform high-intensity physical activity tasks. However, recent research in this area has established that motivation and task understanding can be controlled and are primarily related to the use of proper testing methodologies. Researchers have developed a comprehensive familiarization protocol used prior to actual testing to ensure that participants are comfortable with the laboratory procedures and can understand what is expected of them (12,22,28,30). Thus, with appropriate familiarization, poor motivation and task understanding do not explain the low aerobic power often reported.

LACK OF PHYSICAL ACTIVITY

It is generally assumed that most children, adolescents, and adults with MR (with and without DS) do not engage in regular physical activity, and thus lack of activity contributes to the poor cardiovascular fitness reported in the literature (12,28,29). However, few objective data exist on physical activity patterns of individuals with MR.

An abstract by Frey et al. (31) reported low physical activity levels measured by activity monitors in a small number of adults (four males and one female) with MR. However, children with MR do not appear to differ from their peers without MR. Using the doubly labeled water technique to measure energy expenditure, Luke et al. (32) reported that the total daily energy expenditure in children with DS did not differ from that seen in their nondisabled peers. Lorenzi et al. (33) found that children with and without MR exhibited similar activity levels during school recess (activity was measured by direct observation). Their findings (33) were recently supported by those of Horvat and Franklin (34), who used HR and activity monitors. However, a study by Johnson et al. (35) reported no relationship between laboratory-assessed $\dot{V}O_{2peak}$ and intensity (measured by HR monitors) of spontaneous physical activity in 16 adolescents (12 males and 4 females) with MR. Thus, it is unclear if their daily physical activity levels are lower, especially those of adults with MR.

The work by Frey et al. (13) and Guerra et al. (26) does imply, however, that individuals with MR who are very active (compared with individuals with MR who are presumed sedentary) demonstrate higher cardiovascular fitness. Frey et al. (13) reported high $\dot{V}O_{2peak}$ levels (56.3 mL·kg^{-1}·min^{-1}) in well-trained runners with MR, which is considerably better than the values of 30–40 mL·kg^{-1}·min^{-1} reported in studies that described their participants with MR as "sedentary." Similarly, Guerra et al. (26) found that trained individuals with DS had higher $\dot{V}O_{2peak}$ values than their sedentary peers (34.3 vs. 27.4 mL·kg^{-1}·min^{-1}, respectively). These two studies strongly suggest that lifestyle (i.e., active vs. sedentary) has a similar impact on the cardiovascular fitness of persons with MR and those in the general population (36,37).

LEG STRENGTH AND CARDIOVASCULAR FITNESS

Muscle strength is not generally a limiting factor for aerobic performance, except in some populations with severely reduced muscle strength, such as heart failure patients (38). Pitetti and Boneh (39) demonstrated a significant relationship between isokinetic leg strength and $\dot{V}O_{2peak}$ in adults with MR, especially in those with DS. Pitetti and Fernhall's study (40) showed similar findings in children and adolescents with MR. Furthermore, leg strength contributes to endurance run performance in youth with MR, and the relationship between leg strength and run performance was similar to that of $\dot{V}O_{2peak}$ and run performance (41). Although indirect, these data suggest that leg strength is a significant contributor to $\dot{V}O_{2peak}$ for persons with MR.

Studies comparing the leg strength of persons with MR with that of their nondisabled peers reported the following: (*a*) isokinetic leg strength of adults with MR, with and without DS, was significantly weaker than that of nondisabled adults (42,43), (*b*) adults with DS had lower leg strength than their peers with MR but without DS (42), and (*c*) leg and back strength of children and adolescents with MR was lower than that of their peers without disabilities (44,45). Given that reportedly leg strength is significantly related to $\dot{V}O_{2peak}$ and run performance for adults and youths with MR and that leg strength of persons with MR is lower, it is possible that poor leg strength is a limiting factor to $\dot{V}O_{2peak}$ in this population.

CHRONOTROPIC INCOMPETENCE

The chronotropic response to maximal exercise is reduced in persons with MR, especially in those with DS. This is similar to chronotropic incompetence (a low maximal or peak HR) observed in several clinical populations (46), thus the term *chronotropic incompetence* has been applied to the HR response of persons with MR (6). A number of investigators have suggested that chronotropic incompetence is a possible limitation to $\dot{V}O_{2peak}$ in persons with MR (5,6,14), especially persons with DS, because a low HR_{peak} would limit maximal cardiac output. Fernhall et al. (5) provided support for this notion, showing that the difference in $\dot{V}O_{2peak}$ between groups with and without DS disappeared when differences in HR_{peak} were controlled.

Exercise Testing

Motivation, task understanding, attention deficits, and poor motor capacities can cause wide variability in test results. Therefore, practice sessions must be scheduled before the actual test to help control for these factors. Practice sessions will (*a*) familiarize the participant with the test protocol, environment, and staff and (*b*) allow staff members to adjust the protocol to ensure safety of the participant and validity of test results. The latter becomes especially important for treadmill testing. Walking protocols are strongly recommended for treadmill testing, and the speed should be selected on the basis of the participant's ability. Selecting a walking speed that is too fast can result in early termination of the test due to trepidation, rather than fatigue. In addition, the practice session may reveal that the participant cannot perform the intended protocol or exercise mode. For instance, ambulatory limitations and/or poor coordination could prevent a participant from performing a treadmill test and/or keeping the proper cadence/rhythm in pedaling/stepping-type tests. More practice time or a different mode of testing may be necessary to ensure valid results.

Chronotropic incompetence of persons with MR results in peak HRs 15 to 30 bpm below that obtained from age-predicted formulas (e.g., 220 − age) used for the general population. Therefore, these general formulas cannot be used to predict maximal/peak HR for persons with MR. Fernhall and colleagues (14) developed a population-specific formula for predicting HR_{peak}

in persons with MR, including those with DS:

$$HR_{max} = 210 - 0.56 \, (age) - 15.5 \, (DS)$$
$$(R = .57, SEE = 11.8, \, P < .01) \, (46)$$

For persons with DS, DS would be coded 2; for a person with MR but without DS, DS would be coded 1.

The age range of the participants used to develop the formula (14) was limited to 8 to 46 years. Thus, this formula should only be used to predict maximal/peak HR in individuals with MR between these ages. This formula may help as a guide during maximal and submaximal exercise testing and could provide a basis for exercise prescription when testing is not feasible.

CARDIOVASCULAR TESTING

Treadmill
One must select a walking speed between 2.0 and 3.5 mph (3.2 to 5.6 km·h^{-1}) to allow the participants to walk briskly and in control (i.e., without the need to hold onto hand rails). Begin at a grade of 0%, with 2.5% increases every 2 min until a grade of 12.5% is reached. If participants can continue, keep the grade at 12.5% while increasing speed 0.5 mph (0.8 km·h^{-1}) every minute until they can no longer continue. This protocol can be used to evaluate children, adolescents, and/or adults with MR, with and without DS (5,12,20), as well as adolescents and young adults with multiple disabilities (e.g., MR and concomitant disabilities such as blindness, deafness, Asperger's disorder, speech and language impairments) (47).

Combined Arm and Leg Cycle Ergometry
Ambulatory limitations due to physical disabilities (e.g., cerebral palsy) that can accompany MR and/or poor coordination may limit the walking capacity of some individuals with MR. A combined arm and leg cycle ergometer, such as the Schwinn Air-Dyne, can elicit peak HR and $\dot{V}O_{2peak}$ values similar to, or higher than, those obtained with a treadmill test for persons with MR without physical disabilities (48) and for persons with cerebral palsy (49). The protocol recommended for this mode is an initial power output of 25 W, with increases of 25 W every 2 min. Unfortunately, most combined arm and leg ergometers are built to accommodate adults and older adolescents (15–18 years) but not young adolescents (11–14 years) or children.

Leg Cycle Ergometry
Leg cycle ergometry can also be used for cardiovascular evaluation of persons with MR. The limiting factor for persons with MR using this method is their inability to maintain the proper cycle speed. Leg protocols on mechanically braked ergometers require a constant pedal speed, which is difficult for many persons with MR to maintain. Electronically braked cycle ergometers automatically adjust resistance to the pedal speed to keep the power output (W) constant, which circumvents this limitation. The other limiting factor of leg cycle ergometry is similar to that mentioned for the combined arm and leg cycle ergometry—most models cannot accommodate young adolescents or children. The protocol recommended for leg cycle ergometry is the same as for combined leg and arm cycle ergometry: an initial power output of 25 W, with increases of 25 W every 2 min. However, these types of cycling protocols have not been validated in populations with MR.

Field Testing
In all field-testing procedures presented in this section, the use of a *pacer* is essential to ensure validity and reliability of the test performance by the participants with MR. A pacer runs alongside or slightly in front of the participant to (a) provide constant verbal support and encouragement (to minimize the effect of poor motivation) and (b) prevent having the participant start the test at too fast a pace (to ensure that the participants will run/walk at a pace that will measure their aerobic, rather than anaerobic, capacity).

The following factors should also be considered when using these field tests: (a) the age population from which these tests are corroborated were either young adults (19–40 years) or children and adolescents (8–18 years); (b) only a modest number of participants (20–40) were involved in each of the studies; (c) the 1.5-mile run/walk test (50,51) and the 1-mile walk test (Rockport fitness walking test) (9,10) studies involved only adults, whereas the 20-meter shuttle run test (20 MST) (17,18) studies involved only children and adolescents; (d) the 1-mile Rockport fitness walking test (9,10) involved only males; and *(e)* although all the field tests are reliable, only one (the 20 MST) has been shown to be valid through both validation and cross-validation studies (17,18).

1.5-Mile Run/Walk. These studies (50,51) were performed on a 220-yard indoor track housed in a temperature-controlled building. In the first study (50), the prediction equation from bivariate regression analysis was: $\dot{V}O_{2peak}$ (mL·kg^{-1}·min^{-1}) $= 49.9 - 1.0(x)$, where $x =$ time in minutes for completion of 1.5-mile run/walk. The second study (51) produced a second prediction equation: $\dot{V}O_{2peak}$ (mL·kg^{-1}·min^{-1}) $= 47.5 - 0.919(x)$. Given the same time (x) to complete the test, only a 3% difference was found between formulas.

1.0-Mile Rockport Fitness Walking Test. This test was performed in an indoor temperature-controlled facility using a 1/8-mile course that was marked with cones. The first study (9) used a multiple regression analysis to develop the following equation for predicting cardiovascular fitness: $\dot{V}O_{2peak}$ (mL·kg^{-1}·min^{-1}) $= 101.92 - 2.35$(mile time in min) $- 0.42$(weight in kg). The second study (10) was an attempt to cross-validate the formula developed from the initial study (9). However, the equation developed in the first study (9) significantly underestimated the measured $\dot{V}O_{2peak}$ values for most participants in the second study (10), suggesting that the formula may not be statistically valid. Also, the participants in both studies (9,10) were male.

20-Meter Shuttle Run Test (20 MST) for Children and Adolescents. The 20 MST has been validated and cross-validated as a valid and reliable field test to determine the cardiovascular fitness of children and adolescents (8–18 years) with MR without DS (17,18). The 20 MST can be administered on either a tennis court surface or gymnasium floor, with the distance marked by painted or taped stripes and also marked by cones, as described by Fernhall et al. (17). Prudential Fitnessgram (52) tapes must be used for proper pacing, along with a pacer. The formula used to estimate cardiovascular fitness (17) is as follows:

$$\dot{V}O_{2peak}(mL \cdot kg^{-1} \cdot min^{-1}) = 0.35 \,(\text{No. of laps})$$
$$-0.59 \,(\text{body mass index } [BMI])$$
$$-4.61(\times 1, \text{male}; \times 2, \text{female}) + 50.6$$

Using the formula for a 10-year-old male with a BMI of 20 who stops on lap 35 gives him a predicted $\dot{V}O_{2peak}$ of 46.5 mL·kg^{-1}·min^{-1}. This formula should not be used for children and adolescents with DS because it significantly overestimates their actual $\dot{V}O_{2peak}$ (27).

STRENGTH TESTING

Isotonic Strength Testing
Weight machines (e.g., Nautilus) rather than free weights should be used for safety purposes when testing muscle strength. One repetition maximum (1RM) weight measurement can be reliably determined using the following guidelines (53): *(a)* allow practice time for each movement at the lightest weight until participants can perform the movement properly and *(b)* increase weight by 2 1/2 to 5 lb (1.1–2.3 kg) for upper-body strength tests and 5 to 10 lb (2.3–4.5 kg) for trunk and lower-body strength tests for each trial until a weight is reached that cannot be lifted. Use the last weight successfully lifted as 1RM.

Isokinetic Strength Testing
When measuring isokinetic strength with an isokinetic dynamometer (e.g., Cybex) of persons with MR, tests should be performed on at least two separate days because *(a)* over 40% of the time, the best effort (i.e., strongest effort) is performed on the second test day and *(b)* differences between the best effort on the two separate testing days can range from 10 to 19% (54).

Participants must be allowed enough practice time for each movement with no resistance to ensure that they will complete the full range of motion (ROM) for the joint to be measured (e.g., elbow/knee flexion and extension). There is a tendency for persons with MR to shorten their ROM during the movement.

Once proper ROM has been established, the participant should then perform 10 practice repetitions, starting with little effort on the first two repetitions and gradually building to maximal effort on the final repetition. The following verbal coaching is recommended: *(a)* first two repetitions, "okay, lets start really easy now"; *(b)* repetitions 3–6, "okay, a little harder now"; *(c)* repetitions 7–8, "harder, harder"; and *(d)* repetitions 9–10, "go for it, give me your best." Allow a 2-min rest period, followed by two sets of three maximal efforts, with 30 sec between each set. The slower recommended angle speeds for each movement should be used. For instance, Pitetti and colleagues used angle speeds of 60 and $90°·sec^{-1}$ to measure elbow and knee flexion and extension of adolescents and young adults with MR, with and without DS (41,42, 54–56).

Isometric Strength Testing

Laboratory Testing. Most isokinetic machines can be used for isometric strength testing, and the protocol used to measure isometric strength for the general population can be used for persons with MR if familiarization and practice procedures discussed above are followed.

Field Testing. It is not realistic to use sophisticated, laboratory-based equipment to assess strength of individuals with MR in field-based settings. However, lightweight, portable, and affordable techniques have been used to measure isometric strength of children, adolescents, and adults with MR accurately and objectively (56–60). These include

1. Handgrip strength: Handgrip strength can be measured using the handgrip dynamometer. Participants should be seated with the elbow of their testing arm resting on a table and bent at approximately 90°, shoulder in neutral position. They should squeeze the handle of the handgrip dynamometer as hard as possible for 5 sec. Two trials should be performed, with the better of the trials recorded as the maximal effort for each hand.

2. Elbow flexion and extension strength: A hand-held dynamometer can be used to measure elbow flexion and extension. Participants should lie supine on a table with their elbow flexed at 90°, shoulder in a neutral (relaxed) position. The forearm should be in full supination during flexion and full pronation during extension. The hand-held device should be placed 1 in. below the styloid process of the ulna during the testing. Once participants are positioned, a "make" test is performed. In a "make" test, participants apply maximal force against the contact plate while the tester provides resistance to prevent the participant's arm from moving for 5 sec. The

better of two trials should be recorded as maximal effort.

3. Knee flexion and extension strength: A hand-held dynamometer should be used. Participants should be seated in an upright position on a table with their knees at the edge and feet freely hanging above the floor. The tester should kneel in front of them, stabilizing the contact plate of the device on the distal anterior (for knee extension) or posterior tibia (for knee flexion) 3 in. above the lateral malleolus. Once participants are positioned, a "make" test (described above for elbow flexion and extension) is performed. Two maximal efforts for both right and left knee flexion and extension with a 1-min rest period between efforts should be performed and the better of the two efforts used as maximal effort.

4. Combined back and leg strength: Combination isometric back and leg strength can be measured using a back-and-leg dynamometer. The chain length on the dynamometer should be adjusted so that participants are squatted over the dynamometer with knees flexed approximately 30°. Grasping the handle bar, back straight, participants should pull up, while pushing from the legs, at a maximal effort for 5 sec. Two measurements should be taken, with the stronger effort used as maximal effort.

The above movement is a test only for leg strength. For back strength, the legs are straight and the back is flexed to allow the bar to be at the level of the patella. Subjects are then asked to try to straighten their backs (i.e., stand upright) without bending their knees.

Exercise Prescription

CARDIOVASCULAR EXERCISE PRESCRIPTION

The general guidelines for exercise programing are found in Table 26-1.

Adults without DS
Research has demonstrated that the same principles established by the American College of Sports Medicine for the proper frequency, intensity, time, mode and progression of exercise training needed to improve the cardiorespiratory condition of the

TABLE 26-1 EXERCISE PROGRAMMING FOR PERSONS WITH MENTAL RETARDATION

Modes	Brisk walking; walk/jogging; jogging; bicycle ergometer; combined arm/leg ergometers (e.g., Schwinn Air-Dyne)
Goals	Lose or maintain body weight; improve cardiovascular fitness
Intensity	60–80% peak HR reserve
Frequency	3–5 days/weeks
Duration	20–60-min/session
Special consideration	Because of motivation problems, constant supervision and encouragement is necessary

general population are also true for adults with MR but not DS (12, 13, 28, 60–67), but with some important modifications:

- Exercise should be supervised, since it is unlikely that most persons with MR will exercise on their own at the proper frequency, intensity, and duration.
- It may take longer than anticipated to produce an improvement in $\dot{V}O_{2peak}$ (i.e., 16–35 weeks may be necessary); improvements in *maximal power output* (e.g., peak watts) have occurred with programs of shorter duration.
- Without continual reinforcement and supervision, persons with MR are unlikely to continue to participate in exercise/activity programs through their lifetime.

Adults with DS

In two of the most-controlled exercise studies concerning young adults with DS, Millar et al. (25) and Varela et al. (68) both demonstrated improvements in work performance (i.e., time to exhaustion in graded exercise test, distance covered in walk/run test, and peak work level, in watts) but no significant improvement in $\dot{V}O_{2peak}$. However, these exercise regimens lasted only 10 weeks (25) and 16 weeks (68). As noted above, a longer training period may be needed to elicit improvements in $\dot{V}O_{2peak}$. For instance, Guerra et al. (26) reported that the DS participants who trained all year at a frequency of 5 + hours per week, demonstrated a significantly higher $\dot{V}O_{2peak}$ than their sedentary peers (34.3 vs.

27.4 mL·kg^{-1}·min^{-1}, respectively). Thus, more information on the cardiovascular training response of individuals with DS is needed. However, since a standard exercise prescription improves exercise capacity, following standard guidelines is appropriate.

RESISTANCE/STRENGTH TRAINING

Thera-Band

Croce and Horvat (69) trained three young adults for 12 weeks, three times per week, using Theraband tubing. The exercises worked only the upper body and concentrated on elbow extension, elbow flexion, shoulder transverse adduction, and shoulder abduction strength. Participants performed three sets of 8 to 12 repetitions for each movement. Results demonstrated increased isometric strength for each individual; however, the participants were supervised very closely.

Weight Machines

Rimmer and Kelly (53) trained 12 adults with MR without DS with a program that incorporated the following exercises: leg extension, leg curl, bench press, shoulder press, latissimus dorsi pull, biceps curl, and triceps extension. Participants exercised twice weekly for 9 weeks, worked in pairs, were grouped according to abilities, and were supervised by a graduate student and an activity specialist. Six training sessions preceded the actual training period to ensure that participants used the equipment correctly. The participants performed three sets of exercise on each machine in a progressive manner (i.e., 30, 60, and 70% of 1RM) and completed 8 to 10 repetitions per set. After 9 weeks of training the participants in this study (53) exhibited dramatic improvements in strength ranging from 25% to over 100% in each of the movements outlined above.

Suomi and colleagues (70,71) showed significant improvements in knee extension (70,71) and hip flexion (71) strength ranging from 25 to 177% in adult (25–35 years) males following 12 weeks of training. Hydraulic weight machines were used, with a frequency of exercise of three times per week. A subject-to-instructor ratio of 1:1 or 1:2 was maintained during the 12 weeks. In one of these studies (71), a 1-year self-directed component was added following the initial 12 weeks. The significant strength improvements seen after the 12-weeks training regimen were maintained during this 1-year self-directed training period.

Effects of Training on Mental Retardation

Three criteria are used to diagnose MR; low IQ, limited adaptive skills, and time of onset. Exercise training cannot significantly improve IQ nor overcome the event that caused MR. However, exercise training can improve some adaptive skills. Adaptive skills concerned with health, leisure, and work responsibilities/opportunities are directly related to cardiovascular and muscle strength and endurance (1,2).

For instance, persons with MR cannot live independently in our communities unless they are gainfully employed. The types of jobs that most persons with MR can be trained to perform include *(a)* working as a janitor; *(b)* working in supermarkets loading and unloading merchandise, stacking shelves, and collecting grocery carts; *(c)* working in storehouses of large companies loading and unloading merchandise; and *(d)* working on assembly lines. In conjunction with organizations whose main thrust is helping persons with MR find employment, these authors have found that the main factor limiting their employment opportunities is not their mental capacity, but rather their physical capacity. That is, because of their low physical fitness profiles (as outlined in this chapter), the number of hours they can work at these jobs and, therefore, their weekly earnings are greatly limited.

Summary

- Along with employment opportunities, improving the physical fitness profiles of persons with MR carries obvious health and leisure skill implications.
- Establishing guidelines allows evaluation of cardiovascular and muscle fitness of persons with MR.
- Exercise training, by improving physical capacities of persons with MR, assists in improving the

adaptive skills of these persons and, therefore, the condition of MR.

REFERENCES

1. Luckasson R, Coulter D, Polloway E, et al. Mental Retardation: Definition, Classification, and Systems of Support. 9th ed. Washington, DC: American Association of Mental Retardation, 1992.
2. Sherrill C. Adapted Physical Activity, Recreation and Sport: Cross Disciplinary and Lifespan. 5th ed. Dubuque, IA: Brown & Benchmark, 1998.
3. Kirk SA, Gallagher JJ. Educating Exceptional Children. Boston: Houghton Mifflin, 1972.
4. Shapiro BL. Down syndrome: a disruption of homeostasis. Am J Med Genet. 1983;14:241–269.
5. Fernhall B, Pitetti KH, Rimmer JH, et al. Cardiorespiratory capacity of individuals with mental retardation including Down syndrome. Med Sci Sports Exerc 1996; 28:366–371.
6. Fernhall B, Pitetti KH. Limitations to physical work capacity in individuals with mental retardation. Clin Exerc Physiol 2001;3:176–185.
7. Pitetti KH, Climstein M, Mays MJ, et al. The isokinetic arm and leg strength of adults with Down syndrome: a comparative study. Arch Phys Med Rehabil 1992;73:847–850.
8. Kittredge JM, Rimmer JH, Looney M. Validation of the Rockport fitness walking test for adults with mental retardation. Med Sci Sports Exerc 1994; 26: 95–102.
9. Rintala P, Dunn JM, McCubbin JA, et al. Validity of a cardiovascular fitness test for men with mental retardation. Med Sci Sports Exerc 1992;24:941–945.
10. Rintala P, McCubbin JA, Downs SB, et al. Cross validation of the 1-mile walking test for men with mental retardation. Med Sci Sports Exerc 1997;29:133–137.
11. McCubbin JA, Rintala P, Frey GC. Correlation study of three cardiorespiratory fitness tests for men with mental retardation. Adapt Phys Act Q 1997;14:432–450.
12. Pitetti KH, Rimmer JH, Fernhall B. Physical fitness and adults with mental retardation: an overview of current research, future directions and widespread applicability. Sports Med 1993;16:23–56.
13. Frey GC, McCubbin JA, Hannington-Downs S, et al. Physical fitness of trained runners with and without mental retardation. Adapt Phys Act Q 1999;16:126–137.
14. Fernhall B, McCubbin JA, Pitetti KH, et al. Prediction of maximal heart rate in individuals with mental retardation. Med Sci Sports Exerc 2001;33:1655–1660.

15. Fernhall B, Pitetti KH, Stubbs NS, et al. Validity and reliability of the $1/2$ mile run-walk as an indicator of aerobic fitness in children with mental retardation. Pediatr Exerc Sci 1996;8:130–142.

16. Pitetti KH, Fernhall B. Aerobic capacity as related to leg strength in youths with mental retardation. Pediatr Exerc Sci 1997;9:223–236.

17. Fernhall B, Pitetti KH, Vukovich M, et al. Validation of cardiovascular fitness field tests in children with mental retardation. Am J Ment Retard. 1998;102:602–612.

18. Fernhall B, Pitetti KH, Millar L, et al. Cross validation of the 20-m shuttle run in children with mental retardation. Adapt Phys Act Q 2000;17:402–412.

19. Teo-Koh SM, McCubbin JA. Relationship between $\dot{V}O_2$ and 1-mile walk test performance of adolescents with mental retardation. Pediatr Exerc Sci 1999;11:144–157.

20. Pitetti KH, Millar AL, Fernhall B. Reliability of a peak performance treadmill test for children and adolescents with and without mental retardation. Adapt Phys Act Q 2000;17:322–332.

21. Wasserman K, Hansen JE, Sue KY, et al. Principles of exercise testing and interpretation. 2nd ed. Philadelphia: Lea & Febiger, 1994.

22. Pitetti KH, Millar L, Fernhall B. Reliability of a peak performance treadmill test for children and adolescents with and without mental retardation. Adapt Phys Act Q 2000;17:322–332.

23. Fernhall B, Tymeson G, Millar L, et al. Cardiovascular fitness testing and fitness levels of adolescents and adults with mental retardation including Down syndrome. Educ Train Ment Retard 1989;24:133–138.

24. Pitetti KH, Climstein M, Campbell KD, et al. The cardiovascular capacities of adults with Down syndrome: a comparative study. Med Sci Sports Exerc 1992;24:13–19.

25. Millar AL, Fernhall B, Burkett LN, et al. Effect of aerobic training in adolescents with Down syndrome. Med Sci Sports Exerc 1993;25:260–264.

26. Guerra M, Roman B, Geronimo C, et al. Physical fitness levels of sedentary and active individuals with Down syndrome. Adapt Phys Act Q 2000;17:310–321.

27. Guerra M, daSilva A, Pitetti KH, et al. Predicted aerobic capacity in children and adolescents with Down syndrome. Med Sci Sports Exerc 2002;34(Suppl.):S16.

28. Fernhall B. Physical fitness and exercise training of individuals with mental retardation. Med Sci Sports Exerc 1993;25:442–450.

29. Seidl C, Reid G, Montgomery DL. A critique of cardiovascular fitness testing with mentally retarded persons. Adapt Phys Act Q 1987;4:106–116.

30. Fernhall B, Tymeson G. Graded exercise testing of mentally retarded adults: a study of feasibility. Arch Phys Med Rehabil 1987;68:363–365.

31. Frey GC. Objective assessment of physical activity in adults with mental retardation. Med Sci Sports Exerc 1997;29(Suppl):S244.

32. Luke A, Roisen NJ, Sutton M, et al. Energy expenditure in children with Down syndrome: correcting metabolic rate for movement. J Pediatr 1994:125:829–838.

33. Lorenzi DG, Horvat M, Pellegrini AD. Physical activity of children with and without mental retardation in inclusive recess settings. Educ Train Ment Retard Dev Disab 2000;35:160–167.

34. Horvat M, Franklin C. The effects of the environment on physical activity patterns of children with mental retardation. Res Q Exerc Sport 2001;71:189–195.

35. Johnson TL. Peak $\dot{V}O_2$ measures and heart rates during spontaneous physical activity: is there a correlation in youths with mental retardation. Masters thesis, Wichita State University, 1997.

36. Pate R, Pratt M, Blair SN, et al. Physical activity and public health. A recommendation from the Centers of Disease Control and Prevention and the American College of Sports Medicine. JAMA 1995;273:402–407.

37. Blair SN, Kohl HW, Paffenbarger RS, et al. Physical activity and all cause mortality: a prospective study of healthy men and women. JAMA 1989;262:2395–2401.

38. Volterraini M, Clark AL, Ludman PF, et al. Predictors of exercise capacity in chronic heart failure. Eur Heart J 1994;15:801–809.

39. Pitetti KH, Boneh S. Cardiovascular fitness as related to leg strength in adults with mental retardation. Med Sci Sports Exerc 1995;27:423–428.

40. Pitetti KH, Fernhall B. Aerobic capacity as related to leg strength in youths with mental retardation. Pediatr Exerc Sci 1997;9:223–236.

41. Fernhall B, Pitetti, KH. Leg strength is related to endurance run performance in children and adolescents with mental retardation. Pediatr Exerc Sci 2000;12:324–333.

42. Pitetti KH, Climstein M, Mays MJ, et al. The isokinetic arm and leg strength of adults with Down syndrome: a comparative study. Arch Phys Med Rehabil 1992;73:847–850.

43. Croce RV, Pitetti KH, Horvat M, et al. Comparison of peak torque, average power, and hamstrings/quadriceps ratio in non-disabled adults and adults with mental retardation. Arch Phys Med Rehabil 1996;77:369–372.

44. Horvat M, Croce R, Pitetti KH, et al. Comparison of

isokinetic peak force and work parameters in youth with and without mental retardation. Med Sci Sports Exerc 2000;31:1190–1195.

45. Pitetti KH, Yarmer DA. Lower body strength of children and adolescents with and without mild mental retardation: a comparison. Adapt Phys Act Q 2002; 129:68–81.

46. Cahalin LP. Exercise tolerance and training for healthy persons and patients with cardiovascular disease. In: Hansson SM, ed. Clinical Exercise Physiology. St. Louis: Mosby-Year Book, 1993:81–94.

47. Pitetti KH, Jongmans B, Fernhall B. Feasibility of a treadmill test for adolescents with multiple disabilities. Adapt Phys Act Q 1999;16:362–371.

48. Pitetti KH, Tan DM. Cardiovascular responses of mildly mentally retarded adults to air-brake ergometry and treadmill exercise. Arch Phys Med Rehabil 1990;71:318–321.

49. Fernandez JE, Pitetti KH, Betzen MT. Physiological capacities of individuals with cerebral palsy. Hum Factors 1990;32:457–466.

50. Fernhall B, Tymeson G. The relationship between cardiovascular fitness and field tests with mild and moderate mental retardation. Presented at the 15th national conference of Physical Activity for the Exceptional Individual. Woodland Hills, CA, 1986.

51. Fernhall B, Tymeson G. Validation of a cardiovascular fitness field test for adults with mental retardation. Adapt Phys Act Q 1988;5:49–59.

52. Cureton KJ. Aerobic capacity. In: Morrow JR, Falls HB, Kohl HW, eds. Fitnessgram technical reference manual. Dallas: Cooper Institute for Aerobics Research, 1994:33–56.

53. Rimmer JH, Kelly LE. Effects of a resistance training program of adults with mental retardation. Adapt Phys Act Q 1991;8:146–143.

54. Pitetti KH. A reliable isokinetic strength test for arm and leg musculature for mildly mentally retarded adults. Arch Phys Med Rehabil 1990;71:669–672.

55. Horvat M, Pitetti KH, Croce RV. Arm peak torque, average power, and flexion/extension ratios in nondisabled adults and adults with mental retardation. J Orthop Sports Phys Ther 1997;25:395–399.

56. Croce RV, Horvat M, Pitetti KH. Prediction of dynamic strength in individuals with mental retardation. Clin Kinesiol 1998;52:79–86.

57. Pitetti KH, Yarmer DA. Lower body strength of children and adolescents with and without mild mental retardation: a comparison. Adapt Phys Act Q 2002;19:68–81.

58. Horvat M, Croce RV, Roswal G. Intratester reliability of the Nicholas manual muscle tester on individual

and intellectual disabilities by a tester having minimal experience. Arch Phys Med Rehabil 1994;75:808–811.

59. Horvat M, Croce R, Roswal G, et al. Single trial versus maximal or mean values for evaluating strength in individuals with mental retardation. Adapt Phys Act Q 1995;12:52–59.

60. Pitetti KH, Fernandez JE, Pizarro DC, et al. Field testing: assessment of the physical fitness of mild to moderate mentally retarded individuals. Adapt Phys Act Q 1988;5:318–331.

61. Andrew GM, Reid G, Beck S, et al. Training of the developmentally handicapped young adult. Can J Appl Sport Sci 1979;4:289–293.

62. Beasley CR. Effects of jogging program on cardiovascular fitness and work performances of mentally retarded persons. Am J Ment Defic 1982;86:609–613.

63. Bundschuh EL, Cureton KJ. Effect of bicycle ergometer conditioning on the physical work capacity of mentally retarded adolescents. Am Correct Ther J 1982;36:159–163.

64. Nordgren B. Physical capacity and training in a group of young adult mentally retarded persons. Acta Paediatr Scand 1971;217(suppl):119–121.

65. Schurrer R, Weltman A, Brannel H. Effects of physical training on cardiovascular fitness and behavior patterns of mentally retarded adults. Am J Ment Defic 1985;90:167–170.

66. Tomporowski PD, Ellis NR. The effects of exercise on the health, intelligence, and adapted behavior of institutionalized severely and profoundly mentally retarded persons: a systemic replication. Appl Res Ment Retard 1985;6:465–473.

67. Tomporowski PD, Jameson LD. Effects of a physical fitness training program on the exercise behavior of institutionalized mentally retarded adults. Adapt Phys Act Q 1985;2:197–205.

68. Varela AM, Sardinha L, Pitetti KH. Effects of an aerobic rowing training program in young adults with Down syndrome. Am J Mental Retard. 2001;106:135–144.

69. Croce R, Horvat M. Effects of reinforcement based exercise on fitness and work productivity in adults with mental retardation. Adapt Phys Act Q 1992;9:148–178.

70. Suomi R, Surburg PR, Lecius P. Effects of hydraulic resistance strength training on isokinetic measures of leg strength in men with mental retardation. Adapt Phys Act Q 1995;12:377–387.

71. Suomi R. Self-directed strength training: its effect on leg strength in men with mental retardation. Arch Phys Med Rehabil 1998;79:323–328.

Index

In this index, page numbers in *italics* designate figures; page numbers followed by "t" designate tables; *see also* indicates related topics or more detailed lists